Pharmacology **Success**

NCLEX®-Style Q&A Review

FOURTH EDITION

Christi Doherty, DNP, MSN, RNC-OB, CNE, CHSE, CDP

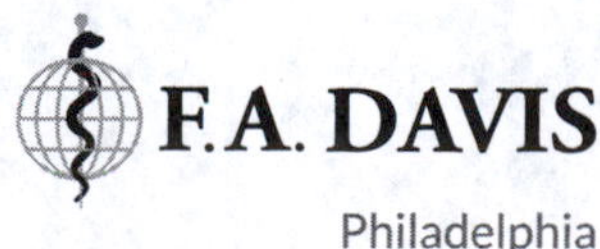

Philadelphia

F.A. Davis Company
1915 Arch Street
Philadelphia, PA 19103
www.fadavis.com

Printed in the United States of America
Last digit indicates print number: 10 9 8 7 6 5 4 3 2 1

Acquisitions Editor: Jacalyn Sharp
Content Project Manager: Veronica Neff
Electronic Project Editor: Sandra A. Glennie
Design and Illustrations Manager: Carolyn O'Brien

Library of Congress Cataloging-in-Publication Data

Names: Doherty, Christi D. author. | Colgrove, Kathryn Cadenhead. Pharmacology success.
Title: Pharmacology success : NCLEX-style Q & A review / Christi Doherty.
Description: Fourth edition. | Philadelphia, PA : F.A. Davis, [2023] | Preceded by Pharmacology success : NCLEX-style Q & A review / Kathryn Cadenhead Colgrove, Christi Doherty. Third edition. [2019]
Identifiers: LCCN 2022006611 (print) | LCCN 2022006612 (ebook) | ISBN 9781719646017 (paperback) | ISBN 9781719648448 (ebook)
Subjects: MESH: Pharmacology | Examination Questions | Nurses Instruction
Classification: LCC RT48 (print) | LCC RT48 (ebook) | NLM QV 18.2 | DDC 616.07/5—dc23/eng/20220617
LC record available at https://lccn.loc.gov/2022006611
LC ebook record available at https://lccn.loc.gov/2022006612

I would like to recognize

Ray Ann Hargrove-Huttel
and
Kathryn Cadenhead Colgrove

for their contributions to the previous
Pharmacology Success *editions.*

For my Dad

Contributing Authors

Kevin D. Doherty, BS, RDCS, RDMS, RVT
Cardiovascular Sonographer
Baylor Scott & White Heart and Vascular Hospital
Dallas, Texas

Kris Skalsky, EdD, MSN, RN
Chair, Research and Scholarship and Professor
American Sentinel College of Nursing & Health Sciences at Post University
Waterbury, Connecticut

Nancy T. Wilkins, DNP, RN-BC
Ferrum College
Ferrum, Virginia

Preface

NEW TO THE 4TH EDITION

Pharmacology Success, 4th edition, has been revised and updated to better prepare nursing students for pharmacology testing in nursing courses and the NCLEX-RN® examination. Revisions include the addition of new FDA approved medications and removal of drugs that have been discontinued in the U.S. market. Medication administration records, flow sheets, and graphs have been enhanced to provide the nursing student with real-life documents, typical of what they will encounter in clinical practice. Additionally, Next Generation NCLEX®-style questions have been included to provide students the opportunity to practice and enhance their clinical judgment skills.

NEXT GENERATION NCLEX (NGN)® EXAMINATION

The goal of the NCLEX-RN® examination has always been to measure the knowledge and skills required by entry-level nurses to care for clients safely. With demographic shifts and technological advances, nurses must make increasingly complex decisions using clinical judgment and incorporate leadership, collaboration, and evidence-based practice into their nursing practice. The National Council of State Boards of Nursing (NCSBN) is currently researching and designing a better way to assess clinical judgment directly and evaluate minimal competency. The Next Generation NCLEX examination, expected to launch earliest in 2023, will include a variety of question types to address critical nursing skills such as recognizing cues, analyzing those cues, prioritizing hypothesis, generating solutions, taking action, and evaluating outcomes (NCSBN, 2018).

The new question types include unfolding case studies, enhanced hot spots, CLOZE questions, extended drag and drop, extended multiple responses, and other question formats.

- The *unfolding case study* includes a narrative describing a client situation. It contains assorted data, and the test taker must discern the relevant information. Then, additional data is revealed, culminating in a complete picture of the client's clinical presentation and associated interventions. The learner makes clinical judgment decisions throughout the case study, adapting the process to the evolving client information. Each unfolding case study has a group of six questions associated with the case.
- *Enhanced hot spots* involve highlighting relevant information contained in a case study.
- *CLOZE questions* are fill-in-the-blank questions with drop boxes that provide four available options for the test taker to select for the blank.
- *Extended drag and drop questions* originate from a brief client scenario or case study. In these questions, the test taker must complete several blanks within a sentence by selecting from a list of seven to eight choices. Another format for extended drag and drop questions is the ranking or sequencing of interventions or processes.
- *Extended multiple responses* are select-all-that-apply questions with more than the traditional five answer options or questions requiring the learner to identify relevant or irrelevant items from a data set of no less than six options.
- *Matrix/grid questions* are charts with multiple rows and columns requiring the learner to select one or more answer options for each row and/or column.

- *Bow-tie questions* require the learner to select actions to take, potential conditions, and parameters to monitor based on a specific client scenario.
- *Trend questions* include client data over a specific time period. The data can include laboratory results, intake and output, vital signs, medications, or other information. The learner must make a decision about the client's care based on the trending data.

Table of Contents

Basic Concepts in Medication Administration

1

Always laugh when you can, it is cheap medicine.

—Lord Byron

INTRODUCTION

Pharmacology is the scientific study of the origin, use, effects, and actions of medications. The administration of medicine is an essential component of nursing care and tested on the NCLEX-RN® examination. Safely and accurately administering medications is of paramount importance and is fundamental to client safety and optimal client outcomes.

RIGHTS OF MEDICATION ADMINISTRATION

Nurses have a responsibility to follow the "rights" of medication administration. In the past, five "rights" were necessary to follow for safe medication administration. However, the rights have evolved to include all responsibilities of the professional nurse role.

Right Client. The nurse should check the client's identity, using a minimum of two identifiers, primarily name and date of birth, before administering medication.

Right Medication. The nurse should check the medication order against the medication label a minimum of three times before administering the drug.

Right Dosage. The nurse is responsible for confirming that the dosage order is appropriate for the client's age, weight, and vital signs. In addition, the nurse should verify any mathematical calculations.

Right Route. Nurses should ensure the client takes medications by the prescribed route. If a route is not identified on an order from a health-care provider (HCP), the nurse should confirm the method of medication delivery.

Right Time. The nurse should confirm the timing of the medication, frequency of administration, and the time the last dose was given. Nursing judgment may lead to some variations in timing and should be approved by the HCP.

Right Documentation. Accurate documentation of medication administration is fundamental to client safety and optimal client outcomes.

Right Reason. A review of the client's history and rationale for appropriateness of the medication for a patient are essential components of safe medication administration.

Right Response or Evaluation. Continual assessment of any desired or undesired client responses to medication is essential.

Right to Refuse. The nurse must always respect the client's right to refuse medication. The nurse should document the reason and take appropriate actions, such as notifying the HCP.

Right Education. Nurses should always be prepared to share information regarding the rights mentioned here with the client.

PHARMACOLOGY TEST-TAKING HINTS

The test taker must know their medications. Additionally, memorization is part of administering medications safely. This chapter contains some tips to assist the test taker in learning about medications. These tips apply to all questions in this book.

First, learn the specific medication classifications, including medication actions, side effects, and adverse effects. Also, learn how to administer medication in its classification safely. Generally speaking, medications in a classification share characteristics, but be sure not to be too broad in your descriptions. For example, do not combine all drugs administered for hypertension in the same category. Angiotensin-converting enzyme (ACE) inhibitors, beta blockers, and calcium channel blockers do not work in the same manner and are not in the same classification, even though they may all be used to treat hypertension. Similarly, diabetes mellitus and diuretics medications fall into several classification groups, and the facts about each specific classification must be learned. This knowledge will assist the nurse in administering medications, because drugs in a specific class will have similar safety requirements, effects, and side effects. For example, **all** beta blocker medications require the nurse to monitor the blood pressure and apical pulse (AP) before administering the medication.

The NCLEX-RN® examination requires the test taker to recognize a medication and its actions and side effects by the generic name. In this book, all medications in the stems of the questions will list only the generic names. The classification and trade names of the medications will be provided in the answers section so the test taker will become familiar with the ways other HCPs and clients may describe the drugs. The exception is when the test taker is required to use a medication administration record (MAR). MARs contain the generic names and trade names of the medications in some clinical facilities, so some MARs will include both in this book.

When administering medications for a group of clients, the test taker must realize that time is a real issue. It is not feasible for the nurse to look up 50 to 60 medications and administer them all within the dosing time frame. Therefore, the nurse must learn about the most common medications.

One tip for learning about medications is for the test taker to complete drug cards. Writing the cards by hand is often better than buying ready-made cards. Handmade drug cards require the test taker to use more than one method of learning—reading, deciding which information to put on the card, and writing the pertinent information on the card. All of this assists the test taker in memorizing the information.

When the test taker decides which information is most important to write on a drug card, the following questions can be used as a guide. The five questions are essential to critical thinking.

1. What classification is the medication that the nurse is administering to the client, and why is this client receiving this medication? What action does the medication have on the body?

Many medications are categorized in one classification group, but the client receives the medication for a different reason. For example, the medication trazodone is labeled as an antidepressant. However, it is often prescribed as a sedative medication for sleep because its sedating effects are more powerful than its antidepressant effects. The action on the body is known as the scientific rationale for administering the medication.

Example #1:
digoxin (Lanoxin) 0.25 mg po generic name (Trade Name)

- The classification of this medication is a cardiac glycoside.
- The medication is administered to clients with congestive heart failure (CHF) or rapid atrial fibrillation.
- Cardiac glycosides increase the contractility of the heart and decrease the heart rate. (In heart failure, the medication is administered to increase the contractility of the heart, but in atrial fibrillation, the medication is administered to slow the heart rate.)

Example #2:
furosemide (Lasix) 40 mg IV push (IVP) generic name (Common Trade Name)

- The classification of the medication is a loop diuretic.
- The medication is administered to clients with essential hypertension or CHF or any other condition in which excess fluid is in the body.
- This medication helps remove excess fluid from the body.
- Loop diuretics remove water from the kidneys along with potassium.

2. When should the nurse question administering this medication? Does the medication have a therapeutic serum level? Which vital signs must be monitored? Which physiological parameters should be monitored during administration?

Example #1:
digoxin (Lanoxin)

- Is the AP less than 60 beats per minute (bpm)?
- Is the digoxin level within the therapeutic range?
- Is the potassium level within normal range?

Example #2:
furosemide (Lasix)

- Is the potassium level within normal range?
- Does the client have signs/symptoms of dehydration?
- Is the client's blood pressure below 90/60?

3. What interventions must be taught to the client to ensure the medication is administered safely in the hospital setting? What interventions must be taught for taking the medication safely at home?

Example #1:
digoxin (Lanoxin)

- Explain the importance of having serum levels checked regularly.
- Teach the client to take his or her radial pulse and not to take the medication if the pulse is less than 60 bpm.
- Inform the client to take the medication daily and to notify the HCP if not taking the medication.

Example #2:
furosemide (Lasix)

- Teach about orthostatic hypotension.
- Instruct the client to drink a limited amount of water to replace insensible fluid loss.
- Because the medication is IVP, inform the client about how many minutes the medication should be pushed, what primary IV is hanging, and whether the IV is compatible with Lasix.

4. What are the side effects and potential adverse reactions? Side effects are undesired effects of the medication, but they do not warrant discontinuing or changing the medication. Adverse reactions are any situations that would require notifying the HCP or discontinuing the medication.

Example #1:
digoxin (Lanoxin)

- There is a decrease in heart rate to below 60 bpm.
- Signs of toxicity are present—nausea, vomiting, anorexia, and yellow haze.

Example #2:
furosemide (Lasix)

- Side effects include dizziness, lightheadedness.
- Adverse effects are hypokalemia; tinnitus if administered too quickly in IVP.

5. How does the nurse know the medication is effective?

Example #1:
digoxin (Lanoxin)

- Have the signs/symptoms of CHF improved?
- Is the client able to breathe easier? How many pillows does the client have to sleep on when lying down? Is the client able to perform activities of daily living (ADLs) without shortness of breath? What do the lung fields sound like?

Example #2:
furosemide (Lasix)

- Is the client's urinary output greater than the intake?
- Has the client lost any weight?
- Does the client have sacral or peripheral edema?
- Does the client have jugular vein distention?
- Has the client's blood pressure decreased?

SAMPLE DRUG CARDS

Front of Card

Classification of Drug	Route
Action of Drug:	
Uses:	
Nursing Implications (When would I question giving the medication?)	
How will I monitor to see if it is working?	

Back of Card

Side Effects:
Teaching Needs:
Drug Names:

It is suggested that the test taker complete these cards from a pharmacology textbook and not a drug handbook because most test questions come from a pharmacology book.

Digoxin Cardiac Glycosides **PO/IV**

Action: Positive inotropic action, increases force of ventricular contraction and thereby increases cardiac output; slows heart, allowing for increased filling time

Uses: CHF and rapid atrial cardiac dysrhythmias

Nursing Implications: Check AP for 1 full minute; hold if <60. Check digoxin level (0.5–2.0 normal, >2.5 = toxic). Check K+ level (hypokalemia is most common cause of dysrhythmias in clients receiving digoxin [3.5–5.0 mEq/L]). Monitor for S/S of CHF, crackles in lungs, I > O, edema. Question if the AP < 60 or abnormal lab values.
IVP—over 5 minutes: maintenance dose .125–.25 mg q day

Effectiveness: S/S of CHF improve, output > intake, weight decreases, breathing improves, activity tolerance improves, atrial rate decreases

Side Effects: Toxic = yellow haze or nausea and vomiting; ventricular rate decreases. If given along with a diuretic, increased risk of hypokalemia.

Teaching needs: To take radial pulse and hold if <60 and notify HCP.
K+ replacement—eat food high in K+ or may need supplemental K+.
Report weight gain of 3 lbs or more.

Drug names: Digoxin (generic)
Lanoxin
Lanoxicap

Sample Card for Furosemide

Furosemide Loop Diuretic **PO/IVP/IM**

Action: Blocks reabsorption of sodium and chloride in the loop of Henle = prevents the passive reabsorption of water = diuresis

Uses: CHF, fluid volume overload, pulmonary edema, HTN

Nursing Implications: I & O, monitor K+ level, check skin turgor, monitor for leg cramps, provide K+-rich foods or supplements, give early in the day to prevent nocturia. If giving IVP, give at prescribed rate (Lasix, 20 mg/min); ototoxic if given faster.

Effectiveness: Decrease in weight, output > intake, less edema, lung sounds clear.

Side Effects: Hypokalemia, muscle cramps, hyponatremia, dehydration.

Teaching Needs: Take early in the day.
Eat foods high in K+.

Drug names: Furosemide (Lasix)
Bumetanide (Bumex)
Torsemide (Demadex)
Ethacrynic acid (Edecrin)

The test taker is encouraged to use these guidelines/test-taking hints when answering the questions about medications in the following chapters. The questions cover medications prescribed for many different disease processes. The book, which is not all-inclusive, is intended to cover the most commonly occurring health-care problems. New medications are approved for use every month. There are medication questions for specific disease processes and a comprehensive test in each chapter that may have some questions regarding less common disease processes and the medications prescribed to treat these problems.

POPULATION-SPECIFIC INFORMATION

Pediatric Clients

The nurse must be aware that pediatric clients have specific prescribing and drug administration needs. The weight of the child's body directly affects the amount of medication that can be administered safely. In addition, possible effects on the liver and brain, which are not fully mature in pediatric clients, must be considered. Pediatric dosing is frequently prescribed in mg/kg. The nurse must have the mathematical ability to convert pounds to kilograms and grams to milligrams. A kilogram is equal to 2.2 pounds.

Elderly Clients

The nurse must be aware that as the body ages, the body processes slower and does not function as it once did. The liver and kidneys are responsible for processing medications and eliminating excess from the body. These are two of the most important organs to monitor when administering medications. The client's reaction to the medicines prescribed, laboratory studies, and potential toxicities all must be carefully monitored. In the elderly, lower doses of medications may be needed to account for the body's decreased ability to process and detoxify drugs.

Females of Childbearing Age

Any time a female client is mentioned in a question and an age is given that indicates the client is of childbearing age and could be pregnant, the test taker must determine if the medication is safe to administer to two clients—the female client and a potential fetus.

COMMON ABBREVIATIONS & TERMINOLOGY

The test taker must know commonly used abbreviations and their meanings. Examples include PRN, an abbreviation for *pro re nata*, a Latin term meaning "as needed" or "as circumstances require," and b.i.d., an abbreviation for *bis in die*, a Latin term meaning "twice a day." Many such abbreviations are used in medical prescribing and the nurse must be knowledgeable about them. Certain previously accepted abbreviations have been banned (Table 1-1). Two of these are q.d. and q.i.d., "once a day" and "four times a day," respectively. The reason is the potential for confusion and incorrect medication administration.

This book and the NCLEX-RN® examination assume the test taker knows common terminology such as *efficacy*, which means "effectiveness," and *teratogenic*, which means "causing developmental malformations." Different medications affect different body organs and may affect different laboratory values. The nurse should know which body organs and laboratory values may be affected by a specific problem or by a specific medication and monitor accordingly. For example, if there is a problem with the pancreas, the nurse might monitor blood glucose levels or lipase and amylase levels.

As stated earlier, the two major organs of the body responsible for detoxifying and eliminating excess substances from the body are the liver and the kidney; therefore, the nurse must monitor liver function tests, blood urea nitrogen (BUN) levels, and creatinine levels. Medications can alter the homeostatic balance of the body, and certain laboratory values

Table 1–1. The Joint Commission's "Do Not Use" Abbreviation List*

Do Not Use	Potential Problem	Use Instead
U (unit)	Mistaken for "0" (zero), the number "4" (four), or "cc"	Write "unit."
IU (International Unit)	Mistaken for "IV" (intravenous) or the number "10" (ten)	Write "International Unit."
Q.D., QD, q.d., qd (daily) Q.O.D., QOD, q.o.d, qod (every other day)	Mistaken for each other; period after the "Q" mistaken for "I" and the "O" mistaken for "I"	Write "daily." Write "every other day."
Trailing zero (X.0 mg)** Lack of leading zero (.X mg)	Decimal point is missed.	Write "X mg." Write "0.X mg."
MS MSO4 and MgSO4	Can mean morphine sulfate or magnesium sulfate; confused for one another	Write "morphine sulfate." Write "magnesium sulfate."

*Applies to all orders and all medication-related documentation that is handwritten (including free-text computer entry) or on preprinted forms.

**Exception: A "trailing zero" may be used only where required to demonstrate the level of precision of the value being reported, such as for laboratory results, imaging studies that report size of lesions, or catheter/tube sizes. It may not be used in medication orders or other medication-related documentation.

indicate a potential threat to the client's life or health status. The NCLEX-RN® examination provides reference values for many of the laboratory tests; however, the nurse should be familiar with reference values for many of the common laboratory tests.

The nurse must always be aware of the effects of medications on the body to determine if a drug is effective. The medication is effective if the signs and symptoms of the disease process for which the medication is being administered are improving. For example, if an antibiotic is being administered to a client with an infection caused by an agent sensitive to that antibiotic, the white blood cell count should decrease. Similarly, if furosemide or digoxin is given to a client with heart failure, the lung fields should be clear if the medication is effective.

All medications have side effects. A side effect is an untoward reaction to the medication. Side effects are not uncommon and are not necessarily a reason for discontinuing the medication. Frequently the nurse must teach the client how to manage a side effect. For example, anticholinergic drugs have the side effect of drying secretions. The client can be taught to chew sugarless gum or hard candies to alleviate this problem.

Adverse effects of medications, however, could be life-threatening, and the HCP should be notified of any problem. For example, an adverse effect of many medications is agranulocytosis, or bone marrow suppression that results in a decreased production of white blood cells and increased susceptibility to infections. Agranulocytosis often manifests with flu-like symptoms. The medication will need to be discontinued.

When reading a question in this book or on the NCLEX-RN® examination, the test taker can assume that if the option is in the question, the nurse has an HCP's order for that option. The test taker should not eliminate an option because they do not think there is an HCP order for the intervention.

Medication Memory Jogger

In each chapter, some comments are available that provide basic medication administration guidelines. These memory joggers are designed to "jog" the test taker's critical thinking ability. Pay particular attention when one of these comments appears in a chapter.

2 Neurological System

A prudent question is one half of wisdom.

—Francis Bacon

QUESTIONS

Head Injury

1. The client diagnosed with a head injury is experiencing increased intracranial pressure. The neurosurgeon prescribes mannitol. For each intervention, specify if the intervention is **indicated or not indicated** for the client's care.

Potential Nursing Intervention	Indicated	Not Indicated
1. Monitor the ABGs during administration.		
2. Do not administer if blood pressure <90/60.		
3. Use a filter needle when administering the medication.		
4. Monitor the serum osmolarity during administration.		
5. Monitor neurological status.		
6. Assess IM injection site for phlebitis.		

2. Which discharge instructions should the emergency department nurse discuss with the client diagnosed with a concussion? **Select all that apply.**
1. "Do not drink any type of alcoholic beverage unless allowed by the HCP."
2. "Take two acetaminophen up to every 6 hours for a headache."
3. "If experiencing a headache, take one hydrocodone every 8 hours."
4. "It is all right to take a couple of aspirin if experiencing a headache."
5. "Notify the HCP if the medication does not relieve your headache."

3. The following clients have a head injury. Which clients should the nurse **question** administering mannitol? **Select all that apply.**
1. The 34-year-old client diagnosed with HIV
2. The 84-year-old client diagnosed with glaucoma
3. The 68-year-old client diagnosed with cor pulmonale
4. The 16-year-old client diagnosed with cystic fibrosis
5. The 58-year-old client diagnosed with congestive heart failure (CHF)

4. The client has an open laceration on the right temporal lobe secondary to being hit on the head with a baseball bat. The emergency department (ED) HCP sutured the laceration; the computed tomography (CT) scan is negative. Which instruction should the nurse discuss with the client?
   1. "Do not put anything on the laceration for 72 hours."
   2. "Use hydrocortisone cream 0.5% on the laceration."
   3. "Cleanse the area with alcohol three times a day."
   4. "Apply a topical antibiotic ointment to the sutured area."

5. The client diagnosed with a head injury is ordered a CT scan of the head with contrast dye. Which statements by the client warrant **immediate** intervention? **Select all that apply.**
   1. "I take atenolol for my high blood pressure."
   2. "I am allergic to many types of fish."
   3. "I get nauseated whenever I take aspirin."
   4. "I am taking metformin for my diabetes."
   5. "I had about three beers before I fell and hit my head."

6. The nurse is preparing to administer medications to the following clients. Which medication should the nurse **question** administering?
   1. Furosemide to a client with a serum potassium level of 4.2 mEq/L
   2. Mannitol to a client with a serum osmolality of 280 mOsm/kg
   3. Digoxin to a client with a digoxin level of 2.4 ng/dL
   4. Phenytoin to a client with a phenytoin level of 14 mcg/mL

7. The client diagnosed with a head injury is admitted into the intensive care unit (ICU). Which HCP medication order should the ICU nurse **question? Select all that apply.**
   1. Morphine
   2. Mannitol
   3. Methylprednisolone
   4. Phenytoin
   5. Oxygen

8. The client has increased intracranial pressure, and the HCP orders a bolus of 0.5 g/kg IV of 25% osmotic diuretic solution. The client weighs 165 pounds. How much medication should the nurse administer to the client?

   ____

Seizures

9. The client diagnosed with a seizure disorder is prescribed phenytoin. Which statement indicates the client **understands** the medication teaching?
   1. "If my urine turns a reddish-brown color, I should call my doctor."
   2. "I should take my medication on an empty stomach."
   3. "I will use a soft-bristled toothbrush to brush my teeth."
   4. "I may get a sore throat when taking this medication."

10. The client diagnosed with a seizure disorder and taking carbamazepine tells the clinic nurse, "I am taking evening primrose oil for my premenstrual (PMS) cramps, and it is really working." Which statement is the nurse's **best** response?
    1. "You should inform your HCP about taking this herb."
    2. "It is very dangerous to take both the herb and carbamazepine."
    3. "Herbs are natural substances. I am glad it is helping your PMS."
    4. "Are you sure you should be taking herbs along with carbamazepine?"

11. Which data should the nurse assess for the client diagnosed with a seizure disorder taking valproate?
    1. Creatinine and BUN levels
    2. White blood cell (WBC) count
    3. Liver enzymes
    4. Red blood cell (RBC) count

12. The nurse is preparing to administer the following anticonvulsant medications. Which medication should the nurse **question** administering?
    1. Carbamazepine for the client with a carbamazepine serum level of 8 mcg/mL
    2. Clonazepam for the client with a clonazepam serum level of 0.06 mcg/mL
    3. Phenytoin for the client with a phenytoin serum level of 26 mcg/mL
    4. Ethosuximide for the client with an ethosuximide serum level of 45 mcg/mL

13. The client diagnosed with a seizure disorder is prescribed fosphenytoin. Which interventions should the nurse discuss with the client? **Select all that apply.**
    1. Instruct the client to wear a medical alert bracelet and carry identification.
    2. Tell the client not to self-medicate with over-the-counter (OTC) medications.
    3. Encourage the client to decrease drinking any type of alcohol.
    4. Discuss the importance of maintaining good oral hygiene.
    5. Explain the importance of maintaining adequate nutritional intake.

14. The client is diagnosed with status epilepticus and is prescribed IV diazepam. The client has an IV of D_5W 75 mL/hr in the right arm and a saline lock in the left arm. Which intervention should the nurse implement?
    1. Dilute the diazepam and administer over 5 minutes via the existing IV.
    2. Do not dilute the medication and administer it at the port closest to the client.
    3. Question the order because diazepam cannot be administered with D_5W.
    4. Inject 3 mL of normal saline (NS) in the saline lock and administer diazepam undiluted.

15. The client diagnosed with epilepsy tells the nurse, "I am very scared to get pregnant because I am taking medication for my epilepsy." Which statement is the nurse's **best** response?
    1. "You are scared because you take medication for your epilepsy."
    2. "Please tell me more about what is concerning you?"
    3. "You should not get pregnant when you are taking anticonvulsants."
    4. "Have you discussed your concerns with your significant other?"

16. The client newly diagnosed with epilepsy is prescribed an anticonvulsant medication. Which information should the nurse tell the client?
    1. "The medication dosage will start low and gradually increase over a few weeks."
    2. "The dosage prescribed initially will be the dosage prescribed for the rest of your life."
    3. "The HCP will prescribe a loading dose and decrease the dosage gradually."
    4. "The medication dose will be adjusted monthly until a serum drug level is obtained."

17. The nurse is preparing to administer phenytoin IV push (IVP). The client has an IV of D_5W 0.45 NS at 50 mL/hr. Which intervention should the nurse implement?
    1. Administer the phenytoin undiluted over 5 minutes via the port closest to the client.
    2. Dilute the medication with NS and administer over 2 minutes.
    3. Flush tubing with NS, administer diluted phenytoin, and then flush with NS.
    4. Insert a saline lock in the other arm and administer the medication undiluted.

Cerebrovascular Accident

18. The 55-year-old client presents to the ED with blurred vision, slurred speech, and left-sided weakness. The client has a history of hypertension (HTN) and benign prostatic hypertrophy (BPH). Which statement regarding the client's medications should the nurse ask at this time?
1. "Have you been taking OTC herbs to treat your BPH?"
2. "Do you take an aspirin every day to prevent heart attacks and strokes?"
3. "Do you eat green, leafy vegetables frequently?"
4. "Have you been taking medications routinely to control hypertension?"

19. The nurse in the ED is preparing to administer alteplase to the client diagnosed with a stroke 2 hours after initial symptoms began. Which interventions should the nurse implement? **Select all that apply.**
1. Check the client's armband for allergies.
2. Hang the medication via IV piggyback (IVPB) and infuse over 90 minutes.
3. Check results of the client's CT scan of the brain.
4. Teach the client that this medication dissolves clots.
5. Monitor the client's partial thromboplastin time (PTT) during drug administration.

20. The long-term–care facility nurse is caring for a client diagnosed 6 months ago with a cerebrovascular accident (CVA) and residual cognitive deficits. The HCP has ordered alprazolam to be administered at bedtime. For each intervention, specify if the intervention is **indicated or not indicated** for the client's care.

Potential Nursing Intervention	Indicated	Not Indicated
1. Offer toileting every 2 hours.		
2. Move the client close to the nurse's station.		
3. Administer the medication at 2100.		
4. Administer the medication with a full glass of water.		
5. Do not administer if the client's apical pulse is <60 bpm.		

21. The client diagnosed with a stroke is prescribed phenytoin. Which statement explains the scientific rationale for prescribing this medication?
1. Some damage to cerebral tissue caused the client's stroke.
2. The stroke caused damage to the brain tissue, resulting in seizures.
3. Hemorrhagic strokes leave residual blood in the brain that causes seizures.
4. This medication can help the client diagnosed with cognitive deficits think more clearly.

22. The 44-year-old client presents to the ED diagnosed with a stroke. Which of the client's current medications from the following list is a risk factor for developing a stroke?

Mary Anne P. Medication List

Medication	Time Taken
Propranolol	At night
Furosemide	Before breakfast
Estradiol and norgestimate	Before breakfast
Metformin	At night

1. Propranolol
2. Furosemide
3. Estradiol and norgestimate
4. Metformin

23. The client diagnosed with chronic HTN is prescribed furosemide and enalapril. The client's blood pressure readings for the last 3 weeks have averaged 178/95, and the HCP has added atenolol to the client's current medication regimen. Which statement is the scientific rationale for including this medication in the client's regimen?
1. Achieving a lower average blood pressure will help prevent a stroke.
2. The other medications are not effective without the addition of atenolol.
3. Atenolol will potentiate the effects of loop diuretics.
4. The HCP will taper off the enalapril and eventually discontinue it.

24. The elderly client diagnosed with a stroke is being discharged. When preparing the discharge instructions, the nurse notes many medications ordered to be taken at different times of the day. Which intervention should the nurse implement **first**?
1. Complete a comprehensive chart for the client to use.
2. Refer the client to a home health-care agency for follow-up.
3. Teach the client to return to the HCP office for follow-up.
4. Discuss the multiple medications and times with the HCP.

25. The nurse is caring for a client diagnosed with a hemorrhagic stroke. Which medication should the nurse **question** administering?
1. Clopidogrel
2. Mannitol
3. Nifedipine
4. Levothyroxine

26. The nurse is preparing to administer oral medications to a client diagnosed with a stroke. Which interventions should the nurse implement? **Select all that apply.**
1. Crush all oral medications and place them in pudding.
2. Elevate the head 30 degrees.
3. Ask the client to swallow a drink of water.
4. Have suction equipment at the bedside.
5. Insert a nasogastric tube to administer medications.

27. The nurse in the ICU is caring for a client diagnosed with a left cerebral artery thrombotic stroke after receiving thrombolytic medication in the ED. Which intervention should be implemented?
1. Administer oral ticlopidine.
2. Place the client in the Trendelenburg position.
3. Keep the client turned to the right side and high Fowler's position.
4. Monitor heparin infusion.

Brain Tumor

28. The nurse is caring for a client diagnosed with a malignant brain tumor. Which medication should the nurse anticipate the HCP ordering?
    1. Cyclophosphamide
    2. Octreotide
    3. Erythropoietin
    4. Phenytoin

29. The client diagnosed with a pituitary tumor has vasopressin prescribed. Which statement by the client indicates the medication is **effective**?
    1. "My headaches are much better since I have been on this medication."
    2. "My nasal drainage was initially worse, but now I don't have any."
    3. "I am not so thirsty when I take this medication."
    4. "My seizures have been eliminated."

30. The client diagnosed with a brain tumor is being admitted to the medical oncology unit at 2000. Which order from the HCP should be implemented **first**?
    1. Regular soft diet with between-meal snacks
    2. Dexamethasone every 6 hours IVP
    3. Prochlorperazine before meals
    4. CBC and chemistry panel laboratory tests

31. The client diagnosed with a brain tumor is prescribed mannitol intravenously. Which interventions for this medication should the nurse implement? **Select all that apply.**
    1. Inspect the bottle for crystals.
    2. Record intake and output every 8 hours.
    3. Auscultate the client's lung fields.
    4. Perform a neurological examination.
    5. Have calcium gluconate at the bedside.

32. The 6-year-old client diagnosed with a brain tumor has returned from the post-anesthesia care unit (PACU) to intensive care. Which medication should the nurse **question**?
    1. Meperidine IVP every 2 hours
    2. Methylprednisolone IVPB every 8 hours
    3. Acetaminophen PO or rectal every 4 hours PRN
    4. Ondansetron IVP every 6 hours PRN

33. The client diagnosed with a brain tumor has been placed on narcotic analgesic medications to control the associated headaches. For each intervention, specify if the intervention is **indicated or not indicated** for the client's care.

Potential Nursing Intervention	Indicated	Not Indicated
1. Instruct the client to increase fluids while taking the medications.		
2. Talk to the client about taking bulk laxatives daily.		
3. Teach the significant other to perform a neurological assessment.		
4. Discuss limiting the amount of medication allowed per day.		
5. Explain safety issues when taking narcotic medications.		

34. The client diagnosed with a brain tumor is undergoing radiation therapy. Which medication should the home health nurse suggest that the HCP order to assist the client in managing side effects of the radiation therapy?

1. An antiemetic to be taken before meals and as needed
2. An increase in the narcotic pain medication
3. A topical medicated lotion for the scalp
4. An antianxiety medication to control anxiety during treatments

35. The client diagnosed with a pituitary tumor has acromegaly. The HCP has prescribed octreotide. Which intervention should the nurse implement regarding this medication?

1. Implement fall precautions.
2. Administer calcium tablets to replace the lost calcium.
3. Have the client discuss acne-like skin problems with a dermatologist.
4. Contact the client's insurance provider to determine if the medication is covered.

36. The 8-year-old client has been diagnosed with a benign tumor in the anterior pituitary gland. Surgery has resulted in inadequate production of growth hormone (GH). The nurse is teaching the client's parents about GH therapy. Which statement indicates the parent **understands** the medication?

1. "If I give too much, then my child will grow to be a giant."
2. "After a few months, I can taper my child off the growth hormone."
3. "If I don't give the hormone, my child will be intellectually disabled."
4. "I should monitor my child's blood glucose levels."

37. The client diagnosed with a brain tumor tells the clinic nurse about having seizures more frequently. The client is taking phenytoin, the oral liquid form of morphine sulfate, acetaminophen, and alprazolam. Which question should the nurse ask next about the client's medications?

1. "How often do you need to take the alprazolam?"
2. "Do you take any vitamins that might cause the seizures?"
3. "What was your last phenytoin level?"
4. "Have you had any x-rays to determine the cause of the seizures?"

Parkinson's Disease

38. The client diagnosed with Parkinson's disease has been prescribed the combination medication carbidopa and levodopa. Which factor indicates the medication is **effective**?

1. The client has cogwheel motion when swinging the arms.
2. The client does not display emotions when discussing the illness.
3. The client can walk upright without stumbling.
4. The client eats 30% to 40% of meals within 1 hour.

39. Which statement made by the wife of a client diagnosed with Parkinson's disease (PD) indicates the medication teaching is **effective**?

1. "The medications will control all the symptoms of PD if they are taken correctly."
2. "The medications provide symptom management, but the effects may not last."
3. "The medications will have to be taken for about 6 months and then stopped."
4. "The medications must be tapered off with improvement, or he will have a relapse."

40. Which statement is the scientific rationale for the combination drug carbidopa and levodopa prescribed to a client diagnosed with Parkinson's disease?
    1. Carbidopa delays the breakdown of the levodopa in the periphery, so more dopamine gets to the brain.
    2. The medication is less expensive when combined, so it is more affordable to clients on a fixed income.
    3. Carbidopa breaks down in the periphery and causes vasoconstriction of the blood vessels.
    4. Carbidopa increases the action of levodopa on the renal arteries, increasing renal perfusion.

41. The client diagnosed with Parkinson's disease has been on long-term levodopa. Which data supports the rationale for placing the client on a "drug holiday"?
    1. The medication is expensive and difficult to afford for clients on a fixed income.
    2. Therapeutic effects have diminished, and adverse effects have increased.
    3. The client has developed HTN that is uncontrolled by medication.
    4. An overdose was taken, and the medication needs to clear the system.

42. The client diagnosed with early-stage Parkinson's disease has been prescribed pramipexole. Which side effects of this medication should the nurse discuss with the client? **Select all that apply.**
    1. Daytime somnolence
    2. On–off effect
    3. Excessive salivation
    4. Pill-rolling motion
    5. Stiff muscles

43. Which statement is an **advantage** of administering entacapone to a client diagnosed with Parkinson's disease?
    1. Entacapone increases the vasodilating effect of levodopa.
    2. Levodopa can be discontinued while the client is taking entacapone.
    3. There are no side effects of the drug to interfere with treatment.
    4. Entacapone causes blood levels of levodopa to be smoother and more sustained.

44. A client diagnosed with Parkinson's disease (PD) is prescribed amantadine. Which information should the nurse teach the client?
    1. "Do not get the flu vaccine because there may be interactions."
    2. "If the symptoms return, you should notify the HCP."
    3. "The dose should be decreased if you are taking other PD medications."
    4. "If a dry mouth develops, discontinue the medication immediately."

45. Which client diagnosed with Parkinson's disease should the nurse **question** administering benztropine?
    1. The client diagnosed with CHF
    2. The client diagnosed with myocardial infarction
    3. The client diagnosed with glaucoma
    4. The client undergoing hip replacement surgery

46. The nurse is caring for a client newly diagnosed with Parkinson's disease receiving levodopa. Which interventions should the nurse implement? **Select all that apply.**
    1. Instruct the client to rise slowly from a seated or lying position.
    2. Teach about on–off effects of the medication.
    3. Discuss taking the medication with meals or snacks.
    4. Tell the client that sweat and urine may become darker.
    5. Inform the client about having routine blood levels drawn.

47. The client diagnosed with Parkinson's disease has been on carbidopa and levodopa for 2 years, and now the symptoms have increased. The HCP added prescription safinamide to the client's daily routine. Which information should the nurse teach the client?
    1. Discontinue the carbidopa and levodopa.
    2. Rise slowly from a lying or sitting position.
    3. Take the medication on an empty stomach.
    4. There are no side effects of this medication as there are for carbidopa and levodopa.

Alzheimer's Disease

48. The family member of a client diagnosed with early-stage Alzheimer's disease who was prescribed donepezil but has not had improvement asks the nurse, "Can anything be done to slow the disease because this medication does not work?" Which statement is the nurse's **best** response?
1. "I am sorry that the medication did not help. Would you like to talk about it?"
2. "You need to prepare for long-term care because confusion is inevitable now."
3. "Your loved one may respond to a different medication of the same type."
4. "No, nothing is going to slow the disease now. Have the client make a will."

49. Which statement is the scientific rationale for prescribing and administering donepezil?
1. Donepezil binds dopamine at neuron receptor sites to increase ability.
2. Donepezil increases availability of acetylcholine at cholinergic synapses.
3. Donepezil decreases acetylcholine in the periphery to increase movement.
4. Donepezil delays transmission of acetylcholine at the neuronal junction.

50. The client diagnosed with Alzheimer's disease is prescribed rivastigmine. Which medication should the nurse **question** administering to the client?
1. Amitriptyline
2. Warfarin
3. Phenytoin
4. Prochlorperazine

51. The nurse caring for clients on a medical psychiatric unit has received the morning shift report. Which client diagnosed with Alzheimer's disease should the nurse administer the medication to **first**?
1. The client with a PO cardiac glycoside daily
2. The client needing a PRN for nausea
3. The client with a cholinesterase inhibitor ordered three times a day
4. The angry and disoriented client with an antipsychotic PRN

52. The registered nurse (RN) is completing an admission assessment on a client being admitted to a medical unit diagnosed with pneumonia. The client's list of home medications are populated in the following list:

John D. Medication List

Medication	Time Taken
Furosemide	Before breakfast
Metamucil	Before breakfast
Galantamine hydrobromide	Before breakfast
Melatonin	At night

Which intervention should the nurse implement **first**?
1. Make sure the client has a room near the nursing station.
2. Check the client's WBC count and potassium level.
3. Have the UAP get ice chips for the client to suck on.
4. Determine the client's usual bowel elimination pattern.

53. The home health-care nurse is caring for a client taking donepezil. Which finding indicates the medication is **effective**?
1. The client is unable to relay their name or birthdate.
2. The client is discussing an upcoming event with the family.
3. The client is wearing underwear on the outside of their clothes.
4. The client is talking on a telephone that signals a dial tone.

54. The daughter of an elderly client diagnosed with Alzheimer's disease (AD) asks the nurse, "Is there anything I can do to prevent getting this disease?" Which statement is the nurse's **best** response?
1. "Not if you are genetically programmed to get Alzheimer's disease."
2. "Yearly brain scans may determine if you are susceptible to getting AD."
3. "There are some medications, but research has not proven that they work."
4. "Hormone replacement therapy may prevent the development of AD."

55. The client diagnosed with Alzheimer's disease is taking vitamin E and ginkgo biloba. Which information should the nurse teach the client?
1. Take the medications on an empty stomach.
2. Have regular blood tests to assess for toxic levels.
3. The medications only slow the progression of the disease.
4. Use a sunscreen with an SPF of 15 or greater when in the sun.

56. Which statement represents the **advantage** of prescribing donepezil over other cholinesterase inhibitors?
1. The dosing schedule for donepezil is only once a day.
2. Donepezil is the only drug that can be given with an NSAID.
3. Donepezil enhances the cognitive protective effects of vitamin E.
4. There are no side effects of donepezil.

57. The client diagnosed with Alzheimer's disease is prescribed galantamine. Which interventions should the nurse implement? For each intervention, specify if the intervention is **indicated or not indicated** for the client's care.

Potential Nursing Intervention	Indicated	Not Indicated
1. Inform the client to take the medication with food.		
2. Check the client's BUN and creatinine levels.		
3. Teach the client to wear a medical alert bracelet with drug information.		
4. Assess the client's other routine medications.		
5. Discuss not abruptly discontinuing the medication.		

Migraine Headache

58. The client presents to the ED reporting a migraine headache. They are prescribed medication. Which scientific rationale is **most appropriate** for administering the medication by the parenteral route?
1. The client requests the medication be given IVP.
2. Migraine headaches do not respond to oral medications.
3. Migraine headaches can cause nausea, vomiting, and gastric stasis.
4. The client is not as likely to develop an addiction to the medications.

59. The 29-year-old female client is taking tanacetum parthenium for chronic migraine headaches. Which information should the nurse teach the client?
1. "Decrease the dose of prescription NSAIDs while taking this herb."
2. "Do not breastfeed, and avoid getting pregnant while taking tanacetum parthenium."
3. "The medication will immediately relieve a migraine headache."
4. "Menstrual problems will become worse while taking this medication."

60. The client diagnosed with chronic migraine headaches who has been taking medications daily for years to prevent migraines from recurring tells the clinic nurse they have a headache "all the time, no matter what I take." Which situation should the nurse suspect is occurring?
1. The client has developed a resistance to pain medication.
2. The client is addicted and wants to increase the narcotics prescribed.
3. The client has developed medication overuse headaches.
4. The client may have a complication of therapy and possibly a brain tumor.

61. The client diagnosed with a migraine headache rates the pain at a 4 on a 1 to 10 scale. Which medication should the nurse administer?
1. Ibuprofen orally
2. Butorphanol intramuscularly
3. Dihydroergotamine intranasally
4. Sumatriptan subcutaneously

62. The nurse is caring for a client diagnosed with migraine headaches. Which information should the nurse teach regarding abortive medication therapy?
1. Use the medication every day, even if there is no headache.
2. Take the radial pulse for 1 minute before taking the medication.
3. The medication can cause severe HTN.
4. Limit use of the medication to 1 or 2 days a week.

63. The client is prescribed sumatriptan, 6 mg subcutaneously, for a migraine headache. The medication comes as 12 mg/mL. How many milliliters should the nurse administer?

____

64. The client diagnosed with migraine headaches that occur every 2 to 3 days is placed on preventive therapy with propranolol. Which data indicate the medication is **effective**?
1. The client has had only one headache in the past week.
2. The client's apical pulse is 78 beats per minute (bpm).
3. The client has developed orthostatic hypotension.
4. The client supplemented propranolol with sumatriptan four times.

65. The client presents to the outpatient clinic reporting headaches that occur suddenly. The client describes a throbbing in the right orbital area and on the right side of the forehead that lasts for an hour or longer and has been occurring regularly for the past 2 weeks. Which medications should the nurse anticipate being prescribed?
1. Propranolol and almotriptan
2. Prednisone lithium
3. Amitriptyline and an estradiol/levonorgestrel patch
4. Ibuprofen and metoclopramide

66. The nurse in an HCP's office is assessing a female client diagnosed with a tension headache. Which question should the nurse ask the client **first**?
1. "Have you been sunbathing recently?"
2. "Do you eat shellfish or other iodine-containing foods?"
3. "Is there a chance you might be pregnant?"
4. "What OTC medications have you tried?"

67. The nurse is administering medications at 1600. Which medication should the nurse administer **first**?
1. Humalog insulin to a client with a blood glucose level of 200 mg/dL
2. Morphine to a client diagnosed with a headache rated an 8
3. Divalproex to a client diagnosed with migraine headaches
4. Metoclopramide to a client diagnosed with gastric stasis

ANSWERS AND RATIONALES

The correct answer number and rationale are in **boldface blue type.** Rationales for why other answer options are incorrect are also given.

Head Injury

1.

Potential Nursing Intervention	Indicated	Not Indicated
1. Monitor the ABGs during administration.		X
2. Do not administer if blood pressure <90/60.		X
3. Use a filter needle when administering the medication.	X	
4. Monitor the serum osmolarity during administration.	X	
5. Monitor neurological status.	X	
6. Assess IM injection site for phlebitis.		X

1. **The client's arterial blood gases (ABGs) are not affected by administering the osmotic diuretic mannitol (Osmitrol); therefore, there is no need to monitor them.**
2. **The client's blood pressure does not affect the administration of the osmotic diuretic mannitol (Osmitrol).**
3. **The nurse must use a filter needle when administering the osmotic diuretic mannitol (Osmitrol) because crystals may form in the solution and syringe and be inadvertently injected into the client if a filter needle is not used.**
4. **The normal serum osmolality is 275 to 295 mOsm/kg. The osmotic diuretic mannitol (Osmitrol) is held if the serum osmolality exceeds 320 mOsm/kg.**
5. **The clients being treated for intracranial pressure should have their neurological status monitored.**
6. **Mannitol (Osmitrol) is administered IV, not intramuscularly (IM). The nurse should evaluate the IV site for signs of phlebitis or infection.**

MEDICATION MEMORY JOGGER: The nurse must know accepted standards of practice for medication administration, including which client assessment data and laboratory data should be monitored before administering the medication.

2. **Correct answers are 1, 2, and 5.**
   1. **Traumatic brain injuries impair many brain functions that can be significantly worsened by alcohol, so the client should not drink alcoholic beverages until allowed by the HCP.**
   2. **Acetaminophen (Tylenol), a nonnarcotic analgesic, can be taken to relieve a headache for a client diagnosed with a concussion. If the Tylenol does not relieve the headache, the client should contact the HCP.**
   3. Hydrocodone (Vicodin), a narcotic analgesic, should not be taken after a head injury because medication such as this may further depress neurological status.
   4. Aspirin could lead to bleeding; therefore, a client diagnosed with a concussion does not want to risk a chance of increased bleeding.
   5. **If acetaminophen (Tylenol) does not relieve the client's headache, the client should notify the HCP because this may indicate a worsening condition, such as increased intracranial pressure.**

3. **Correct answers are 3 and 5.**
   1. The osmotic diuretic mannitol (Osmitrol) would not be contraindicated for a client diagnosed with HIV.
   2. The osmotic diuretic mannitol (Osmitrol) would not be contraindicated for a client diagnosed with glaucoma.
   3. **Cor pulmonale is right-sided heart failure, often secondary to chronic obstructive pulmonary disease. Because mannitol pulls fluid off the brain, it may lead to a circulatory overload, which the**

heart with right-sided failure could not handle. This client would need an order for a loop diuretic to prevent serious cardiac complications.

4. The client is 16 years old, and even with cystic fibrosis, the client's heart should handle the fluid volume overload.
5. **Because the osmotic diuretic mannitol (Osmitrol) pulls fluid off the brain, it may lead to a circulatory overload, which the client in CHF could not handle. This client would need an order for a loop diuretic to prevent serious cardiac complications.**

4. 1. The sutured area may get infected; therefore, the client should keep the wound clean and apply antibiotic ointment.
2. Hydrocortisone cream is an anti-inflammatory medication and would not be applied to a laceration.
3. Alcohol would be very painful and should not be used to clean the laceration.
4. **The sutured area must be cleansed with soap and water and patted dry, and an antibiotic ointment, such as Neosporin, should be applied to prevent infection.**

5. Correct answers are 2 and 4.
1. Atenolol (Tenormin), a beta blocker antihypertensive medication, would not interfere with the contrast dye used when performing a CT scan.
2. **The contrast dye used in a CT scan is iodine-based. An allergy to shellfish suggests an allergy to iodine and would warrant the nurse notifying the HCP to cancel the contrast part of the CT scan. Further assessment would be needed.**
3. Aspirin would not interfere with the contrast dye used when performing a CT scan.
4. **Metformin (Glucophage), a biguanide medication used for the control of diabetes, must not be taken because the kidneys remove metformin; contrast medium can significantly increase the level of metformin in the blood because damaged kidneys are not as effective at eliminating metformin from the body.**
5. Alcohol is not contraindicated when performing a CT scan.

MEDICATION MEMORY JOGGER: The nurse must be knowledgeable about accepted standards of practice for disease processes and conditions. If the nurse administers a medication the HCP has prescribed, and it harms the client, the nurse could be held accountable. Remember, the nurse is a client advocate.

6. 1. The normal serum potassium level is 3.5 to 5.3 mEq/L. The nurse has no reason to question this medication order because the client's potassium level is within normal range.
2. The normal serum osmolality is 275 to 295 mOsm/kg. Because the client's level is within this range, the nurse would have no reason to question administering this medication.
3. **The normal digoxin level is 0.5 to 2 ng/dL. A digoxin level of 2.4 ng/dL would warrant the nurse questioning administration of this medication. The trade name for digoxin is Lanoxin, and the classification is a cardiac glycoside.**
4. The therapeutic serum level of phenytoin (Dilantin), an anticonvulsant, is 10 to 20 mcg/mL. Because the client's level is within this range, the nurse should not question administering this medication.

7. Correct answers are 1 and 3.
1. **Administering narcotics to clients diagnosed with head injuries may mask findings of increased intracranial pressure, so the nurse questioning this medication would be appropriate.**
2. An osmotic diuretic, mannitol (Osmitrol), is the treatment of choice to help decrease intracranial pressure that occurs with a head injury.
3. **Research supports the finding that clients diagnosed with head injuries treated with anti-inflammatory corticosteroids are 20% more likely to die within 2 weeks after the head injury than those not treated with anti-inflammatory corticosteroids. The nurse should question this medication.**
4. Seizures are a common complication of head injuries; therefore, an order for an anticonvulsant medication would be appropriate.
5. There is no reason for the nurse to question an order for oxygen—which is considered a medication—for a client diagnosed with a head injury.

8. **37.5 g. To determine this, first find the client's weight in kilograms (165 pounds ÷ 2.2 = 75 kg). Then, multiply 0.5 g by weight in kilograms (0.5 × 75 kg = 37.5 kg).**

Seizures

9. 1. Phenytoin (Dilantin), an anticonvulsant, may cause the client's urine to turn a harmless pinkish-red or reddish-brown; therefore, the client does not need to call the HCP.

2. The client should take phenytoin (Dilantin), an anticonvulsant, at the same time every day with food or milk to prevent gastric upset.

3. The client should use a soft-bristled toothbrush to prevent gum irritation and bleeding. Gingival hyperplasia (overgrowth of gums) is a side effect of this medication.

4. A sore throat, bruising, or nosebleeds should be reported to the HCP because this may indicate a blood dyscrasia.

10. 1. Evening primrose oil may lower the seizure threshold, and the dose of carbamazepine (Tegretol), an anticonvulsant, may need to be modified. Therefore, the client should notify the HCP.

2. Evening primrose oil is not dangerous, and the nurse should not scare the client.

3. Although evening primrose oil may help the client's premenstrual syndrome, the nurse should inform the client that because she is also taking carbamazepine (Tegretol), an anticonvulsant, she should inform her HCP because the dose of Tegretol may need to be adjusted.

4. The nurse needs to give factual information to the client—not ask the client a question.

11. 1. Valproate (Depakote), an anticonvulsant, does not cause nephrotoxicity.

2. Valproate (Depakote), an anticonvulsant, does not cause blood dyscrasia.

3. Hepatotoxicity is one of the possible adverse reactions to Valproate (Depakote), an anticonvulsant; therefore, liver enzymes should be monitored.

4. Valproate (Depakote), an anticonvulsant, does not affect RBC count.

MEDICATION MEMORY JOGGER: The nurse must know accepted standards of practice for medication administration, including which client assessment data and laboratory data should be monitored before administering the medication.

12. 1. The therapeutic serum level of carbamazepine (Tegretol), an anticonvulsant, is 4 to 12 mcg/mL. Because the client's level is within that range, the nurse has no reason to question administering the drug.

2. The therapeutic serum level of clonazepam (Klonopin), an anticonvulsant, is 0.02 to 0.08 mcg/mL. Because the client's level is within that range, the nurse has no reason to question administering the drug.

3. The therapeutic serum level of phenytoin (Dilantin), an anticonvulsant, is 10 to 20 mcg/mL. The nurse should question administering this medication because the client's level is above that range.

4. The therapeutic serum level of ethosuximide (Zarontin), an anticonvulsant, is 40 to 100 mcg/mL. Because the client's level is within that range, the nurse has no reason to question administering the drug.

13. Correct answers are 1, 2, and 5.

1. The client should wear a MedicAlert bracelet and carry identification so that an HCP and others involved in the client's care know that the client has a seizure disorder.

2. The client should not take any OTC medications without first consulting with the HCP or pharmacist because many medications interact with fosphenytoin (Cerebyx), an anticonvulsant.

3. Alcohol and other central nerve depressants can cause an added depressive effect on the body and should be *avoided*, not just decreased.

4. Gingival hyperplasia (overgrowth of gums) is a side effect of phenytoin (Dilantin), not fosphenytoin (Cerebyx).

5. Fosphenytoin (Cerebyx) may cause anorexia, nausea, and vomiting; therefore, the client should maintain an adequate nutritional intake.

14. 1. Diazepam (Valium), a benzodiazepine, is oil-based and should not be diluted.

2. Diazepam (Valium), a benzodiazepine, is oil-based and should not be administered in an existing IV line if another option is available.

3. Diazepam (Valium), a benzodiazepine, should not be administered in an existing IV line, but the nurse does not need to question the order because there is an existing saline lock.

4. The nurse should administer the diazepam (Valium), a benzodiazepine, undiluted through the saline lock.

15. 1. This is a reflective therapeutic response that encourages the client to verbalize feelings, but the nurse should provide factual information to this client.

2. The nurse should explore the reasons for the client's fear to relay information to help the client decide to become pregnant or not, as many anticonvulsant medications can have teratogenic properties.
3. A female client diagnosed with epilepsy can take medications when pregnant and give birth to an infant without major congenital malformations.
4. The client should discuss a potential pregnancy with the significant other, but this is not addressing the client's concerns.

16. **1. Anticonvulsant dosages usually start low and gradually increase over several weeks until the serum drug level is within therapeutic range or the seizures stop.**
2. It is incorrect to state that the dosage prescribed will be the dosage for the rest of the client's life, but it is correct to state that the client will most likely remain on the medication for the rest of their life.
3. This is incorrect information. The medication is started in low dosages and gradually increased.
4. The dose of medication will be adjusted until a serum drug level is reached, but it will be more frequent than monthly.

17. 1. Phenytoin (Dilantin), an anticoagulant, cannot be administered with dextrose because it will cause precipitation.
2. Dextrose solutions should be avoided because of drug precipitation.
3. Phenytoin (Dilantin), an anticoagulant, should be diluted in a saline solution, and the IV tubing should be flushed before and after administration, because a dextrose solution will cause drug precipitation.
4. There is no reason for the nurse to cause more pain to the client by starting a saline lock because the IV tubing is already in place and can be flushed before and after the administration of phenytoin (Dilantin), an anticoagulant.

MEDICATION MEMORY JOGGER: Any time a nurse administers an IVP medication the nurse should dilute the medication. This causes less pain for the client, helps prevent infiltration of the vein, and allows the nurse to administer the medication over the correct amount of time if it is diluted to a 10-mL bolus.

Cerebrovascular Accident

18. 1. The nurse should ask all clients about taking OTC preparations when being admitted, but this question would have no bearing on the client's presenting stroke symptoms.
2. The client has symptoms of a stroke. Taking aspirin to prevent a potential problem is irrelevant. The client has a problem at this time.
3. Green, leafy vegetables are high in vitamin K, the antidote for Coumadin. The client has no reason to be taking an anticoagulant at this time.
4. Many medications for HTN have the adverse effect of causing erectile dysfunction, which many men are hesitant to discuss with their HCP. So a client may simply stop taking the medication to avoid this side effect. The nurse should assess how the client has controlled his HTN and ask specifically about erectile dysfunction related to hypertensive medicines. HTN is a risk factor for developing other cardiovascular diseases, including stroke.

19. **Correct answers are 1, 2, 3, 4, and 5.**
1. The nurse should always check the client's armband before administering medication.
2. This is the correct procedure when hanging the medication.
3. There are three types of strokes: thrombotic, embolic, and hemorrhagic. Before hanging a medication that destroys clots, the nurse must know that the client has not had a hemorrhagic stroke. Administering alteplase (Activase), a thrombolytic medication, to a client diagnosed with a hemorrhagic stroke can result in death.
4. Teaching the client can be done after the medication has been administered.
5. The client will be receiving heparin to prevent reclotting of the thrombus along with thrombolytic medication; therefore, the nurse should monitor the PTT.

20.

Potential Nursing Intervention	Indicated	Not Indicated
1. Offer toileting every 2 hours.	X	
2. Move the client close to the nurse's station.	X	
3. Administer the medication at 2100.	X	
4. Administer the medication with a full glass of water.		X
5. Do not administer if the client's apical pulse is <60 bpm.		X

1. **Alprazolam (Xanax), an antianxiety medication, has a side effect of drowsiness, which is why the HCP chose this medication for the client—to help the client rest at night. The client has cognitive deficits and should be on fall precautions, so assisting the client to the bathroom every 2 hours may prevent the client from falling while trying to get to the bathroom alone.**
2. **The client at risk for falling should be near the nursing station, if possible. This allows the staff to keep a closer watch on the client.**
3. **The medication is ordered for bedtime, usually 2100 in most health-care facilities.**
4. **Giving the medication with a full glass of water would increase the client's need to get up during the night to use the bathroom, increasing the risk of falling.**
5. **This medication does not require the apical pulse being monitored before administering the medication.**

21.
1. Strokes cause damage to the cerebral tissue; the brain does not cause damage to itself.
2. **Stroke-caused loss of function in areas of the brain leads to a problem with nerve impulse transmission; this blocked transmission can initiate a seizure. Phenytoin (Dilantin) is an anticonvulsant.**
3. If the client survives a hemorrhagic stroke, the body will reabsorb the blood. There should not be any residual blood.
4. Anticonvulsants do not increase cognitive ability.

22.
1. Propranolol (Inderal), a beta blocker, is administered for cardiac dysrhythmias and HTN and migraine headache prophylaxis. The medication could help prevent a stroke by lowering blood pressure.
2. Furosemide (Lasix) is a loop diuretic. Loop diuretics have an indirect ability to lower blood pressure by decreasing the volume of fluid in the body. This would decrease the risk of a stroke.
3. **Estradiol and norgestimate (Ortho-Cyclen) is a combination hormone used to prevent conception. Combination oral contraceptives have been associated with venous and arterial thromboembolism, pulmonary embolism, myocardial infarction, and thrombotic stroke.**
4. Adverse reaction to metformin Glucophage, a biguanide, is lactic acid buildup, not stroke.

23.
1. **HTN is a risk factor for developing a stroke. Some clients require multiple medications to control their HTN.**
2. If this were true, then atenolol (Tenormin) would be the only medication the client needs. Beta blockers are frequently used in combination with other antihypertensive medications to control a client's blood pressure.
3. Atenolol (Tenormin), a beta blocker, does not potentiate the effectiveness of loop diuretics.
4. Beta blockers, not ACE inhibitors such as enalapril (Vasotec), must be tapered off when discontinuing them to prevent rebound cardiac dysrhythmias. The HCP is adding a beta blocker to the current medications.

MEDICATION MEMORY JOGGER: Typically, medications ending in "ol" or "al" are in the beta blocker classification. Typically, medications ending in "il" are ACE inhibitors; verapamil, a calcium channel blocker (CCB), is an exception to the rule.

24.
1. This could be done if the nurse and HCP cannot simplify the medication routine.
2. This may need to be done based on the nurse's evaluation of the client's situation, but it is not the first intervention.
3. This should be done, but it is not the first intervention and does not address the problem of many medications and multiple administration times.
4. **The client has had a stroke and may have difficulty complying with multiple medications and different administration times. Research (for all clients) indicates that the fewer medication**

administration times during the day, the better the compliance with taking the medication as ordered. The nurse should discuss simplifying the medication regimen with the HCP.

25. **1. The client has experienced a bleed into the cranium. Clopidogrel (Plavix), an antiplatelet, interferes with the client's clotting ability. This medication should be held and discussed with the HCP.**

2. There is no reason to question giving a medication to decrease intracranial pressure. Osmitrol (Mannitol) is the diuretic of choice for this client. It is an osmotic diuretic, which should have the best effect on the cranial tissues.
3. Nifedipine (Procardia) is a CCB that will decrease the client's blood pressure, which is elevated in clients diagnosed with increased intracranial pressure.
4. Levothyroxine (Synthroid) is not contraindicated in hemorrhagic stroke; however, hypothyroidism is associated with an increased risk of ischemic stroke.

26. Correct answers are 1, 3, and 4.

1. Some medications can be crushed and administered in pudding if the client has difficulty swallowing, but the nurse needs to be aware that enteric-coated or timed-release medications should not be crushed.

2. The head of the bed should be elevated to 90 degrees when the client is swallowing food or medications.

3. The client's ability to swallow must be assessed before administering any oral medication. Water is the best fluid to use because it will not damage the lungs if aspirated.

4. The client who has experienced a stroke should have safety equipment at the bedside when determining if the client can swallow oral medications.

5. The client's medications are being administered orally; therefore, the nurse should not insert a nasogastric tube.

27. 1. Ticlopidine (Ticlid), an antiplatelet, may be ordered in the future once the cause of the thrombus is determined, but this would not be ordered in the ICU.

2. The Trendelenburg position is head down and would increase intracranial pressure.
3. There is no reason to restrict the client to lying on the right side, and high Fowler's is sitting upright. This would be a difficult position for the client to maintain. The client should have the head of the bed elevated approximately 30 degrees to decrease intracranial pressure by gravity drainage.

4. The anticoagulant medication heparin is administered to prevent clot reformation after lysis of the clot by the thrombolytic. Its infusion should be monitored.

Brain Tumor

28. 1. Most drugs do not cross the blood–brain barrier, so most antineoplastic agents, such as cyclophosphamide (Cytoxan), an alkylating antineoplastic agent, are not effective against cancers in the brain.

2. Octreotide (Sandostatin), a pituitary suppressant, is a growth hormone (GH) suppressant and is useful in treating acromegaly, not malignant tumors of the brain.
3. Brain tumors rarely metastasize outside of the skull cavity to cause systemic disease manifestations, such as anemia, for which erythropoietin (Epogen, Procrit), a hematopoietic growth factor, would be prescribed. Brain tumors, malignant or benign, kill by occupying space and causing increased intracranial pressure.

4. A brain tumor can cause erratic stimulation of the neurons in the brain, resulting in seizures. The nurse should expect the HCP to order phenytoin (Dilantin), an anticonvulsant, to prevent or control seizures.

29. 1. Vasopressin (DDAVP) is the antidiuretic hormone produced by the pituitary gland that is instrumental in the body's ability to conserve water. It does not affect headaches or any other type of pain. Diabetes insipidus is caused by a lack of vasopressin.

2. DDAVP is given intranasally, and the nurse should be alert to rhinitis symptoms, but lack of nasal drainage does not indicate that the medication is effective.

3. DDAVP is a synthetic form of the antidiuretic hormone vasopressin. Without vasopressin, the body does not conserve water, and a large amount of very dilute urine is excreted. The body will attempt to have the client replace the fluid by producing a symptom of extreme thirst. Lack of thirst indicates the medication is effective.

4. DDAVP will not affect seizure activity.

MEDICATION MEMORY JOGGER: The nurse determines the effectiveness of medication by assessing for the symptoms, or lack thereof, for which the medication was prescribed.

30. 1. The diet is not a priority over preventing increased intracranial pressure resulting from the tumor. It is 2000, or 8 p.m., and meals are usually served in hospitals around 0800, 1200, and 1700. The next meal will be served at 0800.

2. Dexamethasone (Decadron) is the glucocorticoid of choice for brain swelling. The client is at risk for increased intracranial pressure as a result of the tumor and edema caused by the tumor. The nurse should administer the steroid first to initiate the positive effects of the medication.

3. Prochlorperazine (Compazine) is an antiemetic. This medication is ordered a.c., which means "before meals." The next dose of this medication is not until 0730.

4. These are routine laboratory tests and will not be drawn until the next morning.

31. Correct answers are 1, 2, 3, and 4.

1. Mannitol (Osmitrol), an osmotic diuretic, can crystallize in the containers in which it is packaged, and the crystals must not be infused into the client. The nurse should inspect the bottle for crystals before beginning the administration.

2. Any client receiving a diuretic should be monitored for intake and output to determine if the client is excreting more than the intake.

3. Mannitol (Osmitrol) is an osmotic diuretic and works by pulling fluid from the tissues into the blood vessels. Clients diagnosed with heart failure or at risk for heart failure may develop fluid volume overload. Therefore, the nurse should assess lung sounds before administering this medication.

4. Neurological examinations should be performed when administering this medication for a brain tumor.

5. Calcium gluconate will not affect this medication, nor is it an antidote.

32. 1. Meperidine (Demerol), a narcotic opioid, metabolizes into normeperidine in the body, and accumulation of this substance can cause seizures. It is not recommended to give Demerol to children, and the schedule may be excessive. The nurse should not automatically administer narcotics to a client diagnosed with neurological impairment. The nurse should determine the client's neurological status before administering a medication that can mask symptoms.

2. There is no reason to question prescription of a steroid to a client with a brain tumor.

3. The client may need this medication to control mild pain or fever until the body has a chance to readjust its thermoregulatory mechanism.

4. An antiemetic can prevent the child from vomiting and increasing intracranial pressure during that activity. The vomiting center is in the brain and can become irritated due to increased intracranial pressure.

33.

Potential Nursing Intervention	Indicated	Not Indicated
1. Instruct the client to increase fluids while taking the medications.	X	
2. Talk to the client about taking bulk laxatives daily.	X	
3. Teach the significant other to perform a neurological assessment.		X
4. Discuss limiting the amount of medication allowed per day.		X
5. Explain safety issues when taking narcotic medications.	X	

1. The client is at risk for constipation because of the effects of narcotics on the gastrointestinal tract. The client should be encouraged to increase the amount of fluid intake.

2. The client is at risk for constipation. A bowel regimen should be instituted, including bulk laxatives as part of the regimen.

3. The significant other does not need to be taught to perform a neurological assessment for this medication. They should be instructed to hold the next dose and notify the HCP if the client becomes excessively drowsy. It may be necessary to allow the drowsiness to control the pain.

4. **The medication may need to be increased, not limited, to control the pain. The amount of pain medication required should be provided.**
5. **The client should not drive motor vehicles or use machinery and should be careful ambulating and climbing stairs. These are safety issues.**

34. 1. **Radiation therapy may cause nausea. An antiemetic should be ordered so the client can maintain nutritional status and comfort.**
2. As the tumor shrinks from the radiation, the pain associated with the tumor should decrease, not increase, so the medication is not needed.
3. The skin in the radiation field should be cleaned with mild soap and water, being careful not to obliterate the markings. Medicated lotions can irritate the skin.
4. The therapy sessions take from 5 to 10 minutes and require the client to lie still, but usually, antianxiety medications are not needed.

35. 1. Octreotide (Sandostatin), a pituitary suppressant, does not increase the risk of falls.
2. Octreotide (Sandostatin), a pituitary suppressant, does not cause bone resorption, so calcium replacement is not needed.
3. Octreotide (Sandostatin), a pituitary suppressant, does not cause acne or acne-like problems.
4. **Octreotide (Sandostatin), a pituitary suppressant, can cost thousands of dollars a year (about $8,000). Before beginning the treatment, the nurse and HCP must know that the client can afford the medication.**

36. 1. The HCP will regulate the dose to achieve a normal growth rate for the child. Heights and weights are taken monthly to determine the effectiveness of the medication. This therapy continues until the epiphyseal closure occurs or until about 20 to 24 years.
2. Tapering is not needed.
3. Lack of growth hormone (GH) can result in dwarfism, but will not cause intellectual disability.
4. **Human GH is diabetogenic and can cause hyperglycemia.**

37. 1. Alprazolam (Xanax), an antianxiety medication, does not cause seizures; the client has a brain tumor that is most likely the cause of the seizures.
2. The client would not know if a vitamin was causing a seizure. The most probable cause of the seizure is the brain tumor.
3. **Therapeutic levels of phenytoin (Dilantin), an anticonvulsant, are needed to control aberrant brain activity. The therapeutic level is 10 to 20 mcg/dL.**
4. The client may need a CT scan or magnetic resonance imaging to determine if tumor growth is causing the increase in frequency of seizures, but the nurse should determine if a therapeutic level of phenytoin (Dilantin), an anticonvulsant, is being maintained first.

Parkinson's Disease

38. 1. Cogwheel motion is a symptom of PD. Displaying cogwheel motion does not indicate the medication is effective.
2. Carbidopa and levodopa (Sinemet) is an anti-Parkinson's drug that is a combination medication designed to delay the breakdown of levodopa (dopamine) in the periphery. A flat affect or no emotions would not indicate the medication is effective.
3. **One of the symptoms of PD is a forward shuffling gait, so being able to walk upright without stumbling would indicate that the medication is effective.**
4. The client should be encouraged to consume at least 50% of the meals provided. Meal times that last 1 hour are not encouraged because the client becomes fatigued and the food temperature changes. Hot foods become cold and cold foods become lukewarm. The client should be served frequent, small meals each day.

39. 1. All the symptoms may not be controlled even if the client adheres to a strict medication regimen.
2. **PD is treated with medications and surgery. The medications have side effects and adverse effects, so effectiveness may be reduced over time.**
3. The client diagnosed with PD will need to take the medications for life unless surgery is performed and a significant improvement is achieved.
4. The medications do not have to be tapered when discontinued.

40. 1. **In PD, there is decreased dopamine in the brain. Carbidopa delays the breakdown of levodopa (dopamine) in the periphery so that more of the levodopa crosses the blood–brain barrier and reaches the brain.**
2. The expense of the medication is not the reason for the drug combination.

3. Levodopa breaking down in the periphery is why the medications are combined.
4. Carbidopa does not increase levodopa's action; it delays the breakdown of the compound in the periphery.

41. 1. The medication is not interrupted for this reason.
2. With long-term use of levodopa (L-Dopa), an anti-Parkinson's medication, the adverse effects tend to increase, and the client may develop a drug tolerance where therapeutic effects decrease. A short hiatus from the medication (10 days) may result in beneficial effects being achieved with lower doses.
3. Early in treating PD with levodopa, the client may have postural hypotension, but HTN is not associated with levodopa.
4. An overdose was not taken; the client's tolerance to the medication has changed.

42. Correct answers are 1 and 5.
1. Daytime somnolence is seen in about 22% of clients taking pramipexole (Mirapex), a dopamine agonist medication. A few clients experience overwhelming and irresistible sleepiness that comes on without warning.
2. The on–off effect with levodopa occurs when the therapeutic effects of the medication wear off.
3. Salivation is not a side effect of pramipexole (Mirapex), a dopamine agonist medication.
4. Pill-rolling motion is a symptom of PD, not a side effect of a medication.
5. Stiff muscles are a finding of an adverse side effect of pramipexole (Mirapex), a dopamine agonist medication, indicating a need to discontinue the medication.

43. 1. Increased vasodilatation causes hypotension. This is not a reason to administer this drug.
2. Entacapone (Comtan) is a catechol-O-methyltransferase (COMT) inhibitor. Entacapone is given in conjunction with levodopa to inhibit the metabolism of levodopa in the intestines and peripheral tissues. There is no substitute for dopamine. Medications can increase the relative availability of dopamine present in the body or can be a form of dopamine itself.
3. Many side effects may interfere with treatment, including hallucinations, postural hypotension, dyskinesias, and sleep disturbances.
4. Entacapone (Comtan) is a catechol-O-methyltransferase (COMT) inhibitor that increases the half-life of levodopa by 50% to 75%, thereby causing levodopa blood levels to be smoother and more sustained. This delays the "off" effects and prolongs the "on" effects of levodopa.

44. 1. Clients diagnosed with chronic illnesses should receive the flu vaccination. There is no reason not to get the flu vaccine when receiving amantadine.
2. The effectiveness of amantadine (Symmetrel) may diminish in 3 to 6 months. If clinical manifestations of PD recur, the client should notify the HCP.
3. Amantadine (Symmetrel), a PD medication, can enhance the response of the other PD medications and is given in the same dosage as if given alone.
4. A dry mouth is a side effect, not an adverse effect. The client should be taught to chew sugarless gum or hard candies to relieve the dry mouth.

45. 1. Anticholinergic medications are not contraindicated for clients diagnosed with heart failure.
2. Anticholinergic medications are not contraindicated for clients diagnosed with myocardial infarction.
3. Anticholinergic medications, such as benztropine (Cogentin), block cholinergic receptors in the eye and may precipitate or aggravate glaucoma.
4. Anticholinergic medications are not contraindicated for clients undergoing surgery.

MEDICATION MEMORY JOGGER: Glaucoma is affected by any medication that has the effect of drying secretions.

46. Correct answers are 1, 2, and 4.
1. Initially, levodopa can cause orthostatic hypotension. The client should be taught to rise slowly to prevent falls.
2. The client may experience an "on" effect of symptom control when the medication is effective and an "off" effect near the time for the next dose of medication.
3. Food can decrease the absorption of levodopa; administration with meals should be avoided, if possible.
4. Clients should be warned that darkening of the urine and sweat is a harmless side effect of this medication.
5. Routine blood levels of levodopa are not drawn.

47. 1. Safinamide (Xadago), a monoamine oxidase B (MAO-B) inhibitor, is added to the carbidopa and levodopa (Sinemet) regimen.

2. The nurse should teach the side effects of the medications that the client is prescribed. Safinamide (Xadago) side effects include orthostatic hypotension, dyskinesia, worsening of PD symptoms, falls, insomnia, anxiety, cough, cataracts, and indigestion. The client should notify the HCP if these occur. The medication is started at 50 mg per day for 2 weeks and can be increased to 100 mg per day after that.

3. Safinamide (Xadago) can be administered at any time of the day or night and with or without food.

4. There are side effects with any medication. This is a false statement.

MEDICATION MEMORY JOGGER: The test taker can eliminate option "4" because all medications have side effects. Just because the medication is newer on the market does not mean it has fewer side effects.

Alzheimer's Disease

48. 1. Donepezil (Aricept) is a cholinesterase inhibitor. There are other medications in the classification of cholinesterase inhibitors that may be tried because the medications are not identical. Additionally, vitamin E in large doses, selegiline, and gingko biloba have been shown to slow progression of AD. This answer on the part of the nurse is not providing information and is not directly answering the family member's question.

2. The progression of AD is inevitable at some point. Cholinesterase inhibitors are prescribed for clients diagnosed with mild to moderate symptoms of AD, and they can delay progression of AD. This is not the time to discuss long-term care.

3. If the client does not respond to one of the cholinesterase inhibitors, then another may be tried because the drugs are not identical. The client may be responsive to a different medication in the same classification.

4. There are more options to discuss regarding treatment of AD.

49. 1. Donepezil (Aricept) is a cholinesterase inhibitor that does not bind dopamine.

2. Cholinesterase inhibitors increase availability of acetylcholine at cholinergic synapses, resulting in increased transmission of acetylcholine by cholinergic neurons that have not been destroyed by AD.

3. Donepezil (Aricept) is a cholinesterase inhibitor and does not decrease acetylcholine in the periphery.

4. Donepezil (Aricept) is a cholinesterase inhibitor and enhances availability of acetylcholine at the receptor sites.

50. 1. Tricyclic antidepressants, first-generation antihistamines, and antipsychotics can reduce the client's response to cholinesterase inhibitors. Antipsychotics are useful for clients with erratic and uncontrollable behavior in end-stage disease. The cholinesterase inhibitor rivastigmine (Exelon) would not be helpful at this stage of the disease.

2. Warfarin (Coumadin), an anticoagulant, interacts with several medications but not cholinesterase inhibitors.

3. Cholinesterase inhibitors do not interact with phenytoin (Dilantin), an anticonvulsant.

4. Prochlorperazine (Compazine), an antiemetic, may be used to control nausea produced by rivastigmine (Exelon). There is no reason to question administering this medication.

51. 1. This is a daily medication and could be administered at any time.

2. This client is nauseated and should be given medication after protecting the client at risk for injury.

3. This medication can be administered after the client's nausea medication in option #2, but it is not a priority at this time.

4. This client is at risk of harming themself or others. Antipsychotic medications are used to control this type of behavior.

52. 1. Galantamine hydrobromide (Reminyl) is a cholinesterase inhibitor and is prescribed for mild to moderate AD. The client's safety should be the nurse's first concern. Moving the client to a room where they can be observed more closely is one of the first steps in a fall prevention protocol.

2. This should be done, but it is not prioritized over client safety.

3. The medications do not cause dry mouth. The UAP can provide water for the client, provided there is no reason not to. Clients

taking bulk laxatives should increase fluid intake, but this is not the first intervention.
4. The RN should assess for effectiveness of all medications, including laxatives, but this is not the first concern.

53. 1. This may not indicate a decrease in abilities, but it does not indicate an improvement in cognitive abilities, which is what the question is asking.
2. Cholinesterase inhibitors are prescribed to increase the cognitive ability for clients diagnosed with AD. Discussing an upcoming event indicates the client can focus on a topic and remember that something will happen in the future.
3. This may not indicate a decrease in abilities, but it does not indicate an improvement in cognitive abilities, which is what the question is asking.
4. This may not indicate a decrease in abilities, but it does not indicate an improvement in cognitive abilities, which is what the question is asking.

54. 1. There are medications that can be taken to reduce the risk of developing AD. There is a genetic link to developing AD.
2. Brain scans are not recommended to determine if neuronal damage is occurring and lead to AD development.
3. Research has proved the efficacy of hormone replacement therapy (HRT) and NSAIDs in preventing AD.
4. HRT has been proven to reduce the risk of developing AD by 30% to 40% in postmenopausal women. Other medications that have been proven to aid in preventing AD are NSAIDs.

55. 1. The medications may be taken at any time.
2. There is no reason for routine blood tests to determine toxicity.
3. Medications used to treat AD only slow the progression of AD. Currently, no medications, prescribed or OTC, have been proven to reverse or permanently prevent the progression of neuronal destruction.
4. The medications do not produce photosensitivity. The client should use sunscreen, but not because of the medications.

56. 1. An advantage of donepezil (Aricept), a cholinesterase inhibitor, is once-a-day dosing. Research has proven that the more doses required each day, the less actual compliance with the medication regimen. Additionally, donepezil (Aricept) is not hepatotoxic and is better tolerated than some cholinesterase inhibitors.
2. There is no contraindication to administering NSAIDs and cholinesterase inhibitors simultaneously.
3. Donepezil (Aricept), a cholinesterase inhibitor, does not enhance vitamin E.
4. There are side effects with any medications. The common side effects of Aricept are nausea, diarrhea, and bradycardia.

57.

Potential Nursing Intervention	Indicated	Not Indicated
1. Inform the client to take the medication with food.	X	
2. Check the client's BUN and creatinine levels.	X	
3. Teach the client to wear a MedicAlert bracelet with drug information.		X
4. Assess the client's other routine medications.	X	
5. Discuss not abruptly discontinuing the medication.		X

1. The most common side effect of galantamine (Reminyl), a cholinesterase inhibitor, is gastrointestinal disturbance. This can be minimized if the medication is taken with food.
2. Galantamine (Reminyl), a cholinesterase inhibitor, is excreted by the kidneys. The dose is limited for clients diagnosed with renal or liver impairment and used with caution in clients diagnosed with severe impairment.
3. There is no reason to require the client to wear a MedicAlert bracelet. All clients should keep a list of current medications with them in case of an emergency.
4. Effects of cholinesterase inhibitors may be reduced by first-generation

antihistamine medications, tricyclic antidepressants, and antipsychotics, and the client should not take these medications simultaneously. The nurse should ask the client about other medications taken.

5. **The medication does not have to be tapered off to avoid adverse effects.**

MEDICATION MEMORY JOGGER: Because the hepatic and renal systems are responsible for metabolizing and excreting all medications, monitoring the liver and kidney laboratory values is a pertinent nursing action.

Migraine Headache

58. 1. The client request is not a scientific rationale for prescribing a medication route.
2. Migraine headaches respond to an oral medication when administered prophylactically, but the client is less likely to respond to oral medication after the attack has begun.
3. **Because migraine headaches often cause nausea, vomiting, and gastric stasis, oral medications may not be tolerated or may not be effective once an attack has begun.**
4. Addiction to medications depends on many factors. Depending on the medication in question, the parenteral, IM, IV, or oral route may all be addicting.

59. 1. Feverfew decreases the effectiveness of prescription NSAIDs. The HCP should be notified when a client takes both medications simultaneously so dosage adjustments can be made. The dose of NSAIDs would have to be increased to achieve the same effectiveness.
2. **The client is of childbearing age and should be warned that tanacetum parthenium (Feverfew) crosses the placental barrier and may cause problems with the fetus. The nurse should teach the client to avoid pregnancy and not to breastfeed while taking feverfew.**
3. The client may not see results for 4 to 6 weeks when taking feverfew. The best results are achieved when the medication is taken continuously for prophylaxis of migraine headaches.
4. Feverfew is also given to relieve menstrual problems. It should not increase menstrual difficulties.

MEDICATION MEMORY JOGGER: Whenever the female client is of childbearing age, the nurse must be concerned with possible pregnancy when administering medications. Many medications are teratogenic.

60. 1. These symptoms indicate the client is responding to the long-term use of headache medication, not developing a resistance to the medications.
2. Pain is whatever the client says it is and occurs whenever the client says it does. The client is reporting a subjective symptom and seeking help, not judgment.
3. **Medication overuse headaches occur when clients take headache medication every day. These headaches are also known as rebound or drug-induced headaches. The headache will persist for days to weeks after the medication has been discontinued.**
4. Use of medications for migraine headaches does not cause brain tumors.

61. 1. **The client rates the pain as a 4. NSAIDs are given for mild to moderate migraine pain.**
2. An opioid analgesic should be given only if ergot alkaloids or selective serotonin receptor agonist medications (migraine-specific medications) are not effective in treating the pain.
3. The client reports mild to moderate pain. A migraine-specific drug, such as an ergot alkaloid, should be given for moderate to severe pain.
4. The client reports mild to moderate pain. A migraine-specific drug, such as a selective serotonin receptor agonist, should be given for moderate to severe pain.

62. 1. Abortive therapy is used to treat an actual migraine headache to limit the intensity and duration of the headache. Using the medication more than 1 to 2 days per week can cause medication overuse headaches (MOH).
2. The client should take their radial pulse if receiving preventive therapy with a beta blocker medication—not for the medications used to abort a headache.
3. Common side effects of abortive medications are nausea, vomiting, and diarrhea. Development of HTN is not associated with these medications. Care should be taken to ensure the client is experiencing a migraine because severe HTN can also cause a headache.
4. **Use of abortive medications more than 1 to 2 days per week frequently results in a drug-induced headache, or MOH.**

63. 0.5 mL. To set this problem up algebraically:

The first step is: **6 : X = 12 : 1 (or $\frac{6}{X} = \frac{12}{1}$)**
Then cross-multiply **12 X = 6 to get:**
The next step is **X = $\frac{6}{12}$ to get the X by itself:**
Simplify: **X = 1/2 or 0.5 mL**

64.
1. This indicates an improvement in the number of headaches the client normally experiences and is the only option that indicates an improvement in a condition.
2. This client should be taught to take the radial pulse for 1 minute and to hold the Inderal if the pulse is less than 60 bpm because propranolol (Inderal) is a beta blocker and beta blockers slow the heart rate. This does not indicate the medication is effective.
3. This may be a side effect of the medication because beta blockers are frequently prescribed for HTN, but this effect does not indicate the medication's effectiveness in preventing migraine.
4. Supplementing the Inderal with an abortive medication four times indicates that the Inderal has not been effective in preventing headaches.

65.
1. Propranolol (Inderal), a beta blocker, is used to prevent migraine headaches, and almotriptan (Axert), a triptan, is used to treat migraine headaches. The client's symptoms support the diagnosis of cluster headaches, not migraines.
2. The client's symptoms support the diagnosis of cluster headaches related to migraines but differ in several ways. Cluster headaches are less common than migraines and occur in males 5:1. Cluster headaches do not cause nausea and vomiting; they can be more debilitating than migraines; they do not have an aura; and they are not linked to genetics. The drugs of choice to treat cluster headaches are prednisone, a glucocorticoid, and lithium (Lithobid), a psychotherapeutic agent. High-dose prednisone can reduce symptoms within 48 hours, and lithium can prevent headaches altogether. Lithium takes 1 to 2 weeks before relief is noted.
3. Amitriptyline (Elavil), a tricyclic antidepressant, is useful in preventing migraine headaches, not cluster headaches, and an estrogen patch, estradiol and levonorgestrel (Climara) is useful in preventing menstrual migraine headaches.
4. Ibuprofen (Motrin), an NSAID, is used to treat mild to moderate migraine headaches, and metoclopramide (Reglan), a gastric motility agent, is the antiemetic of choice to treat the nausea and vomiting and relieve the gastric stasis of migraine headaches.

66.
1. Sunbathing does not affect a tension headache. Clients diagnosed with migraine headaches may be sensitive to light.
2. Iodine will not affect a tension headache. Caffeine intake may prevent a headache for some clients.
3. This would be a good question if the client were suffering from a migraine headache because a drug commonly used to treat migraine, ergotamine, should not be taken by a pregnant woman as it may cause uterine contractions. However, this client has a tension headache, not a migraine.
4. Clients will attempt to self-treat with OTC medications before seeking medical attention. The nurse should assess what the client has already tried to relieve the headache.

67.
1. The meal trays are usually served between 1630 and 1700 on most nursing units. Humalog has an onset of action of 5 to 7 minutes. The nurse should not administer this insulin until closer to the meal being served.
2. Morphine may be used to treat severe migraine headaches when other measures have not been effective. This client needs the medication as soon as possible (pain is rated as 8), and this should be the first medication administered.
3. Divalproex (Depakote ER) is used to prevent migraine headaches in the extended-release form. This medication would not be administered before treating a headache that is occurring.
4. Metoclopramide (Reglan), a gastric motility agent, is given for nausea and vomiting and to relieve gastric stasis for clients diagnosed with a migraine headache. The option did not say that the client was vomiting at this time. A headache rated as an 8 would be a priority.

MEDICATION MEMORY JOGGER: Pain is a priority, and pain rated as an 8 indicates severe pain. The test taker should look at the times and know the actions of the medications administered. This eliminates option 1 as a possible answer.

NEUROLOGICAL SYSTEM COMPREHENSIVE EXAMINATION

1. The client diagnosed with urinary retention is receiving bethanechol. For each intervention, specify if the intervention is **indicated or not indicated** for the client's care.

Potential Nursing Intervention	Indicated	Not Indicated
1. Limit the client's fluid intake to 1,000 mL daily.		
2. Have the client's urinal readily available.		
3. Maintain hourly intake and output for the client.		
4. Monitor the client's serum creatinine level.		
5. Instruct the client to take the medication on an empty stomach.		

2. To which client should the nurse **question** administering atropine?
   1. The 69-year-old client diagnosed with glaucoma
   2. The 60-year-old client diagnosed with symptomatic sinus bradycardia
   3. The 55-year-old client being prepped for abdominal surgery
   4. The 28-year-old client diagnosed with severe diarrhea

3. The 28-year-old client diagnosed with obesity is reporting nervousness, irritability, insomnia, and heart palpitations. Which question should the clinic nurse ask the client **first**?
   1. "How much weight have you gained or lost within the last 12 months?"
   2. "Do you make yourself vomit after eating large meals?"
   3. "Is there any history of you taking illegal drugs such as amphetamines?"
   4. "Have you been taking any OTC appetite suppressants?"

4. The client is undergoing electroconvulsive therapy for major depression and is receiving tubocurarine. The client's vital signs are populated in the following vital sign flowsheet.

Vital Sign Flowsheet	Client Values	Reference Values
Temperature	99.8°F/37.6°C	Oral: 98°F (36.7°C)
Pulse	58 bpm	60 to 100 bpm
Respirations	10 breaths/min	12 to 20 breaths/min
Blood Pressure	110/70 mm Hg	100 to 119 mm Hg systolic 60 to 80 mm Hg diastolic

Which data **warrants immediate** intervention by the nurse?
1. Apical pulse
2. Oral temperature
3. Respiratory rate
4. Blood pressure

5. The client diagnosed with epilepsy and prescribed phenytoin calls the clinic and reports a measles-like rash. Which intervention should the nurse implement?
   1. Instruct the client to come to the clinic immediately.
   2. Determine if the client is drinking grapefruit juice.
   3. Encourage the client to apply hydrocortisone cream to the rash.
   4. Explain that this is a common side effect of this medication.

6. The client diagnosed with Parkinson's disease has been taking amantadine. The home health nurse notes a new finding of mottled skin discoloration. Which intervention should the nurse implement?
   1. Ask the client if they have changed soap products.
   2. Prepare the significant other for the client's imminent death.
   3. Notify the HCP to discontinue the medication.
   4. Explain that this is expected and document the finding.

7. The daughter of a client diagnosed with Alzheimer's disease tells the home health nurse that she gives her mother ginkgo biloba. Which intervention should the nurse implement?
   1. Tell her to stop giving her mother the herb because it will not help.
   2. Teach her that herbs have many life-threatening adverse effects.
   3. Explain that the effects may only last 6 to 12 months.
   4. Ask the HCP to prescribe tacrine instead of the herb.

8. The client diagnosed with late-stage Alzheimer's disease is agitated and having delusions. Which medication should the nurse anticipate the HCP prescribing?
   1. Donepezil
   2. Haloperidol
   3. Fluoxetine
   4. Amitriptyline

9. The client diagnosed with Parkinson's disease taking selegiline, had hip surgery, and is being admitted to the orthopedic department. The nurse is verifying the postoperative orders. Which postoperative order should the nurse **question**?
   1. Enoxaparin
   2. Morphine sulfate
   3. Buspirone
   4. Cefazolin

10. The client diagnosed with epilepsy has undergone a spontaneous remission of the epilepsy, a rare but occasional occurrence. What information should the nurse discuss with the client when **discontinuing** antiepileptic drugs?
    1. Discuss the need to taper off the antiepileptic drugs slowly.
    2. Explain the importance of getting routine serum levels.
    3. Teach the client to continue taking the antiepileptic drugs.
    4. Instruct the client to use a soft-bristled toothbrush.

11. The client with a history of gastric ulcers is diagnosed with transient ischemic attack and prescribed a daily 325-mg aspirin. For each intervention, specify if the intervention is **indicated or not indicated** for the client's care.

Potential Nursing Intervention	Indicated	Not Indicated
1. Encourage the client to take aspirin with one glass of water.		
2. Notify the HCP if ringing in the ears occurs.		
3. Instruct the client to take an enteric-coated brand of aspirin.		
4. Notify the HCP if the client has black, tarry stools.		
5. Explain that gastrointestinal distress is expected when taking aspirin.		

12. The client diagnosed with a severe head injury was exhibiting decorticate posturing during the nurse's assessment 2 hours ago. The client is receiving mannitol. Which data indicates the medication is **not effective**?
   1. The client pushes the nurse's hand away in response to pain.
   2. The client's Glasgow Coma Scale score is a 13.
   3. The client cannot state the day of the week.
   4. The client exhibits flaccid paralysis to painful stimuli.

13. The client presents to the ED reporting a migraine headache. The HCP prescribes sumatriptan. When the nurse enters the room to administer the medication, the client is laughing with their significant other. Which intervention should the nurse implement?
   1. Notify the HCP of the client's drug-seeking behavior.
   2. Ask the client how bad the headache is if they can laugh.
   3. Administer the medication after checking for allergies and the ID bracelet.
   4. Discharge the client and recommend taking OTC medication.

14. The client is admitted into the ED reporting profuse salivation, excessive tearing, and diarrhea. The client tells the nurse about currently camping and living off the land. Which medication should the nurse anticipate administering?
   1. Atropine
   2. Diphenhydramine
   3. Magnesium and aluminum hydroxide
   4. Pantoprazole

15. The client diagnosed with epilepsy is seen in the clinic and has a serum phenytoin level of 5.4 mcg/dL. Which intervention should the nurse implement?
   1. Request that the laboratory verify the results of the test.
   2. Ask the client when the dose was taken last.
   3. Instruct the client not to take the phenytoin for 2 days.
   4. Discuss the need to increase the dose of the medication.

16. The client diagnosed with cerebrovascular accident is reporting a headache. Which interventions should the rehabilitation nurse implement? **Rank in order of priority.**
   1. Assess the client's neurological status.
   2. Administer oral acetaminophen.
   3. Have the client swallow a drink of water.
   4. Ask the client to give their date of birth.
   5. Ask the client to rate pain on a scale of 1 to 10.

17. The client is going on a cruise and tells the clinic nurse, "I am worried about getting seasick. What should I do?" Which statement is the nurse's **best** response?
   1. "You are worried about getting seasick. Let's sit down and talk about it."
   2. "Take the motion sickness medication when you start getting nauseated."
   3. "If you get seasick, you should take an antacid to help with nausea."
   4. "I would recommend taking meclizine HCL 30 minutes before your departure."

18. The client is prescribed meclizine HCL for vertigo. Which statement by the client **warrants intervention** by the nurse?
   1. "I have had someone drive my car because I have been getting dizzy."
   2. "I will tell my HCPs about taking this medication."
   3. "I usually have one or two glasses of wine with my evening meal."
   4. "I will chew sugarless gum or suck on hard candy if my mouth is dry."

19. The client diagnosed with a brain tumor is reporting a headache that is a 5 on a scale of 1 to 10. The prescribed medication for administration is in the following medication administration record (MAR).

Client: K.R.	MR# 1234567	Date: Today
Age: 61 years	Allergies: NKDA	Diagnosis: Brain Tumor
Medication	0701-1900	1901-0700
Acetaminophen 325 mg x 2 tablets PO PRN pain		
Hydrocodone 2.5 mg/Acetaminophen 325 mg x 2 tablets PO PRN pain		
Morphine 4 mg IVP every 6 hours PRN pain		
Lorazepam 1 mg IVP every 8 hours PRN		
Nurse Initials/Credentials	DN/RN	NN/RN

Which medication should the nurse prepare to administer?
1. Acetaminophen
2. Hydrocodone and acetaminophen
3. Morphine
4. Lorazepam

20. The nurse is administering mannitol to the client diagnosed with a head injury. The order reads 1,000 mL IVPB over 6 hours. At which rate should the nurse administer the medication via a pump?

____

21. The nurse is caring for a client diagnosed with chronic neuropathic pain requiring round-the-clock administration of an opioid narcotic pain medication. The client tells the nurse about having very hard stools and only every 4 to 5 days. Which medication should the nurse discuss with the client?
1. Tell the client to take magnesium hydroxide every other day.
2. Teach the client to alternate three acetaminophen 500 mg tablets with the opioid every 2 hours.
3. Instruct the client to discuss taking haloxegol with the HCP.
4. Remind the client to take bisacodyl twice a day to prevent constipation.

22. The RN is preparing to administer the client's morning medications. The prescribed medication for administration is in the following MAR.

Client: R.V.	MR# 1234567	Date: Today
Age: 68 years	Allergies: NKDA	Diagnosis: PD with Hallucinations
Medication	**0701–1900**	**1901–0700**
Carbidopa and levodopa 25 mg/100 mg XR PO daily	0900	
Metformin 500 mg PO b.i.d.	0800	
Pimavanserin 17-mg tabs x 2 tablets PO daily	0900	
Enteric-coated aspirin 81 mg PO daily	0900	
Levothyroxine 75 mcg oral daily	0900	
Nurse Initials/Credentials	**DN/RN**	**NN/RN**

Which intervention should the nurse implement?
1. Sit the client up in the bedside chair.
2. Have the UAP check the client's ability to swallow.
3. Ask the client to demonstrate their ability to ambulate.
4. Assess the client's orientation to person, time, place, and surroundings.

23. The nurse is caring for a client diagnosed with partial onset seizures related to epilepsy. The HCP has prescribed brivaracetam. Which should the nurse discuss with the client?
1. "Be sure to see the dentist regularly because the medication can cause gingival hyperplasia."
2. "Regular laboratory work must be obtained to monitor the levels of the drug."
3. "Do not drive or operate heavy machinery until the HCP determines it is safe to do so."
4. "You should take baths only."

NEUROLOGICAL SYSTEM COMPREHENSIVE EXAMINATION ANSWERS AND RATIONALES

1.

Potential Nursing Intervention	Indicated	Not Indicated
1. Limit the client's fluid intake to 1,000 mL daily.		X
2. Have the client's urinal readily available.	X	
3. Maintain hourly intake and output for the client.		X
4. Monitor the client's serum creatinine level.		X
5. Instruct the client to take the medication on an empty stomach.	X	

1. **If the nurse decreases the client's fluid intake, the client could become dehydrated due to the increase of urine output caused by the bethanechol (Urecholine), a muscarinic agonist, as well as sweating, salivation, bronchial secretions, and increased secretions of gastric acid.**
2. **This medication relaxes the urinary sphincters and increases voiding pressure by contracting the detrusor muscle of the bladder; therefore, the client will need to have a urinal available for frequent urination.**
3. **An every-shift intake and output would be sufficient to determine the effectiveness of this medication. An hourly intake and output is not needed.**
4. **The client's kidney function does not need to be evaluated before administering this medication.**
5. **The client should take bethanechol on an empty stomach, at least 1 hour before or 2 hours after a meal.**

2.
1. **Atropine, a muscarinic agent, is contraindicated for a client diagnosed with glaucoma because atropine causes mydriasis and paralysis of the ciliary muscle, which would increase intraocular pressure and may cause blindness.**
2. Atropine, a muscarinic agent, is the medication of choice for the client with light-headedness and dizziness from sinus bradycardia manifested by low apical pulse rate; therefore, the nurse would not question administering this medication.
3. Preoperative treatment with atropine, a muscarinic agent, can prevent a dangerous reduction in heart rate, and it dries secretions, which is needed during surgery. The nurse should not question administering this medication.
4. By blocking the muscarinic receptors in the intestine, atropine can decrease the tone and motility of intestinal smooth muscle, which will decrease episodes of diarrhea.

MEDICATION MEMORY JOGGER: Glaucoma is affected by any medication that has the effect of drying secretions.

3.
1. Asking about weight loss and weight gain is an appropriate question for a client diagnosed with obesity, but this client's physiological clinical manifestations require a more specific question.
2. This is a question the nurse would ask a client suspected of having bulimia, which is not apparent with this client.
3. Asking the client about illegal drug use may be appropriate, but the nurse should first ask about prescribed medications or OTC self-medication. This question likely will cause the client to become defensive.
4. **These physiological clinical manifestations could indicate long-term use of anorexiants (appetite suppressants); therefore, the nurse should discuss this question with the client.**

4.
1. This medication does not affect the apical heart rate.
2. This medication does not affect the client's temperature.
3. **The primary effect of tubocurarine, a nondepolarizing neuromuscular blocker, is the relaxation of skeletal muscles,**

producing a state of flaccid paralysis. Paralysis of the respiratory muscles can cause respiratory arrest; therefore, a respiratory rate of 10 would warrant immediate intervention by the nurse.

4. This blood pressure is within normal limits and, therefore, would not warrant intervention by the nurse.

5. **1. This morbilliform (measles-like) rash may progress to a more serious reaction to phenytoin (Dilantin), an anticonvulsant; therefore, the client should come to the clinic immediately, and the medication should be stopped immediately.**

2. Grapefruit does not cause a measles-like rash; therefore, the nurse should not ask this question.
3. This rash has potentially life-threatening consequences, and hydrocortisone cream will not help the client.
4. This is not a normal side effect of the medication.

MEDICATION MEMORY JOGGER: Grapefruit juice interacts with many medications and causes problems with absorption, but the interaction with medications does not cause a rash.

6. 1. This change in status would not result from soaps. A rash or skin irritation would be expected with soap products.

2. Mottling of the skin is a finding of imminent death in some clients, but the nurse must be aware of the potential side effects of medications. This client is not dying.
3. This side effect is not life-threatening and, as long as the medication is effective, there is no reason to discontinue the medication.
4. **Clients taking amantadine (Symmetrel), an anti-Parkinson's drug, for 1 month or longer often develop a mottled discoloration of the skin called livedo reticularis, a benign condition that will gradually disappear after discontinuation of the drug. This condition is not a reason to discontinue the medication as long as it is effective. The effectiveness of this medication begins to diminish within 3 to 6 months.**

7. 1. This herb can stabilize or improve cognitive performance and social behavior for 6 to 12 months; therefore, it does help the symptoms of uncomplicated AD.

2. Most herbs do not have life-threatening adverse effects. Ginkgo biloba should be taken with caution when taking antiplatelets or anticoagulants because it will increase the risk of bleeding.
3. **Research has determined that ginkgo biloba has biological activity in treating uncomplicated AD for up to 12 months. At this time, medications for AD result in temporary improvement of the symptoms.**
4. Ginkgo biloba extract has proven to be as effective as tacrine (Cognex), a cholinesterase inhibitor agent, so there is no reason to change to this medication. Tacrine has a significant risk of liver damage and is avoided in favor of the other cholinesterase inhibitors.

8. 1. Donepezil (Aricept), a cholinesterase inhibitor, is prescribed in the early stages of AD but would not be effective in the late stages.

2. **Delusions and agitation respond to antipsychotic medications. Haloperidol (Haldol), an antipsychotic medication, has been used and has proven to be effective in treating these symptoms, so the nurse should anticipate this prescription.**
3. Fluoxetine (Prozac), a selective serotonin reuptake inhibitor, is useful in treating the depression of AD, but these symptoms do not indicate depression.
4. Amitriptyline (Elavil) is a tricyclic antidepressant. Tricyclic antidepressants have significant anticholinergic actions and may intensify the symptoms of AD; therefore, the nurse would not anticipate this being prescribed.

9. 1. The nurse would expect the client to be taking a prophylactic anticoagulant to prevent deep vein thrombosis (DVT) secondary to bedrest.

2. Morphine sulfate is an opioid narcotic given frequently for postoperative pain.
3. **Buspirone (BuSpar) is an anxiolytic medication prescribed for anxiety, post-traumatic stress disorder (PTSD), and many other conditions. It does have potential severe interactions with selegiline (Eldepryl), an anti-Parkinson's drug, which the client cannot be abruptly taken off of.**
4. Cefazolin (Ancef) is an antibiotic. Prophylactic antibiotics should be prescribed for a client undergoing surgery; therefore, the nurse would not question this medication.

MEDICATION MEMORY JOGGER: Meperidine (Demerol) metabolizes into normeperidine, which is not readily eliminated from the body and results in the accumulation of toxic substances. The use of Demerol is questioned in many situations and is currently not being used as the first-line medication for pain.

10. **1. The most important rule in discontinuing antiepileptic drugs (AEDs) is that they be withdrawn over 6 weeks to several months to avoid side effects. If the client is taking two AEDs, the drugs should be discontinued sequentially, not simultaneously.**
  2. There is no need to obtain serum levels when the medication is being discontinued.
  3. When the epilepsy is in remission, the client should stop taking the AED because medication should not be taken if it is not necessary.
  4. Soft-bristled toothbrushes are recommended for clients taking phenytoin (Dilantin) because of gingival hyperplasia, but this client will stop taking an AED because of being in remission.

11.

Potential Nursing Intervention	Indicated	Not Indicated
1. Encourage the client to take aspirin with one glass of water.		X
2. Notify the HCP if ringing in the ears occurs.	X	
3. Instruct the client to take an enteric-coated brand of aspirin.	X	
4. Notify the HCP if the client has black, tarry stools.	X	
5. Explain that gastrointestinal distress is expected when taking aspirin.		X

  1. Aspirin, a salicylate and antiplatelet, does not need to be taken with a glass of water. It should be taken with food if it is not enteric-coated.
  2. Tinnitus, ringing in the ears, is a finding of aspirin toxicity, and the client should notify the HCP.
  3. Because the client has a history of a gastric ulcers, the client should take enteric-coated aspirin to ensure that the medication will not dissolve in the stomach and potentially cause gastric irritation leading to bleeding.
  4. If the client has black, tarry stools, the HCP should be notified because this is a finding of gastric bleeding.
  5. Gastrointestinal distress is not expected with taking aspirin and should be reported to the HCP. Gastrointestinal distress can be a serious side effect of aspirin, an antiplatelet.

12. 1. This behavior indicates the client's neurological status is improving; therefore, the medication is effective.
  2. The highest possible score on the Glasgow Coma Scale is 15; therefore, a 13 indicates the client is getting better, and the medication is effective.
  3. If the client is alert, even if unable to identify the day of the week, this indicates the client is getting better, and the medication is effective.
  4. Flaccid paralysis is the client's worst response to painful stimuli, equivalent to a 3 on the Glasgow Coma Scale. Decorticate posturing would receive a 5 on the Glasgow Coma Scale. Therefore, flaccid paralysis indicates the medication is not effective.

13. 1. Clients experiencing chronic pain must adjust to living with the pain and do not always act as the nurse assumes they should. Sumatriptan (Imitrex), a serotonin receptor agonist, is not a narcotic; therefore, this is not drug-seeking behavior.
  2. Laughing may be the client's way of dealing with the pain, and the nurse should not be judgmental.
  3. The nurse must check two forms of identification and allergies before administering any medication. The nurse should not be judgmental when caring for any client. Pain is what the client states it is.
  4. OTC medications are not effective in treating severe vasospasm headaches, which is what a migraine headache is.

14. **1. The client reports living off the land, and the symptoms reported are clinical manifestations of muscarinic poisoning from eating wild mushrooms. Therefore, the nurse should anticipate administering the antidote atropine, a muscarinic agonist.**
  2. An antihistamine, diphenhydramine (Benadryl), would be prescribed for an allergic reaction, not for muscarinic poisoning.

3. Magnesium and aluminum hydroxide (Maalox), an antacid, neutralizes gastric acid and is not used for mushroom poisoning.
4. Pantoprazole (Protonix), a proton-pump inhibitor, decreases gastric acidity, and is not prescribed for muscarinic poisoning.

15. 1. There is no indication for verifying the serum phenytoin (Dilantin) level.
2. This level is below the therapeutic range of 10 to 20 mcg/dL; therefore, the nurse should determine if the client is taking the medication as directed.
3. This is below the therapeutic range; therefore, the medication should not be omitted.
4. Because this level is below the therapeutic range, the nurse must determine how the medication is being taken before discussing the need to increase the dose.

16. Correct order is 1, 5, 4, 3, 2.
1. The nurse should apply the nursing process and always assess the client unless the client is in distress. The nurse must determine if this is routine pain for which the HCP has prescribed acetaminophen or a complication that warrants medical intervention.
5. The nurse must then determine how much pain the client is in to determine the most appropriate medication. The pain scale will also help evaluate the effectiveness of the medication.
4. The nurse must identify the client before administering the medication.
3. Because the client has had a CVA, the nurse must determine if the client can swallow before administering medication. If the client has problems swallowing water, the nurse should thicken liquids to help prevent aspiration.
2. The nurse should administer the medication after all the previous steps are completed.

17. 1. This is a therapeutic response, and the client needs information; therefore, it is not the nurse's best response.
2. Meclizine HCL (Antivert) antivertigo or antimotion-sickness medications are most effective when administered prophylactically rather than after symptoms have begun.
3. Antacids neutralize the gastric acid and will not help nausea experienced with motion sickness.
4. Dimenhydrinate (Dramamine) is the OTC drug of choice for motion sickness. It should be taken 30 to 60 minutes before departure and 30 minutes before meals after that.

18. 1. Because of the illness and its drug treatment, the client should not be driving a car; therefore, this statement does not warrant immediate intervention by the nurse.
2. This client should make sure the HCP knows about this medication; therefore, this statement does not warrant intervention by the nurse.
3. The client should avoid other central nervous system depressants, including alcohol. Therefore, this statement requires intervention and further teaching by the nurse.
4. This medication may cause dryness of the mouth, and chewing sugarless gum or sucking hard candy would be appropriate; therefore, this statement does not warrant intervention.

MEDICATION MEMORY JOGGER: Usually, if there is a question regarding alcohol consumption and medication interaction, the recommendation is to avoid alcohol altogether, not limit the intake.

19. 1. Acetaminophen (Tylenol), a nonnarcotic analgesic, is helpful in the relief of mild to moderate pain, 1–3 on the pain scale.
2. Hydrocodone (Vicodin), a narcotic analgesic, is equivalent to codeine. It is useful for relieving moderate to severe pain, 4–6 on the pain scale. This client has a brain tumor, which would include increasing intracranial pressure and pain; therefore, this would be the most appropriate medication at this time.
3. Morphine, a narcotic analgesic, IVP, is a potent analgesic used to treat severe pain, 7–10 on the pain scale.
4. Lorazepam (Ativan), an antianxiety medication, is not used to treat pain.

20. 167 mL/hr.
The nurse should divide the volume (1,000 mL) by the number of hours (6). This equals 166.6666. The nurse should round up if the number is greater than 5; therefore, the nurse should set the pump at 167 mL/hr.

21. 1. The client is experiencing opioid-induced constipation. Magnesium hydroxide (milk of magnesia) every other day will not be sufficient to treat this issue.
2. The client's concern is constipation. The question's stem did not say the pain control regimen was not working. Acetaminophen has a maximum daily dose of under 4 g of medication. Each tablet contains 500 mg

of medication. Three tablets every dose would be 1,500 mg or 1.5 g. Alternating the dosing of mediation would mean that the client would receive the narcotic every 4 hours and the Tylenol every 4 hours, six doses of each medication per day. The client would be taking 9 g of Tylenol each day.

3. **Haloxegol (Movantik), a mu-opioid receptor agonist, blocks the receptors in the colon from reacting to the narcotic. This medication should be considered to be added to the client's pain control regimen.**
4. Biscodyl (Dulcolax) is a stimulant medication that stimulates peristalsis in the intestines. Over time the colon narrows, and it becomes almost impossible for the stool to pass through.

22. 1. The client should sit upright to take the morning medications, but it is not necessary to make the client get out of bed.
2. The RN should assess the client's swallowing ability, not the UAP. Assessment is beyond the scope of the UAP's abilities.
3. The nurse should perform a full head-to-toe assessment at some time during the shift, but the gait is not needed with regard to the MAR.
4. **The client was admitted for PD with hallucinations. The medications listed on the MAR are carbidopa and levodopa, an anti-Parkinsonian drug, and (Nuplazid), an atypical antipsychotic used to treat the hallucinations associated with PD. The nurse should determine the neurological status of the client.**

23. 1. Phenytoin (Dilantin) causes gingival hyperplasia, not brivaracetam (Briviact). Both medications are anticonvulsants.
2. No blood level monitoring is needed with Briviact. The effects are immediate. The client's response determines dosing.
3. **Brivaracetam (Briviact) has a side effect of causing drowsiness, as do most other anticonvulsant medications. It is prescribed for partial onset seizures related to epilepsy.**
4. Clients diagnosed with epilepsy are encouraged to take showers rather than baths to prevent the risk of drowning in case of a seizure.

3 Cardiovascular System

A love affair with knowledge will never end in heartbreak.

—Michael Garrett Marino

QUESTIONS

Angina and Myocardial Infarction

1. The nurse is teaching the client diagnosed with angina about sublingual nitroglycerin (NTG). Which statement indicates the client **needs more** medication teaching? guidance?
   1. "I will always carry my nitroglycerin in a dark-colored bottle."
   2. "If I have chest pain, I will put a tablet underneath my tongue."
   3. "If my pain is not relieved with one tablet, I will get medical help."
   4. "I should expect to get a headache after taking my nitroglycerin."

2. The nurse is preparing to administer a NTG transdermal patch to the client diagnosed with myocardial infarction (MI). For each intervention, specify if the intervention is **indicated or not indicated** for the client's care.

Potential Nursing Intervention	Indicated	Not Indicated
1. Question applying the patch if the client's blood pressure is less than 110/70.		
2. Use nonsterile gloves when applying the transdermal patch.		
3. Date and time the transdermal patch before applying to the client's skin.		
4. Place the transdermal patch on the site where the old patch was removed.		
5. Hold the patch firmly for 20 to 30 seconds to ensure the patch sticks firmly.		
6. Avoid applying the patch to broken or irritated skin.		

3. The client is reporting severe chest pain radiating down the left arm and is nauseated and diaphoretic. The HCP suspects the client is having an MI and has ordered morphine sulfate for the pain. Which interventions should the nurse implement? **Select all that apply.**
   1. Instruct the client not to get out of the bed without notifying the nurse.
   2. Administer the morphine sulfate intramuscularly (IM) in the ventral gluteal muscle.
   3. Dilute the morphine sulfate to a 10-mL bolus with normal saline.
   4. Administer the morphine sulfate slowly over 5 minutes.
   5. Question the order because morphine sulfate should not be administered to a client diagnosed with an MI.

4. The nurse is administering 0900 medications to the following clients. Which client should the nurse **question** administering the medication?
   1. The client receiving a calcium channel blocker (CCB) after drinking grapefruit juice
   2. The client receiving a beta blocker with an apical pulse of 62 beats per minute (bpm)
   3. The client receiving a NTG patch with a blood pressure of 148/92
   4. The client receiving an antiplatelet medication with a platelet count of 150,000

5. The client diagnosed with angina and prescribed NTG tells the nurse, "I don't understand why I can't take my sildenafil. I need to take it so that I can make love to my partner." Which statement is the nurse's **best** response?
   1. "If you take the medications together, they may cause you to have very low blood pressure."
   2. "You are worried your partner will be concerned if you cannot make love?"
   3. "If you wait at least 8 hours after taking your nitroglycerin, you can take your sildenafil."
   4. "You should get clarification with your HCP about taking sildenafil."

6. The client diagnosed with an MI is receiving thrombolytic therapy. Which factor **warrants immediate** intervention by the nurse?
   1. The client's telemetry has reperfusion dysrhythmias.
   2. The client is oozing blood from the IV site.
   3. The client is alert and oriented to date, time, and place.
   4. The client has no findings of infiltration at the insertion site.

7. The nurse is caring for a client diagnosed with angina when the client reports chest pain after walking in the hall. The client has a saline lock in the right forearm. Which intervention should the bedside nurse implement **first**?
   1. Assess the client's vital signs.
   2. Administer transdermal NTG.
   3. Administer IV morphine sulfate via a saline lock.
   4. Administer oxygen via nasal cannula.

8. The client being discharged after sustaining an acute MI is prescribed lisinopril. Which instruction should the nurse include when teaching about this new medication? **Select all that apply.**
   1. Instruct the client to monitor the blood pressure monthly.
   2. Encourage the client to take medication on an empty stomach.
   3. Discuss the need to rise slowly from lying to a standing position.
   4. Teach the client to take the medication at night only.
   5. Tell the client to avoid salt substitutes.
   6. Advise the client that taste changes should resolve in 3 months.

9. The nurse is administering 0.5 inch of NTG paste. How much paste should the nurse apply to the application paper?

Nitro-Bid Ointment Dose Measuring Application

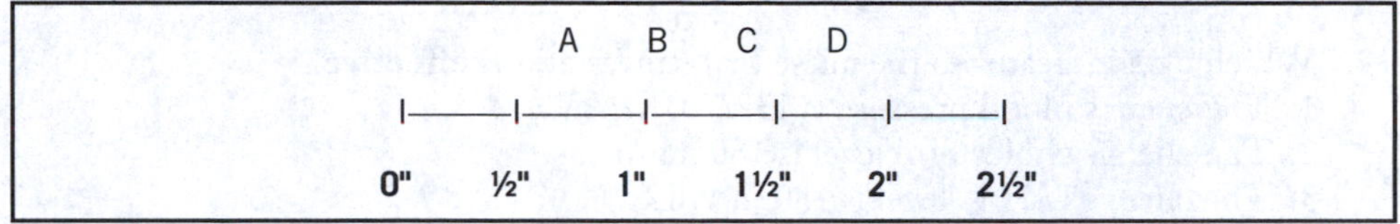

1. A
2. B
3. C
4. D

Coronary Artery Disease

10. The client diagnosed with coronary artery disease (CAD) is prescribed atorvastatin. Which statement by the client **warrants** the nurse notifying the HCP?
1. "I really haven't changed my diet, but I am taking my medication every day."
2. "I am feeling pretty good, except I am having muscle pain all over my body."
3. "I am swimming at the local pool about three times a week for 30 minutes."
4. "I am taking this medication first thing in the morning with a bowl of oatmeal."

11. The client diagnosed with CAD is instructed to take 81 mg of aspirin. Which statement **best** describes the scientific rationale for prescribing this medication?
1. This medication will help thin the client's blood.
2. Daily aspirin will decrease the incidence of angina.
3. This medication will prevent platelet aggregation.
4. Baby aspirin will not cause gastric distress.

12. The client diagnosed with CAD is prescribed cholestyramine. For each intervention, specify if the intervention is **indicated or not indicated** for the client's care.

Potential Nursing Intervention	Indicated	Not Indicated
1. Administer the medication with fruit juice.		
2. Instruct the client to decrease fiber when taking the medication.		
3. Monitor the cholesterol level before giving medication.		
4. Assess the client for upper abdominal discomfort.		
5. Tell client to avoid taking other medications at the same time as cholestyramine.		

13. The elderly client diagnosed with CAD has been taking aspirin daily for more than a year. Which data **warrants** notifying the HCP?
   1. The client has lost 5 pounds in the last month.
   2. The client has trouble hearing low tones.
   3. The client reports having a funny taste in the mouth.
   4. The client has hard, dark, tarry stools.

14. Which data indicates to the nurse that simvastatin is **effective**?
   1. The client's blood pressure is 132/70.
   2. The client's cholesterol level is 180 mg/dL.
   3. The client's LDLC level is 180 mg/dL.
   4. The client's HDLC level is 35 mg/dL.

15. The client diagnosed with CAD is prescribed nicotinic acid. The client reports flushing of the face, neck, and ears. Which **priority** intervention should the nurse implement?
   1. Instruct the client to stop taking the medication immediately.
   2. Encourage the client to take the medication with meals only.
   3. Discuss that this is a normal side effect, and that flushing will decrease with time.
   4. Tell the client to take 325 mg of aspirin 30 minutes before taking the medication.

16. The client with a serum cholesterol level of 320 mg/dL is taking the medication ezetimibe. Which statement by the client indicates the client **needs more** teaching concerning this medication?
   1. "This medication helps decrease the absorption of cholesterol in my intestines."
   2. "I cannot take this medication with any other cholesterol-lowering medication."
   3. "I need to eat a low-fat, low-cholesterol diet even when taking the medication."
   4. "It will take a few months for my cholesterol level to get down to normal levels."

17. The client newly diagnosed with CAD is prescribed a daily aspirin. The client tells the nurse, "I had a bad case of gastritis last year." Which intervention should the nurse implement **first**?
   1. Ask the client if any family members have gastritis.
   2. Explain that regular aspirin could cause gastric upset.
   3. Instruct the client to take an enteric-coated aspirin.
   4. Determine if the client is taking any anti-ulcer medication.

18. The nurse is preparing to administer clopidogrel bisulfate to the client diagnosed with CAD. The client asks the nurse, "Why am I getting this medication?" Which statement by the nurse is **most appropriate**?
   1. "It will help decrease your chance of developing deep vein thrombosis (DVT)."
   2. "Plavix will help decrease your LDLC levels in about 1 month."
   3. "This medication will help prevent blood clotting in the arteries."
   4. "The medication will help decrease your blood pressure if you take it daily."

19. The nurse is assessing the preprinted medication administration record (MAR) for a client admitted with angina. The prescribed medication for administration is in the following MAR.

Client: A.P.	MR# 1234567	Date: Today
Age: 54 years	Allergies: NKDA	Diagnosis: Angina
Medication	0701-1900	1901-0700
Regular insulin SQ ac and hs 0–60: 1 amp D_{50} 61–150: 0 units 151–300: 5 units 301–450: 10 units >450: Call HCP	0730 1130 1630	2100
Metformin 500 mg PO b.i.d.	0800 1700	
Atorvastatin 20 mg PO daily	0900	
Digoxin 0.125 mg PO daily	0900	
Nitroglycerin 0.4 mg on in a.m.	0900	
Nitroglycerin 0.4 mg off in p.m.		2100
Nurse Initials/Credentials	DN/RN	NN/RN

Which medication order should the nurse discuss with the pharmacist?
1. The 1130 regular insulin order
2. The 0800 metformin order
3. The 0900 atorvastatin order
4. The 2100 NTG order

Congestive Heart Failure

20. The home health nurse is caring for a client diagnosed with congestive heart failure (CHF) and prescribed digoxin and furosemide. Which statements by the client indicate the medications are **effective**? **Select all that apply.**
1. "I can walk next door now without being short of breath."
2. "I keep my feet propped up as much as I can during the day."
3. "I have not gained any weight since my last doctor's visit."
4. "My blood pressure has been within normal limits."
5. "I am staying on my diet, and I don't salt my foods anymore."

21. The female client diagnosed with CHF tells the nurse that she has been taking hawthorn extract because the HCP told her that she had heart problems. Which statement by the nurse is **most appropriate**?
1. "You need to take garlic supplements with hawthorn for it to be effective."
2. "You should stop taking this herb immediately because it can cause more problems."
3. "This herb can cause bleeding if you take it with your other medications."
4. "Some clients find this is helpful, but make sure your HCP is aware of the medication."

22. The client diagnosed with stage D CHF has a brain natriuretic peptide (BNP) level greater than 1,500. Which medication should the nurse **anticipate** the HCP prescribing?
    1. Captopril orally
    2. Digoxin IV push (IVP)
    3. Dobutamine IV
    4. Metoprolol orally

23. The client diagnosed with CHF is prescribed enalapril. Which statement explains the scientific rationale for administering this medication?
    1. Enalapril increases the levels of angiotensin II in the blood vessels.
    2. Enalapril dilates arteries, which reduces the workload of the heart.
    3. Enalapril decreases the effects of bradykinin in the body.
    4. Enalapril blocks the intervention of antidiuretic hormone in the kidney.

24. The nurse is providing discharge instructions for a client prescribed hydrochlorothiazide. For each intervention, specify if the intervention is **indicated or not indicated** for the client's care.

Potential Nursing Intervention	Indicated	Not Indicated
1. Drink at least 8 to 10 glasses of water a day.		
2. Weigh yourself monthly and report to HCP.		
3. Eat bananas or oranges regularly.		
4. Try to sleep in an upright position.		
5. Notify the HCP of muscle cramps or weakness.		

25. The nurse in the HCP's office is completing an assessment on a client prescribed digoxin for CHF. Which data indicates the medication has been **effective**?
    1. The client's sputum is pink and frothy.
    2. The client has 2+ pitting edema of the sacrum.
    3. The client's breath sounds bilateral are clear.
    4. The client's heart rate is 78 bpm.

26. Which medication should the nurse **question** administering?
    1. Lisinopril to a client with a blood pressure of 118/84
    2. Carvedilol to a client with an apical pulse of 62
    3. Verapamil to a client diagnosed with angina
    4. Furosemide to a client reporting leg cramps

27. The nurse is administering digoxin to a client diagnosed with CHF. Which interventions should the nurse implement? **Select all that apply.**
    1. Assess the client's carotid pulse for 1 full minute.
    2. Check the client's current potassium level.
    3. Ask the client if they see a yellow haze around objects.
    4. Have the client squeeze the nurse's fingers.
    5. Teach the client to get up slowly from a sitting position.

28. Which medication should the nurse **question** administering to a client diagnosed with stage C CHF?
    1. Ibuprofen
    2. Amlodipine
    3. Spironolactone
    4. Atenolol

29. The HCP prescribed an angiotensin-converting enzyme (ACE) inhibitor for a client diagnosed with CHF. Which instruction should the nurse provide?
1. "Eat a banana or drink orange juice at least twice a day."
2. "Notify the HCP if you develop localized edematous areas that itch."
3. "Expect to have a dry cough early in the morning on arising."
4. "Your symptoms of CHF should improve rapidly."

30. The nurse is administering morning medications. The prescribed medication for administration is in the following MAR.

Client: D.M.	MR# 1234567	Date: Today
Age: 65 years	Allergies: NKDA	Diagnosis: Stage 4 Heart Failure
Medication	**0701-1900**	**1901-0700**
Sacubitril and valsartan 49/51 mg PO daily	0900	
Metformin 500 mg PO b.i.d.	0800 1700	
Atorvastatin 20 mg PO daily	0900	
Nitroglycerin 0.4 mg on in a.m.	0900	
Nitroglycerin 0.4 mg off in p.m.		2100
Captopril 12.5 mg PO three times a day	0900 1300 1700	
Nurse Initials/Credentials	**DN/RN**	**NN/RN**

Which medication would the nurse **question** administering?
1. Metformin
2. Atorvastatin
3. Nitroglycerin
4. Captopril

Dysrhythmias and Conduction Problems

31. The client is exhibiting the following telemetry reading. Which as-needed (PRN) medication should the nurse anticipate the HCP ordering?

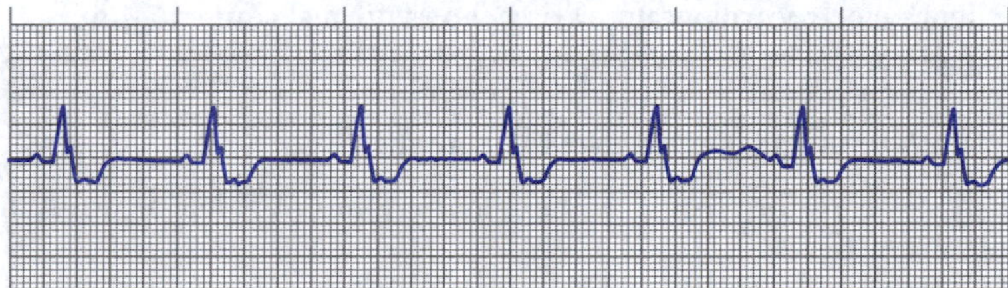

1. Atenolol
2. Verapamil
3. Nitroglycerin
4. Captopril

32. Which assessment data should the nurse obtain **before** administering a calcium channel blocker?
1. The serum calcium level
2. The client's radial pulse
3. The current telemetry reading
4. The client's blood pressure

33. Which medication should the nurse prepare to administer to the client exhibiting the following telemetry strip?

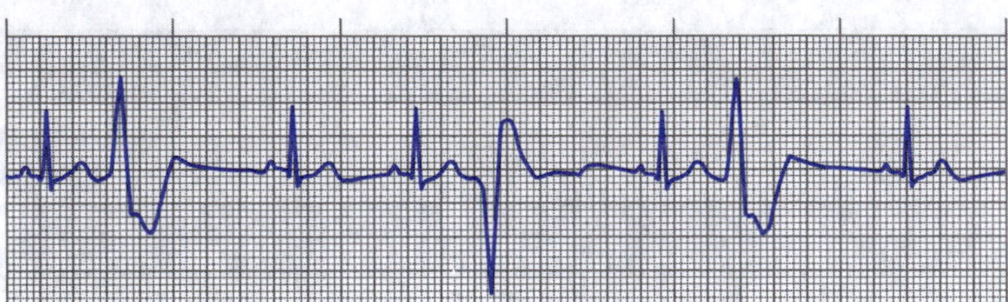

1. Adenosine
2. Amiodarone
3. Digoxin
4. Dopamine

34. The client reports weakness, dizziness, and lightheadedness, and exhibits the following telemetry strip. The nurse administered the antidysrhythmic medication atropine sulfate intravenously. Which data **best** indicates the medication was **effective**?

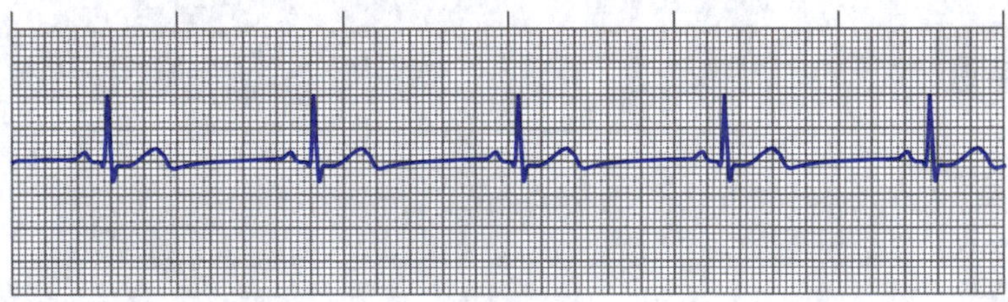

1. The client's apical pulse rate is 68 bpm.
2. The client's blood pressure is 110/70.
3. The client's oral mucosa is moist.
4. The client ambulates to the bathroom safely.

35. The nurse is preparing to administer adenosine for the client diagnosed with supraventricular tachycardia (SVT). Which assessment finding would indicate the medication is **effective**?
1. The client's electrocardiogram tracing shows normal sinus rhythm.
2. The client's apical pulse is within normal limits.
3. The client's blood pressure is above 100/60.
4. The client's serum adenosine level is 1.8 mg/dL.

36. The nurse is caring for clients on the telemetry unit. Which medication should the nurse administer **first**?
1. Digibind to the client with a digoxin level of 1.9 mg/dL
2. Morphine sulfate IVP to the client diagnosed with pleuritic chest pain
3. Lidocaine IVP to the client exhibiting bigeminy
4. Lisinopril to the client with a blood pressure of 170/90

37. The client's 1-day postoperative open-heart surgery is exhibiting the following telemetry strip and has a temperature of 101.6°F, pulse rate of 110 bpm, respiratory rate of 24 breaths/min, and blood pressure reading of 128/92. Which intervention should the nurse implement?

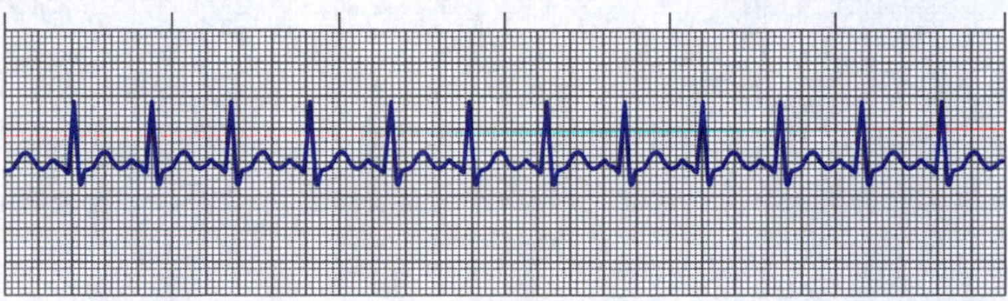

1. Continue to monitor.
2. Administer acetaminophen.
3. Administer quinidine sulfate.
4. Administer disopyramide.

38. The nurse is preparing to administer 2 g/500 mL of lidocaine after administering a 100-mg IV bolus to a client diagnosed with multifocal premature ventricular contractions (PVCs). Which intervention should the nurse implement?
   1. Cover the IV bag and tubing with aluminum foil.
   2. Monitor the brain natriuretic peptide (BNP) daily.
   3. Hold the lidocaine drip if no PVCs are noted.
   4. Obtain an infusion pump to administer the medication.

39. The client exhibiting the following telemetry reading for the last 6 months is being discharged. Which instruction will the nurse discuss with the client?

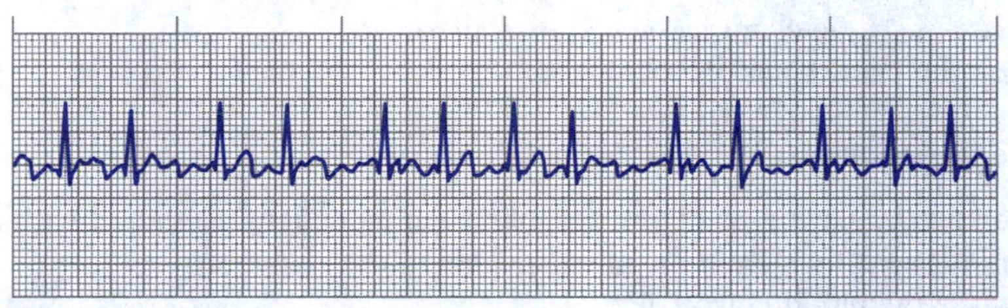

1. The importance of monitoring the client's urinary output
2. The need to monitor the PTT level while taking aspirin
3. Dietary restrictions while taking warfarin
4. The need to take digoxin on an empty stomach

40. The client is exhibiting the following telemetry strip. Which interventions should the nurse implement? **Select all that apply.**

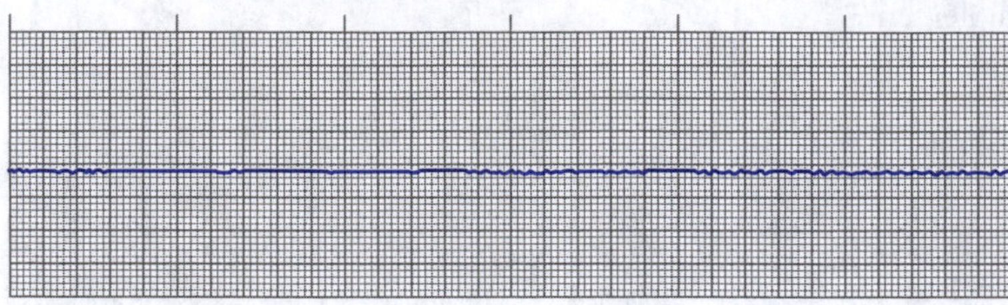

1. Administer atropine.
2. Assess the client's apical heart rate.
3. Administer epinephrine.
4. Initiate cardiopulmonary resuscitation.
5. Administer lidocaine.

Inflammatory Cardiac Disorders

41. The client is diagnosed with subacute bacterial endocarditis (SBE). Which HCP order should the nurse **question**?
1. Initiate intravenous penicillin.
2. Obtain a blood culture and sensitivity (C&S).
3. Administer a positive protein derivative (PPD) intradermally.
4. Place the client on bedrest with bathroom privileges.

42. The nurse is preparing to administer the initial IV antibiotic to a client diagnosed with bacterial endocarditis. Which **priority** intervention should the nurse implement?
1. Determine if the client has any known allergies.
2. Assess the client's peripheral IV site.
3. Monitor the client's vital signs.
4. Take the medication bag out of the refrigerator.

43. The nurse is preparing to administer ibuprofen to a client diagnosed with pericarditis. Which intervention should the nurse include in the plan of care?
1. Monitor the blood glucose level.
2. Have the client sit upright for 30 minutes after taking the medication.
3. Instruct the client to drink a full glass of water.
4. Administer the medication with food.

44. The client diagnosed with pericarditis is taking an NSAID. Which statement by the client **warrants immediate** intervention by the nurse?
1. "I just spit up a small amount of bright red blood."
2. "This medication really doesn't help my pain."
3. "My mother is really allergic to NSAIDs."
4. "My bowel movements have been clay-colored."

45. The client diagnosed with bacterial endocarditis is being discharged home, receiving IV antibiotic therapy. Which interventions should the nurse implement? **Select all that apply.**
1. Refer the client to home health-care services.
2. Teach the client to report an elevated temperature.
3. Explain how to use the IV pump.
4. Contact the hospital pharmacy to provide an IV pump.
5. Discuss the need for prophylaxis before dental procedures.
6. Ensure that the client has adequate support at home.
7. Confirm the patency of the peripherally inserted central catheter (PICC) line.

46. The client diagnosed with bacterial endocarditis develops a rash and reports itching. Which medication should the nurse discuss with the HCP?
   1. IV clindamycin
   2. IV furosemide
   3. Oral prednisone
   4. Oral *lactobacillus acidophilus* (*L. acidophilus*)

47. The client diagnosed with bacterial endocarditis is prescribed gentamicin IV piggyback (IVPB). The IVPB comes in 100 mL of fluid to be administered over 1 hour on an IV pump. At what rate should the nurse administer the medication?

   ____

Arterial Occlusive Disease

48. The client diagnosed with arterial occlusive disease is prescribed pentoxifylline. Which information should the nurse discuss with the client?
   1. Explain that the medication should be taken on an empty stomach.
   2. Instruct the client to avoid smoking when taking this medication.
   3. Discuss that common side effects are flushing of the skin and sedation.
   4. Encourage the client to wear long sleeves and a hat when in the sunlight.

49. The client diagnosed with Raynaud's disease, a peripheral vascular disease, is prescribed isoxsuprine. Which statement indicates the client **understands** the discharge teaching?
   1. "I will probably have palpitations and episodes of low blood pressure."
   2. "I should take the medication when I go outside in the cold weather."
   3. "I need to take an enteric-coated aspirin every morning with food."
   4. "This medication will help increase blood flow to my extremities."

50. The client diagnosed with chronic venous insufficiency has a venous stasis ulcer being treated with autolytic medication for debridement and an occlusive dressing. The nurse notices a foul-smelling odor. Which intervention should the nurse implement?
   1. Assess the client's vital signs, especially the temperature.
   2. Obtain a C&S of the venous stasis ulcer.
   3. Document the finding and take no further intervention.
   4. Ask the HCP to discontinue the medication.

51. The wound care nurse is applying an enzyme debridement ointment to a client diagnosed with a venous stasis ulcer on the left ankle. Which **priority** intervention should the nurse implement?
   1. Cover the wound with damp saline-soaked gauze.
   2. Place dry gauze and a loose bandage over the wound.
   3. Do not allow any ointment on the normal surrounding skin.
   4. Apply the ointment with a sterile tongue blade.

52. The client diagnosed with a venous stasis ulcer has exudate. A calcium alginate dressing is applied to the draining ulcer. The client asks the nurse, "How often will the dressing be changed?" Which statement is the nurse's **best** response?
   1. "The dressing will have to be changed daily."
   2. "It will be changed when the exudate seeps through."
   3. "The doctor will determine when the dressing is changed."
   4. "It will not be changed until the wound is healed."

53. The client diagnosed with arterial occlusive disease is taking clopidogrel. Which statement by the client **warrants intervention** by the nurse?
   1. "I am taking the herb ginkgo to help improve my memory."
   2. "I am a vegetarian and eat a lot of green, leafy vegetables."
   3. "I have not had any blood drawn in more than a year."
   4. "I always use a soft-bristled toothbrush to brush my teeth."

54. The client diagnosed with arterial occlusive disease has been taking 325 mg of aspirin daily for 1 month. The client tells the nurse, "I have been having some stomach pain." For each intervention, specify if the intervention is **indicated or not indicated** for the client's care.

Potential Nursing Intervention	Indicated	Not Indicated
1. Instruct the client to take a nonenteric-coated aspirin.		
2. Encourage the client to take the medication with food.		
3. Discuss the need to take only one 81-mg aspirin a day.		
4. Tell the client to notify the HCP.		
5. Ask the client about their bowel movements.		
6. Perform a gastrointestinal assessment.		

55. The client diagnosed with a venous stasis ulcer is being treated with dextranomer, which are highly porous beads. The nurse notes the beads are a grayish-yellow color. Which intervention should the nurse implement?
1. Flush the beads with normal saline and apply a new layer of beads.
2. Take no intervention because this is the normal color of the beads.
3. Apply a new layer of beads without removing the grayish-yellow beads.
4. Prepare the client for surgical debridement of the wound.

56. The client diagnosed with arterial occlusive disease is postoperative right femoral popliteal bypass surgery. Which HCP order should the nurse **question**?
1. D_5W 1,000 mL to infuse at 75 mL/hr
2. Ceftriaxone 500 mg every 12 hours
3. Dipyridamole 50 mg three times a day
4. Morphine sulfate 2 mg IVP every 4 hours

57. The nurse is preparing to administer the initial IV antibiotic to a client diagnosed with an arterial ulcer on the right ankle. The client has a saline lock in the right forearm. In which order should the nurse prepare to administer the medication? **Rank in order of performance.**
1. Inject 3 mL of normal saline into the saline lock.
2. Check to see if a C&S test has been done.
3. Flush the IV tubing with the antibiotic.
4. Determine if the client has any known allergies.
5. Connect the antibiotic medication to the saline lock.

Arterial Hypertension

58. The client diagnosed with essential hypertension (HTN) is prescribed metoprolol. Which assessment data should make the nurse **question** administering this medication?
1. The client's blood pressure is 112/90.
2. The client's apical pulse is 56 bpm.
3. The client has an occipital headache.
4. The client is reporting a yellow haze.

59. The client diagnosed with arterial HTN is receiving furosemide. Which data indicates the medication is **effective**?
1. The client's 8-hour intake is 1,800 mL, and the output is 2,300 mL.
2. The client's blood pressure went from 144/88 to 154/96.
3. The client has had a weight loss of 1.3 kg in 7 days.
4. The client reports occasional lightheadedness and dizziness.

60. The client diagnosed with high blood pressure is prescribed captopril. Which statements by the client indicate to the nurse the discharge teaching has been **effective**? **Select all that apply.**
1. "I should get up slowly when getting out of bed."
2. "I should check and record my blood pressure once a day."
3. "If I get leg cramps, I should increase my potassium supplements."
4. "If I forget to take my medication, I will take two doses the next day."
5. "I can eat anything I want as long as I take my medication every day."

61. The nurse is preparing to administer the following medications. Which medication should the nurse **question** administering?
1. Hydralazine to the client with a blood pressure of 168/94
2. Prazosin to the client with a serum sodium level of 137 mEq/L
3. Diltiazem to the client with a glucose level of 280 mg/dL
4. Furosemide to the client with a serum potassium level of 3.1 mEq/L

62. The nurse is discussing chlorothiazide with a client diagnosed with essential HTN. Which discharge instruction should the nurse discuss with the client?
1. Encourage the client to eat sodium-rich foods.
2. Instruct the client to drink adequate fluids.
3. Teach the client to keep strict intake and output records.
4. Explain about taking the medication at night only.

63. The client diagnosed with essential HTN is taking bumetanide. Which statement by the client **warrants notifying** the client's HCP?
1. "I really wish my mouth would not be so dry."
2. "I get a little dizzy when I get up too fast."
3. "I usually have one or two glasses of wine a day."
4. "I have been experiencing really bad leg cramps."

64. The male client diagnosed with essential HTN tells the nurse, "I cannot make love to my wife since I started my blood pressure medications." Which statement by the nurse is **most appropriate**?
1. "You are concerned that you cannot make love to your wife."
2. "I will refer you to a psychologist so that you can talk about it."
3. "We need to discuss this with your HCP."
4. "Ask your wife to come in, and we can discuss it together."

65. The HCP prescribed a beta blocker for the client diagnosed with arterial HTN. Which statement is the scientific rationale for administering this medication?
1. This medication decreases the sympathetic stimulation to the heart, thereby decreasing the client's heart rate and blood pressure.
2. This medication prevents calcium from entering the cell, which helps decrease the client's blood pressure.
3. This medication prevents the release of aldosterone, which decreases absorption of sodium and water, decreasing blood pressure.
4. This medication will cause increased excretion of water from the vascular system, decreasing blood pressure.

66. The nurse is preparing to administer a calcium channel blocker, a loop diuretic, and a beta blocker to a client diagnosed with arterial HTN. Which intervention should the nurse implement?
1. Hold the medication and notify the HCP on rounds.
2. Check the client's pulse and blood pressure.
3. Contact the pharmacist to discuss the medications.
4. Double-check the HCP's orders.

67. The nurse is administering the combination medication chlorthalidone and atenolol to a client diagnosed with chronic HTN. Which interventions should the nurse implement? **Select all that apply.**
1. Do not administer if the client's blood pressure is less than 90/60.
2. Do not administer if the client's apical pulse is less than 60 bpm.
3. Teach the client how to prevent orthostatic hypotension.
4. Encourage the client to eat potassium-rich foods.
5. Monitor the client's oral intake and urinary output.

Deep Vein Thrombosis

68. The nurse is preparing to administer warfarin. The client's laboratory values are populated in the chart below.

Laboratory Test	Client Values	Reference Values
Prothrombin time (PT)	38 Control 12.9	10 to 13 seconds
Partial thromboplastin time (PTT)	39 Control 36	25 to 35 seconds
International Normalized Ratio (INR)	5.9	0.9 to 1.1 without anticoagulation therapy 2 to 3 with therapy 2.5 to 3.5 if the client has a mechanical heart valve

Which intervention should the nurse implement?
1. Discontinue the IV bag immediately.
2. Prepare to administer phytonadione.
3. Notify the HCP to increase the dose.
4. Administer the medication as ordered.

69. The nurse is discharging the female client diagnosed with deep vein thrombosis (DVT) and prescribed warfarin. Which statement indicates the client **needs more** teaching concerning this medication?
1. "I should wear a medical alert bracelet in case of an emergency."
2. "If I get cut, I will apply pressure for at least 5 minutes."
3. "I will increase the amount of green, leafy vegetables I eat."
4. "I will have to see my HCP regularly while taking this medication."

70. The nurse is preparing to hang the next bag of heparin for a client diagnosed with DVT. The client's laboratory values are populated in the chart below.

Laboratory Test	Client Values	Reference Values
Prothrombin time (PT)	12.7 Control 12.9	10 to 13 seconds
Partial thromboplastin time (PTT)	62 Control 36	25 to 35 seconds
International Normalized Ratio (INR)	1	0.9 to 1.1 without anticoagulation therapy 2 to 3 with therapy 2.5 to 3.5 if the client has a mechanical heart valve

Which intervention should the nurse implement?
1. Hang the IV bag at the same rate.
2. Obtain an order for a STAT PT, INR, and PTT.
3. Notify the HCP.
4. Assess the client for any abnormal bleeding.

71. The client diagnosed with DVT asks the nurse, "Why do I have to take my warfarin in the evening?" Which statement is the nurse's **best** response?
1. "The medication works more effectively while you are sleeping."
2. "The medicine should be given with the largest meal of the day."
3. "The side effects of the warfarin are less if you take it in the evening."
4. "This allows for a more accurate INR level when morning blood is drawn."

72. The client had a right total hip replacement. Which medication should the nurse anticipate the HCP prescribing?
1. Warfarin
2. Heparin
3. Alteplase
4. Enoxaparin

73. The client has petechiae on the anterior lateral upper abdominal wall. The MAR indicates the client is receiving a daily 81-mg aspirin, an IV narcotic, and a low-molecular-weight heparin. Which intervention should the nurse implement?
1. Request an order to discontinue the 81 mg aspirin.
2. Assess the client's pain level on a 1 to 10 scale.
3. Document the finding and take no intervention.
4. Put cool compresses on the abdominal wall.

74. The client on strict bedrest is prescribed subcutaneous heparin. Which data indicates the medication is **effective**?
1. The client's current PT is 22, the INR is 2.4, and the PTT is 70.
2. The client's calves are normal size, normal skin color, and nontender.
3. The client performs active range-of-motion exercises every 4 hours.
4. The client's varicose veins have reduced in size and appearance.

75. The client is immobile. In which area should the nurse administer the subcutaneous heparin injection?

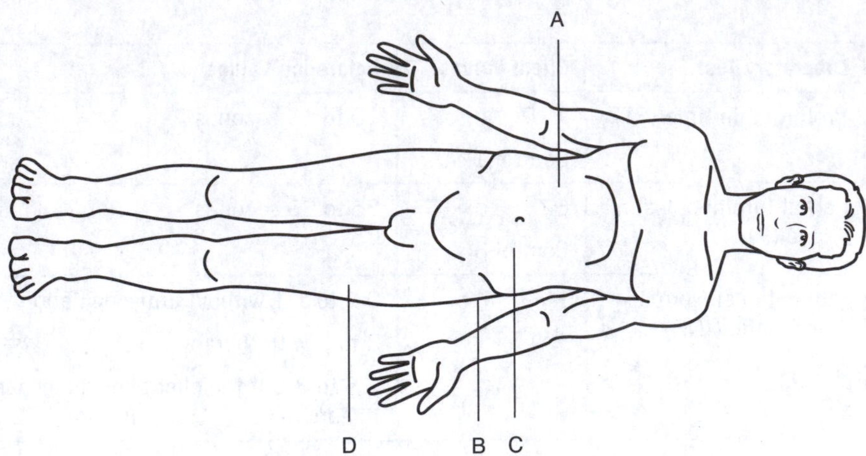

1. A
2. B
3. C
4. D

76. The client is receiving an IV infusion of heparin. The bag hanging has 20,000 units of heparin in 500 mL of D_5W at 22 mL per hour via an IV pump. How many units of heparin is the client receiving every hour?

____

77. The client is receiving an IV infusion of heparin. The bag hanging has 10,000 units of heparin in 100 mL of D_5W. The HCP has ordered the medication to be delivered at 1,000 units per hour. At what rate would the nurse set the IV pump?

____

78. The nurse is reconciling the home medications on a new admit. The HCP has prescribed that the client receive home medications. The client's medication list is populated in the list below.

John D. Medication List

Medication	How Often to Take
Furosemide 40 mg	Daily
Ticagrelor 90 mg	Twice a day
Aspirin 325 mg	Daily
Levothyroxine 0.75 mg	Daily
Digoxin 0.125 mg	Daily
Potassium 20 mEq	Daily
Acetaminophen 650 mg	Every 4 hours as needed
Ibuprofen 400 mg	Every 4 to 6 hours as needed

Which medication(s) should the nurse discuss with the HCP?
1. Furosemide and potassium
2. Ticagrelor and aspirin
3. Levothyroxine and digoxin
4. Acetaminophen and ibuprofen

Anemia

79. The 28-year-old client diagnosed with sickle cell disease (SCD) has been admitted to the medical unit for a vaso-occlusive crisis. Which intervention should the nurse implement **first**?
1. Elevate the head of the client's bed.
2. Administer a narcotic analgesic.
3. Apply oxygen via nasal cannula.
4. Initiate intravenous fluids.

80. The nurse is caring for a client diagnosed with sickle cell disease (SCD). Which medication would the nurse **question**?
1. Morphine sulfate IVP
2. Fentanyl patch
3. Epoetin subcutaneously (SQ)
4. Piperacillin and tazobactam combination medication IVPB

81. The client with gastric bypass surgery asks the nurse, "Why do I need to take vitamin B_{12} injections?" Which statement is the nurse's **best** response?
1. "You have pernicious anemia, and the injections will cure the problem."
2. "Your body cannot absorb the vitamins from the food you eat."
3. "Because of the surgery, you cannot eat enough food to get the amount you need."
4. "You will need to take the injections daily until your body begins to make B_{12}."

82. The client diagnosed with iron-deficiency anemia is being discharged with a prescribed oral iron preparation. For each intervention, specify if the intervention is **indicated or not indicated** for the client's care.

Potential Nursing Intervention	Indicated	Not Indicated
1. Teach the client to perform a fecal occult blood test daily.		
2. Demonstrate how to crush the tablets and mix them with pudding.		
3. Inform the client to take the medication at night.		
4. Tell the client that their stools will be greenish-black.		
5. Instruct the client to avoid caffeinated beverages.		
6. Take antacids and calcium 1 hour before or 2 hours after the iron.		

83. The nurse is administering iron dextran to a client diagnosed with iron-deficiency anemia. Which intervention should the nurse implement?
1. Make sure the client is well hydrated.
2. Give the medication subcutaneously in the deltoid.
3. Check for allergies to fish or other seafood.
4. Administer the medication by the Z-track method.

84. The client diagnosed with polycythemia vera is being discharged. Which discharge instruction should the nurse teach the client?
   1. "Take the warfarin as ordered."
   2. "Do not abruptly stop taking prednisone."
   3. "Rise slowly from a seated position to prevent hypotension."
   4. "Restrict fluids to 1,000 to 1,500 mL per day."

85. The HCP ordered a transfusion to be administered to a client diagnosed with aplastic anemia. Which intervention should the nurse implement? **Rank in order of performance.**
   1. Obtain informed consent to administer blood.
   2. Make sure the client understands the procedure.
   3. Check the blood out from the laboratory.
   4. Perform a pretransfusion assessment.
   5. Start an IV with an 18-gauge catheter.

86. The client is diagnosed with folic acid deficiency anemia and Crohn's disease. Which medication should the nurse anticipate being prescribed?
   1. Oral folic acid
   2. Cyanocobalamin intramuscularly
   3. B complex vitamin therapy orally
   4. Intramuscular folic acid

87. The client at the outpatient clinic was diagnosed with folic acid deficiency anemia and given a sample of oral folic acid. At the follow-up visit, the nurse assessed the client to determine effectiveness of the treatment. Which data indicates the treatment is **effective**?
   1. The client has gained 2 pounds and has pink buccal mucosa.
   2. The client does not have any paresthesia of the hands and feet.
   3. The client stopped drinking any alcoholic beverages.
   4. The client can tolerate eating green, leafy vegetables.

88. The nurse is caring for a client newly diagnosed with immunohemolytic anemia. Which medication should the nurse anticipate the HCP ordering?
   1. Filgrastim
   2. Methylprednisolone
   3. A transfusion of red blood cells (RBCs)
   4. Leucovorin

ANSWERS AND RATIONALES

The correct answer number and rationale are in **boldface blue type.** Rationales for why other answer options are incorrect are also given.

Angina and Myocardial Infarction

1. 1. If the NTG, a coronary vasodilator, is not kept in a dark-colored bottle, it will lose its potency. This statement shows the client's understanding of the medication teaching and that more teaching on that topic is not necessary.

2. Sublingual NTG is placed under the client's tongue when chest pain first occurs. The client understands the teaching.

3. The client should put one tablet under the tongue every 5 minutes and, if the chest pain is not relieved after taking three tablets, the client should seek medical attention. This statement indicates the client needs more teaching about the medication.

4. NTG causes vasodilation and will cause a headache. The client understands this.

2.

Potential Nursing Intervention	Indicated	Not Indicated
1. Question applying the patch if the client's blood pressure is less than 110/70.		X
2. Use nonsterile gloves when applying the transdermal patch.	X	
3. Date and time the transdermal patch before applying to the client's skin.	X	
4. Place the transdermal patch on the site where the old patch was removed.		X
5. Hold the patch firmly for 20–30 seconds to ensure the patch sticks firmly.	X	
6. Avoid applying the patch to broken or irritated skin.	X	

1. NTG, a coronary vasodilator, causes hypotension and the nurse should question administering a transdermal patch if the client's blood pressure is less than 90/60, but not if it is less than 110/70.

2. The nurse should use gloves when applying a transdermal patch to protect the nurse from any accidental exposure and absorption of the medication.

3. The nurse should remove the old patch, wash the client's skin, note the date and time the new patch is applied, and apply it in a new area that is not hairy.

4. The transdermal patch must be rotated so that skin irritation will not occur.

5. The nurse should ensure the patch is firmly applied by pressing for 20 to 30 seconds.

6. The nurse should apply the patch to clean, dry, unbroken skin. Too much drug could be absorbed if the skin is broken or irritated.

3. Correct answers are 1 and 4.

1. The client should not get out of the bed without assistance due to the drowsiness that may occur after receiving morphine sulfate, a narcotic analgesic. Also, the client is having chest pain and should not get out of the bed without assistance.

2. Morphine sulfate, a narcotic analgesic, should not be administered intramuscularly to a client with a suspected MI because it will take longer for the medication to take effect, and it can skew cardiac enzyme results.

3. Morphine sulfate, a narcotic analgesic, is given undiluted.

4. Morphine sulfate, a narcotic analgesic, is the drug of choice for chest pain, and it is administered IV so that it acts as soon as possible, within 10 to 15 minutes.

An IVP also allows the nurse to inject the medication more accurately over the 5-minute administration time.

5. Morphine sulfate, a narcotic analgesic, should not be questioned. It is the medication of choice, and the nurse should know it is always administered intravenously for a client diagnosed with an MI.

4. 1. **The client receiving a CCB should avoid grapefruit juice because it can cause the CCB to rise to toxic levels.**
2. The apical heart rate should be greater than 60 bpm before a beta blocker is administered. Because the apical pulse is 62 bpm, the nurse should administer this medication.
3. The NTG patch should be held if the client's blood pressure is less than 90/60. Because the blood pressure reading is above that, the nurse should not question administering this medication.
4. The client's platelet count is not monitored when administering medication.

MEDICATION MEMORY JOGGER: Grapefruit juice can inhibit the metabolism of certain medications. Specifically, grapefruit juice inhibits cytochrome P450-3A4 found in the liver and the intestinal wall. The nurse should investigate any medications the client is taking if the client drinks grapefruit juice.

5. 1. **Life-threatening hypotension can result from concurrent NTG and sildenafil (Viagra), a peripheral vasodilator erectile agent.**
2. This is a therapeutic response, which is inappropriate because the nurse must make sure the client understands the importance of not taking the medications together.
3. The client should not take sildenafil (Viagra) within 24 hours of taking nitrates. Still, the client should be instructed not to take sildenafil (Viagra) while taking Nitrobid, a vasodilator, an oral medication taken daily.
4. The nurse should provide the client with correct medication information and not rely on the HCP for medication teaching.

6. 1. Reperfusion dysrhythmias indicate that thrombolytic therapy is effective. It indicates that cardiac tissue is being perfused.
2. **Any bleeding from the IV site, gums, rectum, or vagina should be reported to the HCP. The HCP may not be able to intervene to prevent the bleeding during therapy, but any such bleeding warrants notifying the HCP.**
3. Being alert and oriented would not warrant intervention by the nurse. However, the nurse should monitor the client's level of consciousness because cerebral hemorrhage is a major concern when a client is being given thrombolytic therapy.
4. The nurse should monitor the IV site for infiltration findings, which could lead to tissue damage. If there are no infiltration findings, intervention by the nurse is not warranted.

7. 1. The client is having chest pain with activity; therefore, the nurse should treat the client.
2. Administering transdermal NTG ointment, a coronary vasodilator, is used primarily to prevent chest pain. Sublingual NTG would be appropriate.
3. Administering morphine sulfate, a narcotic analgesic, would be appropriate, but the nurse would not have morphine sulfate at the bedside, and it would take time to prepare.
4. **The nurse would have oxygen at the bedside, and applying it would be the first intervention the nurse could implement.**

MEDICATION MEMORY JOGGER: When answering test questions or when caring for clients at the bedside, the nurse should remember that assessing the client may not be the correct intervention to take when the client is in distress. The nurse may need to intervene directly to help the client.

8. Correct answers are 3, 5, and 6.
1. The client is taking lisinopril (Zestril), an ACE inhibitor, to improve survival after an acute MI, and the blood pressure should be monitored daily or weekly, not monthly.
2. The client can take the medication with food to help decrease gastric distress.
3. **This medication causes orthostatic hypotension, and the client should be instructed to rise slowly from lying to sitting to standing position to prevent falls and injury.**
4. There is no reason for the medication to be taken at night; it is usually taken in the morning.
5. **Lisinopril can increase blood potassium levels. Salt substitutes or eating high potassium foods can cause hyperkalemia.**
6. **Lisinopril can cause taste impairment that generally resolves in 8–12 weeks.**

9. 1. **A. The line is in increments of 0.5 inches, and the order is 0.5 inches; therefore, the nurse should apply this much paste.**
2. B. This would be 1 inch, twice the prescribed dose of medication.

3. C. This would be 1.5 inches, not the correct dose.
4. D. This would be 2 inches, not the correct dose.

Coronary Artery Disease

10. 1. The client should adhere to a low-fat, low-cholesterol diet, and the nurse can teach the client about diet; therefore, the HCP does not need to be notified.
2. Atorvastatin (Lipitor) is an HMG-CoA reductase inhibitor, also referred to as a statin. Statins can cause muscle injury, leading to myositis, fatal rhabdomyolysis, or myopathy. Muscle pain or tenderness should be reported to the HCP immediately; usually, the medication is discontinued.
3. Sedentary lifestyle is a risk factor for developing atherosclerosis; therefore, exercising should be praised and not be reported to the HCP.
4. The medication should not be taken in the morning, but the nurse can teach this, and there is no need to notify the HCP.

MEDICATION MEMORY JOGGER: If the client verbalizes a symptom, the nurse assesses data, or if laboratory data indicates that an adverse effect is secondary to a medication, the nurse must intervene. The nurse must implement an independent intervention or notify the HCP because medications can result in serious or life-threatening complications.

11. 1. Aspirin does not thin the blood; it prevents platelet aggregation. The nurse must understand the correct rationale for administering medications even if the client may say it "thins the blood."
2. Angina is a complication of atherosclerosis, and aspirin may help decrease angina, but that is not the scientific rationale for why it is prescribed.
3. When 81 mg of aspirin, a baby aspirin, is taken daily, it helps prevent platelet aggregation, which, in turn, helps the blood pass through the narrowed arteries more easily.
4. Baby aspirin can cause gastric distress, but the question asks for the scientific rationale for taking this medication.

12.

Potential Nursing Intervention	Indicated	Not Indicated
1. Administer the medication with fruit juice.	X	
2. Instruct the client to decrease fiber when taking the medication.		X
3. Monitor the cholesterol level before giving medication.	X	
4. Assess the client for upper abdominal discomfort.		X
5. Tell client to avoid taking other medications at the same time as cholestyramine.	X	
6. Maintain good oral hygiene.	X	

1. Cholestyramine (Questran) is a bile acid sequestrant. This medication should be administered with water, fruit juice, soup, or pulpy fruit (applesauce, pineapple) to reduce the risk of esophageal irritation.
2. The client should increase, not decrease, fiber consumption while taking this medication to help reduce constipation.
3. The cholesterol level is initially monitored monthly and then at longer intervals.
4. There is no reason for the nurse to assess the client for upper abdominal discomfort because this is not a potential complication of this medication.
5. The client should take other medications at least 1 hour before or 4 to 6 hours after taking cholestyramine to minimize possible interference with absorption.
6. Sipping or holding the medication in the mouth for prolonged periods can result in discoloration, erosion of tooth enamel, or tooth decay. The client should maintain good oral hygiene.

13. 1. A 5-pound weight loss in 1 month would not make the nurse suspect the client is experiencing any long-term complications from taking daily aspirin.
2. Elderly clients often have hearing loss, but it is not a complication of long-term aspirin use. Tinnitus is, however, a possible complication of aspirin use.
3. Elderly clients often lose taste buds, which may cause a funny taste in the mouth. But loss of taste buds is not a complication of taking daily aspirin.
4. A complication of long-term aspirin use is gastric bleeding, resulting in dark, tarry stools. This data would warrant further intervention.

14. 1. The client's blood pressure is within normal limits, but that does not indicate that the medication is effective.
2. Simvastatin (Zocor) is an HMG-CoA reductase inhibitor or a statin that lowers cholesterol levels. A cholesterol level less than 200 mg/dL is desirable and indicates the medication is effective.
3. The client's optimal low-density lipoprotein cholesterol (LDLC) is less than 100 mg/dL. Greater than 200 mg/dL is considered very high. A level of 180 mg/dL is high.
4. High-density lipoprotein cholesterol (HDLC) promotes cholesterol removal, and the level should be greater than 60 mg/dL. The client's HDLC is low, less than 40 mg/dL, which indicates the medication is not effective.

15. 1. This is an expected side effect of the medication and there is no need to quit taking the medication.
2. Taking the medication with meals will not stop flushing of the face, neck, and ears.
3. Flushing of the face, neck, and ears may or may not decrease with time, but the nurse should address the client's reported symptoms first.
4. Nicotinic acid (Niacin) is a vitamin preparation used to prevent or treat pellagra, a niacin deficiency disease. Taking aspirin before the medication will help reduce the face, neck, and ears flushing.

16. 1. This is a true statement; therefore, the client does not need more teaching.
2. Ezetimibe (Zetia) is an antihyperlipidemic medication. This is not a true statement; therefore, the client needs more teaching. Zetia acts by decreasing cholesterol absorption in the intestine and is used together with statins to help lower cholesterol for clients with cholesterol levels that cannot be controlled by taking statins alone.
3. This is a true statement; therefore, the client does not need more teaching.
4. This is a true statement; therefore, the client does not need more teaching.

17. 1. Gastritis may be inherited (autosomal dominant), but an underlying genetic cause has not been identified. Although this is part of the client's family history, assessing the client's current health and medications is the first nursing intervention.
2. Teaching is essential, but it is not the first intervention.
3. Enteric-coated aspirin is appropriate for this client to take, but it is not the first intervention.
4. Assessment is the first part of the nursing process, and determining if the client is taking any antiulcer medication is the first question the nurse should ask the client.

18. 1. Anticoagulants, not antiplatelets, help prevent DVT.
2. Plavix decreases platelet aggregation, not LDL cholesterol levels.
3. Clopidogrel (Plavix) is an antiplatelet medication. This medication works in the arteries to prevent platelet aggregation and is prescribed for a client diagnosed with arteriosclerosis.
4. Plavix is not an antihypertensive medication; it is an antiplatelet medication.

19. 1. The nurse has no reason to discuss the insulin order with the pharmacist.
2. There is no reason for the nurse to discuss the Glucophage order with the pharmacist.
3. Lipitor should be administered in the evening (not at 0900) to enhance the enzyme that works in the gastrointestinal system to help eliminate cholesterol. The nurse should notify the pharmacist and request a change in administration time.
4. An NTG patch is removed during nighttime; therefore, the nurse would not discuss the medication with the pharmacist.

Congestive Heart Failure

20. Correct answers are 1 and 3.
1. Digoxin (Lanoxin), a cardiac glycoside, and furosemide (Lasix), a loop diuretic, are administered for clients diagnosed

with CHF to improve the contractility of the cardiac muscle and to decrease the fluid volume overload. A symptom of CHF is shortness of breath. The fact that the client can ambulate without being short of breath is an improvement of clinical manifestations, which shows that the medications are effective.

2. This statement indicates compliance with treatment guidelines, not effectiveness of a medication.
3. **Weight gain would indicate that the client is retaining fluid and the medications are not effective. No weight gain indicates the medication is effective.**
4. A client diagnosed with CHF does not have HTN; therefore, a normal blood pressure does not indicate the medications are effective.
5. This statement indicates compliance with treatment guidelines, not effectiveness of a medication.

MEDICATION MEMORY JOGGER: The nurse determines the effectiveness of a medication by assessing for the symptoms, or lack thereof, for which the medication was prescribed.

21. 1. Garlic does not need to be taken for hawthorn to be effective. Both herbs lower blood pressure, so one or the other should be taken.

2. Many clients use herbs, vitamins, and minerals. The nurse should not be judgmental in response to clients confiding pertinent information. Doses of ACE inhibitors, cardiac glycosides, and beta blockers may need to be modified if they are taken in combination with some herbs.
3. The herb does not interfere with platelet aggregation nor does it have any anticoagulant effect, so it would not cause bleeding.
4. **Hawthorn dilates the peripheral blood vessels, increases coronary circulation, improves cardiac oxygenation, acts as an antioxidant, has a mild diuretic effect, and treats CHF and HTN. Doses of ACE inhibitors, cardiac glycosides, and beta blockers may need to be modified if taken in combination with hawthorn.**

22. 1. Captopril (Capoten) is an ACE inhibitor. ACE inhibitors should be prescribed for clients diagnosed with diabetes, hyperlipidemia, and HTN when in stage A heart failure.

2. Digoxin (Lanoxin), a cardiac glycoside, is prescribed in stage C heart failure.
3. **Dobutamine (Dobutrex), a synthetic catecholamine, is given for short-term IV therapy for clients in stage D CHF and is preferred to dopamine because it does not increase vascular resistance. Dobutamine increases myocardial contractility and cardiac output.**
4. Metoprolol (Lopressor) is a beta blocker. Beta blockers are prescribed in stage C heart failure. The client may not see any improvement of symptoms, but research has demonstrated that beta blockers can prolong life even without clinical improvement.

23. 1. ACE inhibitors decrease the level of angiotensin in the body by blocking the conversion from angiotensin I to angiotensin II.

2. **Enalapril (Vasotec) is an ACE inhibitor. By reducing the levels of angiotensin II, ACE inhibitors dilate blood vessels, reduce blood volume, and prevent or reverse angiotensin II pathological changes in the heart and kidneys.**
3. ACE inhibitors increase bradykinin levels.
4. ACE inhibitors have no effect on the intervention of the antidiuretic hormone.

24.

Potential Nursing Intervention	Indicated	Not Indicated
1. Drink at least 8 to 10 glasses of water a day.		X
2. Weigh yourself monthly and report to HCP.		X
3. Eat bananas or oranges regularly.	X	
4. Try to sleep in an upright position.		X
5. Notify the HCP of muscle cramps or weakness.	X	

1. **The client should drink enough fluid to replace insensible losses (e.g., through perspiration and in feces), or the client will become dehydrated; however, the client should not drink 8 to 10 glasses of water per day. The medication is being given to reduce the amount of fluid in the body.**

2. The client should check their weight daily, while wearing the same amount of clothes and at approximately the same time for accuracy in weight measurement. The client should report a weight gain of 3 pounds or more within a week.
3. Hydrochlorothiazide (Diuril) is a thiazide diuretic. Loop and thiazide diuretics cause the body to excrete potassium in the urine. The client should attempt to replace the potassium by eating potassium-rich foods such as bananas and orange juice.
4. The client does not need to sleep in an upright position if the CHF is being controlled. If the client sleeps upright to breathe, the HCP should be notified.
5. The client should notify the HCP of muscle cramps or weakness that could indicate an electrolyte imbalance.

25. 1. Pink, frothy sputum indicates that the client's lungs are filling with fluid. This indicates the client's condition is becoming worse.
2. Pitting edema of the sacrum would be seen in clients on bedrest. This is a symptom of CHF and would only indicate the client is getting better if the client had 3+ or 4+ edema initially.
3. Digoxin (Lanoxin) is a cardiac glycoside. Clear lung sounds bilaterally indicate the treatment is effective. The nurse assesses for the clinical manifestations of the disease for which the medication is being administered. If the symptoms are resolving, then the medication is effective.
4. The client's heart rate must be 60 bpm or above to administer digoxin safely, but the heart rate does not indicate the client diagnosed with CHF is getting better.

26. 1. Lisinopril (Zestril) is an ACE inhibitor. The blood pressure is above 90/60, so there is no reason for the nurse to question administering an ACE inhibitor in this situation.
2. Carvedilol (Coreg) is a beta blocker. The apical pulse is above 60 bpm, so the nurse would not question administering a beta blocker in this situation.
3. Verapamil (Calan) is a CCB. CCBs are prescribed to treat angina, so there is no reason for the nurse to question the medication.
4. Furosemide (Lasix) is a loop diuretic. Leg cramps may indicate a low blood potassium level. The nurse should hold the medication until the potassium level can be checked. Loop diuretics cause the kidneys to excrete potassium. Hypokalemia can cause life-threatening dysrhythmias.

27. Correct answers are 2 and 3.
1. The client's apical pulse, not the carotid pulse, should be assessed.
2. Digoxin (Lanoxin) is a cardiac glycoside used to treat heart failure. The client's potassium and digoxin levels are monitored because high levels of potassium impair therapeutic response to digoxin, and low levels can cause toxicity. The most common cause of dysrhythmias in clients receiving digoxin is hypokalemia from diuretics that are often given simultaneously.
3. Yellow haze indicates the client may have high serum digoxin levels. The therapeutic range for digoxin is relatively small (0.5 to 1.2), and levels of 2.0 or greater are considered toxic.
4. This is part of a neurological assessment and not needed for digoxin.
5. This would be an intervention to prevent orthostatic hypotension. Digoxin does not affect blood pressure.

28. 1. Ibuprofen (Motrin) is an NSAID. NSAIDs promote sodium retention and peripheral vasoconstriction—interventions that can make CHF worse. Additionally, they reduce efficacy and intensify the toxicity of diuretics and ACE inhibitors. The nurse should question use of this medication.
2. Amlodipine (Norvasc) is a CCB. As a category of medications, CCBs are contraindicated for a client diagnosed with CHF; however, the CCB Norvasc is an exception: it alone among CCBs has been shown not to reduce life expectancy. Norvasc may be given to the client safely.
3. Spironolactone (Aldactone), a potassium-sparing diuretic, is prescribed for clients in stage C CHF in addition to loop diuretics for its diuretic effect without causing potassium loss.
4. Atenolol (Tenormin) is a beta blocker. Beta blockers have been shown to improve life expectancy, although clinical symptoms may not improve. The nurse would not question administering this medication.

29. 1. ACE inhibitors have a side effect of hyperkalemia. The client should not be encouraged to eat potassium-rich foods.

2. A condition with localized edematous areas (wheals), accompanied by intense itching of the skin and mucous membranes, is called angioedema. This is an adverse reaction to an ACE inhibitor and should be reported to the HCP.

3. An intractable dry cough is a reason for discontinuing the ACE inhibitor and should be reported to the HCP.

4. Symptomatic improvement may take weeks to months to develop for a client diagnosed with CHF.

30. 1. Metformin (Glucophage) is an antidiabetic medication normally administered with morning and evening meals. The nurse would not question the administration of this medication.

2. Atorvastatin (Lipitor) is an HMG-CoA reductase inhibitor (statin) used to manage hypercholesterolemia. Most HCPs recommend that statins be taken at night because most cholesterol produced in the body occurs at night. Unlike most statins, atorvastatin (Lipitor) can be taken at any time of the day due to its 14-hour half-life. The nurse would not question administration of this medication.

3. Nitroglycerin (Nitro-Dur) 0.4 mg/hr transdermal patch is indicated for prophylaxis of angina pectoris. It can be administered continuously or intermittently with a 12-hour nitrate-free interval. The nurse would not question administration of this medication.

4. Captopril is an ACE inhibitor used to treat high blood pressure and heart failure. Captopril is best taken on an empty stomach. This medication is contraindicated for clients taking sacubitril and valsartan (Entresto). Taking both medications together may increase potassium levels, causing toxicity. The nurse should question use of this medication.

MEDICATION MEMORY JOGGER: Many new medications are being released for clients each year. Before administering a drug, the nurse must know how ANY medication acts on the body.

Dysrhythmias and Conduction Problems

31. 1. Atenolol (Tenormin) is a beta blocker. Beta blockers are commonly prescribed for CHF, HTN, and tremors. This medication is not ordered PRN because the medication must be tapered off.

2. Verapamil (Calan) is a calcium channel blocker. Calcium channel blockers are usually ordered for HTN or certain dysrhythmias, but not bundle branch block.

3. NTG is a coronary vasodilator. The telemetry reading shows a bundle branch block (BBB) that occurs when the right or left ventricle depolarizes late in the cardiac cycle. BBB commonly occurs in clients diagnosed with CAD. NTG dilates coronary arteries to allow increased blood flow to the myocardium; therefore, the nurse would anticipate the HCP prescribing this medication.

4. Captopril (Capoten) is an ACE inhibitor. ACE inhibitors are prescribed for various conditions, including MI and CHF, and to prevent cardiac or renal damage in clients diagnosed with diabetes, but they are not usually prescribed for BBB.

MEDICATION MEMORY JOGGER: Typically, medications ending in "ol" or "al" are in the beta blocker classification. Typically, medications ending in "il" are ACE inhibitors, but verapamil is the exception to the rule. It is a CCB.

32. 1. The client's serum calcium level is not affected by this medication. Calcium levels would be monitored for clients taking calcium supplements.

2. The nurse should assess the client's apical pulse before administering any medication that affects the heart rate. The client should be taught to check the radial pulse when taking the medication at home.

3. The client's telemetry reading would not affect the nurse administering this medication.

4. The nurse should not administer this medication if the client's blood pressure is less than 90/60 because it will further decrease the blood pressure, resulting in the brain not being perfused with oxygen.

33. 1. Adenosine (Adenocard), an antidysrhythmic agent, treats SVT, not PVCs.

2. Amiodarone (Cordarone) is a potassium channel blocker. This potassium channel blocker slows repolarization of the atria and ventricles and is the drug of choice for preventing and treating ventricular dysrhythmia. The strip shows multifocal PVCs in which two or more areas of the ventricle are initiating beats. This is potentially life-threatening.

3. Digoxin (Lanoxin) is a cardiac glycoside that slows the heart rate and increases the contractility of the cardiac muscle, and is used to treat atrial dysrhythmias or CHF, not PVCs.
4. Dopamine (Intropin) is an ionotropic medication used to increase blood pressure or maintain renal perfusion, but it is not used to treat dysrhythmias.

34. **1. Atropine, an antidysrhythmic medication, decreases vagal stimulation, increases the heart rate, and is the medication of choice to treat symptomatic bradycardia—weakness, dizziness, and lightheadedness. An increased heart rate indicates the medication is effective.**
2. Atropine has little or no effect on the client's blood pressure other than when the pulse increases, the cardiac output should increase.
3. A side effect of this medication is a dry mouth, but a moist oral mucosa would not determine if the medication was effective.
4. The client ambulating safely does not determine if the medication is effective.

MEDICATION MEMORY JOGGER: The nurse determines effectiveness of a medication by assessing for the symptoms, or lack thereof, for which the medication was prescribed.

35. **1 Adenosine (Adenocard) is an antidysrhythmic medication used to reverse SVT. The client diagnosed with SVT must be continuously monitored on telemetry when this medication is being administered. When the SVT converts to normal sinus rhythm, the nurse knows the medication has been effective.**
2. The apical pulse can be monitored, but when administering medications for a dysrhythmia, a change in the electrical conductivity of the heart to normal sinus rhythm is the best way to determine the effectiveness of the medication. The normal apical pulse rate is 60 to 100 bpm.
3. The blood pressure would not indicate if this medication was effective.
4. The client's serum adenosine level would not indicate the medication was effective.

36. 1. The digoxin level is within therapeutic range; therefore, the digitalis antidote, Digibind, would not be administered to this client.
2. Morphine is a narcotic analgesic. Pleuritic pain is pain involving the thoracic pleura and should be addressed, but it is not a priority over a life-threatening dysrhythmia.
3. Lidocaine is a sodium channel blocker. A client diagnosed with bigeminy, a life-threatening ventricular dysrhythmia, must be assessed first and treated. An IV bolus of lidocaine, followed by an IV drip, is the treatment of choice offered in this question. Amiodarone may be given in place of lidocaine.
4. Lisinopril (Zestril) is an ACE inhibitor. This blood pressure is elevated, but it is not at a life-threatening level; therefore, this client would not be assessed or treated first.

37. 1. This client's elevated temperature and sinus tachycardia require intervention by the nurse.
2. Acetaminophen (Tylenol) is an antipyretic medication. Sinus tachycardia may be caused by elevated temperature, exercise, anxiety, hypoxemia, hypovolemia, or cardiac failure. Because the client's temperature is elevated, an antipyretic should be administered.
3. Quinidine (Quindex) is an antidysrhythmic used to treat ventricular or atrial dysrhythmias, and the word "sinus" means the beat originates at the sinoatrial node; therefore, the nurse must treat the cause.
4. Disopyramide (Norpace), a sodium channel blocker, is used to treat PVC, SVT, or ventricular tachycardia, and this telemetry strip is sinus tachycardia.

38. 1. Light does not affect lidocaine, an antidysrhythmic; therefore, the nurse does not have to protect the bag and tubing.
2. The BNP level is monitored for a client diagnosed with CHF and is not monitored for a client receiving lidocaine.
3. The lidocaine drip must be administered even if the client has no PVCs to prevent and stabilize ventricular irritability because the half-life of lidocaine is very short.
4. Lidocaine is a very potent medication and is administered in this concentration by an IV pump to maintain a constant rate of administration. The pump also ensures that too much medication is not administered at one time, which can result in death.

39. 1. The client diagnosed with atrial fibrillation would not necessarily be taking a diuretic, which would require the client to monitor fluid status.
2. The PTT level is monitored for a client receiving heparin intravenously.
3. Atrial fibrillation causes pooling of the blood in the atria, which could lead to

development of a blood clot, and the client is prescribed warfarin (Coumadin), an anticoagulant, to decrease the probability of developing a thrombus or embolus. Green, leafy vegetables are high in vitamin K, which is the antidote for Coumadin overdose and should be limited in the client's diet.

4. Digoxin (Lanoxin), a cardiac glycoside, should be administered after meals or with meals to decrease gastric irritability.

40. Correct answers are 1, 2, 3, and 4.

1. Atropine, an antidysrhythmic, decreases vagal stimulation, increases heart rate, and is the drug of choice for a client exhibiting asystole.

2. The nurse should determine if the telemetry reading is artifact or if the client is in asystole before administering any treatment.

3. IV epinephrine, a sympathomimetic, vasoconstricts the peripheral circulation and shunts the blood to the central circulation (brain, heart, lungs) for clients with no heartbeat.

4. Asystole (no heartbeat) requires the nurse to start CPR.

5. Lidocaine or amiodarone are antidysrhythmic medications that are used for clients diagnosed with ventricular dysrhythmia, but they will not help convert asystole into normal sinus rhythm.

Inflammatory Cardiac Disorders

41. 1. Antibiotics are the mainstay of treatment for SBE, and in most cases, the ideal antibiotic is one of the penicillins. The nurse would not question this order.

2. A positive blood culture is a prime diagnostic indicator of SBE, and both aerobic and anaerobic specimens are obtained for culture. The nurse would not question this order.

3. The nurse would question why the HCP is ordering a PPD, a tuberculosis (TB) skin test. TB is not a risk factor for developing SBE.

4. Complete bedrest is not enforced unless the client diagnosed with SBE has a fever or findings of heart failure; therefore, bedrest with bathroom privileges would not be questioned by the nurse.

MEDICATION MEMORY JOGGER: The nurse must be knowledgeable about accepted standards of practice for disease processes and conditions. If the nurse administers a medication that the HCP has prescribed, and it harms the client, the nurse could be held accountable. Remember, the nurse is a client advocate.

42. 1. This is a priority because if the client is allergic to the antibiotic and the nurse administers it, the client could go into anaphylactic shock and die.

2. Even if the antibiotic infiltrates into the client's tissues, it is not a life-threatening emergency.

3. The client's vital signs should be monitored for elevated temperature and findings of heart failure, but this is not a priority over checking for allergies because this is the first dose of antibiotics to be given.

4. The medication should be administered at room temperature, but this is not a priority over determining if the client is allergic to any antibiotics.

43. 1. Ibuprofen (Motrin) is an NSAID. The blood glucose level is not affected by an NSAID.

2. Ibuprofen (Motrin) is an NSAID. There is no reason the client should have to sit up after taking an NSAID.

3. Drinking a full glass of water will not increase or decrease the efficacy of an NSAID.

4. Ibuprofen (Motrin) is an NSAID. NSAIDs interfere with prostaglandin production in the stomach, resulting in erosion of the protective mucosal barrier, causing an ulcer. This can be prevented by taking the NSAID with food.

44. 1. NSAIDs interfere with prostaglandin production in the stomach, resulting in erosion of the protective mucosal barrier, causing an ulcer. Bright red bleeding requires immediate further assessment.

2. Pericarditis causes pain, which is expected, but hemorrhaging could be an adverse effect of NSAIDs and warrants immediate intervention.

3. A family member's allergy does not affect the client taking the medication.

4. Clay-colored stools are not indicative of an adverse or side effect of NSAIDs and would not warrant immediate intervention.

MEDICATION MEMORY JOGGER: If a client verbalizes a symptom, the nurse assesses data, or if laboratory data indicates that an adverse effect is secondary to a medication, the nurse

must intervene. The nurse must implement an independent intervention or notify the HCP because medications can result in serious or life-threatening complications.

45. **Correct answers are 1, 2, 5, 6, and 7.**
    1. **IV antibiotics are prescribed for up to 6 weeks. The client is discharged home and will receive this therapy with the assistance of a home health-care nurse.**
    2. **The nurse must teach the client self-monitoring for manifestations of endocarditis. The client should take their temperature daily and report an elevated temperature.**
    3. The nurse would not explain how to use the IV pump in the hospital because it probably will not be the same equipment provided by the home health-care agency. The home health-care nurse will be responsible for this intervention.
    4. The home health-care nurse will arrange for the IV pump for home use.
    5. **Prophylactic antibiotics are administered before invasive procedures (such as teeth cleaning) to avoid an exacerbation of the endocarditis.**
    6. **The nurse should ensure that the client has adequate support at home.**
    7. **The nurse should confirm the patency of the peripherally inserted central catheter (PICC) line before the client is discharged home for IV therapy.**

46. 1. **Clindamycin (Cleocin) is an antibiotic. Antibiotics are well-known for causing allergic reinterventions. A rash and itching should make the nurse suspect that the client is experiencing an allergic reintervention.**
    2. Furosemide (Lasix) is a loop diuretic. The nurse should not question a loop diuretic as the first medication causing the clinical manifestations of an allergic reintervention.
    3. Prednisone is a glucocorticoid. The nurse should not question a steroid, a hormone produced by the body, as causing an allergic reintervention.
    4. *L. acidophilus* is used to replace good bacteria destroyed by the antibiotics and to prevent or treat diarrhea or secondary yeast infection.

47. **100 mL. The pump administers medication at a rate per hour; therefore, 100 mL would infuse over 1 hour.**

Arterial Occlusive Disease

48. 1. The medication should be taken with food to prevent gastric upset.
    2. **Pentoxifylline (Trental) is a hemorrheologic agent. The client should avoid smoking because nicotine increases vasoconstriction.**
    3. Flushing of the skin, faintness, sedation, and gastrointestinal disturbances are clinical manifestations of an overdose of this medication, **not common side effects,** and should be reported to the HCP.
    4. This medication does not cause photosensitivity, so there is no need for the client to wear long sleeves and a hat.

49. 1. Adverse effects of this medication are hypotension, tachycardia, and palpitations. The client should notify the HCP so that the medication can be discontinued. This statement indicates the client does not understand the teaching.
    2. This medication should be taken on a regular basis at least three to four times a day, not only when going outside in cold weather. The client does not understand the teaching.
    3. This medication is contraindicated for clients diagnosed with bleeding disorders; therefore, the client should not take daily aspirin, an antiplatelet medication.
    4. **Isoxsuprine (Vasodilan) is a peripheral vasodilator. This medication increases blood flow, which is restricted in peripheral vascular diseases, such as Raynaud's disease and atherosclerosis obliterans. This statement indicates the client understands the discharge teaching.**

50. 1. The foul odor does not indicate an infection; therefore, the client's vital signs do not need to be assessed.
    2. A C&S would only be taken if the nurse suspected infection, and this foul odor does not indicate a wound infection.
    3. **This is an expected result. The foul odor is produced by the breakdown of cellular debris and does not indicate that the wound is infected.**
    4. There is no need to discontinue the medication. The foul odor indicates the medication is working effectively.

51. 1. The wound should be covered with a thoroughly wrung-out, saline-soaked gauze, but this is not the priority intervention.

2. After applying the ointment and then the saline-soaked gauze, a dry gauze should be applied to the wound, but this is not the priority intervention.
3. **The most important intervention is not to allow any of the enzymatic ointment to be placed on the normal surrounding skin because it will cause necrosis of the normal skin.**
4. The ointment should be applied with a sterile tongue blade to prevent any type of bacteria from entering the stasis ulcer, but this is not the priority intervention.

52. 1. The dressing is changed at least every 7 days or when the exudate seeps through the dressing.
2. **The dressing is changed when the exudate seeps through the dressing or at least every 7 days.**
3. The doctor does not determine when the dressing will be changed.
4. The dressing will be changed many times before the wound is healed.

53. 1. **Clopidogrel (Plavix) is an antiplatelet medication. Ginkgo, an herb, can increase bleeding when taken with an antiplatelet medication such as aspirin or Plavix. Therefore, this statement warrants intervention, and the nurse should encourage the client to quit taking ginkgo. Ginkgo has been shown to have a beneficial effect of increasing blood flow to the brain, but in this case, risk of bleeding warrants the nurse's intervention.**
2. Green, leafy vegetables would interfere with warfarin (Coumadin) anticoagulant therapy, not with antiplatelet medications; therefore, this would not warrant intervention by the nurse.
3. Antiplatelet medication does not require routine bloodwork to determine effectiveness; therefore, this would not warrant intervention by the nurse.
4. Soft-bristled toothbrushes should be used to help prevent abnormal bleeding.

MEDICATION MEMORY JOGGER: Some herbal preparations are effective, some are not, and a few can be harmful or even deadly. If a client is taking an herbal supplement and a conventional medicine, the nurse should investigate to determine if there is a possible intervention that could cause harm to the client. The nurse should always be the client's advocate.

54.

Potential Nursing Intervention	Indicated	Not Indicated
1. Instruct the client to take a nonenteric-coated aspirin.		X
2. Encourage the client to take the medication with food.	X	
3. Discuss the need to take only one 81-mg aspirin a day.		X
4. Tell the client to notify the HCP.		
5. Ask the client about their bowel movements.	X	
6. Perform a gastrointestinal assessment.	X	

1. **Aspirin causes gastric irritation and the best way to prevent this is to take enteric-coated aspirin, not a nonenteric-coated aspirin. Enteric-coated aspirin will be absorbed in the intestines and not in the stomach.**
2. **Aspirin is an antiplatelet. The client should take the aspirin with food to help prevent gastric irritation, and the nurse should instruct the client to take an enteric-coated aspirin.**
3. **A baby aspirin or a regular aspirin can cause gastric irritation, so the nurse should instruct the client to take an enteric-coated aspirin.**
4. **The nurse should assess the client and notify the HCP about the client's assessment results and report of stomach pain.**
5. **The nurse should assess the client's bowel movements for signs of bleeding.**
6. **The nurse should perform a gastrointestinal assessment, including inspection, auscultation, and light palpation, to identify any abnormalities.**

55. **1. Dextranomer (Debrisan) is a debriding agent. The grayish-yellow color indicates the beads are saturated, at which point their cleansing intervention stops. The beads should be flushed from the wound with normal saline, and a fresh layer should be applied.**
2. This is not the normal color of the beads.
3. The grayish-yellow beads must be removed before a new layer is applied.
4. This is a debriding agent that is working effectively; therefore, no surgical debridement is necessary.

56. 1. This IV order would be an expected prescription for a client after surgery; therefore, the nurse would not question this order.
2. Ceftriaxone (Rocephin) is an antibiotic that would be expected for a client after surgery; therefore, the nurse would not question this order.
3. Dipyridamole (Persantine) is an antiplatelet medication that should have been discontinued 5 to 7 days before surgery because it may cause bleeding in the postoperative client; therefore, the nurse would question why the client is receiving this medication.
4. Morphine is a narcotic analgesic that would be ordered for a client after surgery; therefore, the nurse would not question this medication.

MEDICATION MEMORY JOGGER: The nurse must be knowledgeable about accepted standards of practice for disease processes and conditions. If the nurse administers a medication prescribed by the HCP that harms the client, the nurse could be held accountable. Remember, the nurse is a client advocate.

57. Correct order is 2, 4, 3, 1, 5.
2. If a C&S has been ordered and the nurse administers the antibiotic, the C&S will be skewed, and an accurate result will not be available.
4. The nurse should always check if a client has any known allergies before administering the initial medication, especially an antibiotic.
3. The nurse should prepare the IV antibiotic in the medication room—not at the bedside—and should always flush the tubing so that air will not be injected into the client's vein.
1. The nurse must determine if the saline lock is patent. This is done by injecting normal saline into the lock.
5. After all the previously listed interventions are completed, the nurse can infuse the medication.

Arterial Hypertension

58. 1. The nurse would question administering a beta blocker if the client's blood pressure was less than 90/60 because this medication would lower blood pressure even more.
2. Metoprolol (Lopressor) is a beta blocker. The nurse would question administering a beta blocker if the client's apical pulse was less than 60 bpm because this medication decreases the heart rate.
3. An occipital headache could signify high blood pressure; therefore, the nurse would administer the medication.
4. A yellow haze is a common symptom of a client exhibiting digoxin (a cardiac glycoside) toxicity.

59. **1. Furosemide (Lasix) is a loop diuretic. The client has had 500 mL (2,300 – 1,800 = 500) excess urinary output. This indicates the medication is effective—the diuretic is causing an increase in urinary output.**
2. Blood pressure has increased; therefore, the medication is not effective.
3. A weight loss of 1.3 kg (2.6 pounds) in 7 days would not indicate a loss of fluid, it could be a loss of fat. Remember, 1,000 mL equals about 1 kg (2.2 pounds).
4. These are findings of orthostatic hypotension and do not indicate the medication is effective.

MEDICATION MEMORY JOGGER: The nurse determines a medication's effectiveness by assessing for the symptoms, or lack thereof, for which the medication was prescribed.

60. Correct answers are 1 and 2.
1. Captopril (Capoten) is an ACE inhibitor. Antihypertensive medications generally cause orthostatic hypotension; therefore, the client should be taught to get up slowly from lying to sitting and standing to help prevent dizziness and lightheadedness.
2. Blood pressure must be checked daily.
3. ACE inhibitors do not require potassium supplements.
4. The client should never make up doses of medication missed, as that may cause hypotension.
5. The client should be on a low-salt, low-fat, low-carbohydrate diet for HTN, along with taking medication.

61. 1. Hydralazine (Apresoline) is a vasodilator. Blood pressure (168/94) is elevated;

therefore, the nurse should administer this medication without questioning it.

2. Prazosin (Minipress) is an alpha blocker. The normal serum sodium level is 135 to 145 mEq/L; therefore, the nurse should administer this medication without questioning.
3. Diltiazem (Cardizem) is a CCB. Glucose level is not pertinent when administering this medication. Although the glucose level is elevated, it would not cause the nurse to question administering this medication.
4. **Furosemide (Lasix) is a loop diuretic. The serum potassium level is low (normal is 3.5–5.3 mEq/L). Therefore, because a loop diuretic will cause further potassium loss, the nurse should question administering this medication and obtain a potassium supplement for the client.**

MEDICATION MEMORY JOGGER: The nurse must know accepted standards of practice for medication administration, including which client assessment data and laboratory data should be monitored before administering the medication.

62. 1. The client should be discouraged from eating sodium-rich foods and be encouraged to increase their intake of potassium-rich food.
2. **Chlorothiazide (Diuril) is a thiazide diuretic. The client should drink adequate amounts of fluids to replace the insensible loss of fluids and to help prevent dehydration.**
3. To ask the client to keep strict intake and output is unrealistic. This would be done in the hospital, but not in the client's home.
4. The medication should be taken in the morning to prevent nocturia.

63. 1. The nurse should instruct the client to increase fluids or suck on hard candy, but the HCP does not need to be notified because dry mouth is an expected side effect of this medication.
2. The nurse should discuss how to prevent orthostatic hypotension, but the HCP does not need to be notified because this is an expected side effect.
3. The client should not be drinking alcohol because it may potentiate orthostatic hypotension, but the nurse should discuss this with the client and not necessarily notify the HCP.
4. **Bumetanide (Bumex) is a loop diuretic. Leg cramps could indicate hypokalemia, which is potentially life-threatening secondary to cardiac dysrhythmias. This needs to be reported to the HCP so that the dosage can be reduced or potassium supplements can be ordered for the client.**

MEDICATION MEMORY JOGGER: If the client verbalizes a concern, the nurse assesses data, or if laboratory data indicates an adverse effect secondary to a medication, the nurse must intervene. The nurse must implement an independent intervention or notify the HCP because medications can result in serious or even life-threatening complications.

64. 1. This is a therapeutic response that helps the client vent feelings, but impotence may be a side effect of the medication, and the HCP should be notified.
2. This may be a side effect of the medication, and the HCP should be notified.
3. **This may be a side effect of the medication and is a reason for noncompliance in male clients. The HCP should be notified so that the HCP can discuss the situation and possibly prescribe a different medication.**
4. This may be a side effect of the medication, and the HCP should be notified.

65. 1. **This is the correct scientific rationale for administering this medication.**
2. This is the scientific rationale for a CCB.
3. This is the scientific rationale for an ACE inhibitor.
4. This is the scientific rationale for a diuretic.

66. 1. Many clients diagnosed with HTN are prescribed multiple medications to help decrease blood pressure. There is no need to hold the medication or notify the HCP.
2. **These medications all work on different parts of the body to help decrease the client's blood pressure. The nurse should realize the HCP is having difficulty controlling the client's blood pressure and should monitor the client's blood pressure before administering.**
3. Multiple antihypertensive medications are prescribed to help control a client's blood pressure; therefore, the nurse would not need to contact the pharmacist.
4. The nurse should not question administering multiple antihypertensive medications that work on different parts of the body. This is an accepted standard of care.

67. Correct answers are 1, 2, 3, 4, and 5.
1. **Tenoretic (chlorthalidone and atenolol in combination) is a thiazide diuretic**

and a beta blocker. If the client's blood pressure is less than 90/60, the medication should be held so that the client will not experience profound hypotension.

2. **Tenoretic (chlorthalidone and atenolol in combination) is a thiazide diuretic and a beta blocker. If the client's apical pulse is less than 60 bpm, the medication should be held so that the client's pulse will not plummet to less than 60 bpm, which is sinus bradycardia.**
3. **Tenoretic (chlorthalidone and atenolol in combination) is a thiazide diuretic and a beta blocker. A side effect of antihypertensive medications is orthostatic hypotension, and the nurse should discuss how to prevent episodes.**
4. **Tenoretic (chlorthalidone and atenolol in combination) is a thiazide diuretic and a beta blocker. Thiazide diuretics do not cause excessive loss of potassium. Still, the client should be encouraged to eat potassium-rich foods to prevent hypokalemia, which may occur due to increased urination.**
5. **Tenoretic (chlorthalidone and atenolol in combination) is a thiazide diuretic and a beta blocker. The nurse should monitor the client's intake and output to determine if the medication is effective.**

Deep Vein Thrombosis

68. 1. Warfarin (Coumadin), an anticoagulant, is administered orally. There is no reason to discontinue an IV.

2. **Warfarin (Coumadin), an anticoagulant, is administered orally. AquaMEPHYTON (vitamin K) is the antidote for Coumadin toxicity. The therapeutic range for the INR is 2 to 3. With an INR of 5.9, this client is at significant risk for hemorrhage and should be given vitamin K.**
3. The dose should not be administered because it is above the therapeutic range. The dose should be held until the therapeutic range is obtained.
4. Administering this medication is a medication error that could possibly result in death of the client.

MEDICATION MEMORY JOGGER: When trying to remember which laboratory value correlates with which anticoagulant, follow this helpful hint: "PT boats go to war (warfarin) and if you cross the small "t's" in "Ptt" with one line it makes an "h" (heparin).

69. 1. The client is at risk for bleeding and should wear a medical alert bracelet to notify HCPs about the anticoagulant; therefore, the client understands the medication teaching.

2. If the client is cut, the client should apply direct pressure for 5 minutes without peeking at the cut. If the cut is still bleeding after this time, the client should continue applying pressure and seek medical attention. This statement indicates the client understands the medication teaching.
3. **Green, leafy vegetables are high in vitamin K, the antidote for warfarin (Coumadin) toxicity. Green, leafy vegetables would interfere with the therapeutic effects of warfarin (Coumadin). This statement indicates the client does not understand the medication teaching.**
4. The client's PT and INR are monitored at routine intervals to determine if the medication is within the therapeutic range: an INR of 2 to 3 should be maintained. The client should regularly see the HCP. This statement indicates the client understands the medication teaching.

70. 1. **The therapeutic range for heparin, an anticoagulant, is 1.5 to 2.0 times the control, or 54 to 72. The client's PTT of 62 indicates the client is within therapeutic range and the next bag should be administered at the same rate.**

2. The client's PTT is within therapeutic range; therefore, there is no need to order any further laboratory studies.
3. The HCP need not be notified of the client's situation because the client's PTT is within therapeutic range.
4. The client's PTT is within therapeutic range. This level does not indicate a potential for abnormal bleeding.

71. 1. This is a false statement. Warfarin (Coumadin), an anticoagulant, is administered orally and does not work better during the night.

2. This medication can be taken on an empty stomach or with food.
3. There are no side effects of Coumadin that would be decreased by taking the medication in the evening.
4. **Warfarin (Coumadin), an anticoagulant, requires blood test monitoring to see if the medication dosage is within the therapeutic range. Routine laboratory tests are drawn in the morning. If Coumadin is administered in the morning,**

the INR will be lower due to the medication's effects wearing off. If the Coumadin is taken in the evening, then the INR level will reflect more accurately the peak blood level.

72. 1. Warfarin (Coumadin) is an anticoagulant. The nurse would not anticipate the HCP prescribing a medication that would cause bleeding for a client after surgery.
2. Heparin is an anticoagulant. The nurse would not anticipate the HCP prescribing a medication that would cause bleeding for a client after surgery. IV heparin is only used to treat clients diagnosed with actual clotting problems.
3. Alteplase (Activase) is a thrombolytic. Thrombolytic medications would destroy thrombus formations and not be prescribed for a surgical client.
4. Enoxaparin (Lovenox) is a low-molecular-weight heparin. Lovenox is prescribed for immobile clients, such as this surgical client, to help prevent DVT; therefore, the nurse should anticipate this medication being prescribed.

73. 1. A baby aspirin would not cause the client to have petechiae.
2. Petechiae have nothing to do with the client's pain level.
3. The petechiae, tiny purple or red spots that appear on the skin due to minute hemorrhages within the dermal or submucosal areas, are secondary to subcutaneous injections of Lovenox, a low-molecular-weight heparin.
4. Cool compresses cause vasoconstriction, but this would not help prevent or treat petechiae.

74. 1. Heparin has a very short half-life, and to achieve a therapeutic level it must be administered intravenously. Subcutaneous heparin is used prophylactically to prevent DVT. Laboratory tests are not monitored for this route.
2. Enoxaprin (Lovenox) is a low-molecular-weight heparin. Subcutaneous heparin is used prophylactically to prevent DVT. Clinical manifestations of DVT include calf edema, redness, warmth, and pain on dorsiflexion. The lack of these symptoms indicates that the client does not have DVT and that the medication is effective.
3. Range-of-motion exercise is an intervention and does not indicate the medication is effective.
4. In most people, appearance of varicose veins will improve when the legs are elevated. Remember, however, that varicose veins are superficial veins and that subcutaneous heparin is not used to treat this condition.

MEDICATION MEMORY JOGGER: The nurse determines effectiveness of a medication by assessing for the symptoms, or lack thereof, for which the medication was prescribed.

75. 1. This is the area called the "love handles," and low-molecular-weight heparin, Lovenox, is administered here to prevent abdominal wall trauma.
2. This is the area where IM injections are primarily administered.
3. Subcutaneous heparin is administered in the lower abdomen for better absorption and should be at least 2 inches away from the umbilicus.
4. If subcutaneous heparin is administered in the thigh area, it could possibly result in large hematoma formation secondary to leg movement.

76. 880 units of heparin are being infused every hour. When determining units, the nurse must first determine how many units are in each mL.

$$\frac{20{,}000 \text{ units}}{500 \text{ mL}} = 40 \text{ units per mL}$$

40 units per mL × 22 mL per hour = 880 mL per hour

77. 10 mL per hour. When setting the IV pump, the nurse must first determine the number of units per mL.

$$\frac{10{,}000 \text{ units}}{100 \text{ mL}} = 100 \text{ units per mL}$$

Then divide the desired number of units per hour by the units per mL.

1,000 ÷ 100 = 10 units per mL

78. 1. Furosemide and potassium are frequently prescribed concurrently because furosemide can cause the client to excrete excessive potassium.
2. Ticagrelor (Brilinta) is prescribed to decrease coagulation, thereby preventing strokes and blood clots; aspirin is also administered for the same reason. The nurse should question the concurrent administration of these two medications.
3. Levothyroxine is a thyroid replacement medication and digoxin is administered

for atrial fibrillation with rapid ventricular response or heart failure. These two medications can be administered concurrently without questioning.

4. Clients frequently use acetaminophen and ibuprofen based on personal preferences. Some may prefer Tylenol, perhaps if having a headache, and ibuprofen when having bone aches, etc. They are not usually taken at the same time, and these are PRN medications, so the client chooses the medication for the symptoms they are experiencing at the time.

MEDICATION MEMORY JOGGER: In this question, the nurse is being asked whether two medications that affect the renin angiotension cycle should be administered concurrently (ticagrelor and aspirin).

Anemia

79. 1. Elevating the head of the client's bed would assist with dyspnea, but would not help the client's pain, which is the priority, along with reversing the sickling process.

2. Pain medication is administered intravenously; therefore, the first intervention would be to initiate IV fluids and then administer pain medication.

3. Oxygen is usually administered, but the best method of promoting oxygenation is the reversal of sickling, which is accomplished by administering IV fluids.

4. IV fluids help reverse the sickling process, which is the priority. This reversal will relieve the pain and increase the oxygenation to the cells.

80. 1. Morphine is a narcotic analgesic. The nurse would not question administering morphine to a client subject to painful infarcts of organs and infiltrations of the joints.

2. Fentanyl (Duragesic) is a narcotic agonist. The nurse would not question administering a sustained-release medication for pain to a client subject to painful infarcts of organs and infiltrations of the joints.

3. Epoetin (Procrit) is a biological response modifier. It stimulates the bone marrow to produce RBCs (erythropoiesis). The client diagnosed with SCD produces RBCs that "sickle," increasing the levels of hemoglobin S. The client does not need more RBCs; therefore, the nurse would question administering this medication.

4. Piperacillin and tazobactam (Zosyn) is an antibiotic combination. Clients diagnosed with SCD may go into a crisis situation for several reasons, including dehydration and infection. The nurse would not question an antibiotic.

MEDICATION MEMORY JOGGER: The nurse must be knowledgeable about accepted standards of practice for disease processes and conditions. If the nurse administers a medication the HCP has prescribed, and it harms the client, the nurse could be held accountable. Remember, the nurse is a client advocate.

81. 1. Pernicious anemia is a disease caused by the body's lack of intrinsic factor needed to absorb vitamin B_{12} from ingested food. There is no cure for the disease; there is only treatment with cyanocobalamin, vitamin B_{12}. This client has not been identified as having pernicious anemia.

2. The rugae in the stomach produce intrinsic factor, which is necessary for the absorption of vitamin B_{12} from the food eaten. A gastric bypass surgery eliminates much of the surface area of the stomach and rugae, so the client cannot absorb vitamin B_{12}. The client will need to replace vitamin B_{12}, which is needed for RBC production.

3. The problem is not in the amount of food eaten; it is the lack of rugae in the stomach lining.

4. Injections are given on a weekly or monthly schedule depending on the severity of the vitamin deficit. The body does not make vitamin B_{12} on its own; it absorbs the vitamin from ingested foods.

82.

Potential Nursing Intervention	Indicated	Not Indicated
1. Teach the client to perform a fecal occult blood test daily.		X
2. Demonstrate how to crush the tablets and mix them with pudding.		X

Potential Nursing Intervention	Indicated	Not Indicated
3. Inform the client to take the medication at night.		X
4. Tell the client that their stools will be greenish-black.	X	
5. Instruct the client to avoid caffeinated beverages.	X	
6. Take antacids and calcium 1 hour before or 2 hours after the iron.	X	

1. **HCPs sometimes ask clients to obtain fecal occult blood test specimens, usually once a year. The client brings the card to the HCP's office to complete the test. This is not a daily test the client performs at home.**
2. **The tablets should not be crushed because they are enteric-coated. If the client cannot swallow tablets, liquid iron preparations are available.**
3. **The medication should not be taken with food if the client can tolerate it, but it does not need to be taken at night.**
4. **Iron causes the stool to turn a greenish-black and can mask the appearance of blood in the stool. The client should know that this will occur.**
5. **Caffeinated beverages, especially tea, interfere with iron absorption.**
6. **Antacids, calcium supplements, H2 receptor blockers, and proton pump inhibitors (PPIs) should be taken 1 hour before or 2 hours after an iron preparation (Society for the Advancement of Blood Management, 2019).**

83. 1. The client's hydration status will not affect the medication.
2. The medication is black and will stain the skin, sometimes permanently. It is never given in the upper extremities or subcutaneously.
3. Knowledge of seafood allergies is important when administering any iodine preparation, not iron.
4. **Iron dextran (Imferon) is an iron preparation. Iron is black and stains the skin. The medication is administered deep IM in the dorsogluteal muscle in adults and the lateral thigh in small children. It is given by the Z-track method to trap the medication in the deep tissues and prevent leakage back into the shallow tissues.**

84. 1. **Warfarin (Coumadin) is an anticoagulant. Polycythemia vera is a malignant overproduction of RBCs. The blood becomes viscous and tends to clot. Anticoagulants are ordered to prevent clot formation.**
2. Prednisone is a glucocorticoid. Steroids are not ordered for polycythemia vera.
3. Clients diagnosed with polycythemia vera develop HTN due to the increased RBC volume. The blood viscosity causes increased resistance in the blood vessels.
4. The blood is "thick" (viscous) so fluids are increased, not limited.

85. Correct order is 2, 1, 4, 5, 3.
2. **The nurse should determine that the client understands the procedure before signing the permission form for receiving blood or blood products. The HCP is responsible for informing the client about the procedure, but the nurse should make sure the client understands before witnessing the signature.**
1. **The administration of blood or blood products requires that the client sign a consent form. If the client does not consent, the procedure is stopped, and resumed if the client agrees.**
4. **A pretransfusion assessment should be performed to determine preexisting conditions or problems. The nurse uses this information to guide the safe administration of the blood.**
5. **An 18-gauge catheter is preferred to administer blood so that the cells are not broken (lysed) during the transfusion.**
3. **The blood is not retrieved from the laboratory until the nurse is ready to transfuse it. The nurse has 30 minutes from the time the blood is checked out**

from the laboratory until initiation of the infusion.

86. 1. Oral folic acid preparations are administered to clients diagnosed with a folic acid deficiency with no malabsorption problem, such as Crohn's disease.
2. A vitamin B_{12} (Cyanocobalamin) deficiency is not the problem for this client.
3. B complex vitamins are not folic acid.
4. Crohn's disease is the second most common cause of folic acid deficiency anemia. Crohn's disease is a malabsorption syndrome of the small intestines. The client must receive the medication via the parenteral route.

87. **1. Clinical manifestations of folic acid deficiency include pallor, pale mucous membranes, fatigue, and weight loss. Weight gain and pink buccal mucosa indicate improvement in the client's condition and effective medication.**
2. Paresthesia of the hands and feet is a symptom of vitamin B_{12}, not folic acid, deficiency. Lack of neurological symptoms is the differentiating factor used to diagnose folic acid deficiency because the anemias share most other clinical manifestations.
3. A leading cause of folic acid deficiency anemia is chronic alcoholism, but abstaining from alcohol would not indicate the anemia is better.
4. The client should be encouraged to eat green, leafy vegetables, but tolerance of foods does not indicate medication effectiveness.

MEDICATION MEMORY JOGGER: The nurse determines the effectiveness of medication by assessing for the symptoms, or lack thereof, for which the medication was prescribed.

88. 1. Filgrastim (Neupogen) is a biologic response modifier. In immunohemolytic anemias, the client's own immune system attacks and destroys RBCs. The client does not have leukopenia (low WBCs) for which Neupogen is administered.
2. Methylprednisolone (Solu Medrol) is a glucocorticoid. The first-line therapy for immunohemolytic anemia is steroids, which are temporarily effective in most clients. Splenectomy followed by immune suppressive therapy usually follows. Plasma exchange therapy may be done if immune suppressive therapy is not successful.
3. RBCs are seen by the body as nonself and are attacked. A transfusion is not indicated for this client.
4. Folic acid (Leucovorin), a blood former, is administered in megaloblastic anemia or as rescue factors for methotrexate toxicity, not for immunohemolytic anemias.

CARDIOVASCULAR SYSTEM COMPREHENSIVE EXAMINATION

1. The client in CHF is prescribed milrinone lactate. Which **priority** intervention should the nurse implement?
   1. Assess the client's respiratory status.
   2. Monitor the client's telemetry strip.
   3. Check the client's apical pulse rate.
   4. Evaluate the BNP.

2. The nurse is preparing to administer medications to the following clients. Which client should the nurse **question** administering the medication?
   1. The client receiving losartan and blood pressure 168/94
   2. The client receiving diltiazem with 1+ nonpitting edema
   3. The client receiving terazosin and reporting a headache
   4. The client receiving hydrochlorothiazide and reporting leg cramps

3. The client taking digoxin has a serum digoxin level of 4.2 ng/mL. Which medication should the nurse **anticipate** the HCP prescribing?
   1. Digitalis binder Fab antibody fragments
   2. Furosemide
   3. The HCP will not prescribe any medications.
   4. Digoxin

4. The nurse is preparing to administer labetalol IVP to a client diagnosed with hypertensive crisis. Which intervention should the nurse implement?
   1. Monitor the client's labetalol serum drug level.
   2. Keep the medication covered with tin foil.
   3. Administer the medication slow IVP over 5 minutes.
   4. Teach the client clinical manifestations of HTN.

5. The nurse is preparing to administer spironolactone. Which **priority** intervention should the nurse implement?
   1. Check the client's potassium level.
   2. Monitor the client's urinary output.
   3. Encourage consumption of potassium-rich foods.
   4. Give the medication with food.

6. The nurse is preparing to administer medication to the following clients. Which medication should the nurse **question** administering?
   1. Metformin to a client diagnosed with type 1 diabetes receiving insulin
   2. Bumetanide to a client diagnosed with essential HTN
   3. Erythropoietin to a client diagnosed with end-stage renal failure
   4. Clonidine to a client diagnosed with heart failure

7. According to the American Heart Association (AHA), which medication should the client suspected of having an MI take **immediately** when having chest pain?
   1. Morphine
   2. Acetaminophen
   3. Acetylsalicylic acid
   4. NTG paste

8. The client diagnosed with CHF is taking digoxin. Which data indicates the medication is **effective**?
   1. The client's blood pressure is 110/68.
   2. The client's apical pulse rate is regular.
   3. The client's potassium level is 4.2 mEq/L.
   4. The client's lungs are clear bilaterally.

9. Which client should the nurse **most** likely suspect will require polypharmacy to control essential HTN?
   1. The 84-year-old Caucasian male client
   2. The 22-year-old Hispanic female client
   3. The 60-year-old Asian female client
   4. The 46-year-old African American male client

10. Which statement indicates to the nurse that the client diagnosed with CAD **understands** the medication teaching for taking aspirin daily?
    1. "I will probably have occasional bleeding when taking this medication."
    2. "I will call 911 if I have unrelieved chest pain, and I will take an aspirin."
    3. "If I have any ringing in my ears, I will call my HCP."
    4. "I should take my daily aspirin on an empty stomach for better absorption."

11. The client is exhibiting the following telemetry reading.

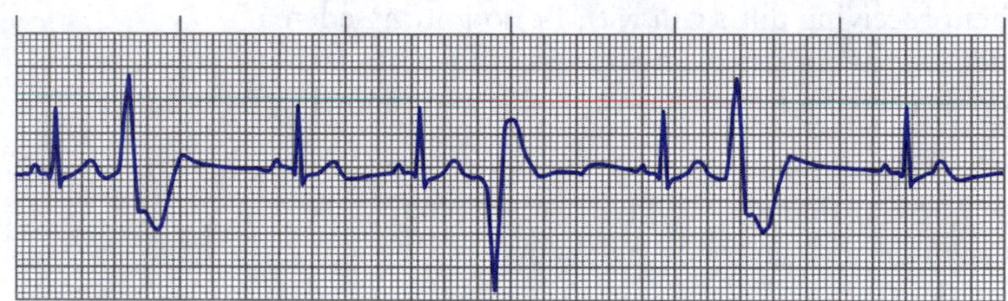

Which antidysrhythmic medication should the nurse administer?
1. Lidocaine
2. Atropine
3. Adenosine
4. Epinephrine

12. The nurse is preparing to administer digoxin to a client diagnosed with CHF. Which area should the nurse assess **before** administering the medication?

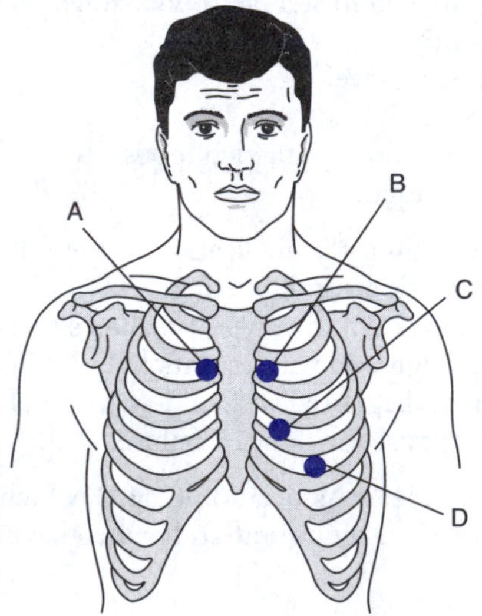

1. A
2. B
3. C
4. D

13. The mother of a child diagnosed with strep throat asks the nurse, "Why do you have to give my child that antibiotic shot?" Which statement is the nurse's **best** response?
1. "You sound concerned. Are you worried about your child getting a shot?"
2. "This injection may keep your child from getting rheumatic fever."
3. "Strep throat always results in children developing heart problems."
4. "I am giving this medication because the throat culture showed a viral infection."

14. The home health-care nurse is visiting the client diagnosed with DVT who is taking warfarin. The nurse assesses a large hematoma on the abdomen and multiple small ecchymotic areas scattered over the body. Which intervention should the nurse implement?
1. Send the client to the emergency department immediately.
2. Encourage the client to apply ice to the abdominal area.
3. Inform the client that this is expected when taking this medication.
4. Instruct the client to wear a medical alert bracelet at all times.

15. The emergency department nurse received a client diagnosed with multiple hematomas and an INR of 7.2. Which medication should the nurse prepare to administer?
1. Protamine sulfate
2. Heparin
3. Phytonadione
4. Vitamin C

16. The nurse is caring for the clients on the telemetry unit. Which medication should the nurse administer **first**?
1. Clopidogrel to the client diagnosed with arterial occlusive disease
2. Digoxin to the client diagnosed with CHF
3. Iron dextran infusion to the pale-skinned client diagnosed with iron-deficiency anemia
4. Amiodarone to the client in ventricular bigeminy on the telemetry monitor

17. The nurse is discharging a client after surgery for a mechanical heart valve replacement. Which statement indicates the client **needs more** discharge teaching?
1. "I will have to take an anticoagulant the rest of my life."
2. "I don't have to take any medications after this surgery."
3. "I must take antibiotics before all dental procedures."
4. "I must go to my HCP for routine bloodwork."

18. The client is being prepared for a cardiac catheterization. Which statement by the client **warrants immediate** intervention by the nurse?
1. "I took my blood pressure medications yesterday."
2. "I broke out in an awful rash after eating oysters."
3. "I have not had my daily aspirin in more than a week."
4. "I am highly allergic to poison ivy or oak."

19. The nurse is preparing to administer an NTG patch to a client diagnosed with CAD. Which interventions should the nurse implement? **Rank in order of performance.**
1. Date and time the NTG patch.
2. Remove the old patch.
3. Clean the site of the old patch.
4. Apply the NTG patch.
5. Check the patch against the MAR.

20. The registered nurse (RN) is preparing to administer nebivolol and valsartan to a client diagnosed with essential HTN. Which intervention should the nurse implement **before** administering the drug? **Select all that apply.**
1. Assess the radial pulse.
2. Take the client's blood pressure.
3. Have the unlicensed assistive personnel (UAP) obtain a complete set of vital signs.
4. Ask the client if they are experiencing a cough.
5. Check the client's apical heart rate.

21. The nurse has just received an order for combination omeprazole and aspirin for a client at risk for an MI. Which is the scientific rationale for the HCP prescribing this medication?
    1. The client requires an antiplatelet medication but has difficulty tolerating the aspirin's effects on the stomach.
    2. The HCP is trying a new concept of managing clients after an MI.
    3. The client cannot afford to take the pills individually because the insurance will not pay for them.
    4. The client is allergic to aspirin and the omeprazole will provide antihistamine properties to prevent a reaction.

22. The nurse is administering morning medications. Which medication should the nurse **question** administering?

Client: W.Z.	MR# 1234567	Date: Today
Age: 50 years	Allergies: NKDA	Diagnosis: Angina
Medication	0701-1900	1901-0700
Regular insulin SQ ac and hs 0–60: 1 amp D_{50} 61–150: 0 units 151–300: 5 units 301–450: 10 units >450: Call HCP	0730 BG 129 1130 1630	2100
Metformin 500 mg PO b.i.d.	0800 1700	
Evolocumab 140 mg SQ for one dose	0900	
Atorvastatin 89 mg PO daily	1700	
Nitroglycerin 0.4 mg on in a.m.	0900	
Nitroglycerin 0.4 mg off in p.m.		2100
Nurse Initials/Credentials	DN/RN	NN/RN

1. Insulin
2. Metformin
3. Evolocumab
4. Torvastatin

CARDIOVASCULAR SYSTEM COMPREHENSIVE EXAMINATION ANSWERS AND RATIONALES

1. 1. The client's respiratory status should be evaluated, but the cardiac status is priority for this medication.
   2. Milrinone lactate (Primacor) is a phosphodiesterase inhibitor. Primacor inhibits the enzyme phosphodiesterase, thus promoting a positive inotropic response and vasodilation. Severe cardiac dysrhythmias may result from this medication; therefore, the client's telemetry should be monitored.
   3. The client's cardiac status, including pulse rate, heart sounds, and blood pressure, should be monitored, but the client's telemetry reading is the priority.
   4. The BNP is a laboratory test that is useful as a marker in the diagnosis of CHF. Normal is less than 100 pg/mL; however, this test is not a priority when giving a client Primacor for already diagnosed CHF.

2. 1. Losartan (Cozaar) is an angiotension receptor blocker. The nurse would want to give this antihypertensive medication to a client diagnosed with elevated blood pressure. The nurse would question the medication if the blood pressure was low, which it is not.
   2. Diltiazem (Cardizem) is a CCB. The client diagnosed with 1+ nonpitting edema would not be affected by a CCB.
   3. Terazosin (Hytrin) is an alpha blocker. Hytrin is not contraindicated for clients with headaches. The apical pulse should be greater than 60 bpm.
   4. Hydrochlorothiazide (HCTZ) is a thiazide diuretic. Leg cramps could indicate hypokalemia, which may lead to life-threatening cardiac dysrhythmias. Therefore, the nurse should question administering this medication until a serum potassium level is obtained.

MEDICATION MEMORY JOGGER: The nurse must know accepted standards of practice for medication administration, including which client assessment data and laboratory data should be monitored before administering the medication.

3. **1. Digoxin (Lanoxin) is a cardiac glycoside. Digitalis binder Fb antibody fragments (Digibind) is a digitalis antibody. When digoxin overdose is suspected, as it would be with a digoxin level of 4.2 ng/mL, Fb antibody fragments bind digoxin and prevent it from acting. The therapeutic range of digoxin is 0.5 to 2 ng/mL.**
   2. This digoxin level is extremely high and requires stopping the medication and prescribing the antidote. Furosemide (Lasix), a loop diuretic, is not an antidote for digoxin.
   3. The nurse should anticipate the HCP prescribing a medication to lower the digoxin level.
   4. The level is above the toxic range, and the nurse should not administer any more digoxin—it could be fatal.

4. 1. Labetalol (Normodyne) is an alpha blocker. It does not have a serum drug level.
   2. Only medications that are inactivated or weakened by exposure to light would have to be covered. This medication is not affected by light.
   3. Medications that directly affect the cardiac muscle or vasculature are administered slowly over a minimum of 5 minutes for safety reasons. Many medications require dilution with normal saline to have sufficient volume for a smooth equal delivery to prevent cardiac dysrhythmias.
   4. The nurse should teach the client about possible clinical manifestations of HTN, but remember, clients diagnosed with HTN are often asymptomatic. HTN is the "silent killer."

5. **1. Spironolactone (Aldactone) is a potassium-sparing diuretic. When preparing to administer a potassium-sparing diuretic, the nurse should check the potassium level because hyperkalemia and hypokalemia can result in cardiac dysrhythmias that are life-threatening. Therefore, checking the potassium level is a priority nursing intervention.**
   2. Monitoring the client's output is more appropriate for determining medication effectiveness. It is not data that would prevent the nurse from administering the medication.

3. The client should not eat potassium-rich foods because this medication retains potassium.
4. This medication can be administered with or without food; therefore, this is not a priority intervention.

6. 1. Metformin (Glucophage), a biguanide, acts on the liver to prevent gluconeogenesis and is often prescribed along with insulin for type 1 or type 2 diabetes.
2. Bumetamide (Bumex) is a loop diuretic. A client diagnosed with HTN would be prescribed a diuretic; therefore, the nurse would not question administering this medication.
3. Erythropoietin (Procrit) is a biologic response modifier. Procrit is administered to stimulate the bone marrow to produce RBCs and is often prescribed for clients diagnosed with chronic kidney disease.
4. Clonidine (Catapres) is an alpha agonist. The nurse would question administering Catapres to a client diagnosed with decreased cardiac output (heart failure), because this medication acts within the brain stem to suppress sympathetic outflow to the heart and blood vessels. The result is vasodilation and reduced cardiac output, both of which lower blood pressure.

7. 1. Morphine is a narcotic analgesic and, in this situation, must be administered IVP to achieve rapid relief of chest pain; therefore, the client could not self-administer this medication.
2. Acetaminophen (Tylenol) is a nonnarcotic analgesic and will not help the client having a "heart attack."
3. The American Heart Association (AHA) recommends that a client having chest pain chew two baby aspirins or one 325-mg tablet immediately to help prevent platelet aggregation and further extension of a coronary thrombosis.
4. NTG is a coronary vasodilator and must be taken sublingually, not as a paste, during acute chest pain to achieve rapid effect of the medication.

8. 1. Digoxin, a cardiac glycoside, does not affect the client's blood pressure; therefore, it cannot be used to determine the effectiveness of the medication.
2. The client's apical pulse must be assessed before administering the medication, but this data is not used to determine the medication's effectiveness.
3. The client's potassium level must be assessed before administering the medication, but it is not used to determine the medication's effectiveness.
4. Clinical manifestations of CHF are crackles in the lungs, jugular vein distention, and pitting edema; therefore, if the client has clear lung sounds, the nurse can assume the medication is effective.

MEDICATION MEMORY JOGGER: The nurse determines medication effectiveness by assessing for the symptoms, or lack thereof, for which the medication was prescribed.

9. 1. The elderly client is often prescribed multiple medications, but Caucasians usually respond well to one antihypertensive medication.
2. A young Hispanic female would not be considered high risk for HTN and would probably not require multiple antihypertensive medications.
3. The Asian diet is high in omega-3 fatty acid, which decreases atherosclerosis, a risk factor for HTN. This population usually does not require multiple antihypertensive medications.
4. Ethnically and racially, African Americans have poorer responses to ACE inhibitors, beta blockers, and other antihypertensive medications than do people of other backgrounds. There is no specific reason known for this, but it is empirically and scientifically documented. Polypharmacy is using multiple medications to medically treat a client, and African Americans often require this to treat HTN.

10. 1. If the client experiences any abnormal bleeding, the HCP should be notified.
2. Aspirin is administered as an antiplatelet to prevent coronary artery occlusion. It is not administered for chest pain. If the client has chest pain that is not relieved with NTG, the client should call the EMS and get medical treatment immediately. Taking an extra aspirin may prevent further cardiac damage.
3. Tinnitus, or ringing in the ears, is a symptom of aspirin toxicity. The client taking one aspirin a day would not be at risk for this.
4. Aspirin is very irritating to the gastric mucosa and should be taken with food to help prevent gastric irritation resulting in ulcers. Enteric-coated aspirin is used to help prevent this complication.

11. 1. The telemetry reading shows multifocal PVCs. Lidocaine, an antidysrhythmic, suppresses ventricular ectopy and is the

first-line drug for the treatment of ventricular dysrhythmias.

2. Atropine, an antidysrhythmic, decreases vagal stimulation, which increases the heart rate and is the drug of choice for asystole, complete heart block, and symptomatic bradycardia.
3. Adenosine, an antidysrhythmic, is the drug of choice for terminating paroxysmal SVT by decreasing the automaticity of the sinoatrial node and slowing conduction through the AV node.
4. Epinephrine, a sympathomimetic medication, constricts the periphery and shunts the blood to the central trunk. It is the first medication administered to a client in a code.

12. 1. This is the second intercostal space right sternal notch, which is one of the two areas used to auscultate the aortic valve, but it is not where the apical pulse is assessed.
2. This is the second intercostal space left sternal notch, which is used to auscultate the pulmonic valve, but it is not where the apical pulse is assessed.
3. This is the fourth and fifth intercostal space to the left of the sternum and is where the tricuspid valve is best heard.
4. The apical pulse located at the fifth intercostal midclavicular space must be assessed for 1 minute before administering digoxin. If the apical pulse is less than 60 bpm, the nurse should hold the medication.

13. 1. This is a therapeutic response and does not answer the mother's question. This type of response is used to encourage the client to ventilate feelings.
2. Antibiotics will treat strep throat, which will decrease the child's fever and pain. If untreated, strep throat can lead to rheumatic fever (although rare), which can result in rheumatic endocarditis in future years.
3. This is a false statement.
4. Strep throat is a bacterial infection, not a viral infection.

14. 1. Abnormal bleeding is a sign of an overdose of warfarin (Coumadin), an anticoagulant. The client needs to be assessed immediately and have a stat INR laboratory test.
2. Ice causes vasoconstriction, but this bleeding is abnormal and will not stop without medical treatment.
3. Abnormal bleeding to this extent is not expected while receiving Coumadin therapy.
4. This is an appropriate teaching intervention for clients receiving Coumadin, but this is not an appropriate intervention at this time.

15. 1. Protamine sulfate is the antidote for heparin toxicity.
2. Heparin is a parenteral anticoagulant and would not be administered for warfarin (Coumadin) toxicity.
3. Vitamin K is the antidote for warfarin (Coumadin) toxicity, which is supported by an INR of 7.2 and bruising. The therapeutic range is 2 to 3.
4. The antidote is vitamin K, not vitamin C.

16. 1. Clopidogrel (Plavix) is an antiplatelet. This medication can be administered after the nurse treats the client diagnosed with a life-threatening dysrhythmia.
2. Digoxin (Lanoxin) is a cardiac glycoside and is not a priority medication over treating a client diagnosed with a life-threatening dysrhythmia.
3. An iron dextran infusion must be closely monitored during administration. The nurse must treat the client diagnosed with a life-threatening dysrhythmia before devoting time to medication administration.
4. Amiodarone (Cordarone) is an antidysrhythmic. Ventricular bigeminy is a life-threatening dysrhythmia that must be treated immediately to prevent cardiac arrest.

17. 1. The client will be taking warfarin (Coumadin), an anticoagulant, the rest of their life. This statement indicates the client understands the teaching.
2. The client with a mechanical heart valve replacement will be taking anticoagulants and periodic antibiotics. The client needs more discharge teaching.
3. If antibiotics are not taken before dental procedures, the client may develop strep infections leading to vegetative growth on cardiac structures. The client understands this.
4. The client must have regular INR blood laboratory tests drawn to determine if anticoagulant levels are within the therapeutic range. Therapeutic INR for a client with a mechanical valve replacement is 2.0 to 3.5.

18. 1. The client should take their blood pressure medication before the cardiac catheterization; therefore, this statement does not warrant intervention.

2. **This may indicate the client is allergic to iodine, a component of the cardiac catheterization dye, and warrants further assessment by the nurse.**
3. The client should stop any medication that interferes with clot formation, so this statement does not require intervention by the nurse.
4. An allergy to poison ivy or oak would not interfere with this procedure.

MEDICATION MEMORY JOGGER: The nurse must be knowledgeable about diagnostic tests and surgical procedures. If the client provides information that would indicate potential harm to the client, the nurse must intervene. Iodine is found in many types of seafood and is used in many diagnostic tests.

19. Correct order is 5, 1, 2, 4, 3.
   5. **The nurse should implement the rights of medication administration, and the first is to make sure it is the right medication and the right client.**
   1. **Before applying the NTG patch, the nurse should date and time the application paper before putting it on the client so that the nurse does not press on the client when writing on the patch.**
   2. **The nurse should have gloves on when removing the old patch.**
   4. **Next, the nurse should administer the NTG patch application paper in a clean, dry, nonhairy place.**
   3. **The nurse should make sure no medication remains on the client's skin.**

20. Correct answers are 2, 4, and 5.
   1. When administering medications, the nurse uses the apical heart rate not the radial pulse.
   2. **Nebivolol (Bystolic) is in the beta blocker classification. Beta blockers relax the blood vessels, reducing the heart rate and the blood pressure. Beta blockers usually have an "ol" or an "al" at the end of their generic names. The nurse should take the blood pressure and hold or notify the HCP if it is less than 90/60. Valsartan (Diovan) is an angiotension receptor blocker (ARB) used to treat HTN and CHF. The trade name of the combination of nebivolol and valsartan is Byvalson.**
   3. The registered nurse (RN) should not ask the UAP to take the apical heart rate and blood pressure. If the nurse is administering the medication, it is the nurse's responsibility. Temperature and respirations are not needed.
   4. **A cough is a side effect of an ARB. The nurse should assess for possible side effects of medications.**
   5. **An apical heart rate is required for any beta blocker medication if the nurse is to administer the medication safely.**

21. 1. **The combination medication of omeprazole and aspirin (Yosprala) is specifically indicated for clients requiring aspirin for secondary prevention of cardiovascular and cerebrovascular events, and at risk of developing aspirin-associated gastric ulcers. Aspirin is an antiplatelet and omeprazole is a PPI.**
   2. Medication combination is not a new concept. The medication is combining different chemicals to achieve desired effects and manage the potential risks.
   3. Aspirin is an old medication that is inexpensive if purchased over the counter. Omeprazole (Prilosec) is a PPI also available over the counter. New medications have a 17-year patent, allowing the pharmaceutical manufacturer to recoup the cost of research and development. This prescription would be much more expensive for the client or insurance company to purchase.
   4. Omeprazole is a PPI, not an antihistamine. $Histamine_1$ blockers are useful in the treatment of allergies. $Histamine_2$ blockers block $histamine_2$ produced in the stomach and do not work on allergies.

22. 1. **The client's blood glucose is within the acceptable range. No insulin should be administered at this time.**
   2. There is no indicated reason to question administering metformin.
   3. Evolocumab (Repatha) is a human monoclonal antibody used to treat heterozygous familial hypercholesterolemia (HeFH) or atherosclerotic cardiovascular disease. It is used in combination with statin medications to reduce high levels of low-density lipoproteins. Evolocumab is administered subcutaneously once every 2 weeks.
   4. Atorvastatin (Lipitor) is administered in combination with Repatha.

4

Pulmonary System

Breathe in the future, breathe out the past.

—Cassie Alston

QUESTIONS

Upper Respiratory Infection

1. The client diagnosed with arterial hypertension develops a cold and plans to take an over-the-counter (OTC) medication. For each teaching intervention, specify if the intervention is **indicated or not indicated** for the client's care.

Potential Nursing Intervention	Indicated	Not Indicated
1. Try to find a medication that will not cause drowsiness.		
2. OTC medications are not as effective as a prescription.		
3. OTC medications are more expensive than prescriptions.		
4. Do not take OTC medication unless approved by the HCP.		
5. OTC medications can be high in sodium.		
6. NSAIDs can increase your blood pressure.		

2. The client diagnosed with the flu is prescribed an OTC cough suppressant dextromethorphan. Which information should the nurse teach regarding this medication?

1. Take the medication every 4 to 8 hours as needed for cough.
2. The medication can cause addiction if taken too long.
3. Do not drive or operate machinery while taking the drug.
4. Do not take a beta blocker while taking this medication.

3. The health-care provider (HCP) prescribed amoxicillin and clavulanate for a client diagnosed with chronic obstructive pulmonary disease (COPD) and a cold. Which intervention should the nurse implement?

1. Discuss the prescription with the HCP because antibiotics do not help viral infections.
2. Teach the client to take all antibiotics as ordered.
3. Encourage the client to seek a second opinion before taking the medication.
4. Ask the client if they are allergic to sulfa drugs or shellfish.

4. The teenager's parent asks the nurse why their child would have many boxes of pseudoephedrine in their room. Which statement is the nurse's **best** response?
   1. "Has your child always had allergy problems?"
   2. "Teenagers will try to take care of their own health problems."
   3. "Has your child's behavior at school or home changed recently?"
   4. "Remove the medication and say nothing to your teenager about it."

5. The client diagnosed with the flu has been taking acetylcysteine. The nurse should assess for which adverse effect?
   1. Bronchospasm
   2. Nausea
   3. Fever
   4. Drowsiness

6. Which OTC herb should the nurse recommend for a client diagnosed with a cold and has mild hypertension?
   1. *Crataegus laevigata* (hawthorn)
   2. *Zingiber officinale* (ginger)
   3. *Allium sativum* (garlic)
   4. *Hydrastis canadensis* (goldenseal)

7. The client using oxymetazoline nasal spray for several weeks reports to the nurse that the spray no longer seems to work to clear the nasal passages. Which information should the nurse teach?
   1. "Increase the number of sprays used until the desired effect has been reached."
   2. "This type of medication can cause rebound congestion if used too long."
   3. "Alternate the oxymetazoline with a saline nasal spray every 2 hours."
   4. "Place the oxymetazoline nasal spray in a vaporizer at night for the best results."

8. Which statement is the scientific theory for prescribing zinc preparations for a client diagnosed with a cold?
   1. Zinc binds with the viral particle and reduces cold symptoms.
   2. Zinc decreases the immune system's response to a virus.
   3. Zinc activates viral receptors in the body's immune system.
   4. Zinc blocks the virus from binding to the epithelial cells of the nose.

9. The client diagnosed with the flu is prescribed the cough medication hydrocodone. For each intervention, specify if the intervention is **indicated or not indicated** for the client's care.

Potential Nursing Intervention	Indicated	Not Indicated
1. Teach the client to monitor bowel movements for diarrhea.		
2. Tell the client to avoid driving or operating machinery while taking this medication.		
3. Instruct client to plan for rest periods, as this medication usually causes insomnia.		
4. Explain that this medication is more effective when taken with a mucolytic.		
5. Encourage the client to take a second dose if the medicine is not working well.		
6. Teach the client to rise slowly from a sitting or lying position.		
7. Tell the client to report tachycardia, anxiety, or muscle spasms to the HCP.		

10. The nurse on a medical unit is administering 0900 medications. Which medication should the nurse **question** administering?
1. Acetylcysteine to a client coughing forcefully
2. Cefazolin IV piggyback (IVPB) to a client diagnosed with the flu
3. Diphenhydramine to a client with congestion
4. Dextromethorphan to a client diagnosed with pneumonia

Lower Respiratory Infection

11. The client diagnosed with COPD tells the nurse about expectorating "rusty-colored" sputum. Which medication should the nurse anticipate the HCP prescribing?
1. Prednisone
2. Nicotine (transdermal)
3. Dextromethorphan
4. Ceftriaxone

12. The female client is being admitted to a medical unit with a pneumonia diagnosis. Which intervention would the nurse implement? **Rank in order of performance.**
1. Start an IV access line.
2. Administer the IVPB antibiotic.
3. Teach the client to notify the nurse of any vaginal itching.
4. Obtain sputum and blood cultures.
5. Place an identity band on the client.

13. The client diagnosed with emphysema is admitted to the surgical unit for a bowel resection. For each intervention, specify whether the intervention is **indicated or not indicated** for the client's immediate postoperative care.

Potential Nursing Intervention	Indicated	Not Indicated
1. Have the client turn, cough, and breathe deeply every 2 hours.		
2. Administer oxygen to the client at 4 L/min.		
3. Assess the surgical dressing every 4 hours.		
4. Medicate frequently with morphine 15 mg IV push.		
5. Use the incentive spirometer every 4 hours.		
6. Keep sequential compression devices in place while the client is in bed.		
7. Give the client a high-fiber diet.		
8. Monitor intake and output closely.		

14. The nurse is discharging a client diagnosed with COPD. Which discharge instructions should the nurse provide regarding the client's prescription for prednisone?
1. Take all prednisone as ordered until the prescription is empty.
2. Take prednisone on an empty stomach with a full glass of water.
3. Stop taking prednisone if noticeable weight gain occurs.
4. Do not abruptly discontinue taking prednisone.

15. The nurse is preparing to administer medications on a pulmonary unit. Which medication should the nurse administer **first**?
1. Prednisone for a client diagnosed with chronic bronchitis
2. Oxygen via nasal cannula at 2 L/min for a client diagnosed with pneumonia
3. Lactic acidophilus to a client receiving IVPB antibiotics
4. Cephalexin to a client being discharged

16. The client diagnosed with COPD is prescribed morphine sulfate continuous release. Which statement is the scientific rationale for prescribing this medication?
1. Morphine will depress the respiratory drive.
2. Morphine dilates the bronchi and improves breathing.
3. Morphine is not addicting, so it can be given routinely.
4. Morphine causes bronchoconstriction and decreased sputum.

17. The client diagnosed with adult respiratory distress syndrome (ARDS) has a disease-causing organism resistant to antibiotics being given. Which intervention should the nurse implement?
1. Monitor the blood levels of the new antibiotic prescribed for treatment.
2. Prepare to administer the glucocorticoid medication ordered intramuscularly.
3. Obtain an order for repeat cultures to identify the resistant organism.
4. Place the client on airborne isolation precautions.

18. The client diagnosed with COPD is prescribed methylprednisolone intravenous push (IVP). The client's laboratory values are populated in the chart below.

Laboratory Test	Client Values	Reference Values
White blood cells (WBC)	9.8	4.5–11.1 (10^3/cells/microL)
Hemoglobin (Hgb)	15.1	Men: 14–17.3 g/dL Women: 11.7–15.5 g/dL
Hematocrit (Hct)	43%	Men: 42%–52% Women: 36%–48%
Glucose	95	Fasting: Less than 100 mg/dL Random: Less than 200 mg/dL
Blood urea nitrogen (BUN)	15	8–21 mg/dL Adult over 90 years: 10–31 mg/dL
Creatinine	0.75	Male: 0.61–1.21 mg/dL Female: 0.51–1.11 mg/dL

Which laboratory test should the nurse monitor?
1. White blood cell (WBC) count
2. Hemoglobin (Hgb)
3. Hematocrit (Hct)
4. Glucose level
5. Blood urea nitrogen (BUN)
6. Creatinine level

19. The nurse is caring for a client diagnosed with bacterial pneumonia. For each finding in the following table, does the result show the medication therapy is **effective or not effective?**

Finding	Effective	Not Effective
1. Thick, green sputum		
2. Frequent cough		
3. Clear lung sounds		
4. No pleuritic chest pain		
5. Bluish color to lips and fingernails		
6. Afebrile		

20. The nurse is preparing to administer an IVPB antibiotic to a client diagnosed with pneumonia; 10 mL of the medication is mixed in 100 mL of saline. At what rate would the nurse set the pump to infuse the medication in 30 minutes?

____

Reactive Airway Disease

21. Which information should the nurse discuss with the client diagnosed with reactive airway disease and prescribed slow-release theophylline?
    1. Instruct the client to take the medication on an empty stomach.
    2. Explain that an increased heart rate and irritability are expected side effects.
    3. Discuss the need to avoid large amounts of caffeinated drinks.
    4. Tell the client to double the next dose if a dose is missed.

22. The client diagnosed with chronic reactive airway disease is taking montelukast. Which statement by the client **warrants intervention** by the nurse?
    1. "I have been having a lot of headaches lately."
    2. "I have started taking an aspirin every day."
    3. "I keep this medication up on a very high shelf."
    4. "I must protect this medication from extreme temperatures."

23. The client diagnosed with reactive airway disease is taking oral metaproterenol three times a day. Which intervention should the nurse implement?
    1. Instruct the client to take the last dose a few hours before bedtime.
    2. Teach the client to decrease fluid intake when taking this medication.
    3. Have the client demonstrate the correct way to use the inhaler.
    4. Encourage the client to take the medication with an antacid.

24. The client is prescribed an albuterol metered-dose inhaler. Which behavior indicates the teaching concerning the inhaler is **effective**?
    1. The client holds their breath for 5 seconds and then exhales forcefully.
    2. The client states the canister is full when it is lying on top of the water.
    3. The client exhales and then squeezes the canister as the next inspiration occurs.
    4. The client connects the oxygen tubing to the inhaler before administering the dose.

25. The client admitted for an acute exacerbation of reactive airway disease is receiving IV aminophylline. The client's serum theophylline level is 28 mcg/mL. Which intervention should the nurse implement **first**?
    1. Continue to monitor the aminophylline drip.
    2. Assess the client for nausea and restlessness.
    3. Discontinue the aminophylline drip.
    4. Notify the HCP immediately.

26. Which assessment data indicates the client diagnosed with reactive airway disease has **"good" control** with the medication regimen? **Select all that apply.**
    1. The client's peak expiratory flow rate (PEFR) is greater than 80% of their personal best.
    2. The client's lung sounds are clear bilaterally, anterior and posterior.
    3. The client has only had three acute exacerbations of asthma in the last month.
    4. The client's monthly serum theophylline level is 18 mcg/mL.
    5. The client is taking the medication as directed by the HCP.

27. The client diagnosed with an acute exacerbation of reactive airway disease is prescribed a nebulizer treatment. Which statement **best describes** how a nebulizer works?
   1. Nebulizers are small, handheld pressurized devices that deliver a measured dose of an antiasthma drug with activation.
   2. A nebulizer is an inhaler that delivers an antiasthma drug in the form of a dry, micronized power directly to the lungs.
   3. A nebulizer is a small machine used to convert an antiasthma drug solution into a mist delivered through a mouthpiece.
   4. Nebulizers are small devices used to crush glucocorticoids so that the client can place them under the tongue for better absorption.

28. The nurse is caring for a client prescribed a glucocorticoid inhaler. For each intervention, specify if the intervention is **indicated or not indicated** for the client's care.

Potential Nursing Intervention	Indicated	Not Indicated
1. Advise client to gargle after each administration.		
2. Instruct client to use the inhaler PRN.		
3. Encourage client to avoid attaching a spacer to the inhaler.		
4. Teach client to check their forced expiratory volume daily.		
5. Tell client to keep the medication in the refrigerator.		

29. The 28-year-old client diagnosed with chronic reactive airway disease is taking montelukast sodium. Which statement by the client indicates the client teaching is **effective**?
   1. "I will not drink coffee, tea, or any type of cola drinks."
   2. "I will take this medication at the beginning of an asthma attack."
   3. "It is all right to take this medication if I am trying to get pregnant."
   4. "I should not decrease the dose or suddenly stop taking this medication."

30. Which medical treatment is recommended for a client diagnosed with mild intermittent asthma?
   1. This classification of asthma requires a combination of long-term control medication plus a quick-relief medication.
   2. Mild intermittent asthma needs a routine glucocorticoid inhaler and a sustained-relief theophylline.
   3. This classification requires daily inhalation of an oral glucocorticoid and daily nebulizer treatments.
   4. Mild intermittent asthma is treated on an as-needed (PRN) basis, and no long-term control medication is needed.

Pediatric Reactive Airway Disease

31. The 8-year-old child diagnosed with reactive airway disease is prescribed a cromolyn inhaler. The child shares with the nurse that they want to play baseball but can't because of asthma. Which intervention should the nurse discuss with the child and parents?
   1. Instruct the child to take the medication as soon as shortness of breath starts.
   2. Teach the child to take a puff of the cromolyn inhaler 15 minutes before playing ball.
   3. Encourage the child to play another sport that does not require running outside.
   4. Inform the parents to notify the pediatrician if the child reports a yellow haze.

32. The 6-year-old child is experiencing an acute exacerbation of reactive airway disease. The child passed out, and the parents brought the child to the emergency department (ED). Which intervention should the nurse implement **first**?
1. Administer subcutaneous epinephrine via a tuberculin syringe.
2. Administer albuterol via nebulizer.
3. Administer IV methylprednisolone.
4. Administer oxygen to maintain oxygen saturation above 95%.

33. The clinic nurse is teaching the parent of a child diagnosed with reactive airway disease about nebulizer treatments. Which statement indicates the teaching has been **effective**?
1. "I will use half the medication in the nebulizer at each treatment."
2. "The nebulizer treatment will take about 30 minutes or longer."
3. "I will use a disinfectant solution weekly when cleaning the nebulizer."
4. "I will rinse the nebulizer in clean water after each breathing treatment."

34. The child diagnosed with an acute asthma attack is prescribed a 7-day course of prednisolone. The parent asks the nurse, "Doesn't this medication cause serious side effects?" Which statement is the nurse's **best** response?
1. "Yes, this medication does have serious side effects, but your child needs the medication."
2. "The doctor would not have ordered a medication that has serious side effects."
3. "A short-term course of steroids will not cause serious side effects."
4. "There may be serious side effects if your child takes the medication for a long time."

35. The child diagnosed with reactive airway disease is prescribed a cromolyn inhaler. The mother asks the nurse to explain how this medication helps control her child's asthma. Which statement is the **best** explanation to give to the mother?
1. This medication diminishes the mediator action of leukotrienes.
2. This medication blocks the release of mast cell mediators.
3. This medication causes relaxation of the bronchial smooth muscle.
4. This medication decreases bronchial airway inflammation.

36. Which statement indicates to the nurse that the 13-year-old child **understands** the zone system for monitoring the treatment of asthma?
1. "When I am in the green zone, it means good control, and I do not need any medication."
2. "If I am in the black zone, it means I should go to the emergency department."
3. "If I am in the red zone, it means I should take my cromolyn and steroid inhaler."
4. "The yellow zone means I tell my mom so she can give me a nebulizer treatment."

37. The pediatric nurse is caring for a 7-year-old child diagnosed with chronic reactive airway disease. The nurse must evaluate the child's breathing capacity to determine the effectiveness of the medication regimen before discharge. For each intervention, specify whether the intervention is **indicated or not indicated** when teaching about a peak flow meter.

Potential Nursing Intervention	Indicated	Not Indicated
1. Instruct the child to lie down on the bed in a supine position.		
2. Tell the child to seal the lips tightly around the mouthpiece.		
3. Note the number on the scale after the client gives a sharp, short breath.		
4. Have the child blow into the peak flow meter one time and obtain the results.		
5. Move the pointer on the peak flow meter to zero.		

38. The 10-year-old child is being prescribed a cromolyn inhaler. Which statement indicates the child **needs more** teaching concerning the cromolyn inhaler?
1. "If I cannot take a deep breath, I will not use my cromolyn inhaler."
2. "I should not exhale into my inhaler after I have finished taking a puff."
3. "I should wait at least 1 hour to rinse my mouth after taking my inhaler."
4. "I should not stop taking my inhaler because I might have an asthma attack."

39. The nurse is teaching the mother of a 9-year-old child diagnosed with severe reactive airway disease. The child is prescribed salmeterol by metered-dose inhaler every 12 hours. Which instruction should the nurse include when discussing the medication with the mother?
1. Instruct the mother to perform and record a daily salmeterol level.
2. Inform the mother to notify the HCP if the child vomits or becomes irritable.
3. Tell the mother to observe the child for a sore throat and respiratory infection.
4. Recommend that the medication be refrigerated at all times.

40. The HCP has ordered theophylline 5 mg/kg/q 6 hours for a child weighing 35 pounds (16 kgs). How much medication would the nurse administer in each dose?

____

Pulmonary Embolus

41. The client diagnosed with deep vein thrombosis (DVT) is experiencing dyspnea and chest pain on inspiration. On assessment, the nurse finds a respiratory rate of 40. Which medication should the nurse anticipate the HCP ordering?
1. Warfarin
2. Aspirin
3. Heparin
4. Ticlopidine

42. The nurse is preparing to administer warfarin. The client's laboratory values are populated in the chart below.

Laboratory Test	Client Values	Reference Values
Prothrombin time (PT)	22	10 to 13 seconds
Partial thromboplastin time (PTT)	39	25 to 35 seconds
International Normalized Ratio (INR)	3.6	0.9 to 1.1 without anticoagulation therapy 2 to 3 with therapy 2.5 to 3.5 if the client has a mechanical heart valve

Which intervention should the nurse implement? **Select all that apply.**
1. Question administering the medication.
2. Prepare to administer vitamin K.
3. Notify the HCP to increase the dose.
4. Administer the medication as ordered.
5. Assess the client for abnormal bleeding.

43. The HCP has ordered streptokinase intravenously for the client diagnosed with a pulmonary embolus. The client has IV heparin infusing at 1,600 units per hour via a 20-gauge angiocath. Which intervention should the nurse implement?
1. Administer the streptokinase via Y-tubing.
2. Start a second IV site to infuse the streptokinase.
3. Discontinue the heparin and infuse streptokinase via the 20-gauge angiocath.
4. Piggyback the streptokinase through the heparin line at the port closest to the client.

44. The client diagnosed with a massive pulmonary embolus is prescribed streptokinase. The nurse notes on the medication administration record (MAR) that the client is allergic to "-mycin" medications, including streptomycin. Which intervention should the nurse implement?
1. Call the HCP to report the allergy.
2. Administer the medication as ordered.
3. Call the pharmacist to substitute medication.
4. Check the bleeding-time laboratory values.

45. The nurse is discharging the client diagnosed with a pulmonary embolism (PE) and prescribed warfarin. Which statement indicates the client **understands** the medication teaching?
1. "I should use a straight razor when I shave."
2. "I will use a hard-bristled toothbrush to clean my teeth."
3. "An occasional nosebleed is common with this drug."
4. "It will be important for me to have regular bloodwork done."

46. The client diagnosed with a PE is receiving IV heparin, and the HCP prescribes 5 mg warfarin orally once a day. Which statement **best** explains the scientific rationale for prescribing these two anticoagulants?
1. Warfarin interferes with the production of prothrombin.
2. It takes 3 to 5 days to achieve a therapeutic level of warfarin.
3. Heparin is more effective when administered with warfarin.
4. Warfarin potentiates the therapeutic action of heparin.

47. The nurse is administering alteplase to a client diagnosed with a massive PE. Which data indicates the medication is **effective**?
1. The client's partial thromboplastin time (PTT) level is within the therapeutic range.
2. The client can ambulate to the bathroom.
3. The client denies chest pain on inspiration.
4. The client's chest x-ray is normal.

48. The nurse is preparing to hang the next bag of heparin. The client's laboratory values are populated in the chart below.

Laboratory Test	Client Values	Reference Values
Prothrombin time (PT)	13.4	10 to 13 seconds
Partial thromboplastin time (PTT)	92	25 to 35 seconds
International Normalized Ratio (INR)	1	0.9 to 1.1 without anticoagulation therapy 2 to 3 with therapy 2.5 to 3.5 if the client has a mechanical heart valve

Which intervention should the nurse implement?
1. Discontinue the heparin infusion.
2. Prepare to administer protamine sulfate.
3. Notify the HCP.
4. Assess the client for bleeding.

49. The client is receiving an IV heparin infusion. The bag hanging has 25,000 units of heparin in 500 mL of D_5W at 14 mL per hour via an IV pump. How many units of heparin is the client receiving every hour?

____

50. The client is receiving an IV heparin infusion. The hanging bag has 40,000 units of heparin in 500 mL of D_5W. The HCP has ordered medication to be delivered at 1,200 units per hour. At what rate would the nurse set the IV pump?

____

51. The client prescribed rivaroxaban after a diagnosis of PE presents to the clinic with reports of dark, tarry stools. Which intervention should the nurse implement **first**?
1. Call 911 and have the paramedics take the client to the ED.
2. Assess the client for any other findings of bleeding.
3. Check the client's prothrombin time (PT) and international normalized ratio (INR) levels.
4. Notify the HCP of the dark, tarry stools.

52. The client is being admitted to the medical unit with an anemia diagnosis. The nurse is reconciling the client's medication list. The client's home medications are populated in the following chart.

Medication List

Medication	Time Taken
Levothyroxine	Daily
Dabigatran	Daily
Digoxin	Daily
Prednisone	Tapering daily (2 days left)
Warfarin	Every evening

Which information should the nurse notify the HCP of **immediately**?
1. Notify the HCP of the levothyroxine and digoxin.
2. Notify the HCP of the dabigatran and warfarin.
3. Notify the HCP of the prednisone tapering schedule.
4. Notify the HCP to request a digoxin antidote.

ANSWERS AND RATIONALES

The correct answer number and rationale are in **boldface blue type.** Rationales for why other answer options are incorrect are also given.

Upper Respiratory Infection

1.

Potential Nursing Intervention	Indicated	Not Indicated
1. Try to find a medication that will not cause drowsiness.		X
2. OTC medications are not as effective as a prescription.		X
3. OTC medications are more expensive than prescriptions.		X
4. Do not take OTC medication unless approved by the HCP.	X	
5. OTC medications can be high in sodium.	X	
6. NSAIDs can increase your blood pressure.	X	

1. **The nurse should inform the client about the dangers of self-medicating with OTC medications. Many OTC medications work by causing vasoconstriction, which will increase the client's hypertension.**
2. **Efficacy of medications depends on the medication and strength. Most OTC medications were one-time prescription medications. There are many variables, and this statement is too general to be true.**
3. **Medication expense is not the relevant point for this client. The problem is to inform the client about the actions of many OTC medications and the effect on the client's hypertension.**
4. **Many OTC medications work by causing vasoconstriction, which will increase the client's hypertension. The client should only take medications (approved by the HCP) that will not affect the client's hypertension.**
5. **Many OTC medications contain sodium, which can raise blood pressure.**
6. **NSAIDs such as ibuprofen and naproxen sodium can increase blood pressure (American Heart Association, 2021).**

2. 1. **OTC dextromethorphan (Robitussin, Delsym), an antitussive, is sold under several names. Dextromethorphan is relatively safe in the recommended dose range of 10 to 30 mg every 4 to 8 hours. At these levels, it does not produce respiratory depression, and side effects are uncommon.**
2. This medication does not cause addiction but is subject to abuse. Inappropriately high doses induce a state of psychosis, including delusions, hallucinations, and paranoia (Martinak et al., 2017).
3. This medication does not produce drowsiness, so driving or operating machinery while taking dextromethorphan is acceptable.
4. The medication does not slow the heart rate, and there is no reason for a client not to take a prescribed beta blocker medication while taking dextromethorphan.

3. 1. Antibiotics do not treat viral infections, but HCPs will frequently prescribe prophylactic antibiotics for clients diagnosed with comorbid conditions (such as COPD) to prevent a secondary bacterial infection.
2. **Amoxicillin and clavulanate (Augmentin) is an antibiotic. Clients prescribed antibiotics should always be taught to take all medication as ordered to prevent resistant strains of bacteria from developing.**
3. There is no reason for a second opinion, as this is standard medical practice.
4. This is a penicillin preparation, not a sulfa medication or iodine.

4. 1. When used legally, these are allergy medications, but they are also the ingredients in illegal methamphetamine production. Quantities of any medication in a teenager's room should be investigated.
2. Teenagers try to develop independence, but it is always the parent or guardian's responsibility to monitor their health.
3. Pseudoephedrine (Sudafed) is an antihistamine and is used in the manufacture of methamphetamines. This situation could indicate the teenager is involved with the drug culture, taking or manufacturing drugs. The nurse should assess for findings of drug involvement.
4. The parent is responsible for determining the teenager's activities. The situation should be discussed with the teenager.

5. 1. Acetylcysteine (Acetadote, Cetylev) is a mucolytic. Acetylcysteine can cause bronchospasm, which will impair the client's breathing, not improve it. An adverse reaction is a reason to discontinue the medication immediately.
2. Nausea is a side effect of many medications and can usually be managed by taking the medication with food. A side effect is not an adverse effect.
3. Fever would result from the cold, flu, or infection, not from the medication.
4. Drowsiness is caused by some cold and flu preparations, usually antihistamines. Acetylcysteine causes the client to expectorate secretions, which will keep the client awake.

6. 1. Hawthorn is used for mild hypertension, congestive heart failure (CHF), and angina, but it does nothing for a cold or the flu.
2. Ginger is used to stimulate digestion and to help ease nausea and motion sickness. It does nothing for hypertension, flu, or colds.
3. Garlic is used for colds and the flu and can also be given for hypertension. It causes mild vasodilation and will not make hypertension worse.
4. Goldenseal is used for respiratory, digestive, and urinary infections, but it increases the effectiveness of some antihypertensive medications, beta blockers, and antidysrhythmics. It should be used with caution for clients diagnosed with cardiovascular disease, diabetes mellitus, or glaucoma.

MEDICATION MEMORY JOGGER: Some herbal preparations are effective, some are not, and a few can be harmful or even deadly. If a client is taking an herbal supplement and a conventional medicine, the nurse should investigate to determine if the combination will cause harm to the client. The nurse should always be the client's advocate.

7. 1. Increasing the number of sprays will only increase the problem. This medication is for short-term use only (i.e., a few days). Longer use can cause rebound congestion that can be difficult to resolve.
2. Oxymetazoline (Afrin) is a nasal decongestant. Afrin is recommended for short-term relief of nasal congestion for clients older than 6 years. Longer use can cause rebound congestion that can be difficult to resolve.
3. Afrin should be used every 10 to 12 hours only. Using it more often increases the chance of developing a dependence on the medication and rebound congestion.
4. Afrin nasal spray is to be used intranasally. It is not an additive for a vaporizer.

8. 1. Zinc does not bind the viral particle. Symptoms are diminished by blocking the ability of the virus to bind with the nasal lining.
2. Zinc is a micronutrient found in the body that helps to increase the body's immune system.
3. Activating viral receptors would increase the symptoms of a cold.
4. Theoretically, zinc blocks viral binding to nasal epithelium. Observation has shown that increased amounts of zinc can prevent the binding and prevent the development of rhinovirus symptoms.

9.

Potential Nursing Intervention	Indicated	Not Indicated
1. Teach the client to monitor bowel movements for diarrhea.		X
2. Tell the client to avoid driving or operating machinery while taking this medication.	X	
3. Instruct the client to plan for rest periods, as this medication usually causes insomnia.		X

Potential Nursing Intervention	Indicated	Not Indicated
4. Explain that this medication is more effective when taken with a mucolytic.		X
5. Encourage the client to take a second dose if the medicine is not working well.		X
6. Teach the client to rise slowly from a sitting or lying position.	X	
7. Tell the client to report tachycardia, anxiety, or muscle spasms to the HCP.	X	

1. **Hydrocodone is an opioid and can slow the peristalsis of the bowel, resulting in constipation, not diarrhea. The client should be aware of this, increase fluid intake, and use bulk laxatives and stool softeners.**
2. **Opioids can cause drowsiness, so driving or operating machinery should be discouraged.**
3. **Opioids usually cause the client to be drowsy, not have insomnia.**
4. **Hydrocodone is a cough suppressant, and a mucolytic is an expectorant. These are opposite-acting medications.**
5. **The medication is habit-forming. The client should notify the HCP if they feel the medication is not working rather than increase the dosage.**
6. **The medication can cause dizziness or fainting when rising suddenly. The nurse should tell the client to get up slowly to help alleviate this problem.**
7. **Tachycardia, anxiety, restlessness, muscle spasms, and sweating could be symptoms of serotonin syndrome and should be reported to the HCP immediately.**

10. 1. **Acetylcysteine is a mucolytic. An adverse effect of acetylcysteine is bronchospasm. This client should be assessed for bronchospasm before administering a dose of Mucomyst.**
    2. Cefazolin (Ancef) is an antibiotic. Antibiotics are frequently administered to clients diagnosed with viral infections to prevent secondary bacterial infections. This client is considered at risk, or the client would not be in a hospital receiving care. There is no reason to question this medication.
    3. Diphenhydramine (Benadryl) is an antihistamine. Antihistamines are prescribed for congestion, so there is no reason to question this medication.
    4. Dextromethorphan (Robitussin) is an antitussive. A symptom of pneumonia is a cough, so there is no reason to question this medication.

Lower Respiratory Infection

11. 1. Prednisone is a glucocorticoid. Clients diagnosed with COPD are commonly prescribed a steroid (glucocorticoid) medication to decrease inflammation in the lungs. This client should already be taking this or a similar medication. The client's "rusty-colored" sputum indicates an infection, and an antibiotic should be ordered.
    2. A transdermal nicotine system, such as Habitrol, would be anticipated. If still smoking, the client should quit smoking, but the client's "rusty-colored" sputum indicates an infection, and an antibiotic should be ordered.
    3. Dextromethorphan (Robitussin) is an antitussive. The client may require an antitussive but more likely a mucolytic to help expectorate the thick tenacious sputum associated with COPD.
    4. **Ceftriaxone (Rocephin) is an antibiotic. The client's "rusty-colored" sputum indicates an infection, and an antibiotic should be ordered. Rocephin is a broad-spectrum antibiotic.**

12. **Correct order is 5, 4, 1, 2, 3.**
    5. **The laboratory technician drawing the blood cultures will need the band to identify the client before drawing the specimen, and the nurse will need the band before administering the medication. Checking for the right client**

is one of the rights of medication administration.

4. Cultures are obtained before the initiation of antibiotics to prevent skewing of the results.
1. An IV line must be initiated before the nurse can administer IV medications.
2. IV antibiotics should be administered within 1 to 2 hours of the order being written. This should always be considered a "now" medication.
3. Superinfections are a potential complication of antibiotic therapy. Vaginal yeast infections occur when the antibiotic kills off the good bacteria. Diarrhea from the destruction of intestinal flora is also a possibility.

13.

Potential Nursing Intervention	Indicated	Not Indicated
1. Have the client turn, cough, and breathe deeply every 2 hours.	X	
2. Administer oxygen to the client at 4 L/min.		X
3. Assess the surgical dressing every 4 hours.	X	
4. Medicate frequently with morphine 15 mg IV push.		X
5. Use the incentive spirometer every 4 hours.	X	
6. Keep sequential compression devices in place while the client is in bed.	X	
7. Provide the client with a high-fiber diet.		X
8. Monitor intake and output closely.	X	

1. Clients undergoing surgery are encouraged to turn, cough, and deep breathe (TC&DB) a minimum of every 2 hours. Clients diagnosed with emphysema should TC&DB more often than every 2 hours.
2. The client should be administered oxygen at 1 to 3 L/min. Clients diagnosed with chronic lung disease have developed carbon dioxide narcosis. High levels of carbon dioxide have destroyed the client's first stimulus for breathing. Oxygen hunger is the body's backup system for sustaining life. Administering oxygen at levels above 2 L/min at rest and 3 L/min during activity may cause the client to stop breathing.
3. Clients diagnosed with chronic lung disease are frequently prescribed long-term steroid therapy. Steroids delay wound healing. The nurse should assess the wound to determine that the surgical incision is healing as desired.
4. Morphine, a narcotic analgesic, can cause respiratory compromise, especially when given frequently and in large doses. Usual doses of morphine are between 1 and 3 mg per dose. This client is already at risk for respiratory complications from emphysema.
5. The client should use the incentive spirometer to help prevent pneumonia. Every 4 hours is an appropriate period.
6. Sequential compression devices are used to prevent DVT and improve blood flow in the legs.
7. The client should not eat in the immediate postoperative period. When audible bowel sounds are present, the client will be ordered a progressive diet. Eating less fiber can improve pain, abdominal cramping, and gas for the client.
8. Intake and output should be monitored closely. Decreased urine output, less than 30 mL/hr, indicates a complication.

14. 1. This is instruction for an antibiotic. Prednisone is not abruptly discontinued because cortisol (a glucocorticoid) is necessary to sustain life, and the adrenal glands will stop producing cortisol while the client is taking it exogenously.
2. Prednisone can produce gastric distress. It is given with food to minimize gastric discomfort.
3. Weight gain is a side effect of steroid therapy, and the client should not stop taking the medication if this occurs. This medication must be tapered off if the client is

to stop the medication—if the client can discontinue the medication at all.

4. **Prednisone is a glucocorticoid steroid. Prednisone is not abruptly discontinued because cortisol (a glucocorticoid) is necessary to sustain life, and the adrenal glands stop producing cortisol while the client is taking it exogenously. The medication must be tapered off to prevent a life-threatening complication.**

15. 1. Prednisone is a glucocorticoid steroid. This is an oral preparation that can be given daily. This is not the first medication to be administered.

2. **Oxygen is considered a medication and should be a priority whenever it is ordered. A client diagnosed with pneumonia will have some amount of respiratory compromise, and the ordered 2 L/min indicates a client diagnosed with chronic lung disease. This is the priority medication.**
3. Lactic acidophilus (Lactinex) is a biologic replacement. It is administered to replace the good bacteria in the body destroyed by the antibiotic, but it does not need to be administered first.
4. Cephalexin (Keflex) is an oral antibiotic, but this client is being discharged, indicating the client's condition has improved. This client could wait until the oxygen is initiated.

MEDICATION MEMORY JOGGER: Oxygen is a medication, and the nurse should remember basic principles that apply to oxygen administration. The test taker could choose the correct answer based on Maslow's Hierarchy of Needs. Breathing and oxygen are the priority.

16. 1. The nurse does not administer medications to decrease the respiratory drive for any client—especially not one diagnosed with pulmonary disease.

2. **Morphine continuous-release (MS Contin), a narcotic analgesic, is a mild bronchodilator. The continuous-release formulation provides a sustained effect for the client.**
3. All forms of morphine can be addicting.
4. Bronchoconstriction would increase the client's difficulty in breathing and trap sputum below the constricted bronchus.

17. 1. **Currently, the medication used to treat resistant bacteria is vancomycin, but gentamycin may also be used. These medications can be toxic to the auditory nerve and the kidneys. The trough concentration should not exceed 10 mcg/mL (mild-moderate infection) or 15–20 mcg/mL (for severe infections). The nurse should monitor the blood levels.**

2. If ordered, the steroid would be given IV, not intramuscularly.
3. The culture does not need to be repeated. This would add unnecessary expense to the client.
4. The client should be placed on contact and possibly droplet precautions. Airborne isolation is required for tuberculosis (TB).

18. Correct answer is 4.

1. WBCs are monitored to detect the presence of an infection, not for steroids.
2. The Hgb and Hct are monitored to detect blood loss, not for steroid therapy.
3. The Hgb and Hct are monitored to detect blood loss, not for steroid therapy.
4. **Methylprednisolone (Solu Medrol) is a glucocorticoid. Steroid therapy interferes with glucose metabolism and increases insulin resistance. The blood glucose levels should be monitored to determine if an intervention is needed.**
5. The BUN and creatinine levels are monitored to determine renal status. The adrenal glands produce cortisol.
6. The BUN and creatinine levels are monitored to determine renal status. Adrenal glands produce cortisol.

MEDICATION MEMORY JOGGER: The nurse must know accepted standards of practice for medication administration, including which client assessment data and laboratory data should be monitored before administering the medication.

19.

Finding	Effective	Not Effective
1. Thick, green sputum		X
2. Frequent cough		X
3. Clear lung sounds	X	
4. No pleuritic chest pain	X	
5. Bluish color to lips and fingernails		X
6. Afebrile	X	

1. **Thick, green sputum is a symptom of pneumonia, which indicates the antibiotic therapy is not effective. If the sputum were changing from thick, green sputum to thinner, lighter-colored sputum, it would indicate an improvement in the condition.**
2. **Frequent cough indicates that antibiotic therapy is not effective.**
3. **The clinical manifestations of pneumonia include crackles and wheezing in the lung fields. Clear lung sounds indicate an improvement in pneumonia and that the medication is effective.**
4. **Pleuritic chest is a symptom of pneumonia, and no chest pain indicates the medication is effective.**
5. **Bluish tint to lips and fingernails indicates the client is not receiving enough oxygen, and the antibiotic therapy is not effective.**
6. **Fever, sweating, and shaking chills are pneumonia symptoms and indicate the medication is not effective.**

MEDICATION MEMORY JOGGER: The nurse determines medication effectiveness by assessing for the clinical manifestations, or lack thereof, for which the medication was prescribed.

20. 220 mL/hour. The nurse should set the pump at 220 mL/hour.
Pumps are set at an hourly rate.
60 minutes divided by 30 equals 2.
100 plus 10 equals 110
110 multiplied by 2 equals 220.

Reactive Airway Disease

21. 1. The client should take the medication with a glass of water or meals to avoid an upset stomach.
2. The client should notify the HCP of a rapid or irregular heartbeat, vomiting, dizziness, or irritability because these are not expected side effects.
3. **Theophylline (Slo-Phyllin) is a bronchodilator. The client should avoid drinking large amounts of caffeine-containing drinks such as tea, coffee, cocoa, and cola.**
4. If a dose is missed within an hour, the client should take the dose immediately, but if it is more than 1 hour, the client should skip the dose and stay on the original dosing schedule. The client should not double the dose.

22. 1. These drugs are generally safe and well tolerated, with a headache being the most common side effect; therefore, this statement would not warrant intervention by the nurse.
2. **Montelukast (Singulair) is a leukotriene receptor inhibitor. This medication interacts with aspirin, warfarin, erythromycin, and theophylline; therefore, this statement warrants further intervention by the nurse.**
3. All medications should be kept out of the reach of children, and keeping the medication on a high shelf would not warrant intervention by the nurse.
4. Montelukast (Singulair) is a leukotriene receptor inhibitor. It does not need to be kept from extreme temperatures; it is the antiasthmatic zafirlukast (Accolate) that must be protected from extremes of temperature, light, and humidity.

MEDICATION MEMORY JOGGER: If the client reports a symptom, the nurse assesses data, or if laboratory data indicates an adverse effect secondary to a medication, the nurse must intervene. The nurse must implement an independent action during intervention or notify the HCP because medications can result in serious or life-threatening complications.

23. 1. **Metaproterenol (Alupent) is a sympathomimetic bronchodilator. The client should take the last dose a few hours before bedtime so that the medication does not produce insomnia.**
2. The client should increase fluid intake, especially water because it will make the mucus thinner and help the medication work more effectively.
3. This medication is taken orally; therefore, there is no reason for the client to demonstrate the correct use of an inhaler.
4. Antacids decrease medication absorption; therefore, the medication should not be taken within 30 minutes before or 2 hours after taking an antacid.

24. 1. The client should hold their breath as long as possible before exhaling to allow the medication to settle before administering another dose; 5 seconds is not long enough.
2. The client can check how much medication is in a metered-dose canister by placing the canister in a glass of water. If the canister stays under water, the canister is full; if it floats on top of the water, it is empty.

3. **Albuterol (Ventolin) is a metered-dose sympathomimetic bronchodilator. This is the correct way to use an inhaler because it will carry the medication into the lungs.**
4. Oxygen is not used when using an inhaler; oxygen is used to deliver the medication when using an aerosol.

25. 1. The therapeutic level for theophylline is 10 to 20 mcg/mL; therefore, the nurse should take action.
2. As the serum theophylline level rises above 20 mcg/mL, the client will experience nausea, vomiting, diarrhea, insomnia, and restlessness. This theophylline level may have serious effects, such as convulsion and ventricular fibrillation; therefore, the client should not be assessed first.
3. **Theophylline (Aminophylline) is a bronchodilator. The client has the potential for having convulsions and ventricular fibrillation because the theophylline level is too high; therefore, the nurse should discontinue the aminophylline drip first.**
4. After discontinuing the aminophylline drip and then assessing the client for potentially life-threatening complications, the nurse should notify the HCP.

MEDICATION MEMORY JOGGER: The nurse must know accepted standards of practice for medication administration, including which client assessment data and laboratory data should be monitored before administering the medication.

26. Correct answer is 1.
1. **The PEFR is defined as the maximal rate of airflow during expiration in a relatively inexpensive, handheld device. If the peak flow is less than 80% of personal best, more frequent monitoring should be done. The PEFR should be measured every morning.**
2. A normal respiratory assessment does not indicate that the medication regimen is effective and has "good" control.
3. Three asthma attacks in the last month would not indicate the client has "good" control of reactive airway disease.
4. A serum theophylline level between 10 and 20 mcg/mL indicates the medication is within therapeutic range, but is not the best indicator of the client's control of clinical manifestations.
5. Taking medication as directed is appropriate for the client, but it does not indicate the medication regimen is effective.

27. 1. This is the description of how a metered-dose inhaler works.
2. This is the description of how a dry-powder inhaler works.
3. **This is the description of how a nebulizer works. Nebulizers take several minutes to deliver the same amount of drug contained in one puff from an inhaler. They are usually used at home but can be used in the hospital.**
4. This is not the description of how a nebulizer works. Glucocorticoids are not used sublingually to treat acute or chronic asthma.

28.

Potential Nursing Intervention	Indicated	Not Indicated
1. Advise the client to gargle after each administration.	X	
2. Instruct the client to use the inhaler on a PRN basis.		X
3. Encourage the client to avoid attaching a spacer to the inhaler.		X
4. Teach the client to check their forced expiratory volume daily.	X	
5. Tell the client to keep the medication in the refrigerator.		X

1. **Gargling after each administration will help decrease development of oropharyngeal yeast infections.**
2. **Glucocorticoids are intended for preventive therapy, not for aborting an ongoing asthma attack, and they should not be taken on a PRN basis.**

3. **A spacer, a device that attaches directly to the metered-dose inhaler, should be used because a spacer increases drug delivery to the lungs and decreases drug deposition on the oropharyngeal mucosa.**
4. **Forced expiratory volume is the most helpful lung function test and can be measured by a home spirometer.**
5. **The medication is stored at room temperature, not in the refrigerator.**

29. 1. This medication does not stimulate the central nervous system (CNS); therefore, the client does not need to avoid caffeinated products. This statement indicates that the teaching is not effective.
2. These medications are not used to treat an acute exacerbation of reactive airway disease. They are adjunctive drugs given as part of an asthma regimen. This statement indicates that teaching is not effective.
3. The safety of these drugs has not been established in pregnancy and breastfeeding. This statement indicates that the teaching has not been effective.
4. **Montelukast (Singulair) is a leukotriene receptor inhibitor. The client should not suddenly stop taking the medication or decrease the dose. This statement indicates the teaching has been effective. Singulair is used with other types of asthma medications and should be continued if the client has an acute asthma attack.**

30. 1. This type of medical treatment would be used for a client diagnosed with mild persistent asthma.
2. This medical treatment would be prescribed for a client diagnosed with moderate persistent asthma.
3. The most severe class, severe persistent asthma, is managed with daily inhalation of a glucocorticoid (high dose), plus salmeterol, a long-acting inhaled agent.
4. **Mild intermittent asthma is treated on a PRN basis; long-term control medication is not needed. The occasional acute attack is managed by inhaling a short-acting beta$_2$ agonist. If the client needs the beta$_2$ agonist more than twice a week, moving to Step 2 (mild persistent asthma) may be indicated.**

Pediatric Reactive Airway Disease

31. 1. Cromolyn is a safe and effective drug for asthma prophylaxis, but it is not helpful for aborting an ongoing attack.
2. **Cromolyn (Intal) is a mast cell stabilizer and can prevent bronchospasm in children subject to exercise-induced asthma. It should be administered 15 minutes before anticipated exertion.**
3. The child diagnosed with a chronic illness should be encouraged to live as normal a life as possible; therefore, discouraging the child from playing ball is inappropriate.
4. Cromolyn is devoid of significant adverse effects and drug interactions. A yellow haze is not an expected side effect or adverse effect of cromolyn.

32. 1. Because the child is unconscious, the nurse should prepare to administer epinephrine, a beta$_2$-adrenergic agonist, but this is not the first action.
2. The client is unconscious; therefore, a nebulizer could not be administered to the child. It would be administered as soon as the child is conscious. Albuterol (Ventolin) is a metered-dose sympathomimetic bronchodilator.
3. A nebulizer treatment could be applied, but if there is no response to the nebulizer, the child should receive an IV glucocorticoid.
4. **The first intervention should be administering oxygen to the child and then administering medication. Oxygen is considered a medication.**

33. 1. All medication in the nebulizer should be used during treatment; medication should not be stored in the nebulizer for later use.
2. Length of treatment is usually 10 to 15 minutes. If it takes longer, the parent should check the nebulizer equipment or compressor for defects or problems.
3. The nebulizer should be cleaned daily (not weekly) using a disinfecting solution or a solution containing one part white vinegar and four parts water.
4. **The nebulizer should be cleaned with water after each treatment and allowed to air dry after loosely covering it with a clean paper towel. Storing the equipment wet promotes the growth of mold and bacteria.**

34. 1. Prednisolone is a systemic glucocorticoid medication. Prolonged glucocorticoid therapy can cause serious adverse effects such as adrenal suppression, osteoporosis, hyperglycemia, and peptic ulcer disease. Short-term use does not cause these adverse effects.
2. Doctors often order medications with serious side effects, but it must be done to treat the client. This statement is false and is not appropriate.
3. This is a true statement and the nurse's best response.
4. This is not the best response to the parent's question about their child's medication use. Prolonged glucocorticoid therapy can cause serious adverse effects, but short-term use does not cause these adverse effects.

35. 1. This is the explanation for administering leukotriene blockers.
2. Cromolyn (Intal) is a mast cell stabilizer. This is the correct explanation for administering a cromolyn inhaler. It prevents asthma attacks by blocking the release of mast cell mediators.
3. This is the explanation for administering theophylline, a bronchial dilator.
4. This is the explanation for administering glucocorticoids, such as prednisone.

36. 1. The zone system is used to help children monitor their treatment. The child uses a peak flow meter that monitors breathing capacity and shows the child's peak flow zone—green, yellow, or red. Treatment, if needed, is then based on which zone the peak flow meter shows. Green zone means all clear; no asthma symptoms are present.
2. There is no such zone as the black zone.
3. The red zone indicates a medical alert—a bronchodilator should be taken, and the child should seek medical attention for severe acute asthma. The cromolyn and steroid inhaler are not used for an acute asthma attack.
4. The yellow zone indicates caution because an acute episode may be present. The control is insufficient. The child should inhale a short-acting beta$_2$ agonist. If this fails to return the child to the green zone, a short course of oral glucocorticoids may be needed.

37.

Potential Nursing Intervention	Indicated	Not Indicated
1. Instruct the child to lie down on the bed in a supine position.		X
2. Tell the child to seal the lips tightly around the mouthpiece.	X	
3. Note the number on the scale after the client gives a sharp, short breath.	X	
4. Have the child blow into the peak flow meter one time and obtain the results.		X
5. Move the pointer on the peak flow meter to zero.	X	

1. The child should be standing up at the bedside, not lying down.
2. This is the correct way to obtain the peak flow meter results.
3. This is the correct way to take a reading from the peak flow meter.
4. The peak flow meter should be repeated three times, waiting at least 10 seconds between each attempt. The highest reading of the three attempts is recorded.
5. The pointer should be at zero every time the child attempts to blow into the peak flow meter.

38. 1. Cromolyn (Intal) is a mast cell stabilizer. The cromolyn inhaler should be taken routinely and is not used for an acute asthma attack; therefore, the child understands the teaching.
2. Moisture (from exhaled air) will interfere with proper use of the inhaler; therefore, the child understands the teaching.
3. The child should rinse their mouth with water immediately after using the inhaler to help prevent throat irritation, dry mouth, and hoarseness. Cromolyn (Intal) is a mast cell stabilizer.

4. Discontinuing the medication quickly can cause the child to have an acute attack of asthma. The child understands this.

39. 1. Serum salmeterol levels are not obtained.
2. This would apply to theophylline, not salmeterol.
3. Salmeterol (Serevent) is a metered-dose bronchodilator inhaler. Salmeterol is used when the client has not been responsive to other medications. Side effects include pharyngitis and upper respiratory tract infections. The parent should be aware of the side effects.
4. Salmeterol does not need to be refrigerated.

40. 79.5 mg. First, convert the child's weight to kilograms: 35 divided by 2.2 equals 15.9 kg. Then, determine how many milligrams should be given with each dose: 15.9 kg multiplied by 5 mg equals 79.5 mg per dose.

Pulmonary Embolus

41. 1. Warfarin (Coumadin) is an oral anticoagulant. An oral anticoagulant would not be prescribed in an acute situation.
2. Aspirin is an antiplatelet useful to prevent myocardial infarction and cerebrovascular accident but not used to treat PE.
3. Heparin is the medication of choice for treating PE, which the nurse should suspect with these clinical manifestations. IV heparin will prevent further clotting.
4. Ticlopidine (Ticlid) is a medication used to treat arterial, not venous, conditions.

MEDICATION MEMORY JOGGER: Remember that antiplatelets work in the arteries and anticoagulants work in the veins.

42. Correct answers are 1, 2, and 5.
1. Warfarin (Coumadin) is an oral anticoagulant. Coumadin requires careful monitoring of laboratory values to maintain the INR between 2 and 3. The INR is above the therapeutic range; therefore, the nurse should question administering this medication.
2. Vitamin K is the antidote for warfarin (Coumadin) toxicity; therefore, the nurse may administer this with an HCP order.
3. There is no reason to notify the HCP to request an increase in the dose because the client is above the therapeutic range.
4. The INR is above therapeutic range; therefore, the nurse should not administer the medication. Coumadin requires careful monitoring of laboratory values to maintain the INR between 2 and 3.
5. The INR is above therapeutic range; therefore, the nurse should assess the client for bleeding.

MEDICATION MEMORY JOGGER: When trying to remember which laboratory value correlates with which anticoagulant, here's a helpful hint: "PT boats go to war (warfarin), and if you cross the small 't's' in 'Ptt' with one line, it makes an 'H' (heparin)."

43. 1. Blood or blood products are the only fluids infused through Y-tubing.
2. Streptokinase (Streptase) is a thrombolytic. Heparin and streptokinase cannot be administered in the same IV line because they are incompatible. The nurse must start a second line to administer the streptokinase simultaneously with the heparin. The nurse does not need an order to do this.
3. The client needs both medications; therefore, the nurse cannot discontinue heparin. Streptokinase is a thrombolytic, which will dissolve the clot in the pulmonary artery, but heparin, an anticoagulant, is prescribed to prevent reformation of the clot.
4. Heparin and streptokinase cannot be administered in the same IV line because they are incompatible. The nurse must start a second line to administer streptokinase simultaneously with heparin. The nurse does not need an order to do this.

44. 1. Streptokinase is a foreign protein extracted from the cultures of streptococci bacteria. Streptomycin is derived from *Streptomyces*. As a result, this could cause the client to have an allergic reaction. The nurse should discuss this allergy with the HCP.
2. The nurse should not administer this medication until determining if the client is at risk for an allergic reaction.
3. The pharmacist is not licensed to change an HCP order.
4. Bleeding times could be assessed after determining that streptokinase will not cause the client to have an allergic reaction.

45. 1. The client is at risk for bleeding and should be encouraged to use an electric razor.
2. The client is at risk for bleeding, and a soft-bristled toothbrush should be used.

3. Any abnormal bleeding, such as a nosebleed, is unexpected and should be reported to the HCP. Unexplained bleeding is a finding of toxicity.
4. **Warfarin (Coumadin) is an oral anticoagulant. The client's INR is monitored at routine intervals to determine if the medication is within therapeutic range, INR 2 to 3.**

46. 1. Warfarin (Coumadin) is an oral anticoagulant. This is the scientific rationale for why Coumadin is prescribed to prevent thrombus formation, but it is not the rationale for why the medications are administered together.
2. **Warfarin (Coumadin) is an oral anticoagulant. Heparin has a short half-life and is prescribed as soon as a PE is suspected. The client must go home having taken an oral anticoagulant such as Coumadin, which has a long half-life and needs at least 3 to 5 days to reach a therapeutic level. Discontinuing the heparin before achieving a therapeutic level of Coumadin places the client at risk for another PE.**
3. Heparin and warfarin work in different steps in the bleeding cascade.
4. This is a false statement. Heparin and warfarin work in different steps in the bleeding cascade.

47. 1. The PTT test is used to monitor the anticoagulant heparin, not the thrombolytic alteplase (Activase).
2. A client diagnosed with a massive PE would be on bedrest; therefore, ambulating would not indicate the medication is effective.
3. **Alteplase (Ativase) is a thrombolytic. To determine if the medication is effective, the nurse must assess for improvement in the clinical manifestations for the condition for which the medication was ordered. Chest pain is one of the most common clinical manifestations of PE. Denial of chest pain would indicate the medication is effective.**
4. In the client diagnosed with a PE, the chest x-ray is usually normal; therefore, it would not be used to determine if the thrombolytic is effective.

48. 1. **This would be the first intervention because the client is above therapeutic range. Therapeutic range for heparin is 1.5 to 2.0 times the control, or 54 to 72. The client's PTT of 92 places them at risk for bleeding; therefore, the nurse must prevent further medication infusion.**
2. Protamine sulfate is the antidote for heparin, but the nurse would not administer this first. Discontinuing the heparin infusion for a few hours may be sufficient to correct the overdose.
3. The HCP should be notified of the client's situation, but it is not the first intervention.
4. Assessment is the first step in the nursing process, but if the client is in "distress" or experiencing a complication, the nurse should first treat the client.

MEDICATION MEMORY JOGGER: When trying to remember which laboratory value correlates with which anticoagulant, here's a helpful hint: "PT boats go to war (warfarin), and if you cross the small 't's' in 'Ptt' with one line, it makes an 'H' (heparin)."

49. **700 units of heparin are being infused every hour. When determining the units, the nurse must first determine how many units are in each milliliter.**

$$\frac{25{,}000 \text{ units}}{500 \text{ mL}} = 50 \text{ units per mL}$$

50 units per mL × 14 mL per hour = 700 mL per hour

50. **15 mL per hour. When setting the IV pump, the nurse must first determine the number of units per milliliter.**

$$\frac{40{,}000 \text{ units}}{500 \text{ mL}} = 80 \text{ units per mL}$$

$$\frac{1{,}200 \text{ units per hour}}{80 \text{ units per mL}} = 15 \text{ mL per hour}$$

51. 1. The client presented to the outpatient clinic, so the nurse should first determine how much bleeding has occurred. The nurse knows the consistency and color of the stools, but not the duration or amount. The nurse should assess the client before arranging for an emergency transfer.
2. **The nurse should first assess the client for clinical manifestations of bleeding such as decreased blood pressure and increased pulse, bruising, hematuria, hemogram, etc. The nurse should then notify the HCP at the clinic, and call 911 if needed. Rivaroxaban (Xarelto) is a Factor Xa inhibitor. PT and INR would not measure the medication's impact on the body.**

3. Rivaroxaban (Xarelto) is a Factor Xa inhibitor. PT and INR would not measure the medication's impact on the body.
4. The nurse should notify the HCP after the nurse has fully assessed the client's bleeding.

MEDICATION MEMORY JOGGER: The test taker should recognize that rivaroxaban and warfarin are anticoagulants. The nurse should at least understand that medications that impact the body similarly will have a risk of overtreating the issue and result in problems for the client.

52. 1. Levothyroxine and digoxin have no contraindications for administering to the client concurrently.

2. Dabigatran (Pradaxa), a direct thrombin inhibitor, and warfarin (Coumadin), an anticoagulant that impacts prothrombin, are anticoagulant medications. This would place the client at high risk for uncontrolled bleeding. The HCP should be notified immediately (STAT). The anemia may be the result of internal bleeding. Coumadin has vitamin K (AquaMEPHYTON) as an antidote. In 2016 the U.S. Federal Drug Administration (FDA) approved idarucizumab (Praxbind) as an antidote for Pradaxa. The HCP should be notified so that the appropriate tests can be performed and treatment can be initiated.

3. The nurse should ensure that the client's prednisone schedule is resumed, but this can be done on routine rounds.
4. The antidote for digoxin is Digibind, but the client has anemia, possibly from bleeding. Digoxin does not affect anemia.

MEDICATION MEMORY JOGGER: The test taker must recognize medications and how they work on the body.

PULMONARY SYSTEM COMPREHENSIVE EXAMINATION

1. The nurse is caring for a client diagnosed with COVID-19. The HCP has prescribed remdesivir IV. For each intervention, specify if the intervention is **indicated or not indicated** for the client's care.

Potential Nursing Intervention	Indicated	Not Indicated
1. Monitor the alanine aminotransferase level (ALT).		
2. Use the mixed remdesivir IV solution within 1 hour.		
3. Do not mix remdesivir with other IV medications.		
4. Assess for hypotension, diaphoresis, and shivering.		
5. Flush IV line with 30 mL NS after infusion is complete.		

2. The client diagnosed with asthma asks the nurse, "Why should I use the corticosteroid inhaler instead of prednisone?" Which statement by the nurse is **most appropriate**?
   1. "The lungs are incapable of using prednisone to decrease inflammation."
   2. "The inhaler costs less than the prednisone."
   3. "The inhaler will not cause the systemic problems that prednisone does."
   4. "Prednisone is not on your insurance formulary and the inhaler is."

3. The pediatric clinic nurse is assessing routine medications for a child diagnosed with cystic fibrosis (CF). Which medication should the nurse **question**?
   1. Tobramycin
   2. Pancrelipase
   3. Benzonatate perles
   4. Dornase alpha

4. The client diagnosed with TB is administered rifampin. Which information should the nurse discuss with the client?
   1. Instruct the client to consume fewer dark green, leafy vegetables.
   2. Explain that the client's urine and other body fluids will turn orange.
   3. Encourage the client to stop smoking cigarettes while taking this medication.
   4. Tell the client to increase fluid intake to 3,000 mL a day.

5. The client is having an acute exacerbation of asthma. The HCP has prescribed epinephrine subcutaneously. Which intervention should the nurse implement when administering this medication?
   1. Administer the medication using a tuberculin syringe.
   2. Dilute the medication to a 5-mL bolus before administering.
   3. Perform a complete respiratory assessment.
   4. Monitor the client's serum epinephrine level.

6. The nurse is preparing to administer the following medications. Which client should the nurse **question** administering the medication?
   1. The client receiving prednisone with a glucose level of 140 mg/dL
   2. The client receiving ceftriaxone with a WBC count of 15,000
   3. The client receiving heparin with a PTT of 68 seconds and a control of 0.35
   4. The client receiving cromolyn inhaler and is having an asthma attack

7. The nurse is discussing health-promotion activities for a client diagnosed with COPD. What information should the nurse discuss with the client?
   1. Instruct the client to get the influenza vaccine semiannually.
   2. Teach the client to continue taking low-dose antibiotics at all times.
   3. Encourage the client to get the pneumococcal vaccine every 5 years.
   4. Discuss the need to receive three doses of the hepatitis B vaccine.

8. The registered nurse (RN) and the unlicensed assistive personnel (UAP) are caring for a client diagnosed with COPD. Which action by the UAP **warrants immediate** intervention by the nurse?
   1. The UAP encourages the client to wear the nasal cannula at all times.
   2. The UAP calculates the client's fluid intake after the lunch meal.
   3. The UAP increases the oxygen to 5 L/min while ambulating the client.
   4. The UAP obtains the client's pulse oximeter reading.

9. The client diagnosed with active TB is prescribed antitubercular medications. Which intervention should the public health nurse implement?
   1. Request the client come to the public health clinic weekly for sputum cultures.
   2. Place the client and family in quarantine while the client takes the medication.
   3. Inform the neighbors and coworkers that the client has been diagnosed with TB.
   4. Arrange for a HCP to observe the client taking the medication daily.

10. Which statement by the nurse **best** describes the scientific rationale for how a nonnarcotic antitussive medication works in the body?
    1. It suppresses the cough reflex by directly acting on the medulla of the brain.
    2. It reduces the cough reflex by anesthetizing stretch receptors in the respiratory passages.
    3. Nonnarcotic antitussives slow down the destruction of sensitized mast cells.
    4. It acts to block receptors for cysteinyl leukotrienes that prevent bronchoconstriction.

11. The client diagnosed with an acute exacerbation of asthma is being treated with asthma medications. For each finding in the following table, does the result show the medication therapy is **effective or not effective?**

Finding	Effective	Not Effective
1. Bilateral wheezing		
2. Clear lung sounds		
3. Pulse oximeter reading of 96%		
4. Chronic dry cough		
5. No shortness of breath		
6. Rapid breathing		

12. A child diagnosed with CF is taking high-dose IV cephalosporin, and is getting progressively worse. Which medication should the intensive care nurse anticipate being added to the medication regimen?
    1. An IV corticosteroid
    2. An IV aminoglycoside antibiotic
    3. An oral proton-pump inhibitor (PPI)
    4. An oral mucolytic agent

13. The client diagnosed with TB is prescribed isoniazid. Which diet selection indicates the client **needs more** teaching?
   1. Tuna fish sandwich on white bread, potato chips, and iced tea
   2. Pot roast, mashed potatoes with brown gravy, and a light beer
   3. Fried chicken, potato salad, corn on the cob, and white milk
   4. Caesar salad with chicken noodle soup and water

14. The client's current arterial blood gas results are populated in the following chart.

Arterial Blood Gas	Client Values	Reference Values
pH	7.48	7.35 to 7.45
PCO_2	30	35 to 45 mm Hg
HCO_3	24	22 to 26 mEq/L
PaO_2	98	80 to 95 mm Hg

   Which intervention is **most appropriate** for this client?
   1. Administer oxygen 10 L/min via nasal cannula.
   2. Administer an antianxiety medication.
   3. Administer 1 amp of sodium bicarbonate IVP.
   4. Administer 30 mL of an antacid.

15. The 3-year-old child is admitted to the ED diagnosed with an acute episode of laryngotracheobronchitis (LTB). The HCP has prescribed racemic epinephrine nebulized with oxygen. Which intervention should the nurse implement?
   1. Administer the epinephrine with a tuberculin syringe.
   2. Ensure that antibiotics are given simultaneously.
   3. Notify the pediatric floor of the child's admission.
   4. Obtain a culture and sensitivity of the throat.

16. Which interventions should the nurse implement when administering IV fluids to a 2-year-old diagnosed with acute epiglottitis? **Select all that apply.**
   1. Label the IV fluid with the client's name.
   2. Obtain the daily weight and post at the head of the bed.
   3. Restrain the client's arm with a soft wrist restraint.
   4. Assess the child's IV site for redness and warmth.
   5. Administer the IV fluids with a volume-control chamber.

17. The 8-year-old male child diagnosed with asthma is prescribed albuterol. The child tells the nurse that if he behaves at the doctor's visit, his mom will get a hamburger, French fries, and a cola for him. Which intervention should the nurse implement?
   1. Encourage the child to be good, so he can get his meal.
   2. Tell the mother not to use food as a reward for visiting the doctor.
   3. Suggest drinking a Sprite or 7-Up with his lunch instead of cola.
   4. Explain that the child should not eat foods high in salt, such as fries.

18. The HCP has ordered theophylline 3 mg/kg/q 6 hours for a child weighing 20 pounds. How much medication would the nurse administer to the child in a 24-hour time period?

   ____

19. The nurse is preparing to administer the first dose of an aminoglycoside antibiotic to the client. Which interventions should the nurse implement? **Select all that apply.**

1. Check the client's peak and trough levels.
2. Administer the medication via a subclavian line.
3. Determine if a culture and sensitivity (C&S) was obtained.
4. Check the client's identification band.
5. Teach the client about suprainfection.

20. The nurse is reading this intradermal positive protein derivative (PPD) skin test 72 hours after it was administered. What should the nurse document based on this result?

1. Significant but not at risk
2. Not significant
3. Undetermined reaction
4. Significant and at risk

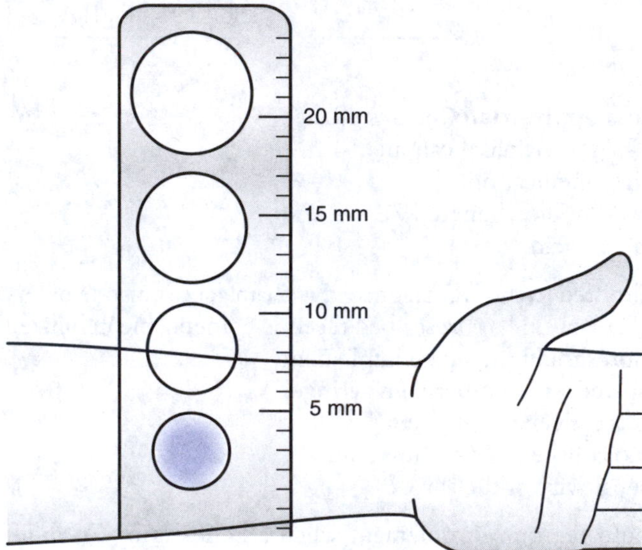

PULMONARY SYSTEM COMPREHENSIVE EXAMINATION ANSWERS AND RATIONALES

1.

Potential Nursing Intervention	Indicated	Not Indicated
1. Monitor the alanine aminotransferase level (ALT).	X	
2. Use the mixed remdesivir IV solution within 1 hour.		X
3. Do not mix remdesivir with other IV medications.	X	
4. Assess for hypotension, diaphoresis, and shivering.	X	
5. Flush IV line with 30 mL NS after infusion complete.	X	

1. **Increased ALT levels have been reported with remdesivir (Veklury). The medication may need to be discontinued if ALT is elevated and symptoms of liver inflammation are present (Gilead, 2021).**
2. **Remdesivir, once mixed, is stable for 4 hours at room temperature or 24 hours in the refrigerator.**
3. **Remdesivir should be given in a separate line. No studies on Y-site administration with other medications are complete at this time (Gilead, 2021).**
4. **Hypotension, diaphoresis, shivering, nausea, and vomiting are signs of an infusion-related reaction, and the medication should be discontinued immediately.**
5. **The infusion line should be flushed with 30 mL of normal saline after the remdesivir infusion is complete.**

2. 1. Prednisone, a glucocorticoid steroid, is a systemic anti-inflammatory medication that has many side effects. The inhaler does not have systemic effects, which is why the inhaler is preferred.
2. The medication cost does not have a bearing on why one route of medication should be used instead of another.
3. **The steroid inhaler does not cause systemic suppression of the adrenal gland and exposure of body cells to excess cortisol. The inhaler delivers the anti-inflammatory medication directly to the lungs, where effects are desired.**
4. Insurance should not be the reason for deciding which medication route a client should be prescribed.

3. 1. Tobramycin (Tobrex) is an aminoglycoside antibiotic. A child diagnosed with CF may be receiving routine daily doses of antibiotics; therefore, the nurse would not question the medication.
2. Pancrelipase (Pancrease) is a pancreatic enzyme. Pancreatic enzymes are administered with every meal and snack to a child diagnosed with CF to aid in digestion, so the nurse would expect this medication to be ordered.
3. **Benzonatate (Tessalon Perles) is an antitussive. An antitussive medication would suppress the cough reflex, which would result in stasis of thick tenacious secretions remaining in the lung and predispose the child to lung infections and possibly respiratory failure. The nurse would question this medication.**
4. Donase alpha (Pulmozyme) is a mucolytic agent used for the treatment of CF. Mucolytic agents are administered to break down the thick sputum and assist the child in expectorating the secretions. The nurse would expect this medication for a child diagnosed with CF.

4. 1. The consumption of dark green, leafy vegetables will not affect this medication.
2. **The client should be informed that Rifampin turns the urine and body secretions orange and can discolor contact lenses. This is not harmful to the client.**
3. The client should be encouraged to stop smoking for general health reasons, but smoking will not affect this medication.
4. Increasing fluid intake has no bearing on taking this medication.

5. 1. **Epinephrine is a bronchodilator nonselective adrenergic agonist and is prescribed in very low doses of 0.2 to 1.0 mg for an adult. The dosage of a**

sympathomimetic must be carefully monitored to prevent tachycardia, decreased or increased blood pressure, nausea, headache, and other CNS symptoms. A tuberculin syringe should be used to help ensure the accuracy of the dosage administered.

2. The epinephrine is being administered subcutaneously; therefore, the nurse will not dilute the medication.
3. The client is in distress with an acute asthma exacerbation; therefore, the nurse should not assess but should treat the client because delaying the medication may result in a respiratory arrest.
4. There is no such laboratory test as a serum epinephrine level.

6. 1. Prednisone is a glucocorticoid. Blood glucose is elevated, but this is an expected side effect of prednisone; therefore, the nurse would not question administering this medication.
2. Ceftriaxone (Rocephin) is an antibiotic. A client receiving an antibiotic would be expected to have an elevated WBC count; therefore, the nurse would not question administering this medication.
3. Heparin is an anticoagulant monitored by aPTT levels. A PTT of 68 seconds is within the range of 1.5 to 2 times the control; therefore, the nurse would not question administering this medication.
4. Cromolyn (Intal) is a mast cell stabilizer used to control the excitability of the mast cells BEFORE they become "excited." Cromolyn is for maintenance only; it does not work for an acute attack. The nurse should administer a beta agonist inhaler for quick response.

MEDICATION MEMORY JOGGER: The nurse must be knowledgeable about accepted standards of practice for disease processes and conditions. If the nurse administers a medication prescribed by the HCP that harms the client, the nurse could be held accountable. Remember, the nurse is a client advocate.

7. 1. The influenza vaccine should be taken yearly, not semiannually (every 6 months).
2. The client may develop resistance to antibiotics if they are taken all the time. Antibiotics will be prescribed during times of infection.
3. The pneumococcal vaccine titers persist in most adults for 5 years. The vaccine protects against pneumonia, and clients diagnosed with COPD should receive it to prevent lung infections.
4. The hepatitis B vaccine is not specifically recommended to promote health for clients diagnosed with COPD.

8. 1. The client should wear the nasal cannula at all times; therefore, the nurse would not need to intervene.
2. The UAP can calculate the fluid intake, but the RN must evaluate it to determine if it is adequate for the client's disease process.
3. Long-term oxygen therapy has been shown to improve the client's quality of life and survival. The oxygen must be kept between 1 and 3 L/min to prevent respiratory failure, which occurs when the oxygen level is increased, and the client's hypoxic drive is no longer active. Carbon dioxide narcosis occurs in clients diagnosed with COPD and eliminates that stimulus for breathing.
4. The UAP can obtain a pulse oximeter reading, but the nurse must evaluate the result to determine if it is normal for the disease process.

9. 1. The client will not have to go to the clinic weekly. Sputum cultures are done to diagnose TB and determine when the client's illness is no longer communicable. Three negative sputum cultures taken for 3 consecutive days 10 to 14 days after starting medication indicate the client's illness is no longer communicable.
2. This medication will be administered for 9 to 12 months, and the client is quarantined for 10 to 14 days until negative sputum cultures are obtained. Family members are not quarantined unless they have active TB.
3. The public health nurse will notify people in contact with the client during the infectious stage. The nurse will not divulge the client's name, which would be a violation of the Health Insurance Portability and Accountability Act. The nurse will explain that the individual may have come in contact with a person recently diagnosed with TB, and the person should receive a PPD skin test.
4. TB is a communicable disease that is a detriment to the community; therefore, the client is mandated to take antitubercular medication and will be observed daily for the regimen's duration, which may be 9 to 12 months. Risk of drug resistance is extremely high if the regimen is not strictly and continuously followed. This will result in multidrug-resistant TB in the community.

10. 1. Narcotic antitussives suppress the cough reflex by acting directly on the cough center in the brain's medulla.

2. Nonnarcotic antitussives reduce the cough reflex at its source by anesthetizing stretch receptors in the respiratory passages, lungs, and pleura and by decreasing their activity.

3. Slowing down the destruction of sensitized mast cells is the scientific rationale for administering cromolyn, a mast cell inhibitor given to prevent asthma attacks.

4. Blocking receptors for cysteinyl leukotrienes is the scientific rationale for administering leukotrienes to reduce asthma symptoms.

11.

Finding	Effective	Not Effective
1. Bilateral wheezing		X
2. Clear lung sounds	X	
3. Pulse oximeter reading of 96%	X	
4. Chronic dry cough		X
5. No shortness of breath	X	
6. Rapid breathing		X

1. Wheezing, a musical respiratory sound made when air is forced out through the small, mucus-lined passages during respiration, does not indicate the medication is effective.

2. Clear lung sounds would indicate that the asthma medications are effective.

3. The client's pulse oximeter indicates the client is adequately being oxygenated and would indicate the medication is effective.

4. A chronic dry cough is a common asthma symptom and indicates the medication is ineffective.

5. An indicator that the medication is effective is no shortness of breath.

6. Rapid breathing is a common sign of asthma and would indicate the medication is not effective.

12. **1. Cephalosporin (Ancef) is an antibiotic. Steroids are sometimes prescribed when pulmonary symptoms are unresponsive to antibiotics because corticosteroids decrease inflammation in the lungs.**

2. Cephalosporin (Ancef) is an antibiotic. The child should have cultures and sensitivities to determine resistance and sensitivity to an antibiotic. Changing an antibiotic depends on C&S results. Based on the information provided, there is no need to change antibiotics.

3. Cephalosporin (Ancef) is an antibiotic. A PPI decreases gastric secretions, but it is not indicated to improve pulmonary symptoms.

4. Cephalosporin (Ancef) is an antibiotic. The client will be receiving inhaled mucolytic therapy in the intensive care unit. There is no reason to add an oral agent.

13. **1. Isoniazid (INH) is an antitubercular medication. Tuna, foods with yeast extracts, aged cheese, red wine, and soy sauce contain tyramine and histamine, which interact with INH and result in headaches, flushing, hypotension, lightheadedness, palpitations, and diaphoresis.**

2. Red wine, not beer, can cause a reaction with INH.

3. Fried foods and whole milk may not be a healthy diet, but they are not contraindicated with INH.

4. Soup is high in sodium content, but it is not contraindicated for clients taking INH.

14. 1. This client is in respiratory alkalosis, which is caused by hyperventilating. Oxygen would not help treat this client.

2. This client is in respiratory alkalosis, which is caused by hyperventilating and could result from anxiety, elevated temperature, or pain. The nurse should assess the cause and administer the appropriate medication.

3. Sodium bicarbonate is the drug of choice for metabolic acidosis, and this is respiratory alkalosis. This medication is an alkaline substance and would increase the client's alkalosis.

4. An antacid would not help treat respiratory alkalosis because it is also an alkaline substance.

15. 1. The child is 3 years old and the medication is being administered with a nebulizer, not via the parenteral route.

2. Antibiotics are not indicated unless a bacterial infection has been confirmed.

3. Racemic epinephrine is delivered by nebulizer treatments. The child taking this medication must be hospitalized to monitor for changes in respiratory status and should not be treated with

epinephrine on an outpatient basis because the effects of epinephrine are temporary and respiratory distress may return.
4. A throat culture is not required before administering epinephrine. This would be appropriate when administering an antibiotic for the first time.

16. Correct answers are 1, 2, 4, and 5.
1. Medications should be labeled appropriately. IV fluids should be considered a medication.
2. The weight is important when administering IV fluids to a child to help prevent fluid volume overload.
3. The child may need an elbow restraint, but the nurse should not restrain the child with wrist restraints because doing so will scare the child.
4. Redness and warmth at the IV site indicate phlebitis, which requires the IV to be discontinued.
5. A volume-control chamber (Buretrol) is a special IV tubing device that allows for 1 hour of fluid to infuse at any one time potentially. It is a safety device to prevent fluid overload in a child.

17. 1. The nurse should teach the child about food preferences because the child has a chronic disease. Caffeinated drinks should be discouraged.
2. The nurse should not be judgmental about the mother's parenting skills.
3. Albuterol (Proventil) is a bronchodilator. The child should avoid drinking large amounts of caffeinated drinks such as tea, cocoa, and cola. Sprite and 7-Up do not contain caffeine.
4. This is an untrue statement. Children rarely have problems with sodium intake.

18. 108 mg/24 hours. First, determine the child's weight in kilograms: 20 pounds divided by 2.2 kilograms equals 9.09 kilograms. Then, determine how many milligrams should be given with each dose: 9.09 kilograms multiplied by 3 milligrams equals 27.27 milligrams. Because it is below 0.5, the nurse should round down to 27. Because the dose is to be given every 6 hours, the child will be receiving four doses in a 24-hour time period: 27 milligrams multiplied by 4 equals 108 milligrams per 24 hours.

19. Correct answers are 3, 4, and 5.
1. The peak and trough level should be monitored when the client is receiving aminoglycosides antibiotics, but not before the first dose. It is usually checked at the fourth, eighth, and 12th doses.
2. The aminoglycoside antibiotic can be administered peripherally and does not have to be administered via a subclavian line.
3. The C&S is obtained before the antibiotic is administered, so the results will not be skewed and useless. This is usually checked at the nurse's station before entering the client's room to give the medication.
4. This should be checked before administering any medication. It is one of the rights in medication administration.
5. The nurse should teach about the antibiotic destroying good flora, resulting in a suprainfection.

20. 1. A wheal 5 mm or greater may be significant in individuals considered at risk.
2. A wheal measuring 5 mm or less is considered not significant, and this client's reaction is less than 5 mm induration.
3. This would indicate the reaction is not readable and could result from poor administration technique of the intradermal injection.
4. A wheal of 10 mm or greater is significant in individuals with normal immunity.

5 Gastrointestinal System

Your life is your story. Write well. Edit often.

—Susan Statham

QUESTIONS

Gastroesophageal Reflux

1. The client reporting "acid" when lying down at night asks the nurse if there is any medication that might help. Which statement is the nurse's **best** response?
   1. "There are no medications to treat this problem, but losing weight will sometimes help the symptoms."
   2. "There are several over-the-counter and prescription medications available to treat this. You should discuss this with your health-care provider."
   3. "Have you had any x-rays or other tests to determine if you have cancer or some other serious illness?"
   4. "Acid reflux at night can lead to serious complications. You need to have tests done to determine the cause."

2. The nurse on a medical unit has received the morning report. Which medication should the nurse administer **first**?
   1. Pantoprazole to a client on call to surgery
   2. Calcium carbonate to a client reporting indigestion
   3. Bismuth to a client diagnosed with an ulcer
   4. Famotidine to a client diagnosed with gastroesophageal reflux disease (GERD)

3. Which statement is the scientific rationale for administering a proton-pump inhibitor (PPI) to a client diagnosed with GERD?
   1. PPI medications neutralize gastric secretions.
   2. PPI medications block H_2 receptors on the parietal cells.
   3. PPI medications inhibit the enzyme that generates gastric acid.
   4. PPI medications form a protective barrier against acid and pepsin.

4. Which statement is an **advantage** to administering a histamine$_2$ (H_2) blocker rather than an antacid to a client diagnosed with GERD?
   1. Antacids are more potent than H_2 blockers.
   2. H_2 blockers have more side effects than antacids.
   3. H_2 blockers are less expensive than antacids.
   4. H_2 blockers require less frequent dosing than antacids.

5. Which side effects should the nurse explain to the male client prescribed cimetidine?
   1. The medication can cause indigestion and heartburn.
   2. The medication can cause impotence and gynecomastia.
   3. The medication can cause insomnia and hypervigilance.
   4. The medication can cause Zollinger-Ellison syndrome.

6. The home health-care nurse is caring for a client diagnosed with a hiatal hernia and reflux. For each finding in the following table, does the result show the medication therapy is **effective or not effective**?

Finding	Effective	Not Effective
Sore throat		
Chronic cough		
Indigestion after eating		
No heartburn at night		
Frequent belching and burping		
Clear lung sounds		

7. The nurse is preparing to administer esomeprazole. Which intervention should the nurse implement? **Select all that apply.**
   1. Select a 22-gauge needle for administration.
   2. Elevate the client's head of the bed.
   3. Check the client's ID with the MAR.
   4. Check for allergies to cephalosporin.
   5. Ask the client for their date of birth.

8. The nurse is discharging a client diagnosed with GERD. Which information should the nurse include in the teaching?
   1. "There are no complications of GERD as long as you take the medications."
   2. "Notify the HCP if the medication does not resolve the symptoms."
   3. "Immediately after a meal, lie down for at least 45 minutes."
   4. "If any discomfort is noted, take an NSAID for the pain."

9. The nurse is discharging a client 2 days postoperative hiatal hernia repair. Which discharge instructions should the nurse include? **Select all that apply.**
   1. "Take all of the prescribed antibiotics."
   2. "Eat six small meals per day."
   3. "Use the legs to bend down, not the back."
   4. "Take esomeprazole twice a day."
   5. "Use the pain medication when the pain is at 8–10."
   6. "Avoid acidic foods like orange juice and soda."
   7. "Wear tight belts or clothes for abdominal support."
   8. "Do not smoke and limit alcohol use."

Inflammatory Bowel Disease (IBD)

10. The client diagnosed with ulcerative colitis is prescribed mesalamine. Which information should the nurse discuss with the client?
    1. Explain to the client that undissolved tablets may be expelled in the stool.
    2. Discuss the importance of taking the medication on an empty stomach only.
    3. Tell the client to avoid drinking any type of carbonated beverage.
    4. Instruct the client not to crush, break, or chew the tablets or capsules.

11. The client diagnosed with severe ulcerative colitis is prescribed azathioprine. Which assessment data concerning the medication **warrants immediate intervention** by the nurse?
 1. Reports of a sore throat, fever, and chills
 2. Reports of 10 to 20 loose stools a day
 3. Reports of abdominal pain and tenderness
 4. Reports of dry mouth and oral mucosa

12. The client diagnosed with IBD taking mesalamine reports nausea, vomiting, and diarrhea. Which intervention should the clinic nurse take?
 1. Instruct the client to quit taking the medication immediately.
 2. Tell the client to take lansoprazole with the medication.
 3. Advise the client to keep taking the medication, but notify the HCP.
 4. Explain that these symptoms are expected and will resolve with time.

13. The nurse is teaching the client diagnosed with Crohn's disease about the newly prescribed medication sulfasalazine. Which information should the nurse discuss with the client? **Select all that apply.**
 1. Advise the client to drink 1,500 mL of water daily.
 2. Teach the client to take the medication once daily with food.
 3. Describe to the client that slight bruising and skin redness is expected.
 4. Inform the client to take an antacid 30 minutes before the sulfasalazine.
 5. Instruct the client to keep a strict record of their intake and output.
 6. Discuss the need to avoid direct sunlight and use sunblock outside.
 7. Indicate that the medication can cause mucus to be present in the stool.
 8. Teach the client that an orange-yellow tint to the skin and urine can occur.

14. The clinic physician is performing laboratory tests for a client diagnosed with IBD and prescribed sulfasalazine 2 weeks ago. The HCP's laboratory orders are in the following order sheet.

Client: P.Z.	MR# 1234567	Date: Today
Age: 45 years	Allergies: NKDA	Diagnosis: IBD routine follow-up
PROVIDER ORDERS:		
Liver function tests		
Serum potassium		
Serum creatinine level		
International normalized ratio (INR)		
Complete blood count with differential		
Sulfapyridine level		
Urinalysis		

Which laboratory data should the nurse question being ordered? **Select all that apply.**
 1. Liver function tests
 2. Serum potassium level
 3. Serum creatinine level
 4. International normalized ratio (INR)
 5. Complete blood count with differential
 6. Sulfapyridine level
 7. Urinalysis

15. A client diagnosed with IBD is prescribed mesalamine suppositories. Which statement indicates the client **understands** the medication teaching?
1. "I should retain the suppository for at least 15 minutes."
2. "The suppository may stain my underwear or clothing."
3. "I should store my medication in the refrigerator."
4. "I should have a full rectum when applying the suppository."

16. The client diagnosed with IBD is prescribed prednisone. Which interventions should the nurse implement? **Select all that apply.**
1. Monitor the client's blood glucose level.
2. Discuss the long-term side effects of prednisone.
3. Administer the medication with food.
4. Explain prednisone will be tapered when being discontinued.
5. Tell the client to notify the HCP if a moon face occurs.
6. Consult with the HCP before receiving any vaccinations.

Peptic Ulcer Disease

17. The nurse is administering 0800 medications. Which medication should the nurse **question**?
1. Misoprostol to a 29-year-old female with an NSAID-produced ulcer
2. Omeprazole to a 68-year-old male with a duodenal ulcer
3. Furosemide to a 56-year-old male with a potassium level of 4.2 mEq/L
4. Acetaminophen to an 84-year-old female with a frontal headache

18. The client diagnosed with severe congestive heart failure (CHF) is reporting indigestion. Which antacid medication should the nurse administer?
1. Sodium bicarbonate
2. Aluminum hydroxide
3. Magaldrate
4. Calcium carbonate and magnesium carbonate

19. The client diagnosed with low back pain has been self-medicating with ibuprofen around the clock. The client calls the clinic and tells the nurse about getting dizzy and lightheaded. Which intervention should the nurse implement?
1. Tell the client to get up from a sitting or lying position slowly.
2. Have the client come to the clinic for laboratory work immediately.
3. Suggest the client take the ibuprofen with food or an antacid.
4. Discuss changing to a different NSAID.

20. The client is diagnosed with a *Helicobacter pylori* (*H. pylori*) infection and peptic ulcer disease (PUD). Which discharge instructions should the nurse teach? **Select all that apply.**
1. Discuss placing the head of the bed on blocks to prevent reflux.
2. Teach never to use NSAIDs again.
3. Encourage the client to quit smoking cigarettes.
4. Instruct the client to eat a soft, bland diet.
5. Take the combination of medications for 14 days as directed.

21. The client diagnosed with PUD has been taking magnesium hydroxide for indigestion. The client reports having diarrhea. Which intervention should the nurse implement?
1. Suggest that the client use magnesium hydroxide with aluminum hydroxide.
2. Encourage the client to discuss the problem with the HCP.
3. Tell the client to take over-the-counter loperamide.
4. Discuss why the client is concerned about experiencing diarrhea.

22. The client diagnosed with PUD is admitted to the medical unit. The client's laboratory values are populated in the chart below.

Laboratory Test	Client Values	Reference Values
Red blood cells (RBC)	2.5 (10^6 cells/microL)	Men: 4.21–5.81 (10^6 cells/microL) Women: 3.61–5.11 (10^6 cells/microL)
White blood cells (WBC)	20 (10^3 cells/microL)	4.5–11.1 (10^3 cells/microL)
Hemoglobin (Hgb)	6.2 g/dL	Men: 14–17.3 g/dL Women: 11.7–15.5 g/dL
Hematocrit (Hct)	18%	Men: 42%–52% Women: 36%–48%

Which intervention should the nurse prepare to implement **first**?
1. Obtain an order for an oral PPI.
2. Instruct the client to save all stools for observation.
3. Initiate an IV with 0.9% normal saline (NS) with an 18-gauge catheter.
4. Place a bedside commode in the client's room.

23. The nurse is preparing to administer pantoprazole IV piggyback (IVPB) in 50 mL of fluid over 20 minutes to a client diagnosed with PUD. The IVPB set delivers 20 drops per mL. At what rate would the nurse set the infusion?

____

24. The nurse is administering 0900 medications to a client diagnosed with PUD. Which medication should the nurse **question**?
1. Metronidazole
2. Bismuth subsalicylate
3. Lansoprazole
4. Sucralfate

25. The client has been on a therapeutic regimen for an *H. pylori* infection. The client reports relief of midepigastric pain and a weight gain of 3 pounds in one week. The client's laboratory values and vital signs are populated in the chart below.

Laboratory Test	Client Values	Reference Values
Hemoglobin (Hgb)	15 g/dL	Men: 14–17.3 g/dL Women: 11.7–15.5 g/dL
Hematocrit (Hct)	44%	Men: 42%–52% Women: 36%–48%
Vital Sign Flowsheet	**Client Values**	**Reference Values**
Temperature	98°F/36.7°C	Oral: 98°F (36.7°C)
Pulse	124 bpm	60 to 100 bpm
Respirations	24 breaths/min	12 to 20 breaths/min
Blood Pressure	92/48 mm Hg	100 to 119 mm Hg systolic 60 to 80 mm Hg diastolic

Which data suggests the medication is **not effective**?
1. Relief of midepigastric pain
2. Laboratory values
3. Weight gain
4. Vital signs

Diverticulosis and Diverticulitis

26. The elderly client diagnosed with diverticulosis is instructed to take psyllium mucilloid. Which question is **most important** for the nurse to ask the client?
   1. "When was your last bowel movement?"
   2. "Do you have any difficulty swallowing?"
   3. "How much fiber do you eat daily?"
   4. "Do you ever notice any abdominal tenderness?"

27. The client is admitted to the medical unit diagnosed with an acute exacerbation of diverticulosis. The HCP has prescribed IV ceftriaxone. Which intervention should the nurse implement **first**?
   1. Monitor the client's white blood cell (WBC) count.
   2. Assess the client's most recent vital signs.
   3. Determine if the client has any known allergies.
   4. Send a stool specimen to the laboratory.

28. The nurse is transcribing orders. The HCP's orders are in the following order sheet. Which orders would the nurse **question**? **Select all that apply.**

Client: D.R.	MR# 1234567	Date: Today
Age: 65 years	Allergies: PCN	Diagnosis: Diverticulitis
PROVIDER ORDERS:		
Administer one bisacodyl PO daily.		
NG tube to intermittent low suction		
Morphine 2 mg IVP q 4 hours PRN pain		
D5 0.45 NS IV at 100/mL per hour		
Fleet enema NOW		

   1. Bisacodyl
   2. Nasogastric tube
   3. Morphine
   4. IV dextrose 5% in water and 0.45 NS
   5. Fleet enema

29. Which information should the nurse discuss with the client diagnosed with diverticulosis and prescribed a bulk-forming laxative? **Select all that apply.**
   1. Teach that mild abdominal cramping can occur.
   2. Explain that results should be evident within 24 hours.
   3. Encourage the client to increase the intake of fluids, especially water.
   4. Instruct the client to decrease fiber intake while taking these medications.
   5. Teach the client to avoid taking other medications at the same time.
   6. Explain that the client should take an oral and a rectal laxative for best results.

30. The 80-year-old client diagnosed with diverticulosis is prescribed docusate sodium. Which assessment data indicates the medication is **effective**?
   1. The client has a bowel movement within 8 hours.
   2. The client has soft, brown stools.
   3. The client has a soft, nontender abdomen.
   4. The client has bowel sounds in all four quadrants.

31. The 62-year-old client suspected of having diverticulosis is scheduled for a colonoscopy and prescribed sodium biphosphate the night before the procedure. Which **priority** intervention should the nurse implement **before** the procedure?
   1. Assess the client's skin turgor and oral mucosa.
   2. Initiate IV therapy for the client.
   3. Determine if the client has iodine allergies.
   4. Monitor the client's bowel movements.

32. The client diagnosed with diverticulosis is taking docusate calcium daily. The client tells the clinic nurse that her daughter has her taking the herb cascara every day. Which intervention should the nurse implement?
   1. Instruct the client to quit taking the herb immediately.
   2. Explain that the herb will help the diverticulosis.
   3. Tell the client to have their daughter call the nurse.
   4. Advise the client to inform their HCP.

33. The client diagnosed with diverticulitis is requesting pain medication. Which intervention should the medical nurse implement **first**?
   1. Administer the client's pain medication as requested.
   2. Check the client's serum sodium and potassium level.
   3. Determine when the last pain medication was administered.
   4. Assess the client's bowel sounds and abdomen for tenderness.

34. The client diagnosed with essential hypertension tells the clinic nurse about taking the OTC medication docusate sodium. Which **priority** action should the clinic nurse implement?
   1. Determine how often the client has a bowel movement.
   2. Discuss the importance of not taking this stool softener.
   3. Ask the client for their last blood pressure reading.
   4. Obtain a stool specimen for an occult blood test.

Liver Failure

35. The client diagnosed with end-stage liver failure has an elevated ammonia level. The HCP prescribes lactulose. Which intervention should the nurse implement to determine the **effectiveness** of the medication?
   1. Monitor the client's intake and output.
   2. Assess the client's neurological status.
   3. Measure the client's abdominal girth.
   4. Document the number of bowel movements.

36. The client diagnosed with end-stage liver failure is prescribed neomycin sulfate. Which statement **best describes** the scientific rationale for administering this medication?
   1. Neomycin sulfate helps lower the hepatic venous pressure.
   2. It helps increase the excretion of fluid through the kidneys.
   3. Neomycin is administered to help prevent a systemic infection.
   4. It reduces the number of ammonia-forming bacteria in the bowel.

37. The client diagnosed with end-stage liver failure is prescribed vitamin K. The client asks the nurse, "Why do I have to take vitamin K?" Which statement is the nurse's **best** response?
   1. "It will help your blood to clot so you won't have spontaneous bleeding."
   2. "It may help prevent eye and skin changes along with night blindness."
   3. "Vitamin K helps prevent skin and mucous membrane lesions."
   4. "It prevents a complication called Wernicke-Korsakoff psychosis."

38. The client diagnosed with end-stage liver failure is experiencing esophageal bleeding. The HCP has prescribed vasopressin. Which statement is the scientific rationale for administering this medication?
   1. It lowers portal pressure by venodilation and decreased cardiac output.
   2. Vasopressin produces constriction of the splanchnic arterial bed.
   3. This medication causes vasoconstriction of the coronary arteries.
   4. Vasopressin causes the liver to decrease in size and vascularity.

39. The nurse is preparing to administer medications. Which client should the nurse **question** administering the medication?
   1. Lactulose to a client with an ammonia level of 100 mcg/dL
   2. Furosemide to a client with a potassium level of 3.7 mEq/L
   3. Spironolactone to a client with a potassium level of 5.9 mEq/L
   4. Vasopressin to a client with a serum sodium level of 137 mEq/L

40. The nurse is reviewing the HCP orders for a client newly admitted to the medical floor. The HCP's orders are in the following order sheet.

Client: L.O.	MR# 1234567	Date: Today
Age: 65 years	Allergies: NKDA	Diagnosis: End-stage liver failure
PROVIDER ORDERS:		
Prepare for paracentesis.		
Vitamin C 100 mg PO daily		
Morphine 2 mg IVP q 4–6 hours PRN pain		
D_5W 0.9 NS IV at 25 mL/hour		

   Which HCP's order should the nurse **question**?
   1. Paracentesis
   2. Vitamin C
   3. Morphine
   4. IV D_5W 0.9 NS

41. The client diagnosed with esophageal varices undergoes endoscopic sclerotherapy. Which postprocedure intervention should the nurse implement?
1. Administer omeprazole.
2. Do not allow the client to eat or drink anything for 24 hours.
3. Administer promethazine.
4. Administer aluminum hydroxide.

42. The client diagnosed with end-stage liver failure is reporting pruritus. Which information should the nurse discuss with the client? **Select all that apply.**
1. Encourage the client to sit in a hot spa before going to bed.
2. Instruct the client to use emollients or lotions on the skin.
3. Explain the need to take the prescribed antihistamine as directed.
4. Apply hydrocortisone 1.0% cream to the affected areas.
5. Tell the client the importance of not scratching the skin.

43. The client diagnosed with end-stage liver failure is taking lactulose. Which statement indicates the client **needs more teaching** concerning this medication?
1. "I will notify my doctor if I have any watery diarrhea."
2. "If I get nauseated, I will quit taking the lactulose."
3. "I will take my lactulose with fruit juice."
4. "I should have two or three soft stools a day."

44. The client diagnosed with end-stage liver failure with ascites is prescribed spironolactone. For each intervention, specify if the intervention is **indicated or not indicated** for the care of the client.

Potential Nursing Intervention	Indicated	Not Indicated
1. Monitor the serum potassium level.		
2. Weigh the client daily.		
3. Assess bowel sounds frequently.		
4. Monitor intake and output.		
5. Monitor abdominal girth.		
6. Assess skin frequently.		

Hepatitis

45. The public health nurse is administering the hepatitis A vaccine to a client. Which statement indicates the client **understands** the medication teaching about the vaccine?
1. "I will not need to have another dose of the vaccine."
2. "I will notify the clinic if there is pain at the injection site."
3. "This vaccine will provide long-term protection against hepatitis A."
4. "This medication will be injected in my buttocks."

46. The employee health nurse is preparing to administer the first dose of the hepatitis B vaccine to an employee. Which question is **most important** for the nurse to ask the employee before administering this medication?
1. "Do you have any known allergies to medications?"
2. "Are you allergic to yeast or any type of yeast products?"
3. "Have you ever had an allergic reaction to egg yolks?"
4. "Are you allergic to any type of milk or milk products?"

47. The client exposed to hepatitis A calls the clinic and wants to know what can be done to prevent getting hepatitis A. Which information should the nurse discuss with the client?
 1. Explain that there is a hepatitis A vaccine available that the client can receive.
 2. Inform the client that there is nothing available to help prevent hepatitis A.
 3. Instruct the client to get an immune globulin injection within 2 weeks.
 4. Tell the client to go to the nearest emergency department (ED) as soon as possible.

48. The client tells the nurse, "I would like to get the vaccine for hepatitis C." Which response is **most appropriate** by the nurse?
 1. "There is no vaccination against hepatitis C."
 2. "The vaccination must be administered in two doses."
 3. "Have you received the hepatitis B vaccination?"
 4. "Why are you interested in receiving this vaccine?"

49. The public health nurse notified a client that one of their sexual contacts was positive for hepatitis B. The client denies ever having hepatitis B or having received the hepatitis B vaccinations. Which information is **most important** for the nurse to discuss with the client?
 1. Instruct the client not to have unprotected sexual intercourse.
 2. Advise the client not to drink any type of alcoholic beverage.
 3. Tell the client to get hepatitis B immune globulin (HBIG).
 4. Encourage the client to get the hepatitis B vaccination.

50. The male client diagnosed with chronic hepatitis C and advanced cirrhosis is prescribed ribavirin in conjunction with ledipasvir and sofosbuvir. Which information should the nurse discuss with the client?
 1. Discuss the importance of using two reliable forms of birth control.
 2. Explain the need to eat a diet high in vitamin K during treatment.
 3. Instruct the client to avoid direct sunlight for long periods.
 4. Teach the client that the medication might cause temporary impotence.

51. The clinic nurse is preparing to administer the hepatitis B vaccine to the client. Which information should the nurse discuss with the client?
 1. Instruct the client to come back to the clinic in 2 months for the last injection.
 2. Teach the client not to wash the injection site for at least 24 hours.
 3. Encourage the client to rotate the arms when receiving the hepatitis B vaccine.
 4. Explain that the client must have two more doses of the vaccine at 1 and 6 months.

52. The homeless client comes to the free clinic. During the interview, the client admits to using illegal IV drugs. Which interventions should the nurse recommend to the client?

Potential Nursing Intervention	Indicated	Not Indicated
1. Recommend the combined Hepatitis A and B vaccine.		
2. Recommend the Hepatitis B vaccination.		
3. Recommend accessing community resources.		
4. Recommend oral testing for the HIV virus.		
5. Recommend a substance abuse treatment center.		
6. Recommend counseling for mental health issues.		

Pediatric Gastroenteritis

53. The pediatric clinic nurse is assessing the 4-year-old child diagnosed with gastroenteritis. The mother tells the nurse about using bilberry herbs to help the child. Which statement assesses the **effectiveness** of the herb?
    1. "Did your child vomit after you administered the bilberry?"
    2. "Does this herb help your child's allergy to milk and milk products?"
    3. "What was the child's temperature when you administered the herb?"
    4. "How many diarrhea stools has your child had since taking the bilberry?"

54. The child diagnosed with infectious gastroenteritis is prescribed trimethoprim sulfa 10 mg/kg/day in divided doses twice a day. The child weighs 60 pounds. The medication comes 100 mg/5 mL. How many milliliters will the nurse administer with the morning dose?

    ____

55. The child diagnosed with chronic kidney infections develops *Clostridium difficile* (*C. difficile*). Which medication should the nurse administer **first** to decrease the amount of diarrhea?
    1. Penicillin
    2. Cholestyramine
    3. Trimethoprim sulfa
    4. Diphenoxylate

56. The 3-year-old child weighing 37.5 pounds is diagnosed with mild to moderate diarrhea and placed on oral replacement therapy (ORT). Which information should the nurse teach the parent?
    1. "Try to get your child to drink about 1,000 mL of Pedialyte over 4 hours."
    2. "The child should drink 100 mL of homemade rice water every 2 hours."
    3. "Get the child to drink apple juice or a lemon-lime soda every 3 to 4 hours."
    4. "Do not let the child eat any solid foods for a few days. Just give the liquids."

57. The HCP wrote an order for "0.33% dextrose solution IV" for a 6-year-old child diagnosed with gastroenteritis. Which interventions should the nurse implement? **Select all that apply.**
    1. Monitor the serum sodium and potassium levels.
    2. Check the fontanels for the hydration status.
    3. Discuss the order with the HCP.
    4. Use a chamber infusion device on the IV pump.
    5. Assess the IV site every hour.

58. The child diagnosed with gastroenteritis is scheduled for an endoscopic examination of the stomach and duodenum. Which intervention is a **priority** for the nurse assisting with the procedure?
    1. Watch the screen for abnormal data.
    2. Hand the physician the instruments.
    3. Monitor the child's respiratory status.
    4. Clean the instruments between clients.

59. The 8-year-old child diagnosed with gastroenteritis is admitted to the pediatric unit. The nurse administered prochlorperazine rectally. Which side effects should the nurse assess for?
    1. Nausea, vomiting, and diarrhea
    2. Tremors, involuntary twitching, and restlessness
    3. Diplopia, ptosis, and urinary retention
    4. Myalgias, hallucinations, and weakness

60. The 10-year-old client is diagnosed with an *Escherichia coli* infection after being at a day camp. Which discharge instructions should the nurse teach the parent?
  1. Give the child an antiemetic suppository before each meal.
  2. Have anyone in contact with the child wear a mask.
  3. Be sure the child takes all the antibiotic medication.
  4. Administer an antidiarrheal after each loose stool.

61. Which is the scientific rationale for administering acidophilus capsules to a child diagnosed with a *Shigella* infection?
  1. The acidophilus capsule will treat the *Shigella* infection.
  2. The acidophilus will help the child develop immunity to *Shigella*.
  3. The acidophilus will prevent a complication of the antibiotics.
  4. The acidophilus is the antibiotic of choice for *Shigella*.

62. The toddler diagnosed with rotavirus is admitted to the hospital. Which intervention should the nurse implement? **Select all that apply.**
  1. Instruct the parents to wash their hands after changing diapers.
  2. Schedule the antibiotic for around-the-clock dosing.
  3. Teach the parents to discard the diapers in a biohazard can.
  4. Initiate IV fluids with a controlled chamber device.
  5. Administer the rotavirus vaccine in the toddler's thigh.

Obesity

63. The client is prescribed orlistat. Which statement by the client indicates the client **requires more** teaching?
  1. "It does not matter what I eat because I will still lose weight."
  2. "I will limit the amount of fat in my diet to 30%."
  3. "I may need to take a fiber supplement daily with the orlistat."
  4. "I will take a daily multivitamin supplement."

64. The client diagnosed with type 2 diabetes mellitus and a body mass index (BMI) of 29 is prescribed semaglutide. Which interventions should the nurse implement?

Potential Nursing Intervention	Indicated	Not Indicated
1. Administer the medication intramuscularly.		
2. Weigh the client daily.		
3. Assess glucose regularly.		
4. Teach to report abdominal pain radiating to the back.		
5. Instruct to mix insulin and semaglutide in one dose.		
6. Advise to have regular thyroid assessments.		

65. Which medication is the **most appropriate** for the obese client trying to quit smoking?
  1. Orlistat
  2. Lorcaserin
  3. Bupropion
  4. Phentermine/topiramate

66. The obese client is participating in a weight loss study using metformin. Which data should the nurse monitor?
1. The Hgb A_1C every 2 months
2. Daily fasting glucose levels
3. The urine ketones every 2 weeks
4. The client's weight every month

Constipation and Diarrhea

67. The older adult client is discussing constipation with the clinic nurse. The client tells the nurse, "I take a laxative every day so that I will have a bowel movement every day." Which statement should the nurse respond to **first**?
1. "Do you have heart problems or diabetes?"
2. "Have you ever had a rash or itching when you took a laxative?"
3. "You should not use laxatives every day."
4. "Most people don't have to have bowel movements daily."

68. The client reports not having a bowel movement in 4 days and is having abdominal discomfort. Which intervention should the nurse **recommend** to the client?
1. Instruct the client to take methylcellulose.
2. Encourage the client to make an appointment with the HCP.
3. Explain to the client the need to take docusate sodium.
4. Tell the client to take castor oil 2 hours after the next meal.

69. The client taking antibiotics calls the clinic and tells the nurse about having diarrhea. Which interventions should the nurse implement?

Potential Nursing Intervention	Indicated	Not Indicated
1. Instruct the client to take lactobacillus.		
2. Report diarrhea to the HCP.		
3. Assess for any intake of bad-tasting or bad-smelling food.		
4. Instruct the client to stop the antibiotic for 24 hours.		
5. Tell the client to take two diphenoxylate and atropine tablets after each loose stool, up to eight tablets a day.		
6. Teach client to avoid alcohol and caffeine.		

70. The client calls the clinic reporting diarrhea and states they just came back from vacation in Mexico. Which intervention should the nurse implement **first**?
1. Instruct the client to take loperamide.
2. Ask how long the client has had diarrhea and when they returned from Mexico.
3. Explain that an antibiotic should be prescribed and that the client needs to see the HCP.
4. Tell the client this is probably traveler's diarrhea and it will run its course.

71. The elderly client calls the clinic and reports loose, watery stools. Which interventions should the nurse implement?

Potential Nursing Intervention	Indicated	Not Indicated
1. Instruct the client to take antidiarrheals as recommended.		
2. Recommend a clear liquid diet.		
3. Assess how long the loose, watery stools have occurred.		
4. Tell the client to go to the ED as soon as possible.		
5. Ask about other medications taken in the past 24 hours.		
6. Question the client about a fever.		
7. Teach client to report loose, watery stools lasting more than 48 hours.		

72. The nurse is working at a senior citizen center and giving a lecture on health-promotion activities for the elderly. Which information should the nurse discuss with the group to help prevent constipation?
1. Dicyclomine taken every morning with the breakfast meal will help prevent constipation.
2. Eating five to six small meals a day, including low-residue foods, will help prevent constipation.
3. Taking a daily stool softener along with daily exercise, increased fluids, and a high-fiber diet will help prevent constipation from developing.
4. Elderly clients must have at least one bowel movement a day to prevent the development of constipation.

73. The client is prescribed senna glycoside for constipation. The client calls the clinic and reports yellow-green feces. Which intervention should the clinic nurse implement?
1. Have the client come to the clinic immediately.
2. Explain that this is a common side effect of senna glycoside.
3. Instruct the client to get a stool specimen to bring to the clinic.
4. Determine if the client has eaten any type of yellow or green food.

Abdominal Surgery with General Anesthesia

74. The day surgery nurse is admitting a client for the repair of an inguinal hernia. Which information provided by the client is **most important** to report to the surgical team? **Select all that apply.**
1. The client has never had surgery before.
2. The client is allergic to shellfish.
3. The client had breakfast this morning.
4. The client had a sinus infection last month.
5. The client has had a productive cough for a week.

75. The client is scheduled for an exploratory laparotomy in the morning. Which health-care order has **priority**?
1. Prepare the preoperative injection for when the operating room notifies the floor.
2. Document the client's Hgb and Hct levels on the checklist.
3. Be sure the client has taken a preoperative hexachlorophene shower.
4. Ambulate the client in the hallway at least two times.

76. The client, after abdominal surgery, returned from the postanesthesia care unit (PACU) with a patient-controlled analgesia (PCA) pump. Which interventions should the nurse implement? **Select all that apply.**
1. Check the PCA setting with another nurse.
2. Administer a bolus by pushing the button.
3. Instruct the client to push the PCA button when in pain.
4. Change the PCA cartridge.
5. Assess the client's IV insertion site.

77. The client had a general anesthetic for abdominal surgery. When reviewing the post-operative orders, the charge nurse notes there is no antiemetic medication ordered. Which action should the charge nurse take?
1. Continue reviewing the orders and do nothing.
2. Ask the anesthesiologist if the client was nauseated during surgery.
3. Contact the surgeon and request an order for an antiemetic.
4. Tell the client's nurse to notify the charge nurse if there is nausea.

78. The client in the PACU has an order for hydromorphone IV push (IVP) every 2 to 3 hours as needed (PRN) for pain. The nurse working in the PACU administers hydromorphone 1 mg IVP. Which statement **best** exhibits how the medication should be entered into the medication administration record (MAR) and in the client's electronic health record (EHR)?
1. Hydromorphone IVP, pain level at "1" on the pain scale
2. Hydromorphone given over 15 seconds IVP
3. Hydromorphone administered, client writhing in pain
4. Respiratory rate: 24 breaths/min, hydromorphone administered by slow IVP

79. The client, after abdominal surgery, has an IV at 150 mL/hr for 12 hours and two IVPBs of 50 mL each. How much fluid would the nurse document on the intake and output record?

____

80. The client is on call for surgery. Which order should the nurse implement when the operating room (OR) nurse notifies the floor that the orderly is on the way to pick up the client?
1. Have the client sign the operative permit.
2. Teach the client to turn, cough, and deep breathe.
3. Notify the family to wait in the OR waiting room.
4. Administer the preoperative antibiotic IVPB.

81. The client postgastrectomy has a PCA pump. Which data requires **immediate intervention** by the nurse?
1. The client reports that the pain is still a "3."
2. The client has serous drainage on the dressing.
3. The client has a T 99.2°F, P 78, R 10, and B/P 110/82.
4. The client splints the incision before trying to cough.

82. The client, after elective cholecystectomy, is receiving a prophylactic antibiotic. Which information indicates the medication is **not effective**?
1. The client's WBC count is 18,000.
2. The client refuses to turn, cough, and deep breathe.
3. The client's sodium level is 139 mEq/L.
4. The client's nasogastric tube has green drainage.

Total Parenteral Nutrition

83. The client diagnosed with full-thickness burns is prescribed total parenteral nutrition (TPN). Which interventions should the nurse implement?

Potential Nursing Intervention	Indicated	Not Indicated
1. Monitor the client's glucose level every 6 hours.		
2. Administer sliding-scale regular insulin.		
3. Assess the peripheral IV site every 4 hours.		
4. Encourage client to eat all food offered at meals.		
5. Change the subclavian dressing per protocol.		
6. Administer the TPN using an IV pump.		
7. Ensure the TPN is tapered off when discontinuing.		

84. Which intervention should the nurse implement **first** for the client receiving TPN bag #8?

1. Check the IV pump that is sounding an alarm.
2. Request TPN bag #9 from the hospital pharmacy.
3. Notify the HCP of the inflamed insertion site.
4. Obtain the client's serum potassium level.

85. The client is receiving TPN bag #4 via a right subclavian line. Which medication should the nurse administer if it is 0730?

Client: M.G.	MR# 1234567	Date: Today
Age: 35 years	Allergies: NKDA	Diagnosis:
Medication	0701-1900	1901-0700
Sliding-scale regular insulin <150 no coverage 151–200 4 units 201–250 6 units 251–300 8 units 301–350 10 units >351 notify HCP	0730 Blood glucose 311	
Nurse Initials/Credentials	DN/RN	NN/RN

1. Administer 4 units of regular insulin.
2. Administer 6 units of regular insulin.
3. Administer 8 units of regular insulin.
4. Administer 10 units of regular insulin.

86. The client's TPN bag #1 has 25 mL in the bag, and bag #2 is not on the unit. The client's IV rate is 68 mL/hr. Which intervention should the nurse implement?
1. Administer D_5W at 68 mL/hr.
2. Decrease the IV rate to 30 mL/hr.
3. Administer dextrose 10% at 68 mL/hr.
4. Notify the HCP.

87. The registered nurse (RN) and unlicensed assistive personnel (UAP) are caring for the client receiving TPN at 70 mL/hr. Which task is **most appropriate** for the RN to delegate to the UAP?
1. Instruct the UAP to weigh the client.
2. Ask the UAP to change the subclavian dressing.
3. Tell the UAP to assist the client with feeding.
4. Request the UAP to assess the client's bowel sounds.

88. The client is receiving TPN bag #3 and TPN bag #4 is brought to the unit by the pharmacy technician. Which intervention should the nurse implement **first**?
1. Place the TPN bag in the refrigerator.
2. Check the TPN bag #4 with the HCP's order.
3. Place new IV tubing on the TPN bag.
4. Obtain the client's glucose level before hanging.

89. The HCP writes an order to decrease TPN rate by 5 mL every hour while discontinuing TPN. The current rate is 77 mL/hr. What rate should the nurse set 3 hours after transcribing the order?

____

90. The nurse is caring for the client receiving TPN with the laboratory values populated in the chart below.

Laboratory Test	Client Values	Reference Values
Potassium	6.2 mEq/L or mmol/L	3.5 to 5.3 mEq/L or mmol/L
Sodium	145 mEq/mL	135 to 145 mEq/L or mmol/L
Glucose	252 mg/dL	Fasting <100 mg/dL Random <200 mg/dL
Protein	7.2 g/dL	6 to 8 g/dL

Which laboratory data requires the nurse to notify the HCP?
1. Potassium
2. Sodium
3. Glucose
4. Protein

Acute Pain

91. At 1030 the client 1 day postoperative for an open cholecystectomy notifies the unit secretary reporting severe pain. After ruling out complications, which intervention should the 0701–1900 nurse implement **first**?

Client: M.R.	MR# 1234567	Date: Today
Age: 55 years	Allergies: Morphine, Keterolac	Diagnosis: Open Cholecystectomy
Medication	0701-1900	1901-0700
Ketorolac IV every 6 hours PRN pain		
Hydromorphone IV by PCA 0.2 mg 10 min lock out	0701 PCA infusing DN	0700 12 mg used during night shift
Ondansetron 4 mg every 4 hours PRN nausea		
Acetaminophen rectal every 4 hours PRN		
Nurse Initials/Credentials	DN/RN	NN/RN

1. Administer the ketorolac IV.
2. Push the PCA button and administer the hydromorphone.
3. Notify the surgeon that the client is not receiving relief from the hydromorphone.
4. Check the PCA and IV tubing to make sure that medication is being delivered.

92. The nurse on a medical floor is caring for a client diagnosed with acute exacerbation of pancreatitis. The client requests a pain medication for pain rated an "8" on a scale of 1–10. Which interventions should the nurse implement? **Select the three options the nurse should implement.**
1. Administer the pain medication intramuscularly only to prevent addiction.
2. Check the MAR to determine when the last pain medication was administered.
3. Check two client identifiers before administering the prescribed pain medication.
4. Assess the client's respiratory and abdomen status.
5. Check the client's amylase level in the EHR.

93. The nurse is preparing to administer pain medication to a client reporting left lower quadrant pain. Which interventions should the nurse implement? **Rank in order of performance.**
1. Evaluate the client's pain level for medication effectiveness.
2. Remove the medication from the narcotics cabinet (PIXYS).
3. Ask the client about allergies to medications.
4. Document the administration in the client's MAR.
5. Administer the medication to the client.

94. The nurse is administering morphine sulfate 2.5 mg IVP to a client after open abdominal surgery. Which intervention should the nurse implement?
1. Administer at the port highest up on the tubing.
2. Administer by slow IVP over 5 minutes.
3. Elevate the client's arm after administration.
4. Ask the client to refrain from coughing.

95. The ED nurse is caring for a 28-year-old client diagnosed with rule-out appendicitis. The client is still undergoing tests to determine if surgery is required but asks for pain medication "NOW!" Which is the nurse's **best** response?
1. "I will get the medication for you now."
2. "Your doctor will have to order some medication, and then I will give it."
3. "I cannot give you narcotic pain medication until a decision is made about surgery."
4. "You seem anxious. Tell me about your pain."

96. The nurse on a medical and surgical unit has received the shift report. Which medication should the nurse administer **first**?
1. Morphine sulfate to a postoperative exploratory laparotomy client with a pain level of 4
2. Hydrocodone to a preoperative client going for a splenectomy
3. Acetaminophen to a client diagnosed with abdominal pain and has a headache
4. Nalbuphine to a client just returning from a lap appendectomy and thrashing in bed

97. The nurse is administering medications on a medical and surgical unit. Which medication should the nurse **question** administering?
1. Acetaminophen with 30 mg of codeine to a 17-year-old client after an appendectomy 2 days ago
2. Meperidine to a 12-year-old after an exploratory laparotomy
3. Morphine to a 38-year-old, 2-day postoperative open cholecystectomy client with a pain level of 6
4. Hydromorphone to a 40-year-old client reporting severe abdominal pain rated a "10" on a scale of 1–10

98. The nurse working in the PACU recovering a client after an exploratory laparotomy administers the prescribed hydromorphone IVP. Five minutes later the nurse assesses respirations of 8. Which intervention should the nurse implement **first**?
1. Ask the anesthesiologist to assess the client.
2. Administer naloxone IVP.
3. Reassess the client's respiratory status in 20 minutes.
4. Use an ambu bag and ventilate the client.

99. The nurse is assessing the pain level of a postoperative abdominal surgery client. The client reports "mild" abdominal pain rated a "4" on a scale of 1–10. Which medication should the nurse prepare to administer?
1. Oxycodone PO
2. Acetaminophen PO
3. Morphine sulfate IVP
4. Ondansetron IVP

ANSWERS AND RATIONALES

The correct answer number and rationale are in **boldface blue type.** Rationales for why other answer options are incorrect are also given.

Gastroesophageal Reflux

1. 1. There are several classifications of medications used to treat acid reflux problems. Sometimes losing weight will help relieve symptoms, but the client did not ask about lifestyle modifications.

2. PPIs, H_2 blockers, and antacids all treat the symptoms of acid reflux. The nurse should encourage the client to discuss which medication is best with the HCP.

3. The symptoms do not indicate cancer. The nurse should not scare the client.

4. Acid reflux can lead to complications, including adult-onset asthma, that should be treated, but most HCPs will empirically treat the symptoms of acid reflux before ordering tests to determine the cause or possible complications.

2. 1. Pantoprazole (Protonix) is a PPI. A medication for a client on call to surgery is a priority; the client's surgery could be delayed if the medication has not been administered when the call to surgery comes.

2. Calcium carbonate (Tums) is an antacid. This would be the second medication to administer, as this client has a report of discomfort.

3. Bismuth (Pepto-Bismol) is an antimicrobial. This medication is a routine medication and could be administered at any time.

4. Famotidine (Pepcid) is an H_2 blocker. This medication is a routine medication and could be administered at any time.

3. 1. Antacids, not PPIs, neutralize gastric secretions.

2. H_2 blockers block receptors on the parietal cells.

3. PPIs inhibit the enzyme that generates gastric acid.

4. Mucosal barrier agents form a protective barrier against acid and pepsin.

4. 1. H_2 blockers block the production of gastric acid and have a more prolonged effect than an antacid.

2. An increase in side effects would not be an advantage.

3. Antacids are usually less expensive than H_2 blockers.

4. H_2 blockers require less frequent administration than antacids, which require regular administration, seven or more times a day, for therapeutic effects. The fewer times a client is expected to take a medication, the more likely the client is to comply with a medication regimen.

5. 1. Cimetidine (Tagamet), an H_2 blocker, is used to treat indigestion and heartburn (pyrosis).

2. Cimetidine (Tagamet) is an H_2 blocker. Over time, Tagamet can cause males to become impotent, have decreased libido, and develop enlarged breast (gynecomastia).

3. Tagamet can cause lethargy and somnolence, not insomnia and hypervigilance.

4. Tagamet is used to treat Zollinger-Ellison syndrome, a syndrome characterized by gastric acid hypersecretion and peptic ulcers.

6.

Finding	Effective	Not Effective
1. Sore throat		X
2. Chronic cough		X
3. Indigestion after eating		X
4. No heartburn at night	X	
5. Frequent belching and burping		X
6. Clear lung sounds	X	

A sore throat, chronic cough, indigestion, and frequent belching and burping indicate that stomach acid is in the esophagus or lungs and indicates the medication is not effective.

An absence of symptoms and lack of wheezing indicates the medication therapy is effective.

MEDICATION MEMORY JOGGER: The nurse determines the effectiveness of a medication by assessing for the symptoms, or lack thereof, for which the medication was prescribed.

7. Correct answers are 2, 3, and 5.
1. Esomeprazole (Nexium), a PPI, is an oral or IV medication. A needle is not needed.
2. **The head of the bed is elevated for the client to swallow the medication.**
3. **The nurse must check the MAR with the client's ID band to ensure the correct client receives the medication.**
4. Esomeprazole (Nexium) is a PPI, not a cephalosporin. The cephalosporins are a class of antibiotics.
5. **The Joint Commission requires that two patient identifiers be used to determine the "right patient." Most health-care facilities use the client's name and date of birth as these identifiers.**

8. 1. There may be several complications of GERD. Adult-onset asthma and Barrett's esophagus leading to cancer of the esophagus are two complications of GERD. The chance of developing these problems is less if the GERD is adequately treated, but there are no guarantees.
2. **The client should always be informed of what symptoms to report to the HCP.**
3. The client should be instructed to sit upright for at least 60 minutes after a meal to prevent reflux from occurring.
4. NSAIDs can increase gastric distress. Ulcers caused by NSAID use may be asymptomatic, or the symptoms may be attributed to GERD. The client should use the prescribed H_2 receptor blocker, PPI, or an antacid to relieve the discomfort associated with GERD.

9. Correct answers are 1, 2, 3, 6 and 8.
1. **Prophylactic antibiotics are frequently prescribed presurgery and postsurgery. The client should be instructed to take all the medication as directed.**
2. **Hiatal hernia repair may not last, and the client should continue the recommended lifestyle modifications, such as eating small meals.**
3. **Part of the lifestyle modifications for hiatal hernia is to limit pressure on the abdominal cavity, especially after a meal. Using the leg muscles to bend down, rather than bending over, should be taught to the client.**
4. Esomeprazole (Nexium) is administered daily, not twice a day.
5. For best relief, pain medication should be taken at the onset of the pain. The client should not wait until the pain is an 8–10 before taking the pain medication.
6. **Acidic foods like orange juice, tomato sauce, and soda can cause acid reflux symptoms.**
7. The client should limit pressure on the abdominal cavity and avoid tight belts or clothes.
8. **Smoking causes heartburn. Alcohol use, vinegar, chocolate, and caffeine should be limited to reduce symptoms.**

Inflammatory Bowel Disease (IBD)

10. 1. Mesalamine (Asacol) is an aspirin derivative. The client should notify the HCP if undissolved tablets or capsules are found in the stool because this is not expected.
2. Mesalamine (Asacol) is an aspirin derivative. This medication can be taken with or without food. Food does not affect the medication effectiveness.
3. Mesalamine (Asacol) is an aspirin derivative. There are no restrictions on foods, beverages, or activities when taking this medication unless the HCP directs otherwise.
4. **Mesalamine (Asacol) is an aspirin derivative. The tablets must be swallowed whole because they are specially formulated to release the medication after it has passed through the stomach.**

11. 1. Azathioprine (Imuran) is an immunosuppressant and can cause a decrease in the number of blood cells in the bone marrow (agranulocytosis). Clinical manifestations that would warrant intervention by the nurse include sore throat, fever, chills, unusual bleeding or bruising, pale skin, headache, confusion, tachycardia, insomnia, and shortness of breath.
2. Ten to 20 loose, watery stools a day are characteristic of an acute exacerbation of ulcerative colitis and would not warrant intervention by the nurse secondary to the medication.
3. Abdominal pain and tenderness are characteristic of an acute exacerbation of ulcerative colitis and would not warrant intervention by the nurse secondary to the medication.
4. Dehydration may occur with ulcerative colitis, but it does not warrant intervention by the nurse secondary to the medication.

MEDICATION MEMORY JOGGER: If a client verbalizes a symptom, the nurse assesses data, or if laboratory data indicates that an adverse effect is secondary to a medication, the nurse must intervene. The nurse must implement an independent intervention or notify the HCP because medications can result in serious or life-threatening complications.

12. 1. Mesalamine (Asacol) is an aspirin derivative. The client should not quit taking the medication abruptly because that would result in an acute exacerbation of IBD.
    2. Lansoprazole (Prevacid) is a PPI. A PPI will not help treat these symptoms.
    3. **Mesalamine (Asacol) is an aspirin derivative. These are side effects of the medication, and the HCP should be notified, but the client should not stop taking the medication.**
    4. Mesalamine (Asacol) is an aspirin derivative. These symptoms will not resolve with time and should be reported to the HCP.

13. **Correct answers are 1, 6, and 8.**
    1. **Sulfasalazine (Azulfidine) is a gastrointestinal anti-inflamatory medication. Increasing fluid intake dilutes the drug, preventing crystalluria (crystals in the urine) from occurring.**
    2. Sulfasalazine is administered every 6 to 8 hours, not daily.
    3. Any type of rash or skin redness should be considered a possible allergic reaction or drug-induced blood disorder (agranulocytosis) and should be reported to the HCP immediately.
    4. Sulfasalazine (Azulfidine) is a sulphonamide antibiotic. The client should not take an antacid with this medication because it will decrease the absorption rate of the medication.
    5. The client should drink several quarts of water a day to prevent the formation of crystals in the urine, but a strict record of urinary output is not required or needed.
    6. **The client should avoid direct sunlight, use sunblock, and wear protective clothing to decrease the risk of photosensitivity reactions to the medication.**
    7. This medication does not cause fat, frothy stools.
    8. **Sulfasalazine can cause an orange-yellow discoloration of the urine and skin, which is not significant. Contact lenses may be permanently stained yellow.**

14. **Correct answers are 1, 3, 5, 6, and 7.**
    1. **Sulfasalazine (Azulfidine) can be hepatotoxic; therefore, liver function tests should be performed before initiating therapy, every second week during the first 3 months, monthly during the second and third months, and every 3 months after while on sulfasalazine therapy.**
    2. The serum potassium level is not affected by sulfasalazine; therefore, the nurse should question this laboratory order as a routine follow-up for sulfasalazine therapy.
    3. **Sulfasalazine (Azulfidine) is a gastrointestinal anti-inflammatory. Sulfasalazine is insoluble in acid urine and can cause crystalluria and hematuria, resulting in kidney damage. Therefore, the nurse should monitor the serum creatinine level, normally 0.61 to 1.21 mg/dL in males and 0.51 to 1.11 mg/dL in females.**
    4. Sulfasalazine (Azulfidine) may cause abnormal bleeding and bruising, but the INR is monitored for clients taking the oral anticoagulant warfarin (Coumadin).
    5. **Complete blood counts with differentials should be performed before initiating therapy, every second week during the first 3 months, monthly during the second and third months, and every 3 months after while on sulfasalazine therapy.**
    6. **Serum sulfapyridine levels can be monitored; concentrations above 50 ųg/mL are associated with adverse reactions (Federal Drug Administration, 2014).**
    7. **Urinalysis can be performed periodically to monitor for crystalluria and urinary calculi formation.**

MEDICATION MEMORY JOGGER: The nurse must be knowledgeable about accepted standards of practice for medication administration, including which client assessment data and laboratory data should be monitored before and during the use of the medication.

15. 1. Mesalamine (Asacol) is an aspirin derivative. The suppository should be retained for 1 to 3 hours, if possible, to get the maximum benefit of the medication.
    2. **Mesalamine (Asacol) is an aspirin derivative. The client should use caution when using the suppository because it may stain clothing, flooring, painted surfaces, vinyl, enamel, marble, granite, and other surfaces. This statement indicates the client understands the teaching.**

3. Mesalamine (Asacol) is an aspirin derivative. The medication should be stored at room temperature, away from moisture and heat.
4. The client should empty the bowel just before inserting the rectal suppository.

16. Correct answers are 1, 2, 3, 4, 5, and 6.

1. Prednisone increases the glucose level; therefore, it should be monitored by the nurse.
2. Long-term side effects occur, and the nurse should teach about these when administering the medication.
3. Steroids are notorious for causing gastric irritation, resulting in peptic ulcers; therefore, administering prednisone with food is a priority.
4. Explaining to the client about tapering the medication is essential.
5. A moon face is an expected sign of prednisone toxicity, but the client should still notify the HCP.
6. Steroids can cause immunosuppression. The client should discuss any vaccinations with the HCP. Live vaccinations may be contraindicated.

Peptic Ulcer Disease

17. 1. Misoprostol (Cytec) is a prostaglandin analog. A 29-year-old female is of childbearing age. The nurse should determine that the client is not pregnant before administering this medication. Misoprostol can be used in combination with mifepristone to produce an abortion.
2. Omeprazole (Prilosec), a PPI, is prescribed to treat duodenal and gastric ulcers; therefore, the nurse would not question this medication.
3. Furosemide (Lasix) is a loop diuretic. The potassium level is within normal range (3.5–5.3 mEq/L); therefore, the nurse would not question this medication.
4. Acetaminophen (Tylenol), a nonnarcotic analgesic, is frequently administered for headaches; therefore, the nurse would not question this medication.

MEDICATION MEMORY JOGGER: Whenever an age is mentioned in the stem of the question or the answer options, one or more of the ages will be important. The only option that gives the test taker a clue regarding the correct answer is the 29-year-old, and the test taker should also note that it is a female client. Twenty-nine-year-old females are of childbearing age, so the nurse has two potential clients to consider.

18. 1. Clients diagnosed with CHF are limited in the amount of sodium they should consume. Sodium bicarbonate has sodium as an ingredient.
2. Aluminum hydroxide (Amphojel), an antacid, is not a low-sodium preparation. This client requires a low-sodium antacid.
3. Magaldrate (Riopan), a low-sodium antacid, is the antacid of choice for clients needing to limit their sodium intake.
4. Calcium carbonate and magnesium carbonate (Mylanta), a combination antacid, is not a low-sodium preparation. This client requires a low-sodium antacid.

MEDICATION MEMORY JOGGER: The nurse must always be aware of comorbid conditions when administering medications. The two keywords or phrases in this question are "severe CHF" and "indigestion."

19. 1. This is information to teach when the client is taking antihypertensive medications, not NSAIDs.
2. Ibuprofen (Motrin) is an NSAID. A life-threatening complication of NSAID use is the development of gastric ulcers that can hemorrhage. Dizziness and light-headedness could indicate a bleeding problem. The client has been taking the medications "around the clock," indicating use during the night when it would be unusual for the client to consume food along with the medication.
3. NSAID medications should be taken with food or something to coat the stomach lining, but this client is symptomatic and should be seen by an HCP.
4. There is no reason to suggest a change in NSAID. The nurse should be concerned that the client has developed an NSAID-produced ulcer.

20. Correct answers are 3 and 5.

1. The client has PUD, not GERD, for which elevating the head of the bed would be recommended.
2. The client's ulcer is caused by a bacterial infection, not NSAID use. The client should limit NSAIDs until the ulcer has healed to prevent complicating the healing process, but the client should be able to use NSAID medications once the *H. pylori* infection has been treated.

3. **Smoking decreases prostaglandin production and results in decreased protection of the mucosal lining. Smoking should be stopped.**
4. A soft, bland diet is not ordered for a client diagnosed with PUD.
5. ***H. pylori* is a bacterial infection that is treated with a combination of medications. At least two antibiotics and an antisecretory medication will be ordered. As with all antibiotic prescriptions, the client should be taught to take all medications as ordered. Resistant strains of *H. pylori* are being documented in clients not compliant with the treatment program.**

21. 1. **Magnesium hydroxide (Milk of Magnesia) is the most potent antacid, but it is usually used as a laxative because of magnesium hydroxide's actions on the bowel. A combination antacid—magnesium hydroxide (produces diarrhea) and aluminum hydroxide (produces constipation)—is preferred to balance the side effects.**
2. The nurse can answer the client's question. It is only necessary to discuss this with the HCP if antacids are not resolving the client's report of indigestion.
3. The Milk of Magnesia is causing the problem, and changing antacids should resolve the situation.
4. Most clients are concerned about diarrhea, and the nurse should be concerned about fluid and electrolyte imbalances resulting from diarrhea.

22. 1. The client would need an IV PPI at first and then later could be changed to an oral PPI. The client may also need a nasogastric tube or to be NPO (nothing by mouth). This client has very low Hgb and Hct levels, indicating active bleeding and the need for a fast route to deliver fluids and medications.
2. The nurse should observe the stool for color (black) and consistency (tarry), indicating blood, but this is not the first action.
3. **This client has very low blood counts; is at risk for shock; and should be assessed for hypotension, tachycardia, and cold, clammy skin. The client will need fluid and blood cell replacement. The nurse should start the IV as soon as possible.**
4. The client should have a bedside commode for safety, but it is not the first intervention. Prevention of or treating shock is the first intervention.

MEDICATION MEMORY JOGGER: The stem listed the client's Hgb and Hct levels, indicating a "crisis" situation. The first step in many crises is ensuring that IV access is available to administer fluids and medications.

23. 50 gtt (drops) per minute. The nurse must first determine the rate per hour:

20 minutes into 60 minutes = 3 (20-minute time segments)
50 mL of fluid × 3 = 150 mL per hour
150 mL ÷ 60 minutes = 2.5 mL/min to infuse
2.5 mL/min × 20 drops per mL = 50 gtt per minute

24. 1. Metronidazole (Flagyl), a gastrointestinal anti-ineffective, is administered in combination with Pepto-Bismol, Prevacid, and one other antibiotic to treat PUD. The nurse would not question this medication.
2. Bismuth subsalicylate (Pepto-Bismol), an antimicrobial, is administered in combination with Flagyl, Prevacid, and one other antibiotic to treat PUD. The nurse would not question this medication.
3. Lansoprazole (Prevacid), a PPI, is administered with a combination of antibiotics to treat PUD. The nurse would not question this medication.
4. **Sucralfate (Carafate) is a mucosal barrier agent and must be administered on an empty stomach for the medication to coat the stomach lining. The nurse should question the medication's administration time and arrange for the medication to be given at 0730.**

25. 1. A lack of epigastric pain would indicate the medication is effective. The question asks which data indicates the medication is not effective.
2. An Hgb level of 15 g/dL and Hct level of 44% are within normal limits and would indicate that the client is not bleeding as a result of the ulcer.
3. Clients diagnosed with a gastric ulcer lose weight because of the pain associated with eating. Weight gain would indicate less pain and the client being able to consume nutrients.
4. **The client has a rapid pulse and low blood pressure, which indicate shock. This could be caused by an ulcer hemorrhage. This client's treatment has not been effective.**

MEDICATION MEMORY JOGGER: The nurse determines medication effectiveness by assessing for the symptoms, or lack thereof, for which any medication was prescribed.

Diverticulosis and Diverticulitis

26. 1. This is a question that the nurse could ask the client, but it is not specific or essential to ask for a client taking psyllium mucilloid (Metamucil); therefore, it is not the most important question to ask the client.

2. Psyllium mucilloid (Metamucil) is a fiber laxative. Bulk laxatives can swell and cause esophagus obstruction; therefore, the most important question to ask the client is if they have difficulty swallowing. If the client answers "yes," the nurse should question the client taking Metamucil.

3. Fiber helps decrease constipation, but fiber does not affect the effectiveness of psyllium mucilloid (Metamucil); therefore, it is not the most important question the nurse should ask the client.

4. Psyllium mucilloid (Metamucil) may cause abdominal cramping, but abdominal tenderness is not pertinent information regarding taking a bulk laxative daily; therefore, it is not the most important question for the nurse to ask the client.

27. 1. The WBC count is monitored to determine the medication's effectiveness and would not be checked before administering the first dose of the antibiotic medication.

2. The nurse should monitor the client's vital signs, especially the temperature, but it would not affect the nurse administering the first dose of antibiotics.

3. Ceftriaxone (Rocephin) is an antibiotic. Antibiotics are notorious for causing allergic reactions, and the nurse should make sure the client is not allergic to any antibiotics before administering this medication. Therefore, this is the first intervention.

4. Stool specimens are sent to the laboratory to detect ova or parasites. Diverticulitis is not the result of ova or parasites; therefore, there is no need for the client to send a stool specimen to the laboratory.

28. Correct answers are 1 and 5.

1. Bisacodyl (Dulcolax) is a stimulant laxative. The client should be NPO and not have any fecal matter going through an inflamed descending and sigmoid bowel; therefore, the nurse would question administering a stimulant laxative, which would cause the client to have a bowel movement.

2. Because the client is NPO, a nasogastric tube is inserted to remove gastric acid and decompress the bowel.

3. The client would have pain medication; therefore, this order would not be questioned.

4. Because the client is NPO, the nurse would not question an order for IV fluids.

5. The client's rectum and sigmoid colon are irritated secondary to the diverticulitis; therefore nothing should be inserted into the rectum to irritate the rectum further. The client is not constipated, so the nurse should question sodium phosphate (Fleet Enema), a saline laxative.

MEDICATION MEMORY JOGGER: The nurse must be knowledgeable about accepted standards of practice for disease processes and conditions. If the nurse administers a medication the HCP has prescribed, and it harms the client, the nurse could be held accountable. Remember, the nurse is a client advocate.

29. Correct answers are 1, 3, and 5.

1. Mild abdominal cramping is expected when this medication is first started; however, there is less risk of cramping or diarrhea that can occur with stimulant laxatives.

2. It takes 2 to 3 days after the initial dose for the medication to work.

3. Bulk-forming laxatives, such as psyllium (Metamucil), polycarbophil (FiberCon), and methylcellulose (Citrucel), absorb water, which adds size to the fecal mass. Esophageal or intestinal obstruction may result if the client does not take adequate fluid with these medications.

4. When taking these medications, the client should increase dietary fiber, such as whole grains, fibrous fruits, and vegetables.

5. Bulk-forming laxatives can impact absorption of other medications. The client should be instructed to avoid taking other medications within 2 hours of taking a laxative.

6. The client should not mix oral and rectal laxatives.

30. 1. A stool surfactant or softener does not stimulate a bowel movement.

2. Docusate calcium (Colace) is a stool softener. If the client has soft brown stools, the medication is effective.

3. The abdomen should be soft and nontender, but this does not indicate that the medication is effective.

4. The client should have bowel sounds in all four quadrants of the abdomen, but this does not indicate the medication is effective.

MEDICATION MEMORY JOGGER: To determine if the medication is effective, the nurse should consider why the medication is being administered. Consider what disease process or condition the medication is being prescribed to treat.

31. 1. Sodium phosphate (Fleet Enema) is an osmotic saline laxative. In addition to being given an osmotic laxative, such as Fleet Phospho-Soda, the client will be NPO. This can lead to dehydration. Skin turgor and the oral mucosa condition should be monitored to assess for dehydration.

2. The client will need an IV line, but it is not a priority over assessing the client.

3. Iodine is not used in a colonoscopy, so the nurse need not ask this question.

4. The client should not have any bowel movements at this time. The bowel should be cleaned out before the colonoscopy.

32. 1. Docusate calcium (Surfak, Colace) is a stool softener. When docusate and certain herbs, such as senna, cascara, rhubarb, or aloe, are taken simultaneously, it will increase their absorption and risk of liver toxicity. The nurse should tell the client to stop taking the herb.

2. The herb will not help the diverticulitis and could cause complications.

3. The nurse cannot talk to the client's daughter because of the Health Insurance Portability and Accountability Act regulations.

4. The nurse can discuss herbs and prescribed medications with the client. There is no specific reason for the client to notify the HCP.

MEDICATION MEMORY JOGGER: Some herbal preparations are effective, some are not, and a few can be harmful or even deadly. If a client is taking an herbal supplement and a conventional medicine, the nurse should investigate to determine if the herb will interact with the conventional medicine or in any way possibly cause harm to the client. The nurse should always be the client's advocate.

33. 1. The nurse should not administer pain medication without first assessing the client for any complications.

2. Electrolyte levels do not need to be monitored before administering pain medication for clients diagnosed with diverticulitis.

3. The nurse should determine when the next pain medication could be administered, but the first intervention is always assessing the client.

4. The nurse must assess the client to determine if this pain should be expected with diverticulitis or if it is a result of a complication of diverticulitis, such as bowel obstruction or bowel perforation. Remember, the first intervention is assessment.

MEDICATION MEMORY JOGGER: Remember, pain may be expected due to the disease process or the condition, but it may also indicate a complication. Assessment is the first intervention when addressing a client's report of pain.

34. 1. Stool softeners do not increase the number of bowel movements; they make the stool softer and easier to pass. Therefore, determining how often the client has a bowel movement is not a priority.

2. Docusate calcium (Surfak, Colace) is a stool softener that contains sodium and calcium. A client diagnosed with essential hypertension would be on a low-sodium diet. Docusate sodium (Colace) should not be given to clients on sodium restriction.

3. The client's current blood pressure should be assessed. The client's last blood pressure reading would not be a priority.

4. There is nothing to indicate that the client is at risk for gastrointestinal bleeding; therefore, this is not a priority intervention.

Liver Failure

35. 1. Lactulose (Cephulac) is an osmotic laxative that functions as an ammonia detoxicant. It will not affect the client's urinary output.

2. Lactulose (Cephulac) is an osmotic laxative that functions as an ammonia detoxicant. An elevated ammonia level affects the client's neurological status. Lactulose is prescribed to remove ammonia through the intestinal tract.

Assessing the client's neurological status will determine the medication's effectiveness.

3. Lactulose (Cephulac) is an osmotic laxative that functions as an ammonia detoxicant. Lactulose is not administered to treat the client's ascites; therefore, measuring the abdominal girth will not help determine lactulose's effectiveness.
4. Lactulose (Cephulac) is an osmotic laxative that functions as an ammonia detoxicant. Lactulose will cause the client to have bowel movements, but the bowel movements will not determine the medication's effectiveness.

MEDICATION MEMORY JOGGER: The nurse determines medication effectiveness by assessing for the symptoms, or lack thereof, for which the medication was prescribed.

36. 1. Neomycin, an aminoglycoside antibiotic, does not help reduce hepatic venous pressure.
2. Diuretics, not the antibiotic neomycin, help increase fluid excretion through the kidneys.
3. Neomycin is an aminoglycoside antibiotic, but it is not administered to help prevent systemic infection.
4. Neomycin, an aminoglycoside antibiotic, is rarely used except in the bowel due to its limited absorbability outside the bowel. Neomycin sulfate is administered to help reduce ammonia by reducing the number of ammonia-forming bacteria in the bowel.

37. 1. End-stage liver failure causes inadequate absorption of vitamins. Vitamin K deficiency results in hypoprothrombinemia, which results in spontaneous bleeding and ecchymosis.
2. Night blindness and eye and skin changes result from a deficiency of vitamin A, not vitamin K.
3. Skin and mucous membrane lesions are caused by a deficiency of riboflavin and pyridoxine, not vitamin K.
4. This psychosis, along with beriberi and polyneuritis, results from a deficiency of thiamine, not vitamin K.

38. 1. Venodilation is the scientific rationale for administering nitrates such as isosorbide (Isordil), not vasopressin.
2. Vasopressin (Pitressin), a pituitary hormone, is prescribed for a client diagnosed with end-stage liver failure because it produces constriction of the splanchnic arterial bed, resulting in decreased portal pressure, which will help decrease esophageal bleeding. Vasopressin is administered IV or by intra-arterial infusion.
3. Coronary arterial vasoconstriction is a side effect of vasopressin. It is treated by administering nitroglycerin combined with vasopressin.
4. Vasopressin does not affect the liver's size or vascularity.

39. 1. Lactulose (Cephulac) is an osmotic laxative that functions as an ammonia detoxicant. The normal plasma ammonia level is 10 to 80 mcg/dL; this client's level is above normal, so the nurse would not question administering this medication, which is prescribed to remove ammonia from the intestinal tract.
2. Furosemide (Lasix) is a loop diuretic. This client's potassium level is within normal limits (3.5 to 5.3 mEq/L); therefore, the nurse should not question the diuretic administration.
3. Spironolactone (Aldactone) is a potassium-sparing diuretic. This client's potassium level is above normal level (3.5 to 5.3 mEq/L); therefore, the nurse should question administering this potassium-sparing diuretic.
4. Vasopressin (Pitressin) is a pituitary hormone. This client's sodium level is within normal limits (135 to 145 mEq/L); therefore, the nurse would not question administering the medication. Clients taking vasopressin may, however, develop hyponatremia or below-normal sodium levels.

MEDICATION MEMORY JOGGER: The nurse must be knowledgeable about accepted standards of practice for disease processes and conditions. If the nurse administers a medication the HCP has prescribed and it harms the client, the nurse could be held accountable. Remember, the nurse is a client advocate.

40. 1. Paracentesis is fluid (ascites) removal from the peritoneal cavity through a small incision or puncture through the abdominal wall under aseptic conditions. This would be an expected procedure for a client in end-stage liver failure.
2. Liver failure causes a decrease in vitamin absorption; therefore, an order for vitamin C to help prevent hemorrhagic lesions of scurvy would be expected.

3. **Morphine is a narcotic analgesic. The client in end-stage liver failure would have hepatic encephalopathy, which affects the client's neurological status. Therefore, sedatives, tranquilizers, and analgesic medications are not administered to the client. The nurse would question this order.**
4. Glucose is administered IV to clients diagnosed with end-stage liver disease to minimize protein breakdown. Because the client is third spacing, the IV rate will be low.

41. 1. Omeprazole (Prilosec) is a PPI. PPIs are not routine medications prescribed after endoscopic sclerotherapy and are not shown to prevent postsclerotherapy complications.
2. The client does not have to be NPO for 24 hours after endoscopic sclerotherapy.
3. Promethazine (Phenergan) is an antiemetic. Endoscopic sclerotherapy does not cause nausea or vomiting; therefore, there is no need to administer an antiemetic.
4. **Aluminium hydroxide (Maalox) is an antacid. Antacids may be administered after the procedure to counteract the gastric reflux effect.**

42. Correct answers are 2, 3, and 5.
1. The client should use warm water rather than hot water when bathing. Hot water increases pruritus.
2. **Emollient or lubricants should be used to keep the skin moist to prevent dry skin.**
3. **Antihistamines are prescribed to help the itching (pruritus) but should be used as directed because decreased liver function increases risk for altered drug responses.**
4. Hydrocortisone cream will not help this type of itching because the itching is not secondary to a rash or skin irritation. Severe jaundice with bile salt deposits on the skin causes pruritus.
5. **The client should not scratch the skin because it will cause bleeding, which may cause infection.**

43. 1. Lactulose (Cephulac) is an osmotic laxative that functions as an ammonia detoxicant. Diarrhea indicates a medication overdose, and the client should call the HCP for a decrease in dosage; therefore, this comment indicates the client understands the teaching.
2. **Lactulose (Cephulac) is an osmotic laxative that functions as an ammonia detoxicant. Although the drug may cause nausea, the client should keep taking it to decrease the ammonia level. The nurse should instruct the client to take the medication with crackers or a soft drink, which may reduce nausea. This statement indicates the client does not understand the medication teaching and needs more instruction.**
3. Lactulose (Cephulac) is an osmotic laxative that functions as an ammonia detoxicant. To mask the sweet taste, lactulose can be diluted with fruit juice. This statement indicates the client understands the medication teaching.
4. Lactulose (Cephulac) is an osmotic laxative that functions as an ammonia detoxicant. Having two to three soft stools a day indicates the medication is working to help decrease the ammonia level.

44.

Potential Nursing Intervention	Indicated	Not Indicated
1. Monitor the serum potassium level.	X	
2. Weigh the client daily.	X	
3. Assess bowel sounds frequently.		X
4. Monitor intake and output.	X	
5. Monitor abdominal girth.	X	
6. Assess skin frequently.	X	

1. **Spironolactone (Aldactone) is a potassium-sparing diuretic. Aldactone addresses one cause of ascites, which is increased aldosterone levels that cause water retention. Because Aldactone is a potassium-sparing diuretic, the client should be monitored for hyperkalemia.**
2. **Spironolactone (Aldactone) is a potassium-sparing diuretic. Diuretics cause excretion of fluid, and a daily weight check is an excellent assessment**

of the medication's effectiveness. Also, 1,000 mL is approximately 1 pound.

3. **Diuretics do not affect the client's gastrointestinal system, so monitoring the client's bowel sounds is unnecessary.**
4. **Diuretics cause excretion of fluid, and intake and output levels evaluate the diuretic therapy's effectiveness.**
5. **Spironolactone (Aldactone) is a potassium-sparing diuretic. Diuretic therapy is prescribed to help decrease ascites, which results from third spacing. Assessing the abdominal girth will help determine if the medication is effective.**
6. **The client's skin should be inspected for a rash and medication discontinued immediately if present because Stevens-Johnson syndrome or toxic epidermal necrolysis could develop.**

Hepatitis

45. 1. Usually, adults achieve immunity after one dose of the vaccine, but two doses are recommended for complete protection.
2. The nurse should inform the client that pain is expected at the injection site. There is no reason to notify the clinic.
3. **Hepatitis A vaccine provides long-term protection against hepatitis A infection, which is transmitted by the fecal-oral route via contaminated shellfish or other food or water and by direct contact with an infected person.**
4. This vaccine is administered intramuscularly into the deltoid muscle.

46. 1. This is a question that a nurse should ask any client before giving a medication, but it is not the most important question when administering the hepatitis B vaccine.
2. **A yeast-recombinant hepatitis B vaccine (Recombivax HB) is used to provide active immunity; therefore, the nurse should specifically ask the client if they are allergic to yeast.**
3. The hepatitis B vaccine is not made with egg yolks; therefore, this would not be an important question.
4. The hepatitis B vaccine is not made with any type of milk; therefore, this would not be an important question.

MEDICATION MEMORY JOGGER: The nurse must be knowledgeable about accepted standards of practice for medication administration, including which client assessment data and laboratory data should be monitored before administering the medication.

47. 1. Once the client has been exposed to the hepatitis A virus; the hepatitis A vaccine will not help prevent the client from getting hepatitis A.
2. This provides incorrect information to the client because there is something available to prevent the client from getting hepatitis A.
3. **This is correct information. An immune globulin injection within 2 weeks of exposure will help prevent the client from getting hepatitis A.**
4. There is no reason for the client to go to the ED. The client can come to the clinic and receive the injection.

48. 1. **At this time, there is no vaccination to prevent hepatitis C; therefore, this is the nurse's best response. Hepatitis C can be cured in 96% to 99% of clients with new treatments. Hepatitis C can go undetected for up to 20 years.**
2. There are vaccines to prevent hepatitis A and B, but there is no vaccination for hepatitis C.
3. This question does not have any relevance to the client's request.
4. This question may be construed as challenging by the client and the nurse should give the client factual information.

49. 1. This is information the client should be told, but it is not a priority at this time. Getting the woman medical treatment for the virus is the priority.
2. This information should be discussed with the client, but the most important intervention is to provide medical treatment.
3. **HBIG provides passive immunity against hepatitis B and is indicated for people exposed to the hepatitis B virus, who never had hepatitis B, and never received the hepatitis B vaccination.**
4. Prompt immunization with the hepatitis B vaccine (within a few hours or days after exposure to hepatitis B) increases likelihood of protection. Because the incubation period for hepatitis B is on average 70 to

80 days, it would be too late for the client to receive the immunization because their partner has just been diagnosed with hepatitis B. The client would have to have been vaccinated within 2 to 3 days after exposure from her partner.

50. 1. **Ribavirin (Virazole) is an antiviral medication. Ledipasvir/sofosbuvir (Harvoni) is also an antiviral that can be taken concurrently with ribavirin for clients with advanced cirrhosis or postliver transplant. The medications can achieve a 97% to 99% cure rate for genotype 1, 4, 5, or 6 hepatitis C. Pregnancy must be ruled out during this combined treatment. Pregnancy and breastfeeding must be avoided by females and by female partners of men taking the antiviral treatment during treatment. Couples should use two reliable forms of birth control to avoid pregnancy during treatment and for 6 months after treatment has been discontinued. The treatment usually lasts for 12 weeks.**
2. There is no vitamin requirement for clients taking antivirals.
3. Sunlight does not cause complications when taking this medication.
4. These medications do not cause impotence in men.

51. 1. This vaccine must be administered in three doses, not two doses; therefore, requesting the client to come back in 2 months and telling the client it is the last dose is incorrect information.
2. There is no reason why the client cannot wash the injection site.
3. There is no reason to rotate arms because there is 1 month and 6 months between injections.
4. **The hepatitis B vaccine must be administered intramuscularly in three doses, with the second and third doses at 1 and 6 months after the first dose. The third dose is essential in producing prolonged immunity.**

52.

Potential Nursing Intervention	Indicated	Not Indicated
1. Recommend combined Hepatitis A and B vaccine.	X	
2. Recommend Hepatitis B vaccination.		X
3. Recommend accessing community resources.	X	
4. Recommend oral testing for the HIV virus.	X	
5. Recommend a substance abuse treatment center.	X	
6. Recommend counseling for mental health issues.		X

1. **The U.S. Food and Drug Administration (FDA, 2001) has approved a combined hepatitis A and B vaccine (Twinrix) for vaccination of persons 18 years of age and older with indications for hepatitis A and B vaccination. The Twinrix vaccination consists of three doses, given on the same schedule as that used for single-antigen hepatitis B vaccine; that is, initial dose, after 1 month, and at 6 months.**
2. **Because the client is homeless and uses illegal IV drugs, the nurse should recommend the hepatitis A and B combined vaccination.**
3. **The client should be referred to community resources for food, shelter, and other needs.**
4. **There is an oral test for HIV. Oral tests detect HIV antibodies in mouth fluid taken from a scraping inside the cheek.**
5. **Recommending the client seek treatment to quit using IV drugs is an appropriate intervention.**

6. **Although an estimated 20% to 25% of the U.S. homeless population suffers from mental illness, nothing in the question indicates this client is experiencing mental illness. The nurse should perform an additional assessment before making this recommendation.**

Pediatric Gastroenteritis

53. 1. Bilberry is used to treat diarrhea in children and is not an emetic.
2. Bilberry does not treat lactose intolerance.
3. Bilberry is not an antipyretic and would not treat a fever.
4. **Bilberry is used to treat diarrhea. This question would assess the herb's effectiveness.**

MEDICATION MEMORY JOGGER: Some herbal preparations are effective, some are not, and a few can be harmful or even deadly. If a client is taking an herbal supplement and a conventional medicine, the nurse should investigate to determine if the herb will cause harm to the client. The nurse should always be the client's advocate.

54. 6.8 mL per dose. The first step is to determine the body weight in kilograms. 60 pounds divided by the 2.2 conversion factor is 27.272, or 27.27 kg. Multiply 27.27 times 10 to find the milligrams, which results in 272.2 or 272 mg of medication every 24 hours. Divide 272 mg by 2 to determine the amount of medication to be administered each dosing time; this equals 136 mg per dose.

To set up the algebraic formula:

$136x = 100$

Then cross multiply:

$100x = 680$

To solve for x, divide each side of the equation by 100:

$x = 6.8$ mL per dose

Trimethoprim sulfa (Bactrim) is a sulfa antibiotic.

55. 1. Penicillin (Ampicillin) is an antibiotic. The most likely cause of the child's developing diarrhea is the administration of antibiotic medications. The antibiotics kill the "good" bacteria in the bowel that are needed for digestion. Penicillin would increase diarrhea.
2. **Cholestyramine (Questran) is an antilipemic. Cholestyramine is used to enhance mucosal recovery and decrease the length of diarrhea.**
3. Trimethoprim sulfa (Bactrim) is a sulfa antibiotic. The most likely cause of the child's developing diarrhea is the administration of antibiotic medications. The antibiotics kill the "good" bacteria in the bowel needed for digestion. Trimethoprim would increase diarrhea.
4. Diphenoxylate is an opioid that contains atropine and is an antidiarrheal. Use of this medication should be limited in children. This would not be the first medication administered.

56. 1. **The American Academy of Pediatrics recommends 50 mL/kg body weight over 4 hours for mild diarrhea and 100 mL/kg for moderate diarrhea. The child is 37.5 pounds, or 17.04 kg (35 ÷ 2.2 = 17.04) or 17 kg; 17 times 50 equals 850 mL and 17 times 100 mL equals 1,700 mL. Pedialyte or Rehydralyte is recommended because they contain electrolytes that should be replaced.**
2. This would only be 200 mL over 2 hours and not enough to treat diarrhea. Homemade rice water does not contain replacement electrolytes.
3. Because juices and soft drinks have high carbohydrate content and because the osmotic effect in the intestine can increase diarrhea, they are not recommended.
4. The child should resume an age-appropriate diet as soon as the fluids have been replaced. Current research indicates that resuming solid food reduces the duration of diarrhea.

57. Correct answers are 1, 3, 4, and 5.
1. **The client is receiving IV fluids, and the nurse should monitor the child's electrolytes.**
2. A 6-year-old child's fontanels have closed. The child is assessed for dehydration by checking skin turgor on the abdomen.
3. **The order is incomplete. No rate has been given. The nurse should clarify the order with the HCP.**
4. **All pediatric IV infusions require safety measures to make sure the child is not fluid overloaded. Using a pump ensures that the rate of infusion is maintained**

and that too much fluid is not infused at one time. Most hospitals also require the simultaneous use of a chambered infusion device (Buretrol).
5. The nurse should assess pediatric IV sites at least every hour.

58. 1. The HCP is responsible for identifying abnormal data noted during the procedure.
2. The instrument being used is a fiberoptic scope, and it will be in the HCP's hands during the procedure. The instrument that might be handed is the biopsy instrument, but this is not a priority over the client's respiratory function.
3. The child will have received conscious sedation. The nurse should monitor the child's respiratory status to ensure that respiratory depression leading to respiratory failure does not occur.
4. The nurse or a technician will clean the instruments after a procedure, but this is not a priority over monitoring the client.

59. 1. Prochlorperazine (Compazine) is an antiemetic and should relieve nausea and vomiting. It is not known to cause diarrhea.
2. Prochlorperazine (Compazine) is an antiemetic. Tremors, involuntary twitching, and restlessness are findings of an extrapyramidal reaction. Children, the elderly, and dehydrated clients are especially susceptible. If these symptoms occur, the medication is held, and the HCP is notified.
3. Prochlorperazine (Compazine) is an antiemetic and does not cause diplopia (double vision), ptosis (drooping eyelids), or urinary retention. It can cause blurred vision.
4. Prochlorperazine (Compazine) is an antiemetic. It does not cause myalgias (muscle aches), hallucinations, or weakness.

60. 1. Antiemetic suppositories are not administered on this schedule for clients diagnosed with gastroenteritis. They are administered on a PRN basis.
2. The bacteria are transmitted by an oral route. The child should be in contact precautions in the hospital. The family should be cautious with handwashing and sharing glasses or eating utensils at home, but wearing a mask is unnecessary.
3. *E. coli* is a bacterium and is treated with antibiotics. The nurse should teach the parents to make sure that the child takes all the antibiotics as prescribed.
4. Current research indicates that taking antidiarrheal medications when an infectious bacterium is present can delay healing because bacteria cannot be eliminated from the body through the stool.

61. 1. Acidophilus is not an antibiotic and will not treat a bacterial infection.
2. Acidophilus will not increase the child's ability to develop immunity to *Shigella.*
3. Acidophilus is a bacterium that replaces the normal intestinal flora and helps to prevent secondary diarrhea caused by destroying this flora.
4. Acidophilus is not an antibiotic.

62. Correct answers are 1 and 4.
1. The mode of transmission for rotavirus is the oral-fecal route; therefore, anyone coming into contact with the child's feces should wash their hands.
2. The rotavirus is a virus, and antibiotics do not treat a virus.
3. The parents should not discard the diapers until the nurse has weighed the diapers to determine the toddler's hydration status.
4. The purpose of admitting a child with rotavirus is to ensure that dehydration is prevented or treated. The nurse should start the IV and use a controlled IV chamber device.
5. Two rotavirus vaccines are available for infants with the first dose at age 2 months; both are administered orally. Vaccines are administered before the infection to prevent an infection from occurring; therefore, they will not help the child at this time.

Obesity

63. 1. Orlistat (Xenical), a lipase inhibitor, inhibits absorption of fats and cholesterol in the gastrointestinal tract. The client should eat a reduced-calorie diet with no more than 30% of the calories coming from fats. Increasing fat intake can result in foul-smelling, frothy, diarrhea stools. The client needs more teaching.
2. The client should eat a reduced-calorie diet with no more than 30% of the calories coming from fats. Increasing the fat intake can result in foul-smelling, frothy, diarrhea stools. This statement does not require intervention.
3. Metamucil will add bulk to the stool and limit diarrhea that can occur with Xenical. This statement does not require intervention.

4. Xenical can interfere with absorption of needed vitamins and minerals. This statement does not require intervention.

64.

Potential Nursing Intervention	Indicated	Not Indicated
1. Administer the medication intramuscularly.		X
2. Weigh the client daily.	X	
3. Assess glucose regularly.	X	
4. Teach to report abdominal pain radiating to the back.	X	
5. Instruct to mix insulin and semaglutide in one dose.		X
6. Advise to have regular thyroid assessments.	X	

1. **Semaglutide (Wegovy) is injected once weekly in subcutaneous tissue, not intramuscularly.**
2. **Semaglutide (Wegovy) is approved by the FDA for chronic weight management for clients with a body mass index of 27 or greater and the presence of at least one weight-related issue. The client's weight should be assessed regularly (FDA, 2021).**
3. **The client taking semaglutide is at risk for hypoglycemia and should assess their glucose regularly.**
4. **Abdominal pain radiating to the back, with or without vomiting, indicates pancreatitis. The client should stop the medication and report the pain to the HCP.**
5. **The client should be instructed not to mix insulin and semaglutide together. They should be two separate injections. They may be given in the same body area but not immediately next to each other.**
6. **Clients taking semaglutide (Wegovy) are at increased risk of benign and malignant thyroid tumors. They should be instructed to report a lump in the neck, hoarseness, or trouble swallowing to the HCP.**

65. 1. Orlistat (Xenical), a lipase inhibitor, will decrease absorption of fats and cholesterol in the gastrointestinal tract, but it will not help the client quit smoking.
2. Lorcaserin (Belviq) can help with weight loss and suppress appetite, but it will not address smoking.
3. **Bupropion (Zyban) is an antidepressant that is used to assist clients in quitting smoking. It has also been shown to suppress the appetite by suppressing the uptake of norepinephrine and serotonin.**
4. Phentermine-topiramate (Qsymia) can help with weight loss and suppress appetite, but it will not address smoking.

66. 1. Glucophage shows modest weight loss in clients with no diabetes. There is no need to monitor the Hgb A_1C. Glucophage acts on the liver to prevent gluconeogenesis; it does not increase insulin levels.
2. Glucophage shows modest weight loss in clients with no diabetes. There is no need to monitor daily fasting blood glucose levels. Glucophage acts on the liver to prevent gluconeogenesis; it does not increase insulin levels.
3. Urine ketones are monitored when a client diagnosed with diabetes has a high glucose level and sometimes by clients on the Atkins diet to monitor if they are having success. Normal diets do not monitor urine ketones.
4. **The medication is being administered for weight loss, so the client's weight should be monitored.**

Constipation and Diarrhea

67. 1. Some laxatives are high in sodium or glucose, and the contents of the laxative should be checked, but this should not be the nurse's first response.
2. Rash or itching indicates an allergic reaction that can occur with laxatives, but because the client has been taking the laxatives daily, this should not be the nurse's first response.
3. **Laxatives are indicated for short-term use only, and laxative overuse robs the bowel of its ability to perform well on its own. Laxative dependency is a very serious and common problem of the elderly; therefore, this should be the nurse's first response. The nurse should teach the client safety.**

4. This is a true statement, but the nurse should first teach the client about safety, specifically the importance of not taking laxatives daily.

68. 1. Methylcellulose (Metamucil) is a bulk laxative. Bulk laxatives add fiber to the diet and should be taken daily, but it may take from 12 hours to 3 days for the laxative to work. Therefore, this should not be recommended to the client.
2. The nurse cannot prescribe medications, but laxatives are OTC medications and the nurse can recommend one to the client. Constipation is not a condition requiring an HCP appointment unless a laxative does not work or if the stool is abnormal.
3. Docusate sodium (Colace) is a stool softener. A stool softener takes from 24 to 48 hours to work, and this client needs something that will work immediately.
4. **Castor oil is a lubricant stimulant laxative. A stimulant laxative usually acts within 6 to 10 hours; however, castor oil acts within 1 to 3 hours. Therefore, this should be recommended because the client has not had a bowel movement in 4 days and is symptomatic.**

69.

Potential Nursing Intervention	Indicated	Not Indicated
1. Instruct the client to take lactobacillus.	X	
2. Report diarrhea to the HCP.	X	
3. Assess for any intake of bad-tasting or bad-smelling food.		X
4. Instruct the client to stop the antibiotic for 24 hours.		X
5. Tell the client to take two diphenoxylate and atropine tablets after each loose stool, up to eight tablets a day.	X	
6. Teach client to avoid alcohol and caffeine.	X	

1. **Lactobacillus (Bacid, Lactinex) is a probiotic. Bacid is a nonprescription product specifically used to treat diarrhea caused by antibiotics. It reestablishes normal intestinal flora and may be used prophylactically for clients diagnosed with a history of antibiotic-induced diarrhea.**
2. **Diarrhea is a side effect of some antibiotics because antibiotics kill the good flora in the bowel. Still, the HCP needs to be notified so something can be done about the diarrhea.**
3. **The nurse should realize that antibiotics can cause diarrhea and should not assess for possible gastroenteritis.**
4. **The client should not quit taking the antibiotic because there may be a relapse of the infection for which the antibiotic was prescribed and the full dosage of antibiotic prescribed should always be taken.**
5. **Diphenoxylate and atropine (Lomotil), an antidiarrheal, may cause serious health problems when overdosed, which is why the client cannot take more than eight tablets in 24 hours.**
6. **Alcohol can cause severe reactions when taking certain antibiotics and should be avoided. Caffeine can make diarrhea worse.**

70. 1. This is known as traveler's diarrhea caused by *E. coli* bacteria. If the client takes an antidiarrheal agent, it will slow peristalsis, delay export of the causative organism, and prolong the infection. Therefore, this should not be the nurse's first intervention. Loperamide (Imodium) is an antidiarrheal.
2. **Tourists are often plagued by infectious diarrhea, known as traveler's diarrhea, caused by the bacteria *E. coli*. As a rule, treatment is not necessary, and the diarrhea is self-limiting. If diarrhea is severe, it is treated with an antibiotic. Therefore, the nurse should assess severity of the diarrhea first.**
3. This is probably traveler's diarrhea, and as a rule, treatment is not necessary because it is self-limiting. If diarrhea is severe, it is treated with an antibiotic. Therefore, the nurse should assess severity of the diarrhea first.
4. This is a possibility, but the nurse should assess severity, length of time of diarrhea, and whether the client is dehydrated before making this statement.

MEDICATION MEMORY JOGGER: When answering test questions or when caring for clients at bedside, the nurse should remember that assessing the client is usually the first intervention, but when the client is in distress, the nurse may need to intervene directly to help the client.

71.

Potential Nursing Intervention	Indicated	Not Indicated
1. Instruct client to take antidiarrheals as recommended.	X	
2. Recommend a clear liquid diet.	X	
3. Assess how long the loose, watery stools have occurred.	X	
4. Tell the client to go to the ED as soon as possible.		X
5. Ask about other medications taken in the past 24 hours.	X	
6. Question the client about a fever.	X	
7. Teach client to report loose, watery stools lasting more than 48 hours.	X	

1. **Some antidiarrheal medications contain habit-forming drugs and should be used as directed only.**
2. **Clear liquids allow the bowel to rest. A client diagnosed with diarrhea should consume clear liquids only for 24 hours, then move on to eating a bland diet, and then progress to eating more solid food if diarrhea does not reoccur.**
3. **If the client has had diarrhea for more than 48 hours, the nurse should recommend the client come to the office because an elderly client is at risk for dehydration.**
4. **The client does not need to go to the ED but may need to be seen in the clinic if diarrhea has occurred for longer than 24 hours or the client shows clinical manifestations of dehydration.**
5. **The nurse should determine what other medications the client is taking because diarrhea is a side effect of digoxin toxicity and may be a side effect of many other medications. The nurse should always ask what other medications the client is taking.**
6. **The nurse should determine if the client is febrile.**
7. **Diarrhea that persists for more than 48 hours should not be self-treated. The HCP should see the client for further evaluation and diagnosis.**

72. 1. Dicyclomine is an antispasmodic. An antispasmodic medication controls spasms of the gastrointestinal tract and may help with irritable bowel syndrome (IBS), but it does not help prevent constipation.
2. Low-residue foods have low fiber and will cause the client to become constipated.
3. **Getting daily exercise, increasing fluid intake, eating a high-fiber diet, and using a stool softener that lubricates the stool lead to regular bowel movements, which, in turn, prevent constipation.**
4. A daily bowel movement is not required to prevent constipation. Some clients have bowel movements every other day, which is fine as long as the bowel movements are regular. Regular bowel movements prevent development of constipation.

73. 1. Senna (Senokot) is a stimulant laxative. Senna may cause the stool to turn this color; therefore, there is no need for the client to come to the clinic.
2. **Senna (Senokot) is a stimulant laxative. Senna (Senokot, Ex-Lax, and Agoral) may cause a yellow or yellow-green cast to feces. It may also cause a red-pink discoloration of alkaline urine or yellow-brown color in acid urine. The nurse should teach the client about this when the medication is prescribed.**
3. Because this change in the color of the stool is common with senna, there is no need for the client to bring a stool specimen to the clinic.

4. Some foods can cause feces discoloration, but yellow-green feces are a medication side effect.

MEDICATION MEMORY JOGGER: If the client verbalizes a symptom, the nurse assesses data, or if laboratory data indicates an adverse effect secondary to a medication, the nurse must intervene. The nurse must implement an independent intervention or notify the HCP because medications can result in serious or even life-threatening complications.

Abdominal Surgery with General Anesthesia

74. Correct answers are 2, 3, and 5.

1. This does not need to be reported to the surgical team.
2. **Shellfish allergy usually indicates an allergy to iodine, the active ingredient in povidone (Betadine) surgical scrub. The nurse should enter an allergy alert in the EHR, put an allergy bracelet on the client, and document the finding on the preoperative checklist.**
3. **If the client has had something to eat, the surgery must be canceled because food can lead to potential aspiration pneumonia.**
4. An infection last month should be cleared by now. This does not need to be reported to the surgical team.
5. **If the client has a productive cough, the surgery may be canceled because coughing postoperatively could cause wound dehiscence.**

MEDICATION MEMORY JOGGER: The nurse must be knowledgeable about diagnostic tests and surgical procedures. If the client provides information that would cause harm to the client, then the nurse must intervene.

75.
1. This is an intervention that will be done the morning of surgery, not the evening before.
2. This is important, but it can be done at any time before surgery. The night nurse or the nurse completing the checklist form in the morning could do this.
3. **Preoperative scrubs are ordered to cleanse the skin of bacteria. This should be done the evening before and also may be done the morning of surgery.**
4. This is an important intervention for postoperative care, but it is not necessary the evening before surgery.

76. Correct answers are 1, 3, and 5.

1. **For safety, the nurse should double-check PCA settings with another nurse. This ensures that the correct dosage is being administered when the client pushes the PCA button.**
2. The initial bolus should have been administered by the PACU nurse. The client and no one else should control the PCA button.
3. **The client is the person to push the PCA button, and it should be pushed when the client is in pain.**
4. The client is returning from the PACU. The cartridge holds 30 mL of medication and should not have been completely used in the PACU.
5. **The PCA pump is administered intravenously, and the nurse should assess the insertion site to ensure it is not inflamed or infiltrated.**

77.
1. The client, after general anesthesia, frequently experiences nausea while effects of the anesthetic agents are wearing off. The charge nurse should anticipate the client's needs and prepare for them.
2. The client would have been "asleep" while under general anesthesia and could not report nausea to the anesthesiologist.
3. **The surgeon may have overlooked the need for an antiemetic while writing the orders. The nurse should contact the surgeon and ask for the order.**
4. The charge nurse should not have to request a primary nurse to keep the charge nurse informed of the client's condition.

78.
1. Administering hydromorphone (Dilaudid) for pain that is a "1" on the pain scale would be overmedicating. Dilaudid is a potent opioid narcotic and should not be administered unless pain is at a moderate to severe level.
2. Hydromorphone is a narcotic analgesic and should be administered over 5 minutes for safety and per manufacturer directions.
3. No directions about how the hydromorphone was administered are listed, and "writhing" is not measurable.
4. **The nurse documented the respiratory rate as 24; this indicates it is safe to administer medications and many facilities accept "slow" for the rate of administration.**

79. 1,900 mL of IV fluid. 150 mL multiplied by 12 equals 1,800 mL, plus 100 mL of IVPB fluid, equals 1,900 mL of IV fluid.

80. 1. The client should have signed the consent form before the call that the orderly is coming to get the client for surgery is placed. Waiting until this point does not give the client time to ask questions and get clarification of concerns.
2. This should have been done the night before or at least earlier on the day of surgery.
3. The family can walk with the client to the operating room entrance and then be escorted or guided to the waiting room.
4. **This is the appropriate time to administer any preoperative medication.**

81. 1. The client's pain level is in the mild range. The nurse can discuss nonpharmacological methods to decrease the pain further, such as distraction or guided imagery, but this level of pain is not a reason for immediate intervention.
2. Serous drainage is expected after surgery and does not warrant immediate intervention.
3. **The client's respiration rate is low, indicating a potential overdose of narcotic medication depressing the respiratory drive. This situation requires immediate intervention.**
4. The client should splint the incision before coughing. The nurse should praise the client.

82. 1. **The WBC count is elevated, indicating an infection. The surgeon would not have performed an elective surgery if the client had an infection at the time. This indicates the antibiotic is not working.**
2. This might indicate that the pain medication is not relieving the client's pain, but it does not provide information about the antibiotic.
3. The sodium level is within normal limits. It does not provide information about the antibiotic.
4. This is the normal color of drainage of a nasogastric tube, but it does not provide information about the antibiotic.

MEDICATION MEMORY JOGGER: The nurse determines medication effectiveness by assessing for the symptoms, or lack thereof, for which the medication was prescribed.

Total Parenteral Nutrition

Potential Nursing Intervention	Indicated	Not Indicated
1. Monitor the client's glucose level every 6 hours.	X	
2. Administer sliding scale regular insulin.	X	
3. Assess the peripheral IV site every 4 hours.		X
4. Encourage client to eat all food offered at meals.		X
5. Change the subclavian dressing per protocol.	X	
6. Administer the TPN using an IV pump.	X	
7. Ensure TPN is tapered off when discontinuing.	X	

83. Correct answers are 1, 2, 5, 6, and 7.
1. **TPN is high in dextrose, which is glucose; therefore, the client's blood glucose level must be monitored closely.**
2. **The client may be on sliding-scale regular insulin coverage for the high glucose level.**
3. **TPN must be administered via a subclavian line because of the high glucose level.**
4. **The client would be NPO to put the bowel at rest, which is the rationale for administering the TPN.**
5. **The TPN must be administered via a subclavian line due to the high glucose level, which can cause a peripheral line to collapse. Dressing changes may be daily, every 3 days, or weekly, depending on the dressing and biopatch.**
6. **TPN should always be administered using an IV pump and not via gravity. Fluid volume resulting from an overload of TPN could cause a life-threatening hyperglycemic crisis.**
7. **TPN should be tapered off when discontinuing to prevent hypoglycemia due to the high dextrose content.**

84. **1. The nurse should first check the IV pump that sounds an alarm because there is something wrong with the IV fluid. Air in the line is a potentially life-threatening complication of TPN.**
2. The nurse should ensure the next bag of TPN is available when the current bag is empty, but it is not a priority over an alarm on the IV pump.
3. The nurse should notify the HCP about an inflamed insertion site, but the nurse should first assess the alarm on the pump to correct a problem immediately.
4. The nurse should monitor the client's serum potassium level, but laboratory results are not prioritized over an IV pump alarm.

85. 1. The client's blood glucose (BG) level is 311; therefore, four units is not the appropriate dose.
2. Six units of regular insulin does not cover a BG level of 311.
3. The HCP order requires 10 units of regular insulin, not eight units.
4. The client has a BG level of 311 per the client's EHR. This requires 10 units of regular insulin, a pancreatic hormone.

86. 1. The client must have the same glucose content as the TPN. The nurse cannot administer D_5W because the client will experience hypoglycemia.
2. The client will experience hypoglycemia if the nurse decreases the rate to 30 mL/hr. The rate should be weaned 5 mL/hr when discontinuing TPN.
3. The nurse must ensure the same glucose content will be administered until TPN bag #2 is ready, so this is the most appropriate intervention.
4. The nurse does not need to notify the HCP because hanging D_{10} is appropriate until TPN bag #2 is ready.

87. **1. The UAP can weigh the client because this task is not assessing, teaching, evaluating, or administering medications.**
2. The subclavian dressing change is a sterile procedure, and the UAP cannot perform sterile procedures.
3. The client receiving TPN should be NPO; therefore, the RN should not delegate this to the UAP.
4. The RN cannot delegate assessment to the UAP.

88. 1. The TPN should be kept in the refrigerator until 1 hour before administering to the client, but this is not the first intervention the nurse should implement.
2. The nurse should first check the TPN bag #4 label with the HCP's order to ensure the prescription is correct. Each TPN bag may have amounts of dextrose, amino acids, lipids, and potassium. TPN should be treated like a medication.
3. The nurse must use new tubing with every bag, but this is not the first intervention. The bag should be spiked just before hanging TPN bag #4.
4. The client's glucose level is checked every 6 hours around the clock, not before administering the TPN bag.

89. **62 mL/hr. The nurse should decrease the rate by 5 mL every hour. In 3 hours, it should be decreased by 15 mL. The nurse should subtract 15 mL from 77 mL to get 62 mL.**

90. **1. The client's potassium level is high and needs immediate intervention because this could cause cardiac problems. A normal potassium level is 3.5 to 5.3 mEq/L.**
2. The normal serum sodium level is 135 to 145 mEq/L, so the nurse does not need to notify the HCP.
3. This glucose level is elevated (normal would be <200 mg/dL), but the nurse has sliding-scale insulin to cover this glucose level. The HCP does not need to be notified.
4. The normal serum total protein level is 6 to 8 g/dL; therefore, the nurse does not need to notify the HCP.

Acute Pain

91. 1. The client's MAR designated ketorolac as an allergy. The nurse would have to know that the client is not allergic to the medication before administering it. Ketorolac (Toradol) is a parenteral NSAID.
2. Only the client should administer hydromorphone (Dilaudid) via the PCA pump for safety to prevent overdosing the client.
3. The nurse should determine the IV patency and pump function before calling the surgeon.
4. The client is receiving hydromorphone (Dilaudid), a narcotic analgesic, that the client can control. According to the MAR, the client has been able to receive medication during the last shift. The first intervention for the nurse is to determine if the IV is patent and the pump is working.

MEDICATION MEMORY JOGGER: A PCA pump is *client controlled*, and the nurse should not call the HCP if the nurse can determine the cause of a problem and intervene to resolve it.

92. Correct answers are 2, 3, and 4.

1. Pain medication is rarely administered intramuscularly anymore because of pain due to another needle, development of indurated tissue from repeated injections, and a longer length of time for the injected medication to become effective. Most parenteral pain medication is administered via IV.
2. **The nurse should check the client's MAR for the last administration time to avoid administering medication too early, increasing risk of respiratory depression.**
3. **The Joint Commission standards for medication administration require that two client-specific identifiers be used before administering any medication.**
4. **Narcotic opioids can cause respiratory depression, so the nurse should assess respiratory status before administering medication. The pancreas is in the abdominal cavity, so the nurse should assess the abdomen to rule out a complication that a narcotic would mask.**
5. Amylase is monitored for a client diagnosed with pancreatitis, but not to administer pain medication.

MEDICATION MEMORY JOGGER: "Select all that apply" questions require the test taker to view each option as a true or false question. One option cannot assist the test taker to eliminate another option.

93. Correct order is 2, 3, 5, 4, 1.

2. **The nurse cannot administer a medication they do not have. First in this list is to obtain the medication.**
3. **Before administering any medication, the nurse should assess for allergies.**
5. **The nurse can administer medication after assessing for complications and rating pain, assessing for allergies, and identifying the client with two client-specific identifiers.**
4. **As soon as a medication is administered, the nurse should document the administration. This is now considered the sixth right of medication administration.**
1. **The client should be evaluated for intervention effectiveness, but the other interventions come first.**

94.
1. The medication should be administered through the lowest port, not the highest. This allows medication to enter the client's body faster and not be lost in the tubing if the tubing comes apart.
2. **Morphine sulfate is a narcotic analgesic. Narcotic analgesics should be administered over 5 minutes so the nurse can observe for drowsiness, lethargy, and respiratory depression, and stop the administration before a full dose is administered.**
3. The client's arm can be elevated after an IVP when the client is in a code to assist the medication entering the body and circulating throughout the system. It is not needed in a nonemergency situation.
4. The client should not be asked to refrain from coughing because they are at risk of developing atelectasis.

95.
1. The client may go to surgery and need to sign a legal document, the operative permit, before doing so. The nurse should not administer a narcotic before asking the client to sign a legal document.
2. Whether or not the HCP writes an order for pain medication, there is still the possibility that the client will need clear thought processes to sign a legal document.
3. **This is the correct statement at this time. The nurse must know about the status of the surgery before administering a narcotic.**
4. This is a therapeutic statement, and the client needs factual information.

96.
1. Morphine is an opioid analgesic. A pain level of "4" is considered mild pain and the nurse should see if a less potent medication is available.
2. Hydrocodone (Vicodin) is an oral opioid narcotic medication. This client should be NPO. The nurse should check to see if parental medication is available.
3. Acetaminophen (Tylenol), a nonnarcotic pain medication, is for mild pain, so this is not the first priority.
4. **Nalbuphine (Nubain) is a synthetic opioid agonist, but it has less potency than morphine sulfate. This client is thrashing in bed, presumably from pain. Continued movement such as "thrashing" could cause other problems such as wound tearing. This medication has priority.**

97. 1. Acetaminophen with 30 mg of codeine (Tylenol #3) is a nonnarcotic pain medication combined with narcotic medication. The medication can be administered without question.

2. Meperidine (Demerol) metabolizes into normeperidine in the body and can accumulate, causing seizures. Because children are especially vulnerable, the nurse should question the order and obtain a suitable medication. Demerol is rarely prescribed now.

3. This pain level is moderately high, so morphine, a narcotic analgesic, is good for this pain.

4. Hydromorphone (Dilaudid) is a potent narcotic analgesic and would be appropriate for a level 10 pain.

98. 1. The nurse should intervene immediately, not wait until the anesthesiologist can get to the client.

2. Hydromorphone (Dilaudid) is a potent narcotic analgesic. Naloxone (Narcan), a narcotic agonist, will reverse effects of an opioid analgesic. This is the first action.

3. This should be implemented after administering naloxone (Narcan), a narcotic agonist, because it has a short half-life, and respiratory depression will return in about 20 minutes.

4. The client is still breathing independently; therefore, this is not necessary at this time.

99. 1. Oxycodone (Percodan), a narcotic analgesic, is an oral medication and appropriate for mild to moderate pain.

2. This medication may not be strong enough for postoperative pain at this level.

3. Morphine is a potent narcotic analgesic and should be given for moderate to severe pain.

4. Ondansetron (Zofran), a 5-HT agonist, is for nausea, not pain.

GASTROINTESTINAL SYSTEM COMPREHENSIVE EXAMINATION

1. The client diagnosed with gastroenteritis was admitted to the medical floor yesterday and has just had another loose, watery stool. Based on the following MAR, which action should the nurse implement?

Client: E.R.	MR# 1234567	Date: Today
Age: 37 years	Allergies: NKDA	Diagnosis: Gastroenteritis
Medication	0701-1900	1901-0700
Acetaminophen 325 mg tablet 1-2 PO PRN temperature or mild pain		
Promethazine 6.25 mg IVP PRN nausea		
Diphenoxylate 5.0 mg PO after each loose stool	0701 DN	0045 NN 0200 NN 0545 NN
0.9 % saline continuous IV at 125 mL/hour	100 DN	0200 NN
Nurse Initials/Credentials	DN/RN	NN/RN

1. Administer a diphenoxylate tablet.
2. Increase the IV fluid rate.
3. Notify the HCP.
4. Send a stool specimen to the laboratory.

2. The client diagnosed with IBD has been prescribed oral prednisone daily. The client has pyrosis. Which statement would be the clinic nurse's **best** response?
   1. "What type of diet are you currently following?"
   2. "When do you take your prednisone?"
   3. "Have you had a change in your weight?"
   4. "Have you discussed this with your HCP?"

3. The mother brought her 3-year-old son to the clinic because the child has had diarrhea since last night. The mother tells the nurse, "My mother was giving my son corn starch in a glass of warm water to help stop diarrhea, but it didn't stop the diarrhea completely." Which statement is the clinic nurse's **best** response?
   1. "Corn starch will not hurt your son, and we need to let the diarrhea run its course."
   2. "You must tell your mother not to give your son anything the doctor has not ordered."
   3. "Why does the grandmother think that corn starch will help your son's diarrhea?"
   4. "I hope that the corn starch has not made your son's diarrhea get worse."

4. The client diagnosed with gastroenteritis is being discharged from the ED with a prescription for promethazine. Which information should the nurse discuss with the client?
   1. Explain that a sore throat and mouth sores are expected side effects.
   2. Tell the client to call the doctor if the urine turns a light amber color.
   3. Encourage the client to drink carbonated beverages.
   4. Instruct the client not to drink alcohol with the medication.

5. The client diagnosed with hepatitis is being treated with interferon alfa. Which information should the clinic nurse discuss with the client?
   1. Explain that if flu-like symptoms occur, the client must stop taking the medication.
   2. Discuss that the client may experience some abnormal bruising and bleeding.
   3. Tell the client that the skin will become yellow while taking this medication.
   4. Recommend taking two tablets of acetaminophen before the injection.

6. Which client should the nurse **question administering** diphenoxylate?
   1. The 68-year-old client diagnosed with glaucoma
   2. The 78-year-old client diagnosed with traveler's diarrhea
   3. The 44-year-old client diagnosed with coronary artery disease
   4. The 28-year-old client receiving aminoglycoside antibiotics

7. The elderly client diagnosed with IBS is prescribed propantheline. Which findings indicate an **adverse reaction** to the medication?
   1. Flatus, abdominal pain, and cramping
   2. Agitation, confusion, and drowsiness
   3. Diarrhea alternating with constipation
   4. Mucus in the stool and low-grade fever

8. The charge nurse notices that the primary nurse is preparing to administer magnesium-aluminum hydroxide to the client receiving routine morning medications. Which intervention should the charge nurse take **first**?
   1. Take no action because this is acceptable standard of practice.
   2. Discuss changing the administration time with the pharmacist.
   3. Inform the primary nurse not to administer the magnesium-aluminum hydroxide.
   4. Instruct the primary nurse to shake the magnesium-aluminum hydroxide container.

9. The nurse is administering the 0900 medications on the following MAR. Which intervention should the nurse implement?

Client: N.O.	MR# 1234567	Date: Today
Age: 61 years	Allergies: NKDA	Diagnosis:
Medication	0701-1900	1901-0700
Omeprazole 40 mg PO daily	0900	
Furosemide 20 mg PO daily	0900	
Acetylsalicylic acid 325 mg PO daily	0900	
Warfarin 5 mg PO daily	1700	
Azithromycin 250 mg PO daily	1800	
Nurse Initials/Credentials	DN/RN	NN/RN

   1. Monitor the client's serum sodium level.
   2. Check the client's INR.
   3. Ensure that the client ate at least 75% of the breakfast meal.
   4. Encourage the client to sit upright for at least 30 minutes after taking omeprazole.

10. The client is scheduled for a bowel resection in the morning. The nurse administered one dose of polyethylene glycol 3350 and electrolyte oral solution. Which task is **most appropriate** for the RN delegate to the UAP?
  1. Remove the client's water pitcher from the room.
  2. Take the client's vital signs every 2 hours.
  3. Place a bedside commode in the client's room.
  4. Administer moisture barrier cream to the anal area.

11. The client diagnosed with end-stage liver failure is taking lactulose. Which assessment data indicates the medication is **effective**?
  1. The client reports a decrease in pruritus.
  2. The client's abdominal girth has decreased.
  3. The client is experiencing diarrhea.
  4. The client's ammonia level is decreased.

12. The client is 2 days postgastric bypass surgery and reports nausea. The nurse is preparing to administer ondansetron IVP. The client has a peripheral IV line infusing normal saline at 100 mL/hr. Which interventions should the nurse implement? **Select all that apply.**
  1. Flush the peripheral IV before administering medication.
  2. Administer the ondansetron undiluted via the port closest to the client.
  3. Start a saline lock in the other arm to administer ondansetron.
  4. Give the ondansetron intramuscularly rather than IV.
  5. Administer the IV medication slowly.

13. Which medication should the nurse **question** administering?
  1. Magnesium hydroxide and aluminum hydroxide to a client diagnosed with chronic kidney disease
  2. Lansoprazole to a client diagnosed with ulcer disease
  3. Docusate to a client diagnosed with diverticulosis
  4. Psyllium to a client diagnosed with diarrhea

14. The home health-care nurse is discussing bowel elimination patterns with an elderly client. The client tells the nurse they must take something to make their bowels move every day. For each intervention, specify if the intervention is **indicated or not indicated** for the client's care.

Potential Nursing Intervention	Indicated	Not Indicated
1. Tell the client to take a cathartic laxative daily.		
2. Encourage the client to take a bulk laxative daily.		
3. Demonstrate how to give a sodium phosphate enema.		
4. Instruct the client to take a daily stool softener.		
5. Recommend the client drink at least 2,000 mL of water daily.		
6. Teach the client to consume high-fiber foods.		

15. The client diagnosed with cancer is not eating and has lost 15 pounds in the past month. The HCP has prescribed dronabinol. Which statement indicates the client **needs more teaching** concerning this medication?
  1. "This medication will help stimulate my appetite."
  2. "It is not uncommon to get drowsy when taking this medication."
  3. "This is marijuana, and I do not want to get addicted to it."
  4. "I should chew sugarless gum when taking this medication."

16. The client diagnosed with lactose intolerance is prescribed lactase. For each intervention, specify if the intervention is **indicated or not indicated** for the client's care.

Potential Nursing Intervention	Indicated	Not Indicated
1. Administer medication on an empty stomach.		
2. Administer medication with a full glass of water.		
3. Administer medication with the client's food.		
4. Administer medication with vitamin D.		

17. The client with an ileostomy is prescribed bismuth subcarbonate tablets orally four times a day. Which statement **best describes** the scientific rationale for administering this medication?
1. This medication will help thicken the ileostomy output.
2. This medication will help decrease the odor in the ileostomy pouch.
3. This medication helps to change the pH of the ileostomy output.
4. This medication coats the lining of the small intestine.

18. The client diagnosed with end-stage liver disease is prescribed hydroxyzine. Which assessment data indicates the medication is **effective**?
1. The client reports a decrease in nausea.
2. The client reports an increase in appetite.
3. The client reports being more alert.
4. The client reports a decrease in itching.

19. The client tells the clinic nurse about getting carsick every time the family goes on a vacation, and the HCP prescribed scopolamine for motion sickness. Which statement indicates the client understands the medication teaching? **Select all that apply.**
1. "I will put the transdermal scopolamine patch behind my ear."
2. "I will put the patch on for 12 hours and take it off at night."
3. "If my car sickness does not go away, I will wear two patches."
4. "I should leave the patch on for 3 days before changing it."
5. "I should take the medication with one glass of water."

20. The nurse is administering rifaximin to a client diagnosed with IBS. Which statement made by the client would cause the nurse to **hold the medication** and check with the HCP?
1. "I have frequent diarrhea with my IBS."
2. "I have not had a bowel movement for 5 or 6 days."
3. "I was diagnosed with IBS when I kept having frequent bowel movements."
4. "IBS makes it difficult to maintain a normal lifestyle."

21. The nurse in the gastroenterology clinic is reviewing client EHRs. The clients have all been prescribed eluxadoline for the treatment of IBS with diarrhea (IBS-D). Which client should the nurse discuss **immediately** with the HCP?
1. The client diagnosed with a history of uncontrolled diarrhea using other medications
2. The client with a laboratory report of liver enzymes within normal range
3. The client after a cholecystectomy 11 years ago
4. The client who takes a social drink every 2 to 3 months

22. The client presents to the outpatient clinic reporting chronic constipation and requesting a medication seen in a commercial on television. Which interventions should the nurse implement? **Rank in order of performance.**

1. Discuss new medications seen on television that are for adults with chronic constipation.
2. Assess which measures the client has tried to alleviate the problem.
3. Have the client complete a 24- to 72-hour food diary to determine which foods could be contributing to the problem.
4. Assist the client in formulating an exercise program to increase activity.
5. Determine how often the client has a bowel movement and have them describe the usual bowel movement.

23. The nurse working on a medical unit is caring for a client requiring large doses of IV antibiotics. As a result, the client has developed *C. difficile* infections. The HCP has prescribed bezlotoxumab. Which intervention should the nurse implement?

1. Determine that the client is still receiving an antibacterial medication to treat the *C. difficile* infection.
2. Remove the client from isolation.
3. Teach the client to take all the prescribed medication after release from the hospital.
4. Notify the dietary department to change the client's diet to clear liquid.

GASTROINTESTINAL SYSTEM COMPREHENSIVE EXAMINATION ANSWERS AND RATIONALES

1. 1. Diphenoxylate is combined with atropine to form Lomotil. Diphenoxylate is an opioid whose only indication is to treat diarrhea, but atropine is added to discourage narcotic abuse. The client cannot have more than eight doses of Lomotil daily.
2. The nurse should not increase the client's IV rate without an HCP's order.
3. The nurse should notify the HCP because the maximum dose of diphenoxylate (Lomotil), an antidiarrheal, is eight doses (20 mg total) in 24 hours.
4. Sending a stool specimen will not treat diarrhea.

2. 1. The client's diet does not have any bearing on the client's heartburn.
2. Prednisone is a glucocorticosteroid and can cause gastric distress. Pyrosis, or heartburn, could be secondary to the client's taking the prednisone on an empty stomach. Prednisone is very irritating to the stomach and must be taken with food to prevent severe heartburn and possible peptic ulcer.
3. A weight change is not significant to the client's report of heartburn.
4. The nurse should assess the client's issues before referring the client to the HCP. If the nurse can give factual information, the nurse should teach the client.

3. 1. Corn starch works by absorbing excess water in the intestines, thus stopping diarrhea. Therefore, this is the nurse's best response. In children, antidiarrheal medication is not prescribed because of possible adverse reactions. Pedialyte is prescribed to prevent dehydration, and diarrhea usually subsides on its own.
2. This statement is judgmental, and many home remedies have produced valid results.
3. A client often interprets a "why" question as judgmental, so this is not the best response.
4. This statement has no factual basis, and even if the nurse were not aware of the effectiveness of corn starch, the nurse should investigate before making the mother worry about her son's condition.

MEDICATION MEMORY JOGGER: Some herbal preparations or alternative therapies are effective, some are not, and a few can be harmful or even deadly. If a client is taking a home remedy, the nurse should investigate. The nurse should always be the client's advocate.

4. 1. A sore throat and mouth sores could indicate that the client is experiencing agranulocytosis, a possible adverse effect of promethazine (Phenergan) and should be reported to the HCP. The HCP would have a complete blood cell count drawn to evaluate for this adverse effect.
2. Urine that is light amber in color indicates the client is no longer dehydrated and would not warrant notifying the HCP.
3. Nonpharmacological measures of alleviating nausea and vomiting, such as flattened carbonated beverages, weak tea, crackers, and dry toast, should be discussed with the client. Drinking carbonated beverages should be discouraged.
4. Promethazine (Phenergan) is an antiemetic. The client should not consume alcohol when taking antiemetics because it can intensify the sedative effect.

MEDICATION MEMORY JOGGER: Drinking alcohol is always discouraged when taking any prescribed or OTC medication because of adverse interactions. The nurse should encourage the client not to drink alcoholic beverages.

5. 1. Flu-like symptoms are expected and should be treated with acetaminophen (Tylenol).
2. Abnormal bleeding and bruising are not expected and should be reported to the HCP.
3. The client may be jaundiced from the hepatitis but not from taking the medication.
4. Interferon alfa (Roferon) is a biologic response modifier used to treat viruses. The body naturally produces interferon in response to a viral infection. Administration of synthetic interferon produces the same flu-like symptoms and should be treated with Tylenol, which will help decrease severity of symptoms from the injection. After multiple interferon injections, the client will no longer have flu-like symptoms.

MEDICATION MEMORY JOGGER: Usually, if a client is prescribed a new medication and has flu-like symptoms within 24 hours of taking the first dose, the client should contact the HCP. These are clinical manifestations of

agranulocytosis, which indicates the medication has caused a sudden drop in WBC count, which, in turn, leaves the body defenseless against bacterial invasion. Biologic response modifiers are the exception to the rule.

6. 1. **The client diagnosed with glaucoma should not receive Lomotil because of the drug's anticholinergic effect, increasing intraocular pressure.**
2. Diphenoxylate (Lomotil) is an antidiarrheal. Lomotil is prescribed for adult clients diagnosed with traveler's diarrhea. In children, diarrhea should be allowed to run its course.
3. Lomotil is not contraindicated for clients diagnosed with coronary artery disease.
4. Antibiotics sometimes cause a suprainfection that kills the normal flora in the bowel, resulting in diarrhea. This client may receive an antidiarrheal medication.

MEDICATION MEMORY JOGGER: Glaucoma is a condition that the nurse should recognize. Its presence precludes the use of many medications.

7. 1. These are the clinical manifestations of IBS.
2. **Propantheline (Pro-Banthine) is an antispasmodic. Agitation, confusion, and drowsiness are clinical manifestations of an adverse reaction in the elderly or debilitated client requiring medication discontinuation.**
3. Diarrhea alternating with constipation is a sign of IBS, not an adverse reaction to the medication.
4. Mucus in the stool is a sign of IBS, but low-grade fever is not. Neither of these indicates an adverse reaction to the medication.

8. 1. Taking antacids with other medications is not an acceptable standard of practice.
2. The charge nurse should discuss changing the times of magnesium-aluminum hydroxide (Maalox) administration to 1 to 2 hours before or after taking other drugs because Maalox could affect the absorption of the other drugs. However, this is not the first intervention.
3. **The client should not receive any oral medications 1 to 2 hours before or after taking an antacid because the antacid may interfere with absorption of other medications.**
4. Magnesium-aluminum hydroxide (Maalox) is a suspension and should be shaken, but this is not the first action the nurse should take.

9. 1. The nurse should monitor the client's serum potassium level, not sodium level, before administering the 0900 furosemide (Lasix).
2. **Omeprazole (Prilosec), a PPI, interacts with warfarin (Coumadin) and may increase the likelihood of bleeding; therefore, the nurse should check the client's INR.**
3. Prilosec can be taken on an empty stomach.
4. The client should sit up after eating a meal, but not after taking Prilosec.

10. 1. The client would not be NPO until midnight. There is no reason for the UAP to remove the water pitcher.
2. There is no reason for the client's vital signs to be taken every 2 hours preoperatively. Vital signs are tasks that can be delegated to a UAP.
3. **Polyethylene glycol 3350 and electrolyte oral solution (GoLYTELY) is an osmotic laxative and electrolyte solution administered to remove stool from the body before bowel surgery. Therefore, the client should have a bedside commode readily available, and the RN can delegate the UAP to perform this task.**
4. The UAP can apply a moisture barrier to excoriated perianal areas, but nothing in the stem indicates the client has this need.

11. 1. Lactulose (Cephulac), an osmotic laxative, is not administered to help with the client's report of itching.
2. Lactulose will not help decrease the client's ascites.
3. Diarrhea is a sign of medication toxicity and would warrant decreasing the medication dose.
4. **Lactulose (Cephulac), an osmotic laxative, is administered to decrease the client's serum ammonia level. The normal adult level is 10 to 80 mcg/dL.**

12. Correct answers are 2 and 5.
1. The primary IV is normal saline; therefore, the nurse does not need to flush the tubing before administering the medication.
2. **Ondansetron (Zofran), an antiemetic, should be administered undiluted.**
3. Ondansetron (Zofran) is compatible with normal saline; therefore, the nurse need not start a saline lock in the other arm, causing the client discomfort.
4. Ondansetron (Zofran) can be given IVP; therefore, the nurse need not give the medication intramuscularly, causing the client discomfort.

5. The nurse must administer the medication slowly over 2 to 5 minutes.

13. **1. Magnesium hydroxide and aluminum hydroxide (Maalox), an antacid, should not be administered to a client diagnosed with chronic kidney disease because it contains magnesium, and diseased kidneys are unable to excrete magnesium, resulting in the client developing hypermagnesemia. If clients need an antacid, they should receive aluminum hydroxide (Amphojel) because it helps remove phosphates.**
2. Lansoprazole (Prevacid) is a PPI. A PPI decreases gastric secretion and would be prescribed for a client diagnosed with PUD.
3. Docusate sodium (Surfak) is a stool softener. A stool softener would be prescribed for a client diagnosed with diverticulosis to help prevent constipation.
4. Psyllium (Metamucil) is a bulk laxative. Promethazine (Phenergan) is an antiemetic. A bulk laxative adds substance to the feces and will help decrease watery stools.

14.

Potential Nursing Intervention	Indicated	Not Indicated
1. Tell the client to take a cathartic laxative daily.		X
2. Encourage the client to take a bulk laxative daily.	X	
3. Demonstrate how to give a sodium phosphate enema.		X
4. Instruct the client to take a daily stool softener.	X	
5. Recommend the client drink at least 2,000 mL of water daily.	X	
6. Teach the client to consume high-fiber foods.	X	

1. A cathartic laxative is a stimulant laxative; daily use can lead to laxative dependence. Elderly clients should be encouraged to use other methods to ensure daily bowel movement.
2. **A bulk laxative is recommended for daily use because it increases fiber and requires the colon to function normally. Stimulant laxatives may cause laxative dependency, which is not healthy for the client.**
3. The client should not be encouraged to take sodium phosphate (Fleet) enemas unless recommended by an HCP because they may cause dependence. The nurse should encourage the use of medications that require the bowel to function normally.
4. **If the client needs to have a bowel movement daily, then a stool softener should be encouraged because it does not stimulate the bowel; it just softens the stool.**
5. **Increasing the client's water intake will help soften the stool.**
6. **Consuming high-fiber foods, such as prunes, wheat bran, apples, and pears, can improve stool consistency and frequency of bowel movements in clients with constipation.**

15. 1. This medication is prescribed to help stimulate the client's appetite; therefore, the client does not need more teaching.
2. A side effect of this medication is drowsiness; therefore, the client does not need more teaching.
3. **The cannabinoid dronabinol (Marinol or Appetrol), the active ingredient in marijuana, is frequently abused like an illegal drug, but it is not addicting.**
4. A side effect of this medication is a dry mouth, so chewing sugarless gum indicates the client understands the medication teaching.

16.

Potential Nursing Intervention	Indicated	Not Indicated
1. Administer medication on an empty stomach.		X
2. Administer medication with a full glass of water.		X
3. Administer medication with the client's food.	X	
4. Administer medication with vitamin D.		X

1. Enzymes break down food; therefore, they must be administered with food.
2. This medication does not need to be administered with water to be effective.
3. **Lactase (Lactaid) is a gastrointestinal enzyme essential for absorbing lactose from the intestines. It must be taken with food.**
4. Vitamin D deficiency results from lack of milk and milk products in the diet. Lactaid is administered so the client can tolerate milk products, but it does not need to be given with vitamin D.

17. 1. Bismuth subcarbonate can darken and thicken the stool but is used primarily to decrease odor.
2. **Decreasing odor is the scientific rationale for administering bismuth subcarbonate to a client with an ileostomy.**
3. This medication does not affect the pH of the ileostomy output.
4. This medication does not coat the lining of the small intestine.

18. 1. Hydroxyzine (Atarax) is frequently prescribed for itching. This medication is being used as an antipruritic; therefore, decreased nausea does not indicate medication effectiveness.
2. Hydroxyzine (Atarax) is often prescribed for itching. This medication does not stimulate the appetite; therefore, appetite assessment does not determine medication effectiveness.
3. Atarax will cause drowsiness and is not administered to increase the client's cognitive ability.
4. **Hydroxyzine (Atarax) is frequently prescribed for itching. The client in end-stage liver disease often has jaundice, which causes pruritus (itching). A decrease in itching indicates the medication is effective.**

MEDICATION MEMORY JOGGER: The test taker must note the drug classification to determine medication effectiveness. Many medications are administered for different reasons, which changes their drug classification.

19. **Correct answers are 1 and 4.**
1. **Scopolamine (Transderm Scop) is a topical anticholinergic. The Transderm Scop patch is applied behind the ears.**
2. The patch can be left on for up to 3 days before changing, but it should not be alternated on and off.
3. The client should not wear two patches at one time because of the anticholinergic effect of the medication.
4. **The patch is effective for up to 3 days; therefore, the client understands the medication teaching.**
5. Transderm should indicate to the nurse the medication is a patch, not a pill to be taken with water.

20. 1. Rifaximin (Xifaxan) is an antibiotic used to treat IBS with diarrhea clinical manifestations. The medication is prescribed for a 2-week course. The nurse would administer the medication.
2. **The medication is administered for a 2-week course of antibiotic treatment, but no bowel movement for 5 to 6 days could indicate destruction of good bacteria. The nurse should hold the medication until the nurse and HCP can discuss the current situation.**
3. Diarrhea associated with the client's diagnosis of IBS is the reason for prescribing rifaximin (Xifaxan).
4. This is a true statement made by the client, but it does not contain any information that would cause the nurse to withhold the medication.

21. 1. Eluxadoline (Viberzi) is a mu-opioid receptor agonist that controls abdominal pain and diarrhea for clients diagnosed with IBS-D. There is no need to discuss this client with the HCP.
2. The nurse would discuss this client with the HCP only if the liver enzymes were higher than the normal range.

3. **Eluxadoline (Viberzi) is a mu-opioid receptor agonist that controls abdominal pain and diarrhea for clients diagnosed with IBS-D. It is a nonnarcotic Schedule IV medication taken twice a day orally. Clients with no gallbladder are at higher risk of developing acute pancreatitis when taking eluxadoline (Viberzi), which can be fatal. The nurse should discuss this situation with the HCP.**
4. Risk of developing acute pancreatitis increases if the client consumes three alcoholic drinks per day. One social drink in 2 to 3 months would not increase the risk of developing pancreatitis.

22. Correct order is 5, 2, 3, 4, 1.

5. **The client is concerned about bowel functioning. Adult clients want their concerns addressed first. The nurse should assess the stools' timing, consistency, and character before addressing any other potential issue. The client will feel the HCP is listening to their concerns.**
2. **Once the nurse has assessed the bowel movement, then they can move on to the issue that the client has already tried to treat. Many OTC remedies and information about the day-to-day treatment of constipation are available on the Internet, in books and magazines, and from persons willing to discuss a client's issues. Most adults will try to self-treat before consulting with a HCP.**
3. **An assessment of foods ingested over time will give the nurse information regarding how the client's diet is either helping the client or making the problem worse.**
4. **A lifestyle change, including increasing physical activity, assists with improving digestive health.**
1. **There are several new medications for chronic constipation in adults. Plecanatide (Trulance), linaclotide (Linzess), and lubiprostone (Amitiza). All may be prescribed for an adult client diagnosed with chronic constipation. These medications are not prescribed until lifestyle changes and other more common remedies have been tried. These medications are in new classifications of cyclase C agonist (Trulance and Linzess) and chloride channel activators (Amitiza).**

23. 1. **The client will be on an antibiotic and bezlotoxumab (Zinplava), a monoclonal antibody, to treat the *C difficile* infection. Bezlotoxumab (Zinplava) binds *C diff* in the gastrointestinal tract and eliminates it through the gut. It is helpful to prevent recurrence.**
2. The client will need to continue to be isolated due to the extreme infectious nature of *C diff*.
3. Bezlotoxumab (Zinplava) is administered IV.
4. There is no dietary restriction associated with bezlotoxumab (Zinplava).

6

Endocrine System

"Happiness" for some – Serotonin, Dopamine, Endorphins . . . for me – "You"

—Kevin Doherty

QUESTIONS

Type 1 Diabetes

1. The nurse administered 25 units of insulin isophane to a client diagnosed with type 1 diabetes at 1600. Which intervention should the nurse implement?
1. Assess the client for hypoglycemia around 1800.
2. Ensure the client eats the nighttime (HS) snack.
3. Check the client's serum blood glucose level.
4. Serve the supper tray to the client.

2. The nurse is teaching the client diagnosed with type 1 diabetes how to use an insulin pen injector. Which information should the nurse discuss with the client?
1. Instruct the client to dial in the number of insulin units needed to inject.
2. Demonstrate the proper way to draw up the insulin in an insulin syringe.
3. Discuss that the insulin pen injector must be used in the abdominal area only.
4. Explain that the traditional insulin syringe is less painful than the injector pen.

3. The nurse is teaching a client with newly diagnosed type 1 diabetes about insulin therapy. Which statements indicate the client **needs more teaching** concerning insulin therapy? **Select all that apply.**
1. "If I have a headache or start getting nervous, I will drink some orange juice."
2. "If I pass out at home, a family member should give me a glucagon injection."
3. "Because I am taking my insulin daily, I do not have to adhere to a diabetic diet."
4. "I will check my blood glucose with my glucometer at least once a day."
5. "I should administer my insulin in my abdomen for best absorption."

4. The nurse administered 12 units of regular insulin to the client diagnosed with type 1 diabetes at 0700. Which meal **prevents** the client from experiencing hypoglycemia?
1. Breakfast
2. Lunch
3. Supper
4. HS snack

5. The client diagnosed with type 1 diabetes is reporting a dry mouth, extreme thirst, and increased urination. For each intervention, specify if the intervention is **indicated or not indicated** for the client's care.

Potential Nursing Intervention	Indicated	Not Indicated
1. Administer one amp of IV 50% glucose.		
2. Prepare to administer IV regular insulin.		
3. Inject insulin isophane subcutaneously in the abdomen.		
4. Hang an IV infusion of D_5W at a keep open rate.		
5. Check the client's blood glucose level via a glucometer.		
6. Provide the client with orange juice to drink.		

6. The client newly diagnosed with type 1 diabetes asks the nurse, "Why should I get an external portable insulin pump?" Which statement is the nurse's **best** response?
1. "It will cause you to have fewer hypoglycemic reactions, and it will control blood glucose levels better."
2. "Insulin pumps provide an automatic memory of the date and time of the last 24 boluses."
3. "The pump injects intermediate-acting insulin automatically into the vein to maintain a normal blood glucose level."
4. "The portable pump is the easiest way to administer insulin to someone with type 1 diabetes and is highly recommended."

7. The nurse in the medical department is preparing to administer insulin lispro to a client diagnosed with type 1 diabetes. Which intervention should the nurse implement?
1. Ensure the client is wearing a MedicAlert bracelet.
2. Administer the dose according to the regular insulin sliding scale.
3. Assess the client for hyperosmolar, hyperglycemic, nonketotic coma.
4. Make sure the client eats the food on the bedside meal tray.

8. Which assessment data **best** indicates the client diagnosed with type 1 diabetes is adhering to the medical treatment regimen? The client's laboratory values are populated in the chart below.

Laboratory Test	Client Values	Reference Values
Glucose (Fasting)	100 mg/dL	Fasting: Less than 100 mg/dL Random: Less than 200 mg/dL
Glucose (Random)	120 mg/dL	Fasting: Less than 100 mg/dL Random: Less than 200 mg/dL
Glycosylated hemoglobin	5.8%	Less than 5.7%
Urinalysis pH Specific gravity Glucose Ketones Hemoglobin Leukocyte esterase	4.9 1.008 Negative Negative Negative Negative	pH 4.5 to 8 1.005 to 1.03 Negative Negative Negative Negative

1. Fasting blood glucose
2. Urinalysis
3. Glycosylated hemoglobin
4. Random blood glucose

9. The nurse is discussing insulin vial storage with the client. Which statement indicates the client **understands** the teaching concerning insulin storage?
   1. "I will keep my unopened vials of insulin in the refrigerator."
   2. "I can keep my insulin in the trunk of my car so that I will have it at all times."
   3. "It is all right to put my unopened insulin vials in the freezer."
   4. "If I prefill my insulin syringes, I must use them within 1 to 2 days."

10. Which statement **best** describes the pharmacodynamics of insulin?
    1. Insulin causes the pancreas to secrete glucose into the bloodstream.
    2. Insulin is metabolized by the liver and muscle and excreted in the urine.
    3. Insulin is needed to maintain colloidal osmotic pressure in the bloodstream.
    4. Insulin lowers blood glucose by promoting use of glucose in the body cells.

Type 2 Diabetes

11. The client diagnosed with type 2 diabetes is prescribed the medication glipizide. Which statement by the client **warrants intervention** by the nurse?
    1. "I have to eat my diabetic diet even if I am taking this medication."
    2. "I will need to check my blood glucose level at least once a day."
    3. "I usually have one glass of wine with my evening meal."
    4. "I do not like to walk every day, but I will if it will help my diabetes."

12. Which statement **best** describes the scientific rationale for prescribing metformin?
    1. This medication decreases insulin resistance, improving blood glucose control.
    2. This medication allows the carbohydrates to pass slowly through the large intestine.
    3. This medication will decrease the hepatic production of glucose from stored glycogen.
    4. This medication stimulates the beta cells to release more insulin into the bloodstream.

13. The nurse is discussing oral glyburide with the client diagnosed with type 2 diabetes. Which information should the nurse discuss with the client?
    1. Instruct the client to take the oral hypoglycemic medication with food.
    2. Explain that hypoglycemia will not occur with oral medications.
    3. Tell the client to notify the health-care provider (HCP) if a headache, nervousness, or sweating occurs.
    4. Recommend that the client check the ketones in the urine every morning.

14. The client diagnosed with type 2 diabetes is receiving the combination oral medication glyburide and metformin. Which data indicates the medication is **effective**?
    1. The client's skin turgor is elastic.
    2. The client's urine ketones are negative.
    3. The serum blood glucose level is 118 mg/dL (fasting).
    4. The client's glucometer level is 170 mg/dL (fasting).

15. The client diagnosed with type 2 diabetes is admitted into the medical department with a wound on the left leg that will not heal. The HCP prescribes sliding-scale insulin. The client tells the nurse, "I don't want to have to take shots. I take pills at home." Which statement is the nurse's **best** response?
    1. "If you can't keep your glucose under control with pills, you must take insulin."
    2. "You should discuss the insulin order with your HCP because you don't want to take it."
    3. "You are worried about having to take insulin. I will sit down, and we can talk."
    4. "During illness, you may need to take insulin to keep your blood glucose level down."

16. The nurse is caring for the client diagnosed with type 2 diabetes. The client is reporting a headache, jitteriness, and nervousness. For each intervention, specify if the intervention is **indicated or not indicated** for the client's care.

Potential Nursing Intervention	Indicated	Not Indicated
1. Check the client's serum blood glucose level.		
2. Give the client a glass of orange juice.		
3. Determine when the last antidiabetic medication was given.		
4. Assess the client's blood pressure and apical pulse.		
5. Administer prescribed insulin via sliding scale.		

17. The overweight client diagnosed with type 2 diabetes reports to the clinic nurse a 35-pound weight loss in the past 4 months. Which intervention should the nurse implement **first**?
1. Determine if the client has had an increase in hypoglycemic reactions.
2. Instruct the client to make an appointment with the HCP.
3. Ask the client if the weight loss is intentional or if it has happened naturally.
4. Check the client's last weight in the electronic health record (EHR) with the weight obtained in the clinic.

18. The client diagnosed with type 2 diabetes tells the clinic nurse about taking ginseng to help improve memory. Which intervention should the clinic nurse implement?
1. Take no action because ginseng does not affect type 2 diabetes.
2. Determine what type of memory deficits the client is experiencing.
3. Explain that herbs are dangerous and the client should not be taking them.
4. Determine if the client is currently taking any type of antidiabetic medication.

19. The school nurse is teaching a class about type 2 diabetes in children to elementary school teachers. Which information is **most** important for the nurse to discuss with the teachers?
1. The importance of not allowing students to eat candy in the classroom
2. An increase in the number of students developing type 2 diabetes
3. Clinical manifestations of hypoglycemia and immediate treatment
4. The need to have the students run or walk for 20 minutes during recess

20. The client newly diagnosed with type 2 diabetes and prescribed an oral hypoglycemic medication calls the clinic and tells the nurse that their sclera has a yellow color. Which intervention should the clinic nurse implement?
1. Ask the client if they have been exposed to someone with hepatitis.
2. Determine if the client has a history of alcohol use or is currently drinking alcohol.
3. Check to see if the client is taking digoxin.
4. Make an appointment for the client to come to the HCP's office.

Pancreatitis

21. The nurse is administering medications. Which medication should the nurse **question** administering?
1. Morphine sulfate to a client diagnosed with pancreatitis
2. Diphenhydramine to a client experiencing an allergic reaction
3. Methylprednisolone to a client diagnosed with type 2 diabetes
4. Vasopressin to a client diagnosed with diabetes insipidus (DI)

22. The nurse has received the morning report. Which medication should be administered **first**?
1. Levothyroxine to a client diagnosed with hypothyroidism
2. Pantoprazole to a client diagnosed with gastroesophageal reflux disease (GERD)
3. Acetaminophen to a client diagnosed with a migraine headache rated 7 on the pain scale
4. Pancreatin to a client diagnosed with chronic pancreatitis

23. The client diagnosed with chronic pancreatitis has a nasogastric tube attached to suction. The charge nurse observes the primary nurse instill a liquid antacid down the tube and then clamp the tube. Which action should the charge nurse take?
1. Tell the nurse to reconnect the tube to suction.
2. Notify the unit manager of the nurse's actions.
3. Do nothing because this is the correct procedure.
4. Instruct the nurse to administer the medication orally.

24. The HCP prescribed chlordiazepoxide for a 55-year-old client diagnosed with chronic pancreatitis. Which statement is the scientific rationale for prescribing this medication?
1. Chlordiazepoxide acts as an adjunct to pain medication.
2. Chlordiazepoxide limits complications related to alcohol withdrawal.
3. Chlordiazepoxide prevents nausea related to pancreatitis.
4. Chlordiazepoxide is used as a sleep aid for nothing-by-mouth (NPO) clients.

25. The client diagnosed with acute pancreatitis is reporting severe abdominal pain. For each intervention, specify if the intervention is **indicated or not indicated** for the client's care.

Potential Nursing Intervention	Indicated	Not Indicated
1. Ask the client to rate the pain on a 1 to 10 scale.		
2. Determine when the client received the last dose of medicine.		
3. Administer hydrocodone pain medicine.		
4. Assist the client to a semi-Fowler's position.		
5. Apply oxygen at 4 L/min via nasal cannula.		

26. The client diagnosed with acute pancreatitis is placed on total parenteral nutrition (TPN). Which interventions should the nurse implement? **Select all that apply.**
1. Monitor blood glucose levels every 6 hours.
2. Assess the peripheral IV site.
3. Check the client's complete blood count.
4. Check the TPN bag with the client's medication administration record (MAR).
5. Change the tubing with every new bag of TPN.

27. The nurse is administering pancreatic secretin to a client to rule out chronic pancreatitis. Which procedure should the nurse follow?
1. Have the client lie on the right side during medication administration.
2. Make sure the client has signed a permit for an investigational procedure.
3. Aspirate gastric and duodenal contents before and after the medication.
4. Place the client in the Trendelenburg position before beginning the medication.

28. Which intervention should be implemented when discharging a client diagnosed with chronic pancreatitis and receiving high doses of hydromorphone for the past 4 weeks?
1. Tell the client to monitor their stools and to avoid constipation.
2. Taper the medication slowly over several days before discharge.
3. Refer the client to a drug withdrawal clinic to stop taking the hydromorphone.
4. Discuss clinical manifestations of drug dependence to report to their HCP.

29. The client diagnosed with pancreatitis is prescribed octreotide. Which data indicates the medication has been **effective**?
1. The client reports that diarrhea has subsided.
2. The client states that they have grown 1 inch.
3. The client has no muscle cramping or pain.
4. The client has no report of heartburn.

30. The client diagnosed with pancreatitis is reporting polydipsia and polyuria. Which medication should the nurse prepare to administer?
1. Insulin lispro intravenously, and then monitor glucose levels
2. Pancrelipase sprinkled on the client's food with meals
3. Regular insulin subcutaneously after assessing the blood glucose level
4. Famotidine orally

Adrenal Disorders

31. The client diagnosed with Addison's disease is being discharged. Which statement indicates the client **needs more** discharge teaching?
1. "I will be sure to keep my dose of steroid constant and not vary."
2. "I may have to take two forms of steroids to remain healthy."
3. "I will get weak and dizzy if I don't take my medication."
4. "I need to notify any new HCP of the medications I take."

32. The client diagnosed with Cushing's disease is prescribed alendronate to prevent osteoporosis. For each intervention, specify if the intervention is **indicated or not indicated** for the client's care.

Potential Nursing Intervention	Indicated	Not Indicated
1. Take the medication and sit upright for 30 minutes.		
2. Take the medication just before going to bed.		
3. Take the medication with an antacid to alleviate gastric disturbances.		
4. Take the medication at least 30 minutes before breakfast.		
5. Take the medication with a full glass of water.		
6. Take the medication with coffee or orange juice.		

33. The client diagnosed with Cushing's disease is scheduled for a bilateral adrenalectomy. Which information regarding the prescribed prednisone should the nurse teach? **Select all that apply.**
1. When discontinuing this medication, it must be tapered.
2. Take the medication regularly; do not skip doses.
3. Stop taking the medication if you develop a round face.
4. Notify the HCP if you start feeling thirsty all the time.
5. Wear a MedicAlert bracelet in case of an emergency.

34. The emergency department nurse is caring for a client diagnosed with an Addisonian crisis. Which intervention should the nurse implement **first**?
1. Draw serum electrolyte levels.
2. Administer methylprednisolone IV.
3. Start an 18-gauge catheter with normal saline.
4. Ask the client what medications they are taking.

35. The client diagnosed with Cushing's disease is prescribed pantoprazole. Which statement is the scientific rationale for prescribing this medication?
 1. Pantoprazole increases the client's ability to digest food.
 2. Pantoprazole decreases the excess amounts of gastric acid.
 3. Pantoprazole absorbs gastric acid and eliminates it in the bowel.
 4. Pantoprazole coats the stomach and prevents ulcer formation.

36. The client is diagnosed with Cushing's syndrome as a result of long-term steroid therapy. Which assessment findings **support** this condition?
 1. The client has dyspnea on exertion and has pale mucous membranes.
 2. The client has a round face and multiple ecchymotic areas on the arms.
 3. The client has pink, frothy sputum and jugular vein distention.
 4. The client has petechiae on the trunk and sclerosed veins.

37. The client is diagnosed with Cushing's syndrome due to ectopic production of adrenocorticotropic hormone (ACTH) by a bronchogenic tumor. Which medication should the nurse anticipate the HCP prescribing?
 1. Ketoconazole
 2. Methylprednisolone
 3. Propylthiouracil
 4. Vasopressin

38. The client diagnosed with iatrogenic Cushing's disease calls the clinic nurse and reports a temperature of 100.1°F (37.8°C). Which intervention should the nurse implement?
 1. Tell the client to take acetaminophen and drink liquids.
 2. Instruct the client to come to the clinic for an antibiotic.
 3. Have the client go to the nearest emergency department.
 4. Encourage the client to discuss their feelings about the disease.

39. The client diagnosed with Addison's disease asks the nurse, "Why do I have to take fludrocortisone?" Which statement is the nurse's **best** response?
 1. "It will keep you from getting high blood sugars."
 2. "Fludrocortisone helps the body retain sodium."
 3. "Fludrocortisone prevents muscle cramping."
 4. "It stimulates the pituitary gland to secrete adrenocorticotropic hormone."

40. The client admitted with primary adrenal insufficiency provides the nurse with a list of home medications. The client's medications are populated in the chart below.

John D. Medication List

Medication	Time Taken
Prednisone	Before breakfast
Ginseng	Before breakfast
Mitotane	Before breakfast
Testosterone	At night

Which medication should the nurse **question**?
 1. Prednisone
 2. Ginseng
 3. Mitotane
 4. Testosterone

Pituitary Disorders

41. The client diagnosed with DI is prescribed desmopressin. Which comorbid condition **warrants** a **change** in medication?
1. Renal calculi
2. Type 2 diabetes
3. Sinusitis
4. Hyperthyroidism

42. The client diagnosed with a pituitary tumor has enlarged viscera and bone deformities. Which medication should the nurse administer?
1. Octreotide
2. Somatrem
3. Ketorolac
4. Corticotropin

43. The client diagnosed with DI is admitted in acute distress. Which interventions should the nurse implement? **Select all that apply.**
1. Start an IV with lactated Ringer's solution.
2. Insert an indwelling catheter.
3. Monitor the urine-specific gravity.
4. Administer furosemide IV push (IVP).
5. Assess the intake and output every shift.

44. The client diagnosed with mild DI is prescribed chlorpropamide. Which discharge instruction should the nurse teach the client?
1. Discontinue the medication if feeling dizzy.
2. Chew sugarless gum to alleviate dry mouth.
3. Take the medication before meals.
4. Discuss clinical manifestations of an insulin reaction.

45. The 30-year-old client is prescribed chorionic gonadotropin. Which intervention should the nurse implement?
1. Have the laboratory draw a follicle-stimulating hormone (FSH) level every week.
2. Schedule regular pelvic sonograms.
3. Discuss not becoming pregnant while taking this drug.
4. Teach to take the medication with food.

46. The HCP ordered furosemide for a client diagnosed with syndrome of inappropriate antidiuretic hormone (SIADH). The client's serum laboratory values are populated in the chart below.

Laboratory Test	Client Values	Reference Values
Sodium	135 mEq/L	135 to 145 mEq/L or mmol/L
Potassium	3.5 mEq/L	3.5 to 5.3 mEq/L or mmol/L
Creatinine	1.0 mg/dL	Male: 0.61 to 1.21 mg/dL Female: 0.51 to 1.11 mg/dL
Adrenocorticotropic hormone (ACTH)	20 pg/mL	Male: 7 to 69 pg/mL Female: 6 to 58 pg/mL

Which laboratory test would be monitored to determine the medication **effectiveness**?
1. Sodium levels
2. Potassium levels
3. Creatinine levels
4. Adrenocorticotropic hormone levels

47. Which medication should the nurse administer to the client diagnosed with nephrogenic DI?
1. Clofibrate
2. Ibuprofen
3. Furosemide
4. Desmopressin

48. The client diagnosed with Hodgkin's disease is prescribed vincristine. Since the last treatment, the client reports the inability to fit into their rings and most shoes because of weight gain. Which intervention should the nurse implement **first**?
1. Administer a diuretic before the vincristine to prevent fluid overload.
2. Monitor the client for findings of infection.
3. Discuss a low-sodium diet with the client.
4. Weigh the client and report the findings to the oncologist.

49. The nurse is administering morning medications. Which medication should the nurse **question**?
1. Black cohosh to a client diagnosed with dysmenorrhea and cramping
2. Desmopressin to a client diagnosed with DI and angina
3. Hydrochlorothiazide to a client diagnosed with syndrome of inappropriate antidiuretic hormone secretion from a head injury
4. Calcitonin to a client diagnosed with hypercalcemia from lung cancer

Thyroid Disorders

50. The client diagnosed with hypothyroidism is prescribed levothyroxine. Which assessment data supports the client's **need** to take **more** medication? **Select all that apply.**
1. The client has a 2-kg weight loss.
2. The client reports being too cold.
3. The client has exophthalmos.
4. The client's radial pulse rate is 90 beats per minute (bpm).
5. The client reports being constipated.

51. Which complication should the nurse assess for in the elderly client newly diagnosed with hypothyroidism and prescribed levothyroxine?
1. Cardiac dysrhythmias
2. Respiratory depression
3. Paralytic ileus
4. Thyroid storm

52. The client diagnosed with hyperthyroidism is administered radioactive iodine (I-131). Which intervention should the nurse implement?
1. Explain that the medication will eradicate the thyroid gland completely.
2. Instruct the client to avoid close contact with children for 1 week.
3. Discuss the need to take the medication at night for 7 days.
4. Administer the radioactive iodine in 8 ounces of cold orange juice.

53. The client diagnosed with hyperthyroidism is prescribed propylthiouracil (PTU). The client's laboratory values are populated in the chart below.

Laboratory Test	Client Results	Reference Values
Arterial blood gases: pH PCO_2 HCO_3 PO_2 O_2 saturation	 7.35 35 22 80 95	 7.35 to 7.45 35 to 45 mm Hg 22 to 26 mmol/L 80 to 95 mm Hg 95% to 99%
Potassium	3.7 mEq/L	3.5 to 5.3 mEq/L or mmol/L
Red blood cell count (RBC)	4.3 (10^6 cells/ microL)	Male: 4.21 to 5.81 (10^6 cells/ microL) Female: 3.61 to 5.11 (10^6 cells/ microL)
White blood cell count (WBC)	4.5 x 10^3/microL	4.5 to 11.1 × 10^3/microL

Which laboratory data should the nurse monitor?
1. Arterial blood gases (ABGs)
2. Serum potassium level
3. Red blood cell (RBC) count
4. White blood cell (WBC) count

54. The nurse is preparing to administer liothyronine to a client diagnosed with hypothyroidism. Which data should cause the nurse to **question** administering the medication?
1. The client reports being nervous.
2. The client's oral temperature is 98.9°F (37.1°C).
3. The client's blood pressure is 110/70.
4. The client reports being tired.

55. The nurse is discussing levothyroxine with the client diagnosed with hypothyroidism. For each intervention, specify if the intervention is **indicated or not indicated** for the client's care.

Potential Nursing Intervention	Indicated	Not Indicated
1. Encourage the client to decrease the fiber in the diet.		
2. Discuss the need to monitor the T3, T4 levels daily.		
3. Tell the client to take the medication with food only.		
4. Instruct the client to report any significant weight changes.		
5. Discuss the importance of not using iodized salt.		
6. Explain the importance of not taking medication with grapefruit juice.		
7. Instruct the client to take the medication in the morning.		
8. Teach the client to monitor daily glucose levels.		

56. The client diagnosed with hyperthyroidism is administered radioactive iodine, I-131, and tells the nurse, "I don't think the medication is working. I don't feel any different." Which statement is the nurse's **best** response?

1. "You should notify your HCP immediately."
2. "You may need to have two or three more doses of the medication."
3. "It may take up to several months to get the full benefits of the treatment."
4. "You don't feel any different. Would you like to sit down and talk about it?"

57. The client diagnosed with hyperthyroidism is prescribed propylthiouracil (PTU). Which statement by the client **warrants immediate** intervention by the nurse?

1. "I seem to be drowsy and sleepy all the time."
2. "I have a sore throat and have had a fever."
3. "I have gained 2 pounds since I started taking PTU."
4. "Since taking PTU, I am not as hot as I used to be."

58. The client diagnosed with hyperthyroidism is prescribed an antithyroid medication. Which interventions should the nurse implement? **Select all that apply.**

1. Monitor the client's thyroid function tests.
2. Monitor the client's weight weekly.
3. Monitor the client for gastrointestinal distress.
4. Monitor the client's vital signs.
5. Monitor the client for activity intolerance.

ANSWERS AND RATIONALES

The correct answer number and rationale are in **boldface blue type.** Rationales for why other answer options are incorrect are also given.

Type 1 Diabetes

1. 1. Insulin isophane (Humulin N) is an intermediate-acting insulin that peaks 6 to 8 hours after administration; therefore, the client would experience findings of hypoglycemia around 2200 to 2400.
2. The nurse needs to ensure the client eats the nighttime (HS) snack to help prevent nighttime hypoglycemia.
3. A serum blood glucose level would have to be done with a venipuncture and the blood sample must be taken to the laboratory. If the client needs the blood glucose checked, it should be done with a glucometer at the bedside.
4. The supper tray would not help prevent a hypoglycemic reaction because the insulin isophane Humulin N is an intermediate-acting insulin that peaks in 6 to 8 hours.

2. 1. The insulin pen injector resembles a fountain pen. It contains a disposable needle and insulin-filled cartridge. When the client operates the insulin pen, the correct dose is obtained by dialing the number of insulin units needed.
2. The insulin pen injector does not require drawing up insulin in a syringe.
3. The insulin pen injector can be used in any subcutaneous site where traditional insulin can be injected.
4. Most clients state that there is less injection pain associated with the insulin pen than there is with the traditional insulin syringe.

3. Correct answer is 3.
1. Headache, nervousness, sweating, tremors, and rapid pulse are findings of a hypoglycemic reaction and should be treated with a simple-acting carbohydrate, such as orange juice, sugar-containing drinks, and hard candy. This statement indicates the client understands the teaching.
2. If a client cannot drink or eat a simple carbohydrate for hypoglycemia, then the client should receive a glucagon injection to treat the hypoglycemic reaction. This indicates the client understands the teaching.
3. Even with insulin therapy, the client should adhere to the American Diabetic Association diet (2021), which recommends "carbohydrate counting." This statement indicates the client needs more teaching.
4. Monitoring and documenting the blood glucose level is encouraged to determine the effectiveness of the treatment regimen. This indicates the client understands the teaching.
5. The abdominal area best absorbs insulin; therefore, the client does not need more teaching.

4. 1. Regular insulin peaks in 2 to 4 hours; therefore, the breakfast meal would prevent the client from developing hypoglycemia.
2. Lunch would cover an 0700 dose of insulin isophane, intermediate-acting insulin, not regular insulin.
3. Supper would cover a 1600 dose of regular insulin, short-acting insulin.
4. The HS (nighttime) snack would cover a 1600 dose of insulin isophane, intermediate-acting insulin, not regular insulin.

5.

Potential Nursing Intervention	Indicated	Not Indicated
1. Administer one amp of IV 50% glucose.		X
2. Prepare to administer IV regular insulin.	X	
3. Inject insulin isophane subcutaneously in the abdomen.		X
4. Hang an IV infusion of D_5W at a keep open rate.		X
5. Check the client's blood glucose level via a glucometer.	X	
6. Provide the client with orange juice to drink.		X

1. **One amp of 50% glucose would be used to treat a severe hypoglycemic reaction, and this client does not have clinical manifestations that indicate hypoglycemia. The client has clinical manifestations of hyperglycemia.**
2. **The client's clinical manifestations indicate the client is experiencing diabetic ketoacidosis (DKA), which is treated with regular IV insulin.**
3. **Insulin isophane, intermediate-acting insulin, is not used to treat hyperglycemia.**
4. **An IV of D_5W would cause the client to have further clinical manifestations of DKA; therefore, the nurse should not administer the IV infusion.**
5. **These are clinical manifestations of DKA; therefore, checking the client's blood glucose level is appropriate.**
6. **The client's clinical manifestations indicate DKA, not hypoglycemia, which could be treated with orange juice.**

6. 1. **A portable insulin pump is a battery-operated device that uses rapid-acting insulin—Lispro, Humalog, or NovoLog. It delivers basal insulin infusion (continuous release of a small amount of insulin) and bolus doses with meals. This provides fewer hypoglycemic reactions and better blood glucose levels.**
2. The pumps provide a memory of boluses, but that is not the nurse's best response to explain why a client should get an external portable insulin pump.
3. External portable insulin pumps are only used to deliver rapid-acting insulin subcutaneously. Intermediate and long-acting insulins are not used with an external portable insulin pump because of unpredictable blood glucose control.
4. The insulin pump is not recommended as the initial way to administer insulin because success depends on the client's knowledge and compliance. Initially, most clients start injecting insulin with a syringe and then graduate to the pumps.

7. 1. Because the client is in the hospital, the client must have a hospital identification band. A MedicAlert bracelet would be needed when the client is not in the hospital.
2. Insulin lispro (Humalog) is not regular insulin; it is fast-acting insulin. It is not administered according to the regular insulin sliding scale. The peak time for insulin lispro is 30 minutes to 1 hour—regular insulin peaks in 2 to 4 hours.
3. A client diagnosed with type 1 diabetes will experience DKA. A client diagnosed with type 2 diabetes will experience hyperosmolar, hyperglycemic, nonketotic coma.
4. **Insulin lispro (Humalog) peaks in 30 minutes to 1 hour; therefore, the client needs to eat when—or shortly after—the medication is administered to prevent hypoglycemia.**

MEDICATION MEMORY JOGGER: Remember that different types of insulin peak at different times, and the nurse must be knowledgeable about peak times to ensure that the client does not experience hypoglycemia. Only the insulin product insulin glargine (Lantus) has no peak time.

8. 1. The fasting blood glucose level is obtained after the client is NPO for 8 hours. Fasting glucose should be less than 100 mg/dL. This blood result does not indicate adherence to the treatment regimen.
2. If the client has no ketones in the urine, it indicates that the body is not breaking down fat for energy, but it does not indicate adherence to the treatment regimen.
3. **A glycosylated hemoglobin (A_1c) gives a blood glucose level average over the past 3 months and indicates adherence to the medical treatment regimen. A glycosylated hemoglobin level of 5.8% is close to normal and indicates that the client is adhering to the treatment regimen. The following table shows blood glucose levels and corresponding glycosylated hemoglobin results:**

Blood Glucose Level	Glycosylated Hemoglobin Result
70 to 110	4.0% to 5.5% normal
135	6%
170	7%
205	8%
240	9%
275	10%
310	11%
345	12%

4. A glucometer reading of 120 mg/dL indicates a normal random blood glucose level (less than 200 mg/dL), but it is a one-time reading. It does not indicate adherence to the medical treatment regimen.

9. 1. This statement indicates the client understands the medication teaching. Keeping insulin in the refrigerator will maintain the insulin's strength and potency. Once the insulin vial is opened, it may be kept at room temperature for 1 month.

2. Insulin vials should not be placed in direct sunlight or in a high-temperature area, such as a car trunk, because it will lose its strength.
3. Insulin should not be kept in the freezer because freezing will cause the insulin to break down and lose its effectiveness.
4. Prefilled syringes should be stored in the refrigerator and should be used within 1 to 2 weeks, not 1 to 2 days.

10. 1. The pancreas does not secrete glucose. It secretes insulin, which is the key that opens the door to allow glucose to enter the body cells. Glucose enters the body through the gastrointestinal system.

2. This statement explains insulin pharmacokinetics and how the body metabolizes and excretes urine. Pharmacokinetics is the process of drug movement to achieve drug interaction.
3. Insulin does not maintain colloidal osmotic pressure. Albumin, a product of protein, maintains colloidal osmotic pressure.
4. **This statement explains pharmacodynamics, which is the drug's mechanism of action or how the body uses insulin. Over time, elevated glucose levels in the bloodstream can cause long-term complications, including nephropathy, retinopathy, and neuropathy. Insulin lowers blood glucose by promoting use of glucose in body cells.**

Type 2 Diabetes

11. 1. Glipizide (Glucotrol) is a sulfonylurea that stimulates the pancreas to secrete more insulin. The client diagnosed with type 2 diabetes must adhere to the prescribed diet to help keep the blood glucose level within the normal range. Delaying or missing a meal can cause hypoglycemia. This statement would not warrant intervention by the nurse.

2. Glipizide (Glucotrol) is a sulfonylurea that stimulates the pancreas to secrete more insulin. The client should check blood glucose levels to determine if the medication is effective; therefore, this statement would not warrant intervention by the nurse.
3. **Glipizide (Glucotrol) is a sulfonylurea that stimulates the pancreas to secrete more insulin. Sulfonylureas and biguanides may cause an Antabuse-like reaction when taken with alcohol, causing the client to become nauseated and vomit. Advise the client to abstain from alcohol and to avoid liquid over-the-counter (OTC) medications that may contain alcohol. Alcohol also increases the half-life of the medication and can cause a hypoglycemic reaction.**
4. The client diagnosed with type 2 diabetes does not need to walk daily to keep the glucose level within normal limits. Walking three times a week will help control stress and help decrease weight if the client is overweight.

12. 1. Metformin (Glucophage) is a biguanide that works to prevent gluconeogenesis in the liver. A thiazolidinedione, pioglitazone (Actos), or rosiglitazone (Avandia), not a biguanide-like metformin, is prescribed to decrease insulin resistance.

2. Metformin (Glucophage) is a biguanide that works to prevent gluconeogenesis in the liver. An alpha-glucosidase inhibitor, acarbose (Precose) or miglitol (Glyset), is administered to allow carbohydrates to pass slowly through the intestine. Glucophage does not do this.
3. **Metformin (Glucophage) is a biguanide that works to prevent gluconeogenesis in the liver. The scientific rationale for administering metformin (Glucophage) is that it diminishes the increase in serum glucose after a meal and blunts the degree of postprandial hyperglycemia by preventing gluconeogenesis.**
4. A meglitinide, repaglinide (Prandin), sulfonylurea, or nateglinide (Starlix) is prescribed to stimulate the beta cells to release more insulin into the bloodstream.

13. 1. Glyburide (Micronase) is a sulfonylurea that stimulates the pancreatitis to secrete more insulin. The oral hypoglycemic medication should be administered with food to decrease gastric upset.

2. Clients receiving oral hypoglycemic medications can experience hypoglycemic reactions, as can clients receiving insulin.
3. These are clinical manifestations of hypoglycemia, and the client should be able to treat this without notifying the HCP.

4. Ketones are a byproduct of fats breaking down, which usually does not occur in clients diagnosed with type 2 diabetes because the client has enough insulin to prevent the breakdown but not enough to keep the blood glucose level within an acceptable level.

14. 1. An elastic skin turgor is expected and normal, but it does not indicate that the antidiabetic medication is effective.
2. Urine ketones should be negative because there should not be a fat breakdown in clients diagnosed with type 2 diabetes, but this does not indicate the medication's effectiveness.
3. **Glyburide and metformin (Glucovance) contain sulfonylurea and a biguanide. The serum blood glucose level should be within normal limits, less than 100 mg/dL (fasting). A 118 mg/dL is close to normal; therefore, the medication can be considered effective.**
4. A self-monitoring blood glucose level of 170 mg/dL (fasting) is above a normal glucose level. This indicates the medication is not effective.

MEDICATION MEMORY JOGGER: The nurse determines a medication's effectiveness by assessing for the symptoms, or lack thereof, for which the medication was prescribed.

15. 1. During illness, the client diagnosed with type 2 diabetes may need insulin to help keep glucose levels under control, but this is a threatening type of statement and is not the nurse's best response.
2. Insulin may need to be prescribed in times of stress, surgery, or serious infection; therefore, the nurse should explain this to the client and not refer the client to the HCP.
3. This is a therapeutic response, and the client needs to have factual information. Therapeutic responses are used to encourage the client to verbalize feelings.
4. **Blood glucose levels elevate during times of stress, surgery, or serious infection. The client diagnosed with type 2 diabetes may need to be given insulin temporarily to help keep the blood glucose level within normal limits.**

16.

Potential Nursing Intervention	Indicated	Not Indicated
1. Check the client's serum blood glucose level.	X	
2. Give the client a glass of orange juice.	X	
3. Determine when the last antidiabetic medication was given.	X	
4. Assess the client's blood pressure and apical pulse.	X	
5. Administer prescribed insulin via sliding scale.		X

1. **The client's serum blood glucose level is checked by drawing a venipuncture blood sample and sending it to the laboratory. This is an appropriate nursing intervention.**
2. **The client is experiencing a hypoglycemic reaction, and the nurse must treat the client by administering simple-acting glucose. This is the first intervention.**
3. **Determining when the last oral hypoglycemic medication was administered is an appropriate intervention.**
4. **The nurse should assess the client's vital signs in any abnormal situation, but these clinical manifestations address diabetes.**
5. **Insulin should be administered if the client is hyperglycemic, not hypoglycemic.**

MEDICATION MEMORY JOGGER: When answering test questions or caring for clients at bedside, the nurse should remember that assessing the client might not be the first action to take when the client is in distress. The nurse may need to intervene directly to help the client.

17. **1. Changes in weight will affect the amount of medication needed to control blood glucose. The nurse should determine if the client's medication dose is too high by determining if the client has increased hypoglycemic reactions. This is the nurse's first intervention.**
2. A significant weight loss may require a decrease or discontinuation of oral hypoglycemic medication. Still, the nurse should first determine if the client has had symptoms of hypoglycemia before referring them to the HCP.
3. Determining if the client was deliberately losing weight or was losing without trying is significant because a 35-pound weight loss in 4 months would warrant intervention, depending on what caused the weight loss. However, this should not be the nurse's first intervention.
4. The nurse should confirm the client's weight loss with the clinic scale and the last weight in the client's EHR, but it is not the clinic nurse's first intervention.

MEDICATION MEMORY JOGGER: Remember that the first step in the nursing process is assessment. Words such as *check*, *monitor*, *determine*, *ask*, *take*, *auscultate*, and *palpate* indicate that the nurse is assessing the client. Before implementing an independent nursing action or notifying the HCP, assessment should be done, except in certain serious or life-threatening situations.

18. 1. The nurse should investigate any herb the client is taking because most herbs affect a disease process or the medication being taken for the disease process.
2. The nurse should determine if ginseng affects the client's type 2 diabetes or medications that the client is taking for the disease process.
3. This is a negative, judgmental statement. Many herbs are beneficial to the client. Before making this type of statement, the nurse should always assess the client and determine if the herb is detrimental to the client's disease process or affects the client's routine medication regimen.
4. **The nurse should determine if the client is taking any medication because many oral hypoglycemics interact with herbs. Ginseng and garlic may increase the hypoglycemic effects of oral hypoglycemics.**

MEDICATION MEMORY JOGGER: Some herbal preparations are effective, some are not, and a few can be harmful or even deadly. If a client is taking an herbal supplement and conventional medicine, the nurse should investigate to determine if the herbal preparation would cause harm to the client. The nurse should always be the client's advocate.

19. 1. Students with type 2 diabetes should not eat candy, but this is not the most important intervention for the school nurse to teach.
2. This is pertinent information, but it is not the most important information.
3. **The most important information for teachers to know is how to treat potentially life-threatening complications secondary to the medications used to treat type 2 diabetes. The school nurse should discuss issues that keep the students safe.**
4. Exercise is important in helping to control type 2 diabetes, but empowering the teachers to be confident when handling complications secondary to medication is the priority for students' safety.

20. 1. Jaundiced sclera may indicate the client has hepatitis, but because the client has been prescribed oral hypoglycemic medications, their possible role in developing jaundice should be assessed.
2. The nurse should not jump to the conclusion that the client is an alcoholic just because the sclera is jaundiced.
3. Digoxin toxicity results in the client seeing a yellow haze, not the client's sclera being yellow.
4. **Oral hypoglycemics are metabolized in the liver and may cause elevations in liver enzymes. The client should be instructed to report the first findings of yellow skin, sclera, pale stools, or dark urine to the HCP.**

Pancreatitis

21. **1. Morphine can cause spasms of the pancreatic ducts and the sphincter of Oddi; therefore, the nurse would question administering this medication. Many clients can tolerate morphine, but if the client experiences abdominal pain soon after a dose of morphine, then the medication should be changed.**
2. Diphenhydramine (Benadryl) is a histamine$_1$ blocker that blocks the release of histamine$_1$ that occurs during allergic reactions. The nurse would not question this medication.

3. Methylprednisolone (Solu-Medrol) is a steroid. Clients diagnosed with type 2 diabetes may at times need steroid medication. The medication may elevate the client's glucose levels; these levels should be monitored. The nurse would not question this medication.
4. Vasopressin is the hormone lacking in clients diagnosed with DI. Desmopressin (DDAVP) is the treatment for DI. The nurse would not question administering this medication.

MEDICATION MEMORY JOGGER: The nurse must be knowledgeable about accepted standards of practice for disease processes and conditions. If the nurse administers a medication the HCP has prescribed, and it harms the client, the nurse could be held accountable. Remember, the nurse is a client advocate.

22. 1. Levothyroxine (Synthroid), a thyroid replacement hormone, is a daily medication that can be administered at any time.
2. Pantoprazole (Protonix), a proton-pump inhibitor (PPI), is a daily medication that can be administered at any time.
3. Acetaminophen (Tylenol), a nonnarcotic analgesic, is for mild to moderate pain. This client would require a more potent analgesic. The nurse should assess the client's medications and discuss other medications with the HCP. This would not be the first medication to administer.
4. Pancreatin (Donnazyme) is a pancreatic enzyme. Pancreatic enzymes are administered with every meal and snack. The nurse should administer this medication so the medication and breakfast foods simultaneously arrive in the small intestine.

23. 1. The nurse is following the correct procedure for administering medications through a nasogastric tube that is connected to suction. The tube should remain clamped for 1 hour before it is reconnected to suction.
2. The nurse followed the correct procedure. There is no reason to notify the manager.
3. The nurse is following the correct procedure for administering medications through a nasogastric tube that is connected to suction. The tube should remain clamped for 1 hour before it is reconnected to suction to allow the medication to be absorbed.
4. The medication is ordered to be administered through the tube, not orally.

24. 1. The chlordiazepoxide (Librium), a sedative-hypnotic, may be an adjunct to pain relief, but this is not the reason for prescribing the medication to this client.
2. The chlordiazepoxide (Librium), a sedative-hypnotic, is helpful in preventing delirium tremens for clients withdrawing from alcohol. Most clients diagnosed with chronic pancreatitis (75%) are middle-aged males diagnosed with chronic alcoholism.
3. The chlordiazepoxide (Librium), a sedative-hypnotic, may have some antiemetic properties, but this is not the reason for prescribing the medication to this client.
4. The chlordiazepoxide (Librium), a sedative-hypnotic, can cause drowsiness, but it is not the drug of choice as a sleep aid for an NPO client.

25.

Potential Nursing Intervention	Indicated	Not Indicated
1. Ask the client to rate the pain on a 1 to 10 scale.	X	
2. Determine when the client received the last dose of medicine.	X	
3. Administer hydrocodone pain medicine.		X
4. Assist the client to a semi-Fowler's position.	X	
5. Apply oxygen at 4 L/min via nasal cannula.		X

1. Clients should be asked to rate their pain on a scale so the nurse can objectively evaluate the effectiveness of interventions.
2. The nurse abides by the rights of medication administration, including the right time. Pain medication is prescribed at specific time intervals. The nurse must make sure the time interval has passed, and it is time for more medication.
3. A client diagnosed with severe acute pancreatitis will be NPO. Hydrocodone is an oral narcotic medication. The nurse would administer an IV medication.

4. **The client should be placed in a semi-Fowler's position to relieve pressure on the abdomen, thereby decreasing the client's pain.**
5. **There is no indication that the client requires oxygenation at this time.**

26. Correct answers are 1, 4, and 5.
1. **Blood glucose levels should be monitored every 4 to 6 hours.**
2. TPN requires a central line for administration, not a peripheral line. The high concentration of dextrose in TPN causes phlebitis in peripheral veins.
3. The client's electrolytes and magnesium levels are monitored, not the complete blood count.
4. **The TPN bag prepared by the pharmacy should be checked with the MAR to ensure the HCP's prescription is correct.**
5. **The TPN solution contains all required nutrients to sustain life. It also makes an ideal medium for bacterial growth. Infection control safety measures include using new tubing with every bag of TPN.**

27. 1. The client will be in a Fowler's or semi-Fowler's position to use gravity to pool secretions near the gastric duodenal tube.
2. This is not an investigational procedure. The general treatment permission form that the client signed when entering the hospital is sufficient.
3. **Gastric and duodenal contents are aspirated and sent to the laboratory for analysis before and after administration of pancreatic secretin, a pancreas secretory hormone that stimulates the pancreas to secrete enzymes.**
4. The client is not placed in a head-down position for this procedure.

28. 1. The nurse should have been monitoring the client for constipation while in the hospital. The client should not be discharged on hydromorphone.
2. **To prevent withdrawal after weeks of administration of hydromorphone (Dilaudid), a narcotic opioid, the client should be tapered off the medication over several days.**
3. The client should be tapered off the medication before leaving the hospital, not sent to a drug withdrawal center.
4. Withdrawal from the medication should be accomplished before discharging the client, so withdrawal symptoms should occur while the client is still in the hospital.

29. 1. Octreotide (Sandostatin), a hormone, stimulates fluid and electrolyte absorption from the gastrointestinal tract and prolongs intestinal transit time, thereby decreasing diarrhea.
2. Octreotide (Sandostatin), a hormone, is prescribed for clients diagnosed with acromegaly to prevent growth, not stimulate it.
3. Octreotide (Sandostatin), a hormone, helps prevent or treat diarrhea and associated abdominal pain, but not muscle cramping or pain.
4. Octreotide (Sandostatin), a hormone, does not treat acid reflux.

MEDICATION MEMORY JOGGER: The nurse determines medication effectiveness by assessing for the symptoms, or lack thereof, for which medication was prescribed.

30. 1. Insulin lispro (Humalog) is not administered intravenously, and glucose levels should be monitored before insulin administration.
2. Pancrelipase (Cotazym) is a pancreatic replacement hormone. The client's symptoms should indicate hyperglycemia to the nurse, not pancreatic enzyme deficiency.
3. **Regular insulin (Humulin R) is administered by a sliding scale to decrease blood glucose levels. Clients diagnosed with pancreatitis should be monitored for development of diabetes mellitus. Polydipsia and polyuria are classic findings of diabetes mellitus.**
4. Famotidine (Pepcid) is a histamine$_1$ blocker. It would not treat the client's symptoms.

Adrenal Disorders

31. 1. The corticosteroid dose may have to be increased during the stress of infection or surgery. It is imperative that under these circumstances, the client receives enough medication to replicate the body's responses to stress (see Table 6-1).
2. The client usually will need to take mineral and glucocorticoid replacement therapy. This statement does not need more teaching.
3. The client will experience symptoms of adrenal insufficiency if not taking the medications. This statement does not need more teaching.
4. Clients should be taught to inform all HCPs of prescribed and OTC medications that they are taking. This statement does not need more teaching.

Table 6-1. Guidelines for Giving Supplemental Doses of Glucocorticoids at Times of Stress Related to Medical Conditions and Surgical Procedures

Medical Condition or Surgical Procedure	Supplemental Glucocorticoid Dosage
MINOR	
Inguinal hernia repair Colonoscopy Mild febrile illness Mild to moderate nausea and vomiting Gastroenteritis	25 mg of hydrocortisone (or 5 mg of methylprednisolone) IV on day of procedure
MODERATE	
Open cholecystectomy Hemicolectomy Significant febrile illness Pneumonia Severe gastroenteritis	50 to 75 mg of hydrocortisone (or 10 to 15 mg of methylprednisolone) IV on day of the procedure Taper quickly over 1 to 2 days to usual replacement dose
SEVERE	
Major cardiothoracic surgery Whipple procedure Liver resection Pancreatitis	100 to 150 mg of hydrocortisone (or 20 to 30 mg of methylprednisolone) IV on day of procedure Rapid taper over 1 to 2 days to usual replacement dose
CRITICAL	
Sepsis-induced hypotension or shock	50 to 100 mg of hydrocortisone IV every 6 to 8 hours (or 0.18 mg/kg/hr as continuous infusion) plus 50 mg of fludrocortisone until shock resolves, which may take several days to a week or more. Then, taper gradually, monitoring vital signs and serum sodium levels.

From Lehne, R. (2016). *Pharmacology for Nursing Care*. Elsevier.

32.

Potential Nursing Intervention	Indicated	Not Indicated
1. Take the medication and sit upright for 30 minutes.	X	
2. Take the medication just before going to bed.		X
3. Take the medication with an antacid to alleviate gastric disturbances.		X
4. Take the medication at least 30 minutes before breakfast.	X	
5. Take the medication with a full glass of water.	X	
6. Take the medication with coffee or orange juice.		X

1. **The client should remain in an upright position for at least 30 minutes after taking alendronate (Fosamax), a bisphosphonate regulator, to prevent esophageal erosion and ulceration.**
2. **The medication is taken first thing in the morning when the stomach is empty. Taking alendronate (Fosamax), a bisphosphonate regulator, and then lying down would cause esophageal reflux, resulting in esophagus erosion and ulceration.**

3. **An antacid will interfere with Fosamax absorption.**
4. **Alendronate (Fosamax) is a bisphosphonate regulator. The medication should be taken at least 30 minutes before food or fluid is consumed for the day to prevent esophageal erosion and ulceration.**
5. **The client should drink a full glass of water with the medication and remain in an upright position for at least 30 minutes after taking alendronate (Fosamax), a bisphosphonate regulator, to prevent esophageal erosion and ulceration.**
6. **The medication should not be taken with mineral water, orange juice, or coffee as these beverages decrease medication absorption.**

33. Correct answers are 2, 4, and 5.
1. The medication cannot be discontinued. A bilateral adrenalectomy means that all the hormones normally produced by the adrenal glands must be replaced. The client now has adrenal insufficiency (Addison's disease).
2. **Prednisone (Deltasone) is a glucocorticoid. The glucocorticoid and mineralocorticoid steroids, and androgens produced by the adrenal glands must be replaced regularly. Doses should not be skipped.**
3. The client cannot stop taking the medication. Doing so could result in a life-threatening situation. Development of a round face is a side effect of glucocorticoids that may indicate that the dose is too high. The client should notify the HCP to review the dosage.
4. **Prednisone (Deltasone) is a glucocorticoid. Excess glucocorticoids may induce diabetes mellitus. The HCP should be notified if the client experiences diabetes symptoms, such as feeling thirsty all the time.**
5. **All clients diagnosed with a chronic medical condition should wear a MedicAlert bracelet or necklace.**

34. 1. The nurse will monitor the client's electrolytes, especially sodium and potassium and glucose levels, but this is not the first action.
2. The nurse should be prepared to replace corticosteroids, but this is not the first action. Methylprednisolone (Solu-Medrol) is a glucocorticoid.
3. **The nurse must treat an Addisonian crisis like all other shock situations. An IV and fluid replacement are imperative to prevent or treat shock. This is the first action.**
4. This is important, but it will not prevent or treat shock.

MEDICATION MEMORY JOGGER: The stem of the previous question told the test taker that the situation is a "crisis." The first step in many crises is ensuring that IV access is available to administer fluids and medications.

35. 1. Pantoprazole (Protonix), a PPI, does not increase the ability to digest food.
2. **Pantoprazole (Protonix), a PPI, decreases production of stomach acid by inhibiting the proton-pump step in gastric acid production.**
3. Pantoprazole (Protonix), a PPI, does not absorb gastric acid; it prevents its production.
4. Sucralfate (Carafate) is a mucosal barrier agent that coats the stomach lining. Protonix does not coat the stomach.

36. 1. Shortness of breath and pale mucous membranes do not indicate long-term steroid use or Cushing's syndrome.
2. **A round face (moon face) indicates a redistribution of fat from steroid therapy. Multiple ecchymotic areas on the arms indicate a redistribution of subcutaneous fats away from the arm (thin extremities). Both are side effects of long-term steroid therapy.**
3. Pink, frothy sputum and jugular vein distention are symptoms of congestive heart failure, not long-term steroid therapy.
4. Petechiae indicate a low platelet count, and sclerosed veins indicate use of IV access for medication administration. These are not findings of steroid therapy.

37. 1. Ketoconazole (Nizoral) is an anti-infective that also suppresses adrenal hormone production. This side effect makes it helpful in treating overproduction of adrenal hormones that results from the secretion of ACTH by tumors that cannot be removed surgically.
2. Methylprednisolone (Solu-Medrol) is a steroid, and ACTH stimulates adrenal hormone production. This would increase the client's symptoms.
3. PTU, a hormone substitute, suppresses production of thyroid hormones, not adrenal hormones.

4. Vasopressin (DDAVP), an antidiuretic, is a pituitary, not adrenal, hormone that prevents diuresis.

38. 1. The client diagnosed with Cushing's disease is at risk for infections because of immune suppression resulting from excess cortisol production. The HCP should see this client.
2. Clients diagnosed with Cushing's disease are at risk for developing infections related to excess production of cortisol by the adrenal glands. The client must be seen by an HCP and antibiotics must be initiated.
3. The client is not in an emergent situation; therefore, the client can be seen at an HCP office or clinic.
4. The client has a physiological, not psychosocial, problem. The client does not need therapeutic conversation.

39. 1. Fludrocortisone (Florinef), a mineral corticosteroid, is not an oral hypoglycemic medication. It is a steroid and may increase blood glucose, not decrease it.
2. Fludrocortisone (Florinef) is a mineral corticosteroid. Mineral corticosteroids help the body maintain the correct serum sodium levels. When sodium wasting occurs, Florinef is the preferred medication for Addison's disease, primary hypoaldosteronism, and congenital adrenal hyperplasia.
3. Fludrocortisone (Florinef) is a mineral corticosteroid. Florinef does not prevent muscle cramps. If the Florinef dose is too high, then potassium wasting will occur, resulting in muscle cramping.
4. Florinef does not stimulate the pituitary gland. The pituitary gland produces hormones that stimulate the adrenal gland. The adrenal gland does not produce hormones that stimulate the pituitary gland.

40. 1. Prednisone (Orasone) is a glucocorticoid. Replacement corticosteroids are necessary for clients diagnosed with adrenal insufficiency. The nurse would not question administering prednisone.
2. Ginseng is an herb that enhances adrenal function. The nurse would not question this medication.
3. Mitotane (Lysodren) is an antineoplastic agent that suppresses cortisone production. The nurse would question this medication for a client with adrenal insufficiency.
4. In males and females, the adrenal glands produce androgens, including testosterone. Replacing this hormone would not be unusual for a client diagnosed with adrenal insufficiency.

MEDICATION MEMORY JOGGER: The nurse must be knowledgeable about accepted standards of practice for disease processes and conditions. If the nurse administers a medication the HCP has prescribed, and it harms the client, the nurse could be held accountable. Remember, the nurse is a client advocate.

Pituitary Disorders

41. 1. Desmopressin (DDAVP) is an antidiuretic hormone and acts on the kidney to concentrate urine, but kidney stones would not warrant a change in the medication.
2. DDAVP is an antidiuretic hormone. Type 2 diabetes would not be a reason to change the medication.
3. DDAVP is an antidiuretic hormone. It is administered intranasally, and a sinus infection could interfere with medication absorption. Vasopressin comes in intramuscular form, and the client may need to take this form of vasopressin until the sinus infection has resolved.
4. Hyperthyroidism would not warrant a change in medication or route.

42. 1. Octreotide (Sandostatin), a hormone, suppresses the pituitary gland's secretion of human growth hormone, which, in adults, causes enlarged viscera, bone deformities, and other clinical manifestations of acromegaly. The nurse would expect to administer this medication. (Acromegaly in children results in gigantism.)
2. Somatrem (Protropin) is a growth hormone and would increase the client's symptoms.
3. Ketorolac (Toradol) is an NSAID. NSAIDs are administered to clients diagnosed with nephrogenic DI to inhibit prostaglandin production.
4. Corticotropin (ACTH) is a pituitary hormone. The client has symptoms of acromegaly, an overproduction of human growth hormone. ACTH would not suppress this production.

43. Correct answers are 1, 2, and 3.
1. The client diagnosed with DI is excreting large amounts of dilute urine because the body cannot conserve water and concentrate the urine. The client

requires fluid-volume replacement. The nurse would insert an IV. The client would have a high sodium level (because of the lack of fluid in the vascular system). Lactated Ringer's solution would be preferred to normal saline.

2. **The client should be on hourly output measurements. An indwelling catheter is needed to measure the client's output. The client requires rest, and voiding many liters of urine every day would leave the client exhausted from lack of sleep.**
3. **The urine specific gravity indicates the client's ability to concentrate urine and should be monitored.**
4. Furosemide (Lasix), a loop diuretic, would increase the client's urinary output. This is the opposite effect of what is needed.
5. In this situation, intake and output measurements are monitored every hour, not every shift.

44. 1. Chlorpropamide (Diabinese), a sulfonylurea, can cause weakness, jitteriness, nervousness, and other findings of a hypoglycemic reaction. The client should be aware of this and be prepared to treat the reaction with a source of simple carbohydrates. This is not a reason to discontinue the medication.
2. Chlorpropamide (Diabinese), a sulfonylurea, is not a cholinergic medication with a side effect of dry mouth.
3. Clients diagnosed with type 2 diabetes usually take the medication before meals. Effects of chlorpropamide (Diabinese), a sulfonylurea, can last 2 to 3 days. This client can take the medication after a meal.
4. **Chlorpropamide (Diabinese), a sulfonylurea, potentiates vasopressin action for clients with residual hypothalamic function. Sulfonylureas are mainly used to treat type 2 diabetes because they stimulate the pancreas to secrete insulin. The client should be aware that an insulin reaction (hypoglycemic reaction) can occur.**

45. 1. Chorionic gonadotropin (Chorigon) is a hormone substitute. This medication is given to cause ovarian follicle maturation and trigger ovulation. An FSH level would have been done before prescribing Chorigon.
2. **Chorionic gonadotropin (Chorigon) is a hormone substitute. This medication is given to cause ovarian follicle maturation and trigger ovulation. The client is monitored for overstimulation of the ovaries by pelvic sonograms.**
3. Chorionic gonadotropin (Chorigon) is a hormone substitute. The medication is a category X medication, which indicates that it is known to cause harm to fetuses, but it is given to stimulate ovulation to achieve a pregnancy. It also is given to maintain the corpus luteum after luteinizing hormone decreases during a normal pregnancy.
4. The medication is given parenterally, not orally.

46. 1. **Furosemide (Lasix) is a loop diuretic. In the syndrome of inappropriate antidiuretic hormone secretion (SIADH), the body retains too much water. Elevated fluid levels in the body result in dilutional hyponatremia. Hyponatremia can cause seizures and other central nervous system dysfunction. The sodium level is monitored to determine the intervention's effectiveness.**
2. The serum potassium level is important to monitor, but it will not measure the effectiveness of Lasix in treating this condition.
3. The problem in SIADH is in the pituitary gland; it is not a kidney problem.
4. The pituitary gland produces ACTH, but ACTH production is not the problem in SIADH. SIADH is an overproduction of vasopressin, an antidiuretic hormone.

MEDICATION MEMORY JOGGER: The nurse must be knowledgeable about accepted standards of practice for medication administration, including which client assessment data and laboratory data should be monitored before administering medication.

47. 1. Clofibrate (Atromid-S) is an antilipemic that has an antidiuretic effect on clients diagnosed with neurogenic DI, but it would not affect a client's neurogenic DI caused by the kidney's inability to respond to the medication.
2. **Ibuprofen (Motrin) is an NSAID. NSAIDs inhibit prostaglandin production and are used to treat nephrogenic DI.**
3. Furosemide (Lasix) is a loop diuretic and would increase urinary output for a client with too much urinary output.
4. Desmopressin (DDAVP) is a form of vasopressin, the antidiuretic hormone, but hormone production is not in question in nephrogenic DI because the pituitary gland is producing the hormone. The problem is that the kidneys are unable to respond to it.

48. 1. The problem is that the client is in fluid-volume overload, probably due to the medication vincristine (Oncovin), an antineoplastic vinca alkaloid. A diuretic may be administered, but as a treatment, not as a prophylactic measure.
2. Weight gain is not a symptom of an infection. These symptoms indicate SIADH.
3. The client's diet is not responsible for fluid weight gain.
4. Vincristine (Oncovin) is an antineoplastic vinca alkaloid. Vincristine, phenothiazines, antidepressants, thiazide diuretics, and smoking stimulate the pituitary gland, resulting in vasopressin overproduction. The client's symptoms indicate SIADH. The nurse should assess weight gain, hold the medication, and notify the HCP.

49. 1. Black cohosh is an OTC herb that is sometimes used to treat dysmenorrhea, premenstrual syndrome, and menopausal symptoms. The nurse would not question this medication.
2. Desmopressin (DDAVP), a pituitary hormone, causes vasoconstriction and is contraindicated for clients diagnosed with angina because of coronary vasoconstriction.
3. Hydrochlorothiazide (Diuril), a thiazide diuretic, would be administered to a client diagnosed with SIADH. SIADH may be caused by a head injury, pituitary tumors, hormone-secreting tumors, medications, and smoking. The nurse would not question this medication.
4. Calcitonin (Cibacalcin), a hormone, is administered to decrease calcium levels. The nurse would not question this medication.

MEDICATION MEMORY JOGGER: The nurse must be knowledgeable about accepted standards of practice for disease processes and conditions. If the nurse administers a medication the HCP has prescribed and harms the client, the nurse could be held accountable. Remember, the nurse is a client advocate.

Thyroid Disorders

50. Correct answers are 2 and 5.
1. The client would have clinical manifestations of hypothyroidism if the client is not taking enough medication. Weight loss is a symptom of hyperthyroidism, which indicates the client is taking too much levothyroxine (Synthroid), a thyroid hormone replacement.
2. Levothyroxine (Synthroid) is a thyroid hormone replacement. The client reports being cold indicates the client has hypothyroidism and needs more thyroid hormone replacement.
3. Exophthalmos (bulging of the eyes) occurs with hyperthyroidism, not hypothyroidism. The client diagnosed with hypothyroidism would be taking Synthroid.
4. A normal radial pulse, 60 to 100 bpm, indicates the medication is effective, and the client would not need to take more medication.
5. Decreased metabolism and constipation indicate that the client is not taking enough thyroid hormone.

51. **1. Levothyroxine (Synthroid) is a thyroid hormone replacement. Synthroid increases basal metabolic rate, which can precipitate cardiac dysrhythmias in clients with undiagnosed heart disease, especially in elderly clients. Synthroid can also cause cardiovascular collapse; therefore, the nurse should assess the client's cardiovascular function.**
2. Respiratory depression is not a complication of thyroid hormone therapy.
3. The client diagnosed with hypothyroidism may experience a paralytic ileus due to decreased metabolism. This would not be an expected complication for a client taking Synthroid.
4. A thyroid storm may occur when the thyroid gland is manipulated during a thyroidectomy, not when the client starts taking Synthroid.

52. 1. The goal of radioactive iodine treatment is to destroy just enough of the thyroid gland so that thyroid function levels return to normal. It does not destroy the entire gland.
2. The client should not be in close contact with children or pregnant women for 1 week after medication administration because the client will be emitting small amounts of radiation.
3. Most clients require a single dose of radioactive iodine; some may need more treatments.
4. Radioactive iodine is a clear, odorless, tasteless liquid that should not be administered with cold orange juice.

53. 1. The client's ABGs are not affected by PTU, a hyperthyroid treatment.

2. The client's potassium level is not affected by PTU, a hyperthyroid treatment.
3. The client's RBC count is not affected by PTU, a hyperthyroid treatment.
4. **The client receiving PTU, a hyperthyroid treatment, is at risk for agranulocytosis; therefore, the client's WBC count should be checked periodically. Because agranulocytosis puts the client at greater risk for infection, efforts to control the invasion of microbes should be strictly observed.**

54. 1. **Liothyronine (Cytomel) is a thyroid hormone. Nervousness, jitteriness, and irritability are clinical manifestations of hyperthyroidism; therefore, the nurse should question administering thyroid hormone.**
2. A normal temperature would indicate the client is in a euthyroid state; therefore, the nurse would not question administering this medication.
3. A normal blood pressure would indicate the client is in a euthyroid state; therefore, the nurse would not question administering this medication.
4. The nurse would not question administering the medication because fatigue is a symptom of hypothyroidism, which is why the client has been prescribed thyroid hormone.

MEDICATION MEMORY JOGGER: If the client verbalizes a symptom, if the nurse assesses data, or if laboratory data indicates an adverse effect secondary to a medication, the nurse must intervene. The nurse must implement an independent intervention or notify the HCP because medications can result in serious or even life-threatening complications.

55.

Potential Nursing Intervention	Indicated	Not Indicated
1. Encourage the client to decrease fiber in the diet.		X
2. Discuss the need to monitor the T3 and T4 levels daily.		X
3. Tell the client to take the medication with food only.		X
4. Instruct the client to report significant weight changes.	X	
5. Discuss importance of not using iodized salt.		X
6. Explain the importance of not taking medication with grapefruit juice.		X
7. Instruct the client to take the medication in the morning.	X	
8. Teach the client to monitor daily glucose levels.		X

1. **Levothyroxine (Synthroid) is a thyroid hormone. The nurse should discuss ways to help cope with hypothyroidism symptoms. The client should increase fiber intake to help prevent constipation.**
2. **T3, T4, and TSH levels are monitored to help determine medication effectiveness, but not done daily by the client. Serum blood levels are monitored monthly initially and then every 6 months.**
3. **The medication should be taken on an empty stomach because thyroid hormones have optimum effect when taken on an empty stomach.**
4. **Levothyroxine (Synthroid) is a thyroid hormone. The client's weight should be monitored weekly. Weight loss is expected due to the increased metabolic rate, and weight changes help determine effectiveness of the drug therapy.**
5. **This would be appropriate if the client is taking antithyroid medication, not thyroid hormones. Iodine increases thyroid hormone production, which is not desirable for clients taking antithyroid medications.**
6. **Grapefruit juice is contraindicated when taking some medications, but not thyroid hormone therapy.**

7. **The medication should be taken in the morning to decrease incidence of drug-related insomnia.**
8. **Thyroid medications do not affect the client's blood glucose level; therefore, there is no need to monitor the glucose level.**

MEDICATION MEMORY JOGGER: Grapefruit juice can inhibit metabolism of certain medications. Specifically, grapefruit juice inhibits cytochrome P450-3A4 found in the liver and the intestinal wall. The nurse should investigate any medications the client is taking if the client drinks grapefruit juice.

56. 1. There is no reason for the client to notify the HCP because it takes several months to attain the euthyroid state.
2. Most clients only need one dose of radioactive iodine, but it takes several months to attain the euthyroid state.
3. **The goal of radioactive therapy for hyperthyroidism is to destroy just enough of the thyroid gland so that thyroid function levels return to normal. Full benefits may take several months.**
4. This is a therapeutic response, which is not appropriate because the client needs factual information.

57. 1. PTU is a hyperthyroid treatment. Antithyroid medications may cause drowsiness; therefore, this statement would not warrant immediate intervention by the nurse.
2. **PTU is a hyperthyroid treatment. The antithyroid medication may affect the body's ability to defend itself against bacteria and viruses; therefore, the nurse should intervene if the client has any sore throat, fever, chills, malaise, or weakness.**
3. As a result of slower metabolism from the PTU, weight gain is expected; therefore, this statement would not warrant intervention by the nurse.
4. This indicates the medication is effective. Symptoms of hyperthyroidism, which include feeling hot much of the time, are decreasing. This would not warrant immediate nurse intervention.

58. Correct answers are 1, 2, 3, 4, and 5.
1. **Thyroid function tests are used to determine drug therapy effectiveness.**
2. **Weight gain is expected as a result of slower metabolism.**
3. **Antithyroid medication may cause nausea or vomiting.**
4. **Changes in metabolic rate will be manifested as changes in blood pressure, pulse, and body temperature.**
5. **Hyperthyroidism results in protein catabolism, overactivity, and increased metabolism, which lead to exhaustion; therefore, the nurse should monitor for activity intolerance.**

ENDOCRINE SYSTEM COMPREHENSIVE EXAMINATION

1. The client diagnosed with Addison's disease tells the clinic nurse about taking licorice every day to help the disease process. Which intervention should the nurse implement?
   1. Tell the client licorice is candy and will not help Addison's disease.
   2. Praise the client because licorice increases aldosterone production.
   3. Ask the client why they think licorice will help the disease process.
   4. Determine if the licorice has caused any mouth ulcers or sores.

2. The client is diagnosed with primary hyperaldosteronism and prescribed spironolactone. The client's laboratory values and vital signs are populated in the chart below.

Laboratory Test	**Client Values**	**Reference Values**
Potassium	4.2 mEq/L	3.5 to 5.3 mEq/L or mmol/L
Sodium	137 mEq/L	135 to 145 mEq/L or mmol/L
Vital Sign Flowsheet	**Client Values**	**Reference Values**
Temperature	99.2°F	Oral: 98°F (36.7°C)
Pulse	100 bpm	60 to 100 bpm
Respirations	20 breaths/min	12 to 20 breaths/min
Blood pressure	140/96 mm Hg	100 to 119 mm Hg systolic 60 to 80 mm Hg diastolic

INTAKE AND OUTPUT RECORD

Day One	**Oral (mL)**	**Intravenous (mL)**	**Urine (mL)**	**Other (Specify) (mL)**
0701 to 1900	NPO	100 mL	460 mL	
1901 to 0700		360 mL	360 mL	
Total	0	460 mL	820 mL	

   Which data supports that the medication is **effective**?
   1. Potassium level
   2. Urinary output
   3. Blood pressure
   4. Sodium level

3. The client diagnosed with DI is receiving desmopressin intranasally. Which assessment data **warrants** the client notifying the HCP? **Select all that apply.**
   1. The client does not feel thirsty all the time.
   2. The client can sleep throughout the night.
   3. The client has gained 2 kg in the past 24 hours.
   4. The client has to urinate 20 to 30 times daily.
   5. The client has elastic skin turgor and moist mucosa.

4. The 2-year-old child is diagnosed with cystic fibrosis (CF). Which interventions should the nurse discuss with the child's parent? **Select all that apply.**
   1. Administer OTC mucolytic agents.
   2. Perform postural drainage and chest percussion.
   3. Administer cough suppressants at night only.
   4. Check the child's blood glucose level four times a day.
   5. Sprinkle pancreatic enzymes on the child's food.

5. The 36-year-old client is prescribed conjugated estrogen tablets after a total abdominal hysterectomy. The client calls the nurse in the health clinic and reports she is producing breast milk. Which intervention should the nurse discuss with the client?
   1. Explain that this is an expected side effect and it will stop.
   2. Determine if the client is having abdominal cramping.
   3. Ask if this mainly occurs during sexual intercourse.
   4. Discontinue taking the estrogen until seen by the HCP.

6. The 10-year-old client is receiving somatropin. Which clinical manifestations **warrant** nurse intervention?
   1. A 3-cm increase in height
   2. A moon face and buffalo hump
   3. Polyuria, polydipsia, and polyphagia
   4. T 99.4°F, P 108, R: 22, and BP 121/70

7. The female client diagnosed with secondary adrenal insufficiency is prescribed ACTH. Which information should the nurse discuss with the client?
   1. Explain that ACTH will increase metabolism.
   2. Instruct the client to limit dietary salt.
   3. Inform the client that an increase in growth may occur.
   4. Tell the client that normal menses is expected.

8. The client is diagnosed with hypothyroidism and is taking levothyroxine. Which data indicates the medication is **effective**?
   1. The client's apical pulse is 84 bpm, and the blood pressure is 134/78.
   2. The client's temperature is 96.7°F (35.9°C), and respiratory rate is 14.
   3. The client reports having a soft, formed stool every 4 days.
   4. The client tells the nurse that the client only needs 3 hours of sleep.

9. The nurse is administering the following medications. Which medication should the nurse **question** administering?
   1. Glyburide to a client diagnosed with type 1 diabetes
   2. Furosemide to a client diagnosed with SIADH
   3. Hydromorphone to a client diagnosed with pancreatitis
   4. Sliding-scale regular insulin to a client diagnosed with type 2 diabetes

10. The client diagnosed with type 1 diabetes is scheduled for a computed tomography (CT) abdominal scan with contrast. The client is taking metformin and 70/30 insulin 24 units at 0700 and 1600. Which instruction should the nurse discuss with the client?
    1. Administer the 70/30 insulin the morning of the test.
    2. Take one-half the dose of the morning insulin on the day of the test.
    3. Do not take metformin after the procedure until the HCP approves.
    4. Take the medications as prescribed because they will not affect the test.

11. The client diagnosed with chronic pancreatitis is prescribed pancrelipase. Which data indicates the dosage should be **increased**?
    1. No bowel movement for 3 days
    2. Fatty, frothy, foul-smelling stools
    3. A decrease in urinary output
    4. An increase in midepigastric pain

12. The client diagnosed with Addison's disease is prescribed prednisone. Which laboratory data should the nurse expect this medication to alter?
    1. Glucose
    2. Sodium
    3. Calcium
    4. Creatinine

13. The client diagnosed with poison ivy is prescribed prednisone. Which information should the nurse discuss with the client? **Select all that apply.**
 1. Take the medication with food.
 2. The medication must be tapered.
 3. Avoid going into the sunlight.
 4. Monitor the blood glucose level.
 5. Do not eat green, leafy vegetables.

14. The client diagnosed with hyperthyroidism undergoes a bilateral thyroidectomy. Which statements indicate the client **understands** the discharge instructions? **Select all that apply.**
 1. "I must take my PTU medication at night only."
 2. "I should not take my medication if I am nauseated."
 3. "I will take my thyroid hormone pill every day."
 4. "I need to check my thyroid level frequently."
 5. "If I have diarrhea, I should contact my doctor."

15. The unlicensed assistive personnel (UAP) notifies the registered nurse (RN) that the client reports being jittery and nervous and is diaphoretic. The client is diagnosed with type 2 diabetes. Which interventions should the RN implement? **Rank in order of performance.**
 1. Have the UAP check the client's glucose level.
 2. Tell the UAP to give the client orange juice.
 3. Check the client's MAR.
 4. Immediately go to the room and assess the client.
 5. Assist the UAP in changing the client's bed linens.

16. The client with type 1 diabetes is diagnosed with diabetic ketoacidosis (DKA). The HCP prescribes regular insulin IV by continuous infusion. Which intervention should the intensive care nurse implement when administering this medication?
 1. Flush the tubing with 50 mL of the insulin drip before administering it to the client.
 2. Monitor the client's serum glucose level every hour and document it on the MAR.
 3. Draw the client's ABG results daily and document them in the client's EHR.
 4. Administer the client's regular insulin drip via gravity at the prescribed rate.

17. The nurse is administering medications to a client diagnosed with type 1 diabetes. The client's 1100 glucometer reading is 310.

Client: Z.A.	MR# 1234567	Date: Today
Age: 38 years	Allergies: NKDA	Diagnosis: Diabetes mellitus
Medication	**0701 to 1900**	**1901 to 0700**
Regular insulin (Humulin R) per sliding scale subcutaneously ac and hs. <60 Notify HCP <150 0 units 151 to 200 2 units 201 to 250 4 units 251 to 300 6 units 301 to 350 8 units 351 to 400 10 units >400 Notify HCP	0730 BG 142 0 units DN	
Nurse Initials/Credentials	DN/RN	NN/RN

Which action should the nurse implement?
 1. Have the laboratory verify the glucose results.
 2. Notify the HCP of the results.
 3. Administer eight units of regular insulin subcutaneously.
 4. Recheck the client's glucometer reading at 1130.

18. The client diagnosed with type 2 diabetes is prescribed sitagliptin. Which information should the nurse discuss with the client?
1. Keep the sitagliptin pen at room temperature after opening.
2. Instruct the client to report any blisters on the skin or pain on the left side.
3. There is no concern if taking sitagliptin concurrently with insulin.
4. Explain that this medication is a type of regular-acting insulin.

19. Which statement by the client diagnosed with type 1 diabetes indicates the client **understands** the medication teaching concerning insulin degludec?
1. "I will throw away my pen in 30 days, even if there is medicine in the pen."
2. "I always keep the needle on my pen, even in the refrigerator."
3. "This medication cost so much I use my pen past the expiration date."
4. "I should not take any other diabetic medication when taking insulin degludec."

20. The client diagnosed with diabetes is prescribed insulin degludec and liraglutide 100/3.6 injection. Which statement indicates the client **needs more** medication teaching?
1. "Low blood glucose levels are no concern with this combination of medications."
2. "The medications work in my body to help control blood glucose levels and my appetite."
3. "I need to monitor my blood glucose levels to make sure they are in range every day."
4. "If I get a cold or stomach virus and cannot keep any food down, I will call my HCP."

ENDOCRINE SYSTEM COMPREHENSIVE EXAMINATION ANSWERS AND RATIONALES

1. 1. This is a false statement, and the nurse should investigate any type of alternative treatment before making this statement.

2. Licorice is a candy flavoring, but it is also used as an herbal medication in tablet, tea, or tincture form. Licorice increases the aldosterone effect, which helps treat Addison's disease.

3. This is an aggressive-type judgmental question; therefore, the client would not owe the nurse an explanation.

4. Licorice is used to treat mouth ulcers; it does not cause them.

MEDICATION MEMORY JOGGER: Some herbal preparations are effective, some are not, and a few can be harmful or even deadly. If a client is taking an herbal supplement and a conventional medicine, the nurse should investigate to determine if the herbal preparation will cause harm to the client. The nurse should always be the client's advocate.

2. 1. Spironolactone (Aldactone) is a potassium-sparing diuretic. Hyperaldosteronism causes hypokalemia, metabolic alkalosis, and hypertension. Spironolactone, a potassium-sparing diuretic, normalizes potassium levels for clients diagnosed with hyperaldosteronism within 2 weeks; therefore, a normal potassium level, which is 4.2 mEq/L, indicates the medication is effective.

2. The urinary output is not used to determine medication effectiveness for a client diagnosed with hyperaldosteronism.

3. The client does have hypertension, but this blood pressure is above normal limits and does not indicate the medication is effective.

4. Serum sodium level is not used to determine medication effectiveness for a client diagnosed with hyperaldosteronism.

MEDICATION MEMORY JOGGER: The nurse determines medication effectiveness by assessing for the symptoms, or lack thereof, for which the medication was prescribed.

3. Correct answers are 3 and 4.

1. The major symptom of DI is polyuria resulting in polydipsia (extreme thirst); therefore, the client's lack of thirst indicates the medication is effective.

2. The client's ability to sleep through the night indicates that they are not getting up to urinate because of polyuria and, thus, that the medication is effective.

3. Desmopressin (DDAVP) is the pituitary antidiuretic hormone. A weight gain of 4.4 pounds indicates the client is experiencing water intoxication, which suggests the client is receiving too much medication, and the HCP should be notified.

4. The client urinating 20 to 30 times a day indicates the medication is ineffective; therefore, the nurse should notify the HCP.

5. The client is well hydrated; therefore, this data does not warrant intervention.

MEDICATION MEMORY JOGGER: If the client verbalizes a symptom, the nurse assesses data, or if laboratory data indicates an adverse effect secondary to a medication, the nurse must intervene. The nurse must implement an independent intervention or notify the HCP because medications can result in serious or life-threatening complications.

4. Correct answers are 1, 2, and 5.

1. Mucolytic medications are administered to help liquefy thick, tenacious secretions characteristic of CF.

2. Postural drainage and chest percussion help cough up mucus from the lungs.

3. The child would not receive cough suppressants (antitussives) because the thick, tenacious secretions need to be expectorated, not suppressed.

4. Eventually, the beta cells will become clogged due to the thick, tenacious secretions in the pancreas, but this would not be a problem in the initial stage after diagnosis.

5. The thick, tenacious secretions clog the pancreatic ducts, decreasing the pancreatic enzymes amylase and lipase in the small intestines. The parent must administer these enzymes with every meal or snack to ensure digestion of carbohydrates and fats.

5. 1. This is not an expected side effect caused by the conjugated estrogen tablets (Premarin), an estrogen replacement hormone stimulating the hypothalamus to produce prolactin. The estrogen dosage must be adjusted or discontinued.

2. Abdominal cramping is a symptom associated with menses, and the client does not have a uterus; therefore, this is not an appropriate question.
3. The breast discharge is unrelated to sexual intercourse.
4. **Conjugated estrogen tablets (Premarin) are an estrogen replacement hormone. The medication should be stopped until the HCP can be seen because this warrants a dosage adjustment or permanent discontinuation. The estrogen stimulates the hypothalamus to produce prolactin, which stimulates the production of breast milk.**

6. 1. The child has grown a little more than 1 inch (2.54 cm equals 1 inch). Because the child has been prescribed the growth hormone to increase growth, this would indicate that the medication is effective and no intervention on the part of the nurse is needed.
2. These are side effects of steroid therapy, not growth hormones.
3. **Somatropin (Humatrope) is a human growth hormone. Growth hormone is diabetogenic; therefore, any clinical manifestations of diabetes mellitus, such as polyuria, polydipsia, and polyphagia, should be reported to the HCP immediately. These are the three Ps of diabetes mellitus.**
4. The nurse must know the normal parameters for these vital signs do not warrant notifying the HCP.

7. 1. Thyroid hormones, not ACTH, would increase the client's metabolism.
2. **ACTH or Acthar, a pituitary hormone, is administered as an adrenal stimulant when the pituitary gland cannot perform this function. This medication will cause sodium absorption and cause edema; therefore, the client should decrease salt intake.**
3. This medication may decrease the client's growth.
4. This medication causes abnormal menses.

8. 1. **Levothyroxine (Synthroid) is a thyroid hormone. If the thyroid medication is effective, the client's metabolism should be within normal limits, and this pulse and blood pressure support this.**
2. These vital signs are subnormal, indicating hypothyroidism.
3. A stool every 4 days indicates constipation, and constipation is a hypothyroidism symptom. This indicates the medication is not effective.
4. Six to eight hours of sleep would be normal. Three hours would indicate hyperactivity, which is a hyperthyroidism symptom. Perhaps a medication dosage adjustment is needed.

9. 1. **Glyburide (Micronase) is a sulfonylurea. The sulfonylureas stimulate beta-cell production of insulin. Clients diagnosed with type 1 diabetes have no functioning beta cells; therefore, they cannot be stimulated. The nurse should question administering this medication.**
2. Furosemide (Lasix) is a loop diuretic. The client diagnosed with SIADH would be receiving a loop diuretic to decrease excess fluid volume.
3. Hydromorphone (Dilaudid) is a narcotic analgesic. Clients diagnosed with pancreatitis have a great deal of pain from the auto-digestion of their pancreas.
4. A client diagnosed with type 2 diabetes is often prescribed insulin during times of stress or illness.

MEDICATION MEMORY JOGGER: The nurse must be knowledgeable about accepted standards of practice for disease processes and conditions. If the nurse administers a medication the HCP has prescribed and harms the client, the nurse could be held accountable. Remember, the nurse is a client advocate.

10. 1. Because the client is NPO for the test, the insulin should be held.
2. Because the client is NPO for the test, the insulin should be held. In addition, the nurse cannot prescribe medication or change the dosage.
3. **Metformin (Glucophage), a biguanide, has a potential side effect of producing lactic acid. Lactic acidosis could result when metformin is administered simultaneously or within a close time span of the contrast dye used for the CT scan. It is recommended to hold the medication 48 hours before and after the CT scan with contrast. The HCP should obtain blood urea nitrogen and creatinine levels to determine kidney function before restarting Glucophage.**
4. Insulin should be held when the client is NPO, and metformin will be held because of the contrast dye.

MEDICATION MEMORY JOGGER: Any time the client is having a diagnostic test the nurse should question administering any medication.

11\. 1. Constipation does not determine Pancrease (pancrelipase) effectiveness.

2. Pancreas enzymes (Pancrease) are replacements for the enzymes normally produced by the pancreas. Steatorrhea (fatty, frothy, foul-smelling stools) or diarrhea indicate a lack of pancreatic enzymes in the small intestines. This would indicate the dosage is too small and needs to be increased.

3\. Urine output does not determine the effectiveness of Pancrease.

4\. An increase in midepigastric pain is a symptom of peptic ulcer disease or GERD and does not indicate pancreatic enzyme effectiveness. The client diagnosed with chronic pancreatitis may have abdominal pain, but the pancreatic enzymes are administered for digestion of food, not to alleviate pain.

12\. **1. Prednisone is a glucocorticoid medication that affects glucose metabolism; therefore, the nurse should expect the glucose level to be altered.**

2\. Sodium is not affected by prednisone.

3\. Calcium is not affected by prednisone.

4\. Creatinine is not affected by prednisone.

13\. **Correct answers are 1 and 2.**

1. Prednisone is very irritating to the stomach and must be taken with food to avoid gastritis or peptic ulcer disease.

2. To avoid adrenal insufficiency or Addisonian crisis, the client must taper the medication.

3\. Prednisone does not cause photosensitivity.

4\. Because prednisone is used short term for treating poison ivy, the blood glucose level would not need to be monitored.

5\. Green, leafy vegetables are high in vitamin K and would be contraindicated in anticoagulant treatment with Coumadin, but not prednisone.

14\. **Correct answers are 3, 4, and 5.**

1\. PTU is an antithyroid medication, and the client has had the thyroid gland removed.

2\. The client must take the thyroid hormone daily or the client may experience clinical manifestations of hypothyroidism.

3. Because the client's thyroid has been removed, the client now has hypothyroidism and must take a thyroid replacement daily for the rest of their life.

4. The thyroid level is checked by a venipuncture test every few months.

5. Diarrhea is a hyperthyroidism symptom. The client should report it to the doctor to determine if it indicates a need to decrease thyroid hormone or is secondary to gastroenteritis.

15\. **Correct order is 4, 1, 2, 3, 5.**

4. These are symptoms of a hypoglycemic reaction, and the nurse should assess the client immediately; therefore, this is the first intervention.

1. Because the registered nurse (RN) is assessing the client in the room, the UAP can take the glucometer reading. The nurse cannot delegate the care of an unstable client but can delegate a task because the nurse is in the room with the client.

2. Treatment of choice for a conscious client experiencing a hypoglycemic reaction is to administer food or a glucose source. Orange juice is a glucose source, and the UAP can get it.

3. The nurse should check the MAR to determine when the last dose of insulin or oral hypoglycemic medication was administered.

5. When the client has been stabilized, then the linens should be changed to make the client comfortable.

16\. **1. Regular insulin adheres to the lining of the plastic IV tubing; therefore, the nurse should flush the tubing with at least 50 mL of the insulin solution so that insulin will adhere to the tubing before the prescribed dosage is administered to the client. If this is not done, the client will not receive the correct insulin dose during the first few hours of administration.**

2\. To monitor serum glucose, the nurse would need to perform an hourly venipuncture. This is painful, more expensive, and takes a longer time to provide glucose results; therefore, a capillary (fingerstick) bedside glucometer will be used to monitor the client's blood glucose level every hour.

3\. The nurse does not draw ABGs. The respiratory therapist or HCP does this.

4\. A regular insulin drip must be administered by an infusion-controlled device (IV pump). It may not be given via gravity because it is a very dangerous medication and could kill the client if not administered correctly.

17. 1. According to the sliding scale, blood glucose results should be verified when less than 60 or greater than 400.
2. The HCP does not need to be notified unless the blood glucose is greater than 400.
3. The client's reading is 310; therefore, the nurse should administer eight units of regular insulin as per the HCP's order.
4. There is no reason for the nurse to recheck the results.

18. 1. Sitagliptin (Januvia) is a dipeptidyl-peptidase 4 inhibitor (DPP-4I) and an oral medication.
2. Side effects with sitagliptin are pancreatitis (pain on the left side) and Stevens-Johnson Syndrome (painful blisters and skin rashes).
3. Sitagliptin slows gastric emptying, so the client could experience hypoglycemic reactions if taken with insulin.
4. Sitagliptin is not a type of insulin.

19. 1. The insulin degludec (Tresiba), an ultralong-acting insulin analog, is in the same classification as glargine and detemir. Any medication remaining after 30 days should be discarded to ensure it has the same potency as when it was first opened.
2. The needle should be removed from the pen when storing the medication in the refrigerator because some medicine may leak from the degludec pen, or air bubbles may form in the cartridge.
3. The degludec pen should not be used after the expiration date printed on the label.
4. Degludec can be used with metformin (Glucophage) or other types of antidiabetic medicine.

20. 1. Administration of any insulin can cause hypoglycemia when combined with medications that act to decrease appetite. Then the client has an even greater risk of developing hypoglycemia. Insulin degludec (Tresiba) and liraglutide (Victoza or Saxenda), incretin mimetics, increase glycemic control by lowering blood glucose level and appetite.
2. The medication works to control blood glucose levels and by providing continuous insulin release and decreasing appetite. It is injected once daily.
3. This is insulin, and the client is still subject to hypoglycemia and hyperglycemia. This statement indicates the client understands the medication regimen.
4. If the client cannot eat and retain food, the HCP should be notified to ensure that the client does not develop complications.

7

Genitourinary System

What lies behind you and what lies in front of you, pales in comparison to what lies inside of you.

—Ralph Waldo Emerson

QUESTIONS

Chronic Kidney Disease

1. The client diagnosed with chronic kidney disease (CKD) is prescribed epoetin. Which statement **best** describes the scientific rationale for administering this medication?
1. This medication stimulates red blood cell (RBC) production.
2. This medication stimulates white blood cell (WBC) production.
3. This medication is used to treat thrombocytopenia.
4. This medication increases urine production.

2. Which intervention should the nurse implement when administering epoetin subcutaneously? **Select all that apply.**
1. Do not shake the vial before preparing the injection.
2. Apply a warm washcloth after administering the medication.
3. Discard any unused portion of the vial after pulling up the correct dose.
4. Keep the medication vials in the refrigerator until preparing to administer.
5. Administer the medication intramuscularly in the deltoid muscle.

3. Complete the sentence by choosing from the list of options.

The nurse knows the scientific rationale for administering aluminum hydroxide to a client diagnosed with CKD is to ______________________________
1. Neutralize gastric acid production.
2. Decrease hyperphosphatemia.
3. Reduce calcium levels.
4. Lessen episodes of constipation.

4. Which statement **best** describes the scientific rationale for administering calcitriol to a client diagnosed with end-stage renal disease (ESRD)?
1. This medication increases the availability of vitamin D in the intestines.
2. This medication stimulates the excretion of calcium from the parathyroid gland.
3. This medication helps the body excrete calcium through the feces.
4. This medication increases serum calcium levels by promoting calcium absorption.

5. The client diagnosed with ESRD is taking calcitriol. Which assessment data **warrants nurse intervention**?
1. The client reports nausea.
2. The client has had two episodes of diarrhea.
3. The client has an increase in serum creatinine level.
4. The client has blood in the urine.

6. The client diagnosed with CKD is taking aluminum hydroxide liquid. Which information should the nurse discuss with the client?
   1. "Drink at least 500 mL of water after taking the medication."
   2. "Do not drink any water for 1 hour after taking the medication."
   3. "Drink 2 to 4 ounces of water after taking the medication."
   4. "Eat 30 minutes before taking the aluminum hydroxide."

7. The client diagnosed with CKD is receiving oral sodium polystyrene. The client's laboratory values are populated in the chart below.

Laboratory Test	Client Values	Reference Values
Phosphorus	4.0 mg/dL	2.5 to 4.5 mg/dL
Sodium	138 mEq/L	135 to 145 mEq/L or mml/L
Potassium	4.2 mg/dL	3.5 to 5.3 mEq/L or mmol/L
Calcium	8.4 mg/dL	8.2 to 10.2 mg/dL

   Which laboratory data indicates the medication is **effective**?
   1. Phosphorus level
   2. Sodium level
   3. Potassium level
   4. Calcium level

8. The nurse is administering hydrochlorothiazide to a client diagnosed with CKD. Which assessment data should cause the nurse to **question** this medication administration? **Select all that apply.**
   1. The client's skin turgor on the upper chest is tented.
   2. The urine output was 90 mL for the last 8 hours.
   3. The client's oral mucosa is moist and pink.
   4. The client has 3+ sacral and peripheral edema.
   5. The client's blood pressure is 90/60 in the left arm.

9. The client diagnosed with CKD on hemodialysis is prescribed lanthanum carbonate. The client's blood laboratory values are populated in the chart below.

Laboratory Test	Client Values	Reference Values
Potassium	5.3 mg/dL	3.5 to 5.3 mEq/L or mmol/L
Sodium	144 mEq/L	135 to 145 mEq/L or mml/L
Blood urea nitrogen (BUN)	18 mg/dL	8 to 21 mg/dL Adult over 90 years: 10 to 31 mg/dL
Phosphorus	4.0 mg/dL	2.5 to 4.5 mg/dL

   Which laboratory data indicates the medication is **effective**?
   1. Potassium level
   2. Sodium level
   3. Blood urea nitrogen (BUN) level
   4. Phosphorus level

10. The client diagnosed with CKD on hemodialysis is prescribed lanthanum carbonate. Which interventions should the nurse discuss with the client? **Select all that apply.**
1. "Chew the tablets completely before swallowing."
2. "Monitor the dialysis graft for bleeding."
3. "Take an over-the-counter proton-pump inhibitor."
4. "Check the radial pulse before taking the medication."
5. "Take the medication with or right after meals."

Urinary Tract Infection

11. The nurse in the long-term care facility is caring for a client with an indwelling catheter. Which preparation should the nurse **order** for the client?
1. Cranberry juice with breakfast daily
2. Nitrofurantoin (100 mg every [q] 12 hours for 7 days)
3. Vitamin C every night at bedtime
4. Goldenseal (2 mL in water two to three times daily)

12. The male client is admitted to the medical floor with a diagnosis of pyelonephritis. Which intervention should the nurse implement **first**?
1. Initiate IV access with a 20-gauge catheter.
2. Administer the IV antibiotic within 2 hours of admission.
3. Obtain a urine specimen for culture and sensitivity.
4. Notify the dietary department to order the client a regular diet.

13. The client diagnosed with glomerulonephritis is receiving trimethoprim sulfa. The client's laboratory values are populated in the chart below.

Urinalysis	**Client Values**	**Reference Values**
pH	6.9	4.5 to 8
Specific gravity	1.010	1.005 to 1.03
Glucose Ketones Hemoglobin Bilirubin Nitrite Leukocyte esterase	Negative	Negative
Protein	Negative	Less than 20 mg/dL
Microscopic		
RBCs	8	Less than 5/hpf (high power field)
WBCs	35	Less than 5/hpf (high power field)
Bacteria	Many	None seen

Which data indicates the medication is **effective**?
1. Urine specific gravity
2. Microscopic WBCs
3. Urine pH
4. Leukocyte esterase

14. The nurse is administering medications to clients on a urology floor. Which medication should the nurse **question**?
1. Ceftriaxone to a pregnant client
2. Cephalexin to a client diagnosed with a penicillin allergy
3. Trimethoprim sulfa to a client postprostate surgery
4. Nitrofurantoin to a client diagnosed with urinary stasis

15. The registered nurse (RN) observes the unlicensed assistive personnel (UAP) performing delegated tasks. Which action by the UAP requires **immediate** intervention?
1. The UAP measures the output of a client after transurethral resection of the prostate.
2. The UAP tells the client with green urine that something must be wrong for the urine to be such an odd color.
3. The UAP encourages the client to drink a glass of water after the nurse administered the oral antibiotic.
4. The UAP assists the client diagnosed with a urinary tract infection (UTI) to the bedside commode every 2 hours.

16. The male client is diagnosed with methicillin-resistant *Staphylococcus aureus* (MRSA) of the urine and is receiving vancomycin IV piggyback (IVPB). Which interventions should the nurse implement when administering this medication? **Select all that apply.**
1. Hold the medication if the trough level is 5 mg/dL.
2. Ask the client if he is allergic to any medication.
3. Administer the medication via an infusion pump.
4. Check the client's BUN and creatinine levels.
5. Assess the client's IV insertion site.

17. The client taking nitrofurantoin for a UTI calls the clinic and tells the nurse the urine has turned dark. Which statement is the nurse's **best** response?
1. "This is a side effect of the medication and is not harmful."
2. "This means that you have cystitis and should come in to see the HCP."
3. "If you take the medication with food, it causes this reaction."
4. "There must be some other problem going on that is causing this."

18. The client diagnosed with a bladder infection is prescribed phenazopyridine. Which statement is the scientific rationale for prescribing this medication?
1. Phenazopyridine is used to treat gram-negative UTI.
2. Phenazopyridine stimulates a hypotonic bladder to increase urine output.
3. Phenazopyridine alleviates pain and burning during urination.
4. Phenazopyridine decreases urinary frequency to control an overactive bladder.

19. The client diagnosed with a UTI is prescribed aztreonam IVPB every 8 hours. For each finding in the following table, does the result show the medication is **effective or not effective**?

Finding	Effective	Not Effective
1. Voids 300 to 400 mL of urine each time		
2. Urinary frequency		
3. Temperature of 99°F		
4. Burning with urination		
5. Pinkish colored urine		

20. The nurse is preparing the client for an indwelling urinary catheter placement. Which statement has **priority** for the nurse to ask the client?
1. "Do you have a preference of which leg the tube is taped to?"
2. "When did you last attempt to void?"
3. "Do you feel the need to void?"
4. "Are you allergic to iodine or Betadine?"

Benign Prostatic Hypertrophy

21. The client diagnosed with mild benign prostatic hypertrophy (BPH) is prescribed finasteride to relieve symptoms of urinary frequency. Which intervention should the clinic nurse implement? **Select three interventions.**
1. Tell the client to drink at least 8 to 10 glasses of water a day.
2. Schedule an appointment with the HCP for a 1-week follow-up examination.
3. Have the laboratory draw a prostate-specific antigen level.
4. Give the client a urinal to measure his daily output of urine.
5. Teach the client to notify the HCP for changes in breasts.
6. Inform the client that erectile dysfunction can occur during therapy.

22. The male client reports urinary frequency and nocturia and tells the nurse he takes saw palmetto herbal supplement. Which statement is the nurse's **best** response?
1. "Use of saw palmetto is an old wives' tale."
2. "This herb does help shrink the prostate tissue."
3. "Have you noticed any itching or rashes?"
4. "Saw palmetto has been known to cause cancer."

23. The client diagnosed with moderate BPH is being treated with tamsulosin. Which intervention should the nurse implement?
1. Check the client's blood pressure.
2. Send a urinalysis to the laboratory.
3. Determine if the client has nocturia.
4. Plan a scheduled voiding pattern.

24. The client diagnosed with BPH had a transurethral resection of the prostate (TURP). The client returns to the unit with a continuous bladder irrigation (CBI) in place. The UAP records emptying the catheter bag of red drainage three times during the shift of 1,500 mL, 2,100 mL, and 1,950 mL. The registered nurse (RN) records infusing 4,100 mL of normal saline irrigation fluid. What is the client's corrected urinary output for the shift?

____

25. Which is the scientific rationale for administering dutasteride to a client diagnosed with BPH?
1. The medication elevates male testosterone levels and decreases impotence.
2. Dutasteride causes a rapid reduction in the size of the prostate and relief of symptoms.
3. The medication decreases the mechanical obstruction of the urethra by the prostate.
4. Dutasteride is as fast as surgery in reducing the obstructive symptoms of BPH.

26. The client, after a TURP procedure, is reporting bladder spasms. The HCP prescribed a belladonna and opiate (B&O) suppository. Which interventions should the nurse implement when administering this medication? **Select all that apply.**
1. Obtain the correct dose of the medication.
2. Lubricate the suppository with K-Y Jelly.
3. Wash hands and put on nonsterile gloves.
4. Check the client's armband for allergies.
5. Ask the client to lie on the left side.

27. The nurse is administering morning medications. Which medication combination should the nurse **question** administering?
   1. Terazosin and captopril
   2. Finasteride and digoxin
   3. Tamsulosin and metformin
   4. *Serenoa repens* and metoprolol

28. Which intervention is a **priority** for a pregnant nurse when administering dutasteride to a client diagnosed with BPH?
   1. Use goggles for personal eye protection.
   2. Protect the nurse's mucosa from contact with liquid.
   3. Ask a male nurse to administer the medication.
   4. Wear gloves while administering the medication.

29. The client diagnosed with BPH has had a TURP. The client is reporting lower abdominal pain. Which interventions should the nurse implement? **Rank in order of performance.**
   1. Administer the prescribed morphine by slow IV push.
   2. Check the urinary catheter for drainage and clots.
   3. Determine if the client has a hard, rigid abdomen.
   4. Adjust the saline irrigation to flush the bladder.
   5. Dilute the morphine with several milliliters of normal saline.

30. The client diagnosed with BPH and congestive heart failure (CHF) is receiving furosemide daily. Which information provided by the UAP **best indicates** to the RN the medication is **effective**?
   1. The UAP recorded the intake as 350 mL and the output as 450 mL.
   2. The UAP stated that the client ambulated to the bathroom without dyspnea.
   3. The UAP emptied a moderate amount of urine from the bedside commode.
   4. The UAP reported that the client lost 1 pound of weight from the day before.

Renal Calculi

31. The client diagnosed with renal calculi was prescribed allopurinol for uric acid stone calculi. Which medication teaching should the nurse discuss with the client? **Select all that apply.**
   1. Inform the client to report chills, fever, and muscle aches to the HCP.
   2. Instruct the client to avoid driving or other activities that require alertness.
   3. Tell the client that the medication must be taken on an empty stomach.
   4. Explain the importance of not eating bread, cereals, and fruits.
   5. Teach the client to drink a full glass of water with each dose of medication.
   6. Advise the client to avoid drinking alcohol with this medication.
   7. Encourage the client to take aspirin instead of acetaminophen for mild pain.

32. Which interventions should the nurse discuss with the client diagnosed with a calcium oxalate renal calculi and prescribed a thiazide diuretic? **Select all that apply.**
   1. Tell the client to increase fluid intake.
   2. Discuss how this diuretic can cause possible kidney stones.
   3. Explain the need to check potassium level daily.
   4. Inform the client to check blood pressure daily.
   5. Instruct the client to take the diuretic in the morning.

33. The client is admitted to the surgical department diagnosed with renal calculi. The HCP prescribes a morphine patient-controlled analgesia (PCA). Which interventions should the RN implement? **Select all that apply.**
   1. Instruct the client to push the control button as often as needed.
   2. Explain the medication will ensure the client has no pain.
   3. Discuss that medication effectiveness is evaluated on a pain scale of 1 to 10.
   4. Inform the client to obtain assistance when getting out of bed.
   5. Instruct the UAP to strain all of the client's urine.

34. The client diagnosed with calcium renal calculi is prescribed cellulose sodium phosphate. The client asks the nurse, "How will this medication help prevent my stones from coming back?" Which statement is the nurse's **best** response?
   1. "It reduces the uric acid level in your bloodstream and the uric acid excreted in your urine."
   2. "This medication will decrease calcium levels in the bloodstream by increasing calcium excretion in the urine."
   3. "It binds calcium from food in the intestines, reducing the amount absorbed in the circulation."
   4. "The medication will help alkalinize the urine, which reduces the amount of cystine in the urine."

35. The client diagnosed with rule-out renal calculi is scheduled for an IV dye pyelogram (IVP). Which interventions should the nurse implement? **Select all that apply.**
   1. Keep the client NPO.
   2. Check the serum creatinine level.
   3. Assess for an iodine allergy.
   4. Obtain informed consent.
   5. Insert an 18-gauge angiocatheter.

36. The client diagnosed with renal calculi has just had an IVP. Which task is **most appropriate** for the registered nurse (RN) to delegate to the UAP?
   1. Hang a new bag of IV fluid.
   2. Discontinue the client's IV catheter.
   3. Assist the client outside to smoke a cigarette.
   4. Maintain the client's intake and output.

Sexually Transmitted Infection

37. The16-year-old female client tells the public health nurse that she thinks her boyfriend gave her a sexually transmitted infection (STI). Which statement is the nurse's **best** response?
   1. "You will need parental permission to be seen in the clinic."
   2. "Be sure and get the proper medications so that you don't become pregnant."
   3. "How would you know that you have a sexually transmitted infection?"
   4. "You need to have tests so you can be started on medications now."

38. The female client is prescribed metronidazole and erythromycin for a persistent *Chlamydia* infection. Which statements by the client indicate the **need for further** teaching? **Select all that apply.**
   1. "I can have a beer or two while taking these medications."
   2. "My boyfriend will have to take the medications too."
   3. "I can develop more problems if I don't treat this disease."
   4. "My birth control pills will still be effective while taking these medications."
   5. "*Chlamydia* is a sexually transmitted infection I got from my boyfriend."

39. The school nurse is teaching a class on STIs to a group of high school students. Which statement provides **accurate** information regarding the treatment of STIs?
 1. Medications are available to cure STIs if the client is not allergic.
 2. Medications will not cure all STIs.
 3. Medications that prevent pregnancy will prevent most STIs.
 4. Medications that treat STIs enhance sexual libido.

40. Which is the preferred treatment for the diagnosis of primary syphilis in a teenage client?
 1. Doxycycline by mouth (PO) every 4 hours for 10 days
 2. Benzathine penicillin G, intramuscularly one time only
 3. Miconazole topical daily for 1 week
 4. Nitrofurantoin twice a day (b.i.d.) for 1 month

41. The male client is diagnosed with herpes simplex 2 viral infection and is prescribed valacyclovir. Which information should the nurse teach?
 1. The medication will dry the lesions within a day or two.
 2. Valtrex may be taken once a week to control outbreaks.
 3. Condom use will increase the spread of herpes.
 4. Even after the lesions have gone, it is still possible to transmit the virus.

42. The male client is diagnosed with pediculosis pubis and is prescribed permethrin rinse. Which data indicate the treatment has been **effective**?
 1. There are no scratches on the client's penis.
 2. The client shaved his head, and his scalp is clear.
 3. The client reports that the intense itching has abated.
 4. The client has no visible lice or nits on his head.

43. The female client has been diagnosed with genital warts and treated with cryotherapy using liquid nitrogen, a freezing agent, on the external genitalia. Which discharge information should the nurse teach?
 1. Wipe the perineum from front to back to prevent cross-contamination of the area.
 2. Encourage the client to use peripads during their menstrual cycle.
 3. Gently cleanse the perineum with a squirt bottle and tepid water after urinating.
 4. Administer daily povidone-iodine douches until the area has healed completely.

44. The client diagnosed with a severe herpes simplex 2 viral infection is admitted to the medical floor. The HCP prescribes acyclovir 10 mg/kg IVPB every 8 hours. The client weighs 220 pounds. How many milligrams will the nurse administer with each dose?

____

ANSWERS AND RATIONALES

The correct answer number and rationale are in **boldface blue type.** Rationales for why other answer options are incorrect are also given.

Chronic Kidney Disease

1. 1. **Epoetin (Epogen, Procrit), a biologic response modifier, is a glycoprotein produced by the kidney that stimulates RBC production in response to hypoxia. It is prescribed to treat anemia that occurs in clients diagnosed with CKD.**
   2. Filgrastim (Neupogen) is the biological response modifier that stimulates WBCs and is not used to treat CKD.
   3. Oprelvekin (Neumega) is the biological response modifier that stimulates megakaryocyte and thrombocyte production, which stimulates platelet production to prevent thrombocytopenia in clients receiving chemotherapy.
   4. No medication increases urine production. Diuretics increase urine excretion but do not affect urine production.

2. **Correct answers are 1, 3, and 4.**
   1. **Do not shake the vial because shaking may denature the biological response modifier, epoetin (Epogen, Procrit), rendering it biologically inactive.**
   2. After administration, the nurse should apply ice to numb the injection site, not a warm washcloth.
   3. **The nurse should only use the vial for one dose. The nurse should not reaccess the vial and should discard any unused portion because the vial contains no preservatives.**
   4. **The medication should be stored in the refrigerator and warmed to room temperature before being administered.**
   5. This injection is administered subcutaneously, not intramuscularly.

3. 1. This is the scientific rationale for administering antacids to clients diagnosed with peptic ulcer disease or gastritis, not clients diagnosed with CKD.
   2. **Clients diagnosed with CKD experience an increase in serum phosphorus levels (hyperphosphatemia), and administering aluminum hydroxide (Amphojel), an antacid, binds with phosphorus to be excreted in the feces.**
   3. Aluminum hydroxide (Amphojel) does not affect the calcium level.
   4. Aluminum hydroxide can cause constipation; it is not used to treat constipation.

4. 1. Calcitriol does not affect vitamin D availability.
   2. Calcitriol is used to treat hypoparathyroidism, but it does not stimulate calcium excretion from the parathyroid gland.
   3. The client in ESRD has hypocalcemia, not hypercalcemia.
   4. **Calcitriol (Rocaltrol), a vitamin D analog, increases serum calcium levels by promoting calcium absorption and thereby helps to manage hypocalcemia, a CKD symptom.**

5. 1. Nausea is a side effect of calcitriol and can also result from ESRD itself.
   2. Diarrhea is an expected side effect of the medication; therefore, it would not warrant intervention from the nurse.
   3. The client in ESRD would have an increased serum creatinine level; therefore, this would not warrant immediate intervention by the nurse.
   4. **Hematuria is an adverse effect of calcitriol (Rocaltrol), a vitamin D analog, and the nurse should notify the HCP. This would warrant taking the client off the medication.**

MEDICATION MEMORY JOGGER: Any time there is blood in the urine, it is cause for concern. The nurse should intervene and investigate what is causing the hematuria.

6. 1. The client should not drink more than 4 ounces of water because water quickens gastric emptying time.
   2. The client should drink some water to ensure the medication gets to the stomach.
   3. **Liquid antacids should be taken with 2 to 4 ounces of water to ensure the medication reaches the stomach.**
   4. Antacids should be taken on an empty stomach and are effective for 30 to 60 minutes before passing into the duodenum.

7. 1. Sodium polystyrene (Kayexalate) is a medication that is administered to decrease an elevated serum potassium level. Therefore, a phosphorus level would not indicate if the medication is effective.
   2. Sodium polystyrene (Kayexalate) is not used to alter the serum sodium level.

3. **Sodium polystyrene (Kayexalate), a cation exchange resin, is a medication that is administered to decrease an elevated serum potassium level. A potassium level within the normal range of 3.5 to 5.5 mEq/L indicates the medication is effective.**
4. Sodium polystyrene (Kayexalate) is used to decrease an elevated potassium level. The medication can decrease the serum calcium level but this would not indicate if the medication is effective.

MEDICATION MEMORY JOGGER: The nurse determines medication effectiveness by assessing for the symptoms, or lack thereof, for which the medication was prescribed.

8. Correct answers are 1 and 5.
   1. **Tented skin turgor indicates the client is dehydrated and the nurse should question administering the thiazide diuretic, hydrochlorothiazide (HydroDIURIL).**
   2. The client diagnosed with CKD would have a less-than-normal urine output, so the nurse would not question giving the client a diuretic.
   3. A moist and pink mucosa indicates the client is hydrated; therefore, the nurse would not question administering this medication.
   4. The medication is being administered to help decrease the sacral edema; therefore, the nurse would not question administering this diuretic.
   5. **Diuretics reduce circulating blood volume, which may cause orthostatic hypotension. Because the client's blood pressure is low, the nurse should question administering this medication.**

MEDICATION MEMORY JOGGER: The nurse must know accepted standards of practice for medication administration, including which client assessment data and laboratory data should be monitored before administering the medication.

9. 1. A normal or decreased potassium level indicates dialysis is effective, but not that the medication is effective.
   2. This medication does not affect sodium level.
   3. A normal or decreased BUN level indicates the dialysis is effective, but not the medication.
   4. **Lanthanum carbonate (Fosrenol), an electrolyte- and water-balancing agent, decreases phosphate absorption in the intestines. Phosphorus is excreted in the feces.**

10. Correct answers are 1 and 5.
    1. **Lanthanum carbonate (Fosrenol), an electrolyte- and water-balancing agent, should not be swallowed. The medication must be chewed for absorption in the intestines.**
    2. Lanthanum carbonate (Fosrenol) may cause graft occlusion, not bleeding.
    3. Lanthanum carbonate (Fosrenol) does not increase gastric acid secretion; therefore, the client would not need to take a proton-pump inhibitor (PPI).
    4. Lanthanum carbonate (Fosrenol) may cause hypotension, and the blood pressure must be checked, but it does not affect the pulse rate.
    5. **Lanthanum carbonate (Fosrenol) should be taken with or right after meals.**

Urinary Tract Infection

11. 1. **Cranberry juice is acidic and will change urine's pH, making it harder for bacteria to survive in the environment. It can be used prophylactically to prevent UTIs. It does not treat infection. The nurse can arrange with the dietitian to include this in the client's dietary plan.**
    2. Nitrofurantoin (Macrodantin), a sulfa drug, is a prescription medication used to treat chronic UTIs, but the nurse could not order this medication.
    3. This over-the-counter (OTC) vitamin would require an HCP order in a long-term care facility.
    4. This is an herb used for UTIs, but it would require an HCP order in a long-term care facility.

MEDICATION MEMORY JOGGER: Nurses do not order medications. Nurses do have latitude in deciding on components and consistency of the meals provided. The dietitian can include cranberry juice in any diet.

12. 1. The IV is essential to initiate therapy, but the nurse should obtain a clean, voided midstream urine for culture and sensitivity before initiating the treatment. If the culture is not obtained before initiating the antibiotic, the laboratory test results will be skewed.
    2. This should definitely be done, but obtaining the culture is the first intervention.
    3. **The nurse should obtain a clean voided midstream specimen for culture and sensitivity before initiating the antibiotics. This is the first intervention to implement.**

4. A diet order is not a priority over getting the treatment started. UTIs in males are difficult to treat and can be life-threatening.

MEDICATION MEMORY JOGGER: The first step in initiating antibiotic therapy is to obtain any ordered culture. Then the nurse must prioritize initiating IV antibiotic therapy in a timely manner, within 1 to 2 hours after the order is written, depending on the facility's standard protocol.

13. 1. A urine specific gravity can indicate dehydration or water intoxication, but it will not provide information about a UTI.
2. A microscopic value of 35 WBCs per high power field (hpf) indicates a UTI, not that the antibiotic is effective. A normal value is less than 5 wbc/hpf.
3. Normal urine pH is 5.0 to 9.0, but the pH does not evaluate a UTI.
4. A negative urine leukocyte esterase indicates that the antibiotic trimethoprim sulfa (Bactrim DS) effectively treats the infection. Leukocytes and nitrates are used to determine bacteriuria and other sources of UTIs.

14. 1. Ceftriaxone (Rocephin), a third-generation cephalosporin, is in pregnancy risk category B. No research has shown harm to the fetus in humans or in animals. The nurse would not question this medication.
2. Some clients have a cross-sensitivity between penicillin and cephalosporins such as cephalexin (Keflex). The nurse should assess the type of reaction that the client experienced when taking penicillin. If the client indicates any symptom of an anaphylactic reaction, the nurse would hold the medication and discuss the situation with the HCP.
3. The nurse has no reason to question trimethoprim sulfa (Bactrim), a sulfa antibiotic, for a client after prostate surgery.
4. The nurse has no reason to question nitrofurantoin (Macrodantin), a sulfa antibiotic, for a client diagnosed with urinary stasis. Nitrofurantoin (Macrodantin) is used to prevent or treat chronic UTIs.

MEDICATION MEMORY JOGGER: The nurse must be knowledgeable of accepted standards of practice for disease processes and conditions. If the nurse administers a medication that the HCP has prescribed and harms the client, the nurse could be held accountable. Remember, the nurse is a client advocate.

15. 1. Urinary output should be measured frequently for a client after a TURP. The client will have bladder irrigation, and the indwelling catheter bag will need to be emptied frequently. The RN would not intervene to stop this action.
2. A green-blue color indicates the client is taking bethanechol (Urecholine), a urinary stimulant used for clients diagnosed with a neurogenic bladder. This is an expected color, and the UAP should not indicate that something is wrong with the client.
3. The client should be encouraged to drink fluids. The nurse would not intervene to stop this action.
4. This action encourages bowel and urine continence and is part of a fall prevention protocol. The nurse would not intervene to stop this action.

16. Correct answers are 2, 3, 4, and 5.
1. The therapeutic range of vancomycin is 10 to 20 mg/dL. The nurse would not hold the medication because the client has not reached a therapeutic range.
2. The nurse should always ask the client if they are allergic to any medication before administering medications, especially an antibiotic.
3. Vancomycin is administered over a minimum of 1 hour. The nurse should obtain an infusion pump to regulate administration speed.
4. Vancomycin is nephrotoxic. The nurse would monitor BUN and creatinine levels, especially in children and the elderly.
5. The nurse should assess the IV insertion site to determine infiltration or inflammation findings. The nurse should not administer vancomycin in an inflamed site.

17. 1. This is a side effect of nitrofurantoin. The client should be warned that the urine might turn brown. This color will disappear when the client is no longer taking the medication. If the client is taking an oral suspension, the nurse should instruct the client to rinse their mouth after taking the medication to prevent teeth staining.
2. This does not indicate cystitis.
3. The client should be instructed to take the medication with food to avoid gastrointestinal upset.
4. This is a side effect of the medication and does not indicate another problem.

18. 1. Phenazopyridine (Pyridium) is not an antibiotic. It will not treat an infection.
2. Phenazopyridine is a urinary analgesic, not a urinary stimulant. It will not increase bladder tone.
3. Phenazopyridine (Pyridium) is a urinary analgesic. It is helpful in treating the pain and burning associated with a UTI.
4. Antimuscarinic and anticholinergic medications control an overactive bladder; urinary analgesic medications do not. Phenazopyridine does help control urinary frequency associated with a UTI.

19. Correct answers are identified in the table.

Finding	Effective	Not Effective
1. Voids 300 to 400 mL of urine each time	X	
2. Urinary frequency		X
3. Temperature of 99°F	X	
4. Burning with urination		X
5. Pink urine	X	

1. The client voiding 300 to 400 mL each time indicates the client cannot void until the bladder is full. This indicates the client is responding to the antibiotic and the medication is effective.
2. Urinary frequency indicates a UTI, which means the medication, aztreonam (Azactam), is not effective.
3. The client is afebrile. This indicates the client is responding to the antibiotic and the medication is effective.
4. Burning upon urination indicates a UTI, which means the medication, aztreonam (Azactam), is not effective.
5. Pinkish urine can result from beet consumption and does not indicate the client has a UTI.

20. 1. This is not a priority. The tubing should be taped to the leg on the side of the bed the bag will be suspended from.
2. This could be asked, but it is not a priority.
3. This could be asked, but it is not a priority.
4. Indwelling catheter kits come prepackaged with povidone-iodine (Betadine) to clean the perineal skin before inserting the catheter. The nurse should assess for allergies to the medication before preparing to cleanse the perineum. Another type of skin cleanser may need to be used.

Benign Prostatic Hypertrophy

21. Correct answers are 3, 5, and 6.
1. The client's intake of water will not affect the medication. Drinking this much water each day until the medication has had an opportunity to shrink the enlarged prostate tissue could cause the client to have difficulty emptying an uncomfortably full bladder.
2. The medication takes 6 to 12 months to have a full effect. There is no reason for the client to be seen in 1 week.
3. Finasteride (Proscar), a 5-alpha-reductase inhibitor, decreases serum prostate-specific antigen (PSA) levels. The client should have a PSA level drawn before beginning finasteride and a level drawn after 6 months. If the PSA level does not drop, the client should be assessed for prostate cancer.
4. Clients do not need to measure their urine outputs daily.
5. The client should notify the HCP for breast changes such as lumps, pain, or nipple discharge.
6. Erectile dysfunction and decreased libido can occur during therapy and after therapy ends.

22. 1. There is documented evidence that this herb effectively treats BPH. Its use is not a folk remedy without a sound basis.
2. Research has proven saw palmetto's efficacy in treating BPH. The exact mechanism of action is unknown, but the herb does shrink prostate tissue, resulting in relief of obstructive urinary symptoms.
3. The client reported that he has been taking the herb. The time to discuss allergies is before or shortly after medication initiation.
4. Research indicates that saw palmetto is as effective as finasteride (Proscar) but has fewer side effects. It is considered a safe and effective treatment for BPH. There is no evidence that the herb causes cancer.

23. 1. The alpha-adrenergic agonist tamsulosin (Flomax) is used to treat hyperplasia of the prostate and was initially developed to treat high blood pressure. The client may develop hypotension when taking these medications. This side effect makes them useful for clients also diagnosed with hypertension.

2. The medication is not given for UTIs, so there is no need for a urinalysis when administering this medication.
3. The client has symptoms of BPH, which could include nocturia, but this is not pertinent when administering the medication.
4. This is an intervention that assists clients diagnosed with incontinence, not BPH.

24. **1,450 mL of corrected urinary output. The drainage in the catheter bag equals 5,550 mL of drainage. 1,500 mL plus 2,100 mL plus 1,950 mL equals 5,550 mL of drainage emptied for the shift. Subtract the 4,100 mL of normal saline irrigation fluid from the 5,550 mL total drainage equals 1,450 mL of corrected urinary output.**

25. 1. Testosterone is converted to dihydrotestosterone (DHT) in the prostate. The 5-alpha-reductase inhibitors reduce DHT, but not testosterone. With a DHT reduction, prostate tissue shrinks. The 5-alpha-reductase inhibitors do not elevate testosterone, nor do they improve impotence problems.
2. The 5-alpha-reductase inhibitors require 6 to 12 months for therapeutic relief of BPH symptoms to occur.
3. **The 5-alpha-reductase inhibitors, such as dutasteride (Avodart), work by reducing the size of the prostate gland, resulting in relief of the obstructive symptoms of urgency, frequency, difficulty initiating a urine stream, and nocturia.**
4. Surgery provides faster relief of symptoms after recovery has taken place. Dutasteride (Avodart) requires a lengthy period for therapeutic effects of the medications and may not provide adequate relief of symptoms if the client has severe BPH.

26. **Correct answers are 1, 2, 3, 4, and 5.**
1. **B&O suppositories come in 15A (1/2 grain) and 16A (1 grain) formulations. When obtaining the medication from the narcotic cabinet, the nurse should obtain the correct dose for the client. B&O suppositories are used to reduce bladder spasms for clients after bladder surgery.**
2. **Lubricating the suppository decreases pain for the client when inserting the suppository.**
3. **Adhering to standard precautions is always an appropriate nursing intervention when caring for the client.**
4. **The nurse should check the armband before opening the medication and preparing to administer it.**
5. **The large intestine and rectum lie on the left side of the body, so placing the client on the left side makes insertion easier and reduces the chance of a ruptured bowel.**

27. 1. **The major adverse effect of terazosin (Hytrin) is hypotension. Most blood pressure–lowering medications can also cause hypotension. The nurse would question administering two medications that can cause the client to become dizzy upon standing, possibly resulting in a fall. The medications that shrink the prostate gland were initially developed to treat high blood pressure. This is a safety issue.**
2. Finasteride (Proscar) does not cause hypotension and does not interact with digoxin. The nurse would not question administering these medications.
3. Tamsulosin (Flomax) is an alpha$_1$-adrenergic agonist but does not cause hypotension. Metformin (Glucophage), a biguanide, does not interact with Tamsulosin (Flomax). The nurse would not question administering these medications.
4. *Serenoa repens* (saw palmetto) has fewer side effects than most prescription medications that treat BPH, and it does not cause hypotension or interact with metoprolol (Toprol XL). The nurse would not question administering these medications.

MEDICATION MEMORY JOGGER: The test taker must know these medications. An alpha blocker usually would have some effect on the cardiovascular system, and an angiotensin-converting enzyme (ACE) inhibitor is used to treat high blood pressure. Most blood pressure medications can cause orthostatic hypotension. Two medications that can cause similar side effects would be questioned.

28. 1. The medication is manufactured in a pill form. The nurse does not need eye protection to prevent exposure.
2. The nurse's mucosa should not be exposed to the medication because it comes only in pill form.
3. The nurse can administer dutasteride safely using the appropriate personal protective equipment. The nurse should not ask for another nurse to administer the medication.
4. **Dutasteride (Avodart) is used to treat BPH and is considered a category X medication, which will cause harm to a developing fetus. The medication can be**

absorbed through the skin. The nurse should wear gloves when administering the medication. Men should not donate blood for at least 6 months after discontinuing the medication to avoid medication administration to a pregnant client through the transfusion.

MEDICATION MEMORY JOGGER: The nurse must remember that some medications can cause harm when administering the medication. A pregnant nurse must be cautious.

29. Correct order is 2, 4, 3, 5, 1.

2. The most obvious reason for a client post-TURP having lower abdominal pain is that the bladder has blood clots that need to be flushed out. Clots that are not flushed from the bladder result in bladder spasms. Assessing urinary drainage would be the first step.

4. The next step is to adjust the irrigation rate to ensure adequate drainage of blood and clots from the bladder.

3. Before administering a narcotic analgesic, the nurse should rule out complications. Assessing for peritonitis (hard, rigid abdomen) is the next step in this situation.

5. Morphine and most other narcotic medications require a very slow IV rate, around 5 minutes, according to the manufacturer's recommendations. Morphine is dispensed in 1-mL tubex syringes or vials. It is difficult to maintain a steady, slow medication administration with only 1 mL over 5 minutes. If the medication is diluted to a total volume of 10 mL, then the nurse can administer the medication at a rate of 1 mL every 30 seconds. Dilution causes less pain for the client and helps decrease vein irritation.

1. The final step in this sequence is actually to administer the analgesic.

30. 1. The client's intake and output measurements are essential, but even accurate intake and output recordings cannot measure insensible losses. An output of 100 mL over the intake may or may not be considered adequate to determine the diuretic's effectiveness.

2. Ambulating to the bathroom without dyspnea is an indicator that the client is not experiencing pulmonary complications related to excess fluid volume, but it is not the best indicator of a diuretic's effectiveness.

3. Terminology such as *small*, *moderate*, and *large* are not objective words. To quantify results, the nurse should use objective data—in this situation, numbers. This would provide an accurate comparison of data to determine medication effectiveness.

4. The most reliable method of determining changes in fluid volume status is to weigh a client in the same type of clothing at the same time each day. One liter (1,000 mL) is approximately 0.9 kg (or 2 pounds). This client has lost approximately 500 mL more fluid than was taken in.

Renal Calculi

31. Correct answers are 1, 5, and 6.

1. The client should notify the HCP if a skin rash or influenza symptoms (chills, fever, muscle aches and pain, nausea, or vomiting) develop because these clinical manifestations may indicate hypersensitivity to allopurinol (Zyloprim).

2. Allopurinol (Zyloprim) does not cause drowsiness, so the nurse does not need to tell the client to avoid activities that require alertness.

3. Allopurinol may be administered with milk or meals to minimize gastric irritation.

4. The client diagnosed with uric acid renal calculi should be eating a low-purine diet. A low-purine diet includes bread, cereals, cream-style soups made with low-fat milk, fruits, juices, low-fat cheeses, nuts, peanut butter, coffee, and tea.

5. The client should take allopurinol (Zyloprim) with a full glass of water and increase fluid intake to prevent renal calculi formation.

6. Large amounts of alcohol increase uric acid concentrations and may decrease effectiveness of allopurinol (Zyloprim).

7. Salicylic acid (aspirin) increases urine acidity. Urine should be alkaline. The nurse should encourage the client to take acetaminophen (Tylenol) instead of salicylic acid to reduce urine acidity.

MEDICATION MEMORY JOGGER: If a client verbalizes a symptom, the nurse assesses data, or if laboratory data indicates an adverse effect secondary to a medication, the nurse must intervene. The nurse must implement an independent intervention or notify the HCP because medications can result in serious or even life-threatening complications.

32. Correct answers are 1 and 5.

1. **The client should drink adequate fluids or increase fluids when taking a thiazide diuretic to help prevent renal calculi formation.**
2. Thiazide diuretics will help prevent renal stones, not increase the chance of developing renal calculi.
3. Thiazide diuretics cause an increase in potassium loss in urine, but not as significant as loop diuretics. In any case, the client would not check the potassium level daily at home.
4. The thiazide diuretic is not being administered to decrease blood pressure; therefore, the blood pressure would not have to be checked daily to ensure medication effectiveness.
5. **Diuretics should be taken in the morning so that the client is not up all night urinating. Thiazide diuretics are prescribed because they decrease the amount of calcium released by the kidneys into the urine by favoring calcium retention in the bone. Most kidney stones (75% to 80%) are calcium stones composed of calcium.**

33. Correct answers are 1, 3, 4, and 5.

1. **The PCA pump automatically administers a specific amount and has a lockout interval time in which the PCA pump cannot administer any morphine. The client can push the control button as often as needed and not receive an overdose of pain medication.**
2. The nurse should inform the client that the pain should be tolerable, not necessarily absent.
3. **Adult clients use the 1 to 10 pain scale, with 0 being no pain and 10 being the worst pain.**
4. **The client receiving PCA morphine should be instructed not to ambulate without assistance due to the chance of falls.**
5. **All the client's urine should be strained by all staff members.**

34. 1. This is the scientific rationale for administering allopurinol (Zyloprim) to help reduce uric stone formation.

2. This is the scientific rationale for administering a thiazide diuretic to help reduce formation of calcium renal calculi. This medication will decrease calcium levels in the bloodstream by increasing calcium excretion in the urine.
3. **This is the scientific rationale for administering cellulose sodium phosphate (Calcibind) to reduce calcium renal calculi formation.**
4. This is the scientific rationale for administering penicillamine to help prevent uric stone formation.

35. Correct answers are 2, 3, and 4.

1. The client does not need to be NPO for this procedure because it is used to diagnose renal abnormalities, not gastrointestinal abnormalities.
2. **The client should not have this diagnostic test if the kidneys are not working correctly. The IV dye could damage the kidneys if normal functioning is not present.**
3. **The nurse would assess for iodine allergy. The nurse should ask if the client is allergic to Betadine or shellfish.**
4. **This is an invasive procedure; therefore, the client must give informed consent.**
5. This diagnostic test does not require blood administration; therefore, the nurse should start a smaller gauge IV catheter, such as a 22- or 20-gauge angiocatheter.

36. 1. IV fluids are medications. The nurse cannot delegate medication administration to the UAP.

2. The UAP may be able to discontinue an IV, but the question asks which is the most appropriate task. The RN should always delegate the least invasive and the simplest task.
3. The UAP should not be assigned to take a client outside to smoke. This is not in the job description of a hospital employee. After the nurse discourages the client from going downstairs to smoke, a family member or friend should escort the client outside.
4. **The UAP can document the client's oral intake and urinary output. Still, the UAP cannot evaluate if urine output is adequate and appropriate for the IVP procedure.**

Sexually Transmitted Infection

37. 1. STIs are considered a public health hazard, and the client can choose to be treated without parental permission.

2. Pregnancy may be a concern, but the client is discussing an STI, and the nurse should address the client's concerns.

3. This is a judgmental statement. The nurse should not impair communication with the client.
4. There are many different STIs. The client needs to have tests run based on her presenting symptoms to initiate appropriate treatment.

38. Correct answers are 1 and 4.
1. Consuming alcohol concurrently with metronidazole (Flagyl) can cause a severe reaction. This statement indicates the need for more teaching.
2. The sexual partners must be treated simultaneously to prevent reinfection from occurring. This statement indicates the client understands the teaching.
3. Untreated STIs can lead to pelvic inflammatory disease, scarred fallopian tubes, and infertility. This statement indicates the client understands the teaching.
4. Antibiotics may interfere with the effectiveness of some birth control pills. The client should use a supplemental form of birth control when taking birth control pills. This statement indicates the client does not understand the teaching.
5. This STI can be transmitted by any male partner; therefore, she understands the teaching.

MEDICATION MEMORY JOGGER: The test taker should realize that consuming alcohol is contraindicated with most medications.

39. 1. Whether the client is allergic or not, there are no medications available to cure herpes simplex 2 virus and HIV. This is a false statement.
2. There are no medications available to cure herpes simplex 2 virus and HIV. There are many medications available to treat the problems associated with these STIs, and they provide hope for the client, but students must be aware of the long-term ramifications of STIs.
3. Birth control medications do not protect against an STI. They may increase the chance of acquiring an STI because the fear of pregnancy is removed, making sexual activity more likely.
4. Antibiotics have side effects, and medications for HIV infections have especially strong associated side effects and adverse reactions. Side effects and adverse reactions are more likely to decrease libido than to enhance it.

40. 1. Syphilis is treated with a penicillin antibiotic unless the client is allergic to penicillin. The dosing schedule of every 4 hours for 10 days would make it difficult to achieve adult compliance, much less compliance of an adolescent.
2. A one-time injection of benzathine penicillin G is the usual treatment for primary syphilis infections.
3. Syphilis is a bacterial infection, and antifungal medications, such as miconazole (Monistat), would not treat a bacterial infection. The antibiotic must be taken internally to treat syphilis.
4. Nitrofurantoin (Macrodantin) is a macrolide antibiotic used primarily for chronic UTIs, not syphilis.

41. 1. Amount of time needed for lesions to heal depends on several factors, including immune status of the infected individual and amount of stress the individual is experiencing at the time. It usually requires several days to more than a week for an outbreak to be healed.
2. Suppressive therapy with valacyclovir (Valtrex) is once daily, every day. This is an advantage over other antiretroviral agents, which require twice-a-day dosing.
3. Condom use may prevent herpes infection spread. It does not increase spread of the virus.
4. It is possible to transmit the virus to a sexual partner with no visible findings of a lesion being present. Valacyclovir (Valtrex), an antiviral, will not prevent spread of the virus. It will treat an outbreak and decrease the risk of transmission.

42. 1. No scratch marks on the penis indicate the client has not scratched himself but does not indicate a lack of infestation in the pubic hair.
2. Pediculosis pubis is pubic lice, not head lice. A clear scalp would not indicate a lack of a pubic infestation.
3. Pediculosis causes intense itching. A lack of itching indicates the treatment with permethrin (Nix), an ectoparasiticide cream rinse, is effective.
4. Pediculosis pubis is pubic lice, not head lice, so no visible lice or nits on the head would not indicate lack of a pubic infestation.

MEDICATION MEMORY JOGGER: The nurse determines medication effectiveness by assessing for the symptoms, or lack thereof, for which the medication was prescribed.

43. 1. Wiping the perineum from front to back is encouraged to prevent a UTI from fecal contamination of the urethral meatus.
2. The procedure should be planned immediately after the menstrual cycle has ended so that protection will not be needed until the client has had time to heal.
3. Liquid nitrogen causes a chemical burn to form, destroying the genital wart. The client should be taught to cleanse the area carefully to decrease pain and risk of infection.
4. Daily Betadine douches would increase pain and discomfort. Betadine is an iodine preparation and could cause the area to sting. The client should be encouraged to limit use of any soap or chemical preparation until released to do so by the HCP.

44. **1,000 mg of medication will be administered with each dose. The client weighs 220 pounds. Convert weight to kilograms by dividing by 2.2 (220 ÷ 2.2 = 100 kg). To find the amount for each dose, multiply 100 kg by 10 mg, which equals 1,000 mg per dose.**

GENITOURINARY SYSTEM COMPREHENSIVE EXAMINATION

1. Which client should the nurse consider at risk for complications when taking sildenafil?
   1. A 56-year-old client diagnosed with unstable angina
   2. An 87-year-old client diagnosed with glaucoma
   3. A 44-year-old client diagnosed with type 2 diabetes
   4. A 32-year-old client diagnosed with an L1 spinal cord injury (SCI)

2. The 33-year-old client is being prescribed an antibiotic for a UTI. Which question is **most important** for the nurse to ask the client when discussing the medication?
   1. "How many UTIs have you had in the past year?"
   2. "What type of underwear do you usually wear?"
   3. "Which way do you clean after a bowel movement?"
   4. "Are you currently using any type of birth control?"

3. The client, 1 day postpartum, is reporting dysuria, urinary urgency, and suprapubic pain. It is 1000; which as-needed (PRN) medications should the nurse administer?

Client: R.M.	MR# 1234567	Date: Today
Age: 25 years	Allergies: NKDA	Diagnosis: Postpartum
Medication	0701–1900	1901–0700
Ondansetron, 8 mg PO q 12 hours PRN		0700
Oxycodone 2.5 mg & acetaminophen 325 mg, 1 to 2 tablets PO q 12 hours PRN		
Phenazopyridine, 200 mg PO q 8 hours PRN		
Acetaminophen 325 mg, 1 to 2 tablets PO q 4 to 6 hours PRN		0700
Nurse Initials/Credentials	DN/RN	NN/RN

   1. Ondansetron
   2. Oxycodone and acetaminophen
   3. Phenazopyridine
   4. Acetaminophen

4. The sexually active 16-year-old client is being seen in the clinic for a Pap test. She has requested to receive the human papillomavirus (HPV) quadrivalent vaccine. Which information should the nurse discuss with the client? **Select all that apply.**
   1. "You must ask your parents if you can take this medication."
   2. "The medication is administered in a series of injections."
   3. "HPV quadrivalent vaccine will guarantee you won't get cervical cancer."
   4. "This medication must be taken for the rest of your life."
   5. "This vaccine will not prevent sexually transmitted diseases."

5. The elderly client is prescribed tolterodine for urge incontinence. Which statement **warrants notifying** the HCP?
   1. "I have to suck on sugarless candy because my mouth is so dry."
   2. "I am so glad I can go all day without having to go to the bathroom."
   3. "I really have problems swallowing the pills whole with water."
   4. "I hate that I had to give up my grapefruit juice, but I know it is best."

6. The nurse is preparing to insert an 18-gauge indwelling urinary catheter in a client diagnosed with a latex allergy. Which intervention is **most important** for the nurse to implement?
   1. Use latex-free gloves when performing this procedure.
   2. Insert a 16-gauge indwelling urinary catheter into the client.
   3. Obtain an appropriate indwelling urinary catheter for the client.
   4. Use a povidone-iodine solution to cleanse the perineal area.

7. The client is diagnosed with *Chlamydia trachomatis* and asks the nurse, "Why must I take an antibiotic when I don't have itching or pain?" Which statement is the nurse's **best** response?
   1. "The itching and pain will start within 2 or 3 days."
   2. "The antibiotics will prevent canker sores on your genitalia."
   3. "If you use a condom, then you don't have to take the antibiotic."
   4. "If it is not treated, you may never be able to have a baby."

8. The 19-year-old client presents to the emergency department with trauma to the flank area resulting from a motor vehicle accident. The client's first urine specimen shows bright red urine. Which intervention should the nurse implement **first**?
   1. Initiate an 18-gauge angiocath with normal saline.
   2. Send a sterile urine specimen to the laboratory.
   3. Type and crossmatch for two units of blood.
   4. Prepare the client for a computed tomography abdominal scan.

9. The 17-year-old athlete tells the nurse about taking anabolic steroids to increase muscle strength. Which action should the nurse implement?
   1. Inform the client's parents about the illegal use of anabolic steroids.
   2. Ask the client where he has been obtaining these anabolic steroids.
   3. Assess the client for moon face, buffalo hump, and weight gain.
   4. Explain that the long-term effects of steroids may cause him never to father a baby.

10. The client diagnosed with CKD is admitted to the medical floor for pneumonia. The admission orders include Zithromax, cyclosporine, and Mylanta. Which question should the nurse ask the client?
    1. "Are you allergic to iodine or any type of shellfish?"
    2. "When was the last time you had your dialysis treatment?"
    3. "Have you had any type of organ transplant?"
    4. "Why don't you take aluminum hydroxide instead of Mylanta?"

11. The nurse is administering medication to a client with a history of kidney transplant and taking cyclosporine. The HCP's medication orders are in the following order sheet.

Client: B.R.	MR# 1234567	Date: Today
Age: 55 years	Allergies: NKDA	Diagnosis: Bronchitis
PROVIDER ORDERS:		
Captopril, 25 mg PO b.i.d.		
Trimethoprim-sulfamethoxazole double strength, 1 tablet PO q 12 hours		
Acetaminophen, 650 mg, PO q 4 to 6 hours PRN pain, not to exceed 3,250 mg/day		
Prochlorperazine, 5 mg IM q 3 to 4 hours PRN for nausea and vomiting		

Which medication should the nurse **question** administering?
1. Captopril
2. Trimethoprim-sulfamethoxazole
3. Acetaminophen
4. Prochlorperazine

12. The client diagnosed with a renal stone is admitted to the medical department. The nurse administers IV morphine over 5 minutes. Which intervention should the nurse implement **first**?
    1. Instruct the client to call for help before getting out of bed.
    2. Tell the client to urinate into the urinal at all times.
    3. Document the time in the MAR and the client's EHR.
    4. Reevaluate the client's pain within 30 minutes.

13. The client diagnosed with renal calculi is receiving morphine via PCA. The client is still reporting excruciating pain and is requesting something else. Which intervention should the nurse implement **first**?
    1. Administer the rescue dose of morphine IV push.
    2. Check the client's urine for color, sediment, and output.
    3. Determine the last time the client received PCA morphine.
    4. Demonstrate how to perform guided imagery with the client.

14. The client diagnosed with stress urinary incontinence is prescribed duloxetine 40 mg PO b.i.d. to relieve symptoms. Which interventions should the nurse discuss with the client? **Select all that apply.**
    1. Mix the medication in water or fruit juice and drink completely.
    2. Avoid taking St. John's wort with duloxetine.
    3. Use caution when driving at the start of therapy.
    4. If nausea occurs, skip the medication for a few days.
    5. Wear sunscreen and a hat when going outdoors.

15. The client diagnosed with overflow incontinence reports incomplete voiding and a weak urine stream. Which medication should the nurse expect to administer?
    1. Bethanechol
    2. Darifenacin
    3. Oxybutynin
    4. Estrogen

GENITOURINARY SYSTEM COMPREHENSIVE EXAMINATION ANSWERS AND RATIONALES

1. 1. **Sildenafil (Viagra), a sexual stimulant, should be used cautiously for clients diagnosed with coronary heart disease. During sexual activity the client could have a myocardial infarction from the extra demands on the heart. Specifically, clients taking nitroglycerin or any nitrate medication should not take Viagra because Viagra's vasodilatation effect may cause hypotension. A client diagnosed with unstable angina would be taking nitrate medication.**

2. Sildenafil (Viagra) is not contraindicated for clients diagnosed with glaucoma.
3. Sildenafil (Viagra) is not contraindicated for clients diagnosed with type 2 diabetes and may help erectile dysfunction.
4. Sildenafil (Viagra) is not contraindicated for clients diagnosed with an SCI and may help erectile dysfunction.

2. 1. The number of UTIs is information the nurse would need to determine if the client is at risk for developing chronic UTIs, but this is not the most important question when discussing antibiotic therapy.

2. Wearing cotton underwear or underwear with a cotton crotch should be encouraged because cotton is a natural material that breathes and allows air to circulate to the area, decreasing UTI risk. It is an appropriate question, but it is not the most important question when discussing antibiotic therapy.
3. Cleaning from back to front after a bowel movement increases risk of fecal contamination of the urinary meatus, but this is not the most important question when discussing antibiotic therapy.
4. **Birth control pills and certain antibiotics may interact, making birth control pills ineffective in preventing pregnancy. This is the most important question for the nurse to ask.**

MEDICATION MEMORY JOGGER: When a client is of childbearing age, the nurse should determine if there is a potential pregnancy or drug interaction with birth control methods.

3. 1. Ondansetron is given for nausea and vomiting.

2. Oxycodone and acetaminophen (Percocet) is given for severe or acute pain and is not indicated by the client's reported symptoms.
3. **Phenazopyridine (Pyridium) is a urinary analgesic designed to relieve the symptoms the client is describing. The nurse should select this medication.**
4. Acetaminophen is an analgesic and antipyretic and can help with suprapubic pain; however, it will not address the urinary urgency and frequency; therefore, it is not the medication the nurse should administer. Additionally, it was administered at 0700 (3 hours prior), and therefore, it is not an option to be given.

4. Correct answers is 2.

1. A sexually active 16-year-old female does not have to have parental permission to be treated for sexually transmitted diseases or to receive a vaccine designed to prevent an STI.
2. **HPV quadrivalent vaccine (Gardasil) is the first vaccine developed to prevent HPV infections and is administered in a series of injections. The nurse must discuss this with the client to ensure that she will return for the entire series.**
3. The Gardasil vaccine can prevent infection from HPV types 6, 11, 16, and 18, but not from every kind of HPV.
4. The Gardasil vaccine is given in a series of injections. It is not an oral medication to be taken for life.
5. The HPV vaccine is effective for many HPV strains but is not helpful in preventing syphilis, gonorrhea, or chlamydia.

5. 1. Anticholinergic medications block the muscarinic receptors on the salivary glands and inhibit salivation, resulting in a dry mouth. This comment would not warrant notifying the HCP.

2. **Inability to void all day long indicates an overdose of tolterodine (Detrol-LA), an anticholinergic, and would require notifying the HCP to decrease the dosage.**
3. Tolterodine (Detrol-LA) is long-acting and should not be crushed. Because the client is swallowing the pill, the HCP would not need to be notified.
4. Grapefruit juice increases the effect of tolterodine (Detrol); therefore, the client not drinking it would not warrant notifying the HCP.

MEDICATION MEMORY JOGGER: Grapefruit juice can inhibit metabolism of certain medications. Specifically, grapefruit juice inhibits cytochrome P450-3A4 found in the liver and the intestinal wall. The nurse should investigate any medications the client is taking if the client drinks grapefruit juice.

6. 1. The nurse should use latex-free gloves when touching the client, but this is not the most important intervention because this is a very short-term exposure to latex for the client.
   2. A smaller catheter does not address the material the catheter is made out of.
   3. The most important intervention is for the client to have a latex-free Foley catheter because this will stay in the client for an extended period.
   4. The solution used to clean the client would not have a bearing on the latex allergy.

7. 1. *Chlamydia* is frequently asymptomatic and is diagnosed with an annual Pap smear.
   2. *Chlamydia* does not cause canker sores. These sores are caused by syphilis.
   3. *Chlamydia* is bacteria and must be treated with an antibiotic. Condoms are used to prevent transmission to a partner.
   4. Untreated *Chlamydia* can lead to pelvic inflammatory disease and long-term effects, including chronic pain, increased risk for ectopic pregnancy, postpartum endometritis, and infertility.

8. **1. The nurse must first initiate steps to prevent the client from developing hypovolemic shock; therefore, the nurse should start a large-bore IV to infuse isotonic normal saline to maintain blood pressure. The nurse should anticipate the client receiving a blood transfusion, which supports the need for an 18-gauge catheter.**
   2. A urine specimen should be sent to the laboratory, but the client's safety and shock prevention are the nurse's first priority.
   3. Ordering blood is a priority, but not a priority over caring for the client at increased risk of hypovolemic shock.
   4. Determining the source of bleeding is important, but caring for the client is a priority.

MEDICATION MEMORY JOGGER: The nurse's first priority is always caring for the client, not a laboratory or diagnostic test.

9. 1. This action would violate the nurse–client relationship. The nurse should encourage the client to tell his parents.
   2. The nurse should not be concerned with where the medications are being obtained. The nurse should strongly discourage use of anabolic steroids because of the long-term effects, including psychological changes.
   3. These are side effects of glucocorticosteroids, not of anabolic steroids.
   4. Anabolic steroids have serious side effects, including low sperm counts and impotence in men, along with permanent liver damage and aggressive behavior. Anabolic steroid use to improve athletic performance is illegal and strongly discouraged by HCPs and athletic associations.

10. 1. Questions about allergies to iodine or shellfish would be appropriate for a client undergoing a test with contrast dye.
    2. The nurse should realize that a client taking cyclosporine has had some type of organ transplant because it is a major immune suppressant drug.
    3. Cyclosporine would not be an expected medication for a client diagnosed with pneumonia or CKD unless the client has had a kidney transplant; therefore, asking this question is appropriate.
    4. Because the client has functioning kidneys, there is no need to take aluminum hydroxide (Amphojel), a phosphate binder.

11. 1. ACE inhibitors, such as captopril (Capoten), would not be questioned for clients with kidney transplants or taking cyclosporine.
    2. The antibiotic trimethoprim-sulfamethoxazole (Bactrim DS) reduces cyclosporine levels, leading to organ rejection; therefore, the nurse should question administering this medication.
    3. The analgesic acetaminophen (Tylenol) is not contraindicated for clients diagnosed with kidney transplants; it is contraindicated for clients diagnosed with liver disorders.
    4. The antiemetic prochlorperazine (Compazine) is not contraindicated for clients with kidney transplants; it is contraindicated for clients diagnosed with liver disorders.

MEDICATION MEMORY JOGGER: The nurse must be knowledgeable of accepted standards of practice for disease processes and conditions. If the nurse administers a medication the HCP has prescribed, and it harms the client, the nurse could be held accountable. Remember, the nurse is a client advocate.

12. 1. Safety of the client is the priority.
2. This is an appropriate intervention, but it is not a priority over safety.
3. The nurse must document the medication in the MAR and the EHR because it is a PRN medication, but it is not the first intervention after administering the medication.
4. The nurse must evaluate the client's pain to determine medication effectiveness, but this is not the first intervention.

13. 1. Administering rescue morphine is an appropriate intervention, but it is not the nurse's first action.
2. Assessing the client and ruling out any complications is the nurse's first intervention.
3. The nurse should determine the last time the client received morphine and the amount of morphine the client has received, but it is not the first intervention.
4. Nonpharmacological interventions are appropriate to address the client's pain, but they should not be implemented first for a client diagnosed with renal calculi.

14. Correct answers are 2, 3, 4, and 5.
1. Duloxetine (Cymbalta) should not be broken, crushed, chewed, or dissolved in fluid.
2. Duloxetine (Cymbalta), a serotonin-norepinephrine reuptake inhibitor (SNRI), combined with St. John's wort, can cause serotonin syndrome characterized by hyperthermia, hypertension, coma, and death.
3. Duloxetine (Cymbalta) can cause drowsiness. The client should use caution when driving or performing activities that require alertness until drowsiness can be determined.
4. The client must taper off the medication after long-term use or the client could experience withdrawal manifestations such as headache, muscle pain, nausea and vomiting, weakness, or abnormal dreams.
5. Photosensitivity can occur with duloxetine (Cymbalta). The client should be taught to wear sunscreen and appropriate clothing outdoors.

15. 1. Overflow incontinence is characterized by incomplete bladder emptying. Bethanechol (Urecholine) is a cholinergic agent that improves bladder contractions and thereby facilitates bladder emptying.
2. Darifenacin (Enablex) is an anticholinergic drug that suppresses involuntary bladder contractions and is helpful for urge incontinence or overactive bladder.
3. Oxybutynin (Ditropan) is an antispasmodic drug that relaxes the smooth muscle of the bladder and is helpful for urge incontinence.
4. Estrogen supplements have shown some benefits for stress incontinence by stimulating the urethra's smooth muscle, but this would not help with improving bladder emptying.

8 Reproductive System

Drug therapy in pregnancy presents a vexing dilemma. When drugs are used during pregnancy, risks apply to the fetus as well as the mother.

—Richard L. Lehne

QUESTIONS

Pregnancy

1. Which medication categories are contraindicated for pregnant clients? **Select all that apply.**
1. Pregnancy category A
2. Pregnancy category B
3. Pregnancy category C
4. Pregnancy category D
5. Pregnancy category X

2. The pregnant client is prescribed ferrous sulfate. Which statement indicates to the nurse the client **needs more** teaching?
1. "I should increase my fluid intake and fiber when taking this medication."
2. "I will take a daily stool softener to prevent becoming constipated."
3. "If I notice that my stool becomes black or dark, I will call my obstetrician."
4. "I should take my iron tablet 2 hours after I eat."

3. At a preconception visit, the nurse instructs the client on the importance of folic acid to prevent serious congenital disabilities. Which statement to the nurse indicates the client **needs more** teaching?
1. "I will increase my intake of spinach, orange juice, and almonds."
2. "I will increase my intake of milk, yogurt, and fish."
3. "I will take my prenatal vitamin with folic acid daily."
4. "I will avoid overcooking my food to prevent vitamin loss."

4. The pregnant client is prescribed metoclopramide to treat hyperemesis gravidarum. Which information should the nurse discuss with the client? **Select all that apply.**
1. "Chew the tablet thoroughly before swallowing."
2. "Take the medication 30 minutes before mealtime."
3. "Do not drink any type of alcoholic beverages."
4. "Muscle spasms are a common side effect."
5. "The medication can cause drowsiness that will make driving unsafe."

5. The nurse is teaching the pregnant client diagnosed with HIV about methods to prevent transmission to the infant. Which information should the nurse discuss with the client? **Select all that apply.**
   1. The client will take zidovudine PO regularly, beginning at 12 to 14 weeks gestation.
   2. The client's newborn should receive oral zidovudine 8 to 12 hours after birth.
   3. Breastfeeding should be encouraged to provide the infant passive immunity to HIV.
   4. If treated in early pregnancy, risk of HIV transmission to the infant is 1% or less.
   5. All clients diagnosed with HIV must have a cesarean delivery at 38 weeks gestation.

6. The client diagnosed with a 32-week pregnancy and preterm labor is prescribed terbutaline. The client's vital signs are populated in the following vital sign flowsheet.

Vital Sign Flowsheet	Client Values	Reference Values
Temperature	98°F/36.7°C	Oral: 98°F (36.7°C)
Pulse	104 bpm	60 to 100 bpm
Respirations	34 breaths/min	12 to 20 breaths/min
Blood pressure	112/60 mm Hg	100 to 119 mm Hg systolic 60 to 80 mm Hg diastolic
Fetal heart rate (FHR)	150 bpm	110 to 160 bpm (at term)

   Which data **warrants intervention** by the nurse?
   1. Respiratory rate
   2. Fetal heart rate (FHR)
   3. Apical heart rate
   4. No contractions noted

7. The nurse is preparing to administer medications in the antepartum unit. Which medication should the nurse **question** administering?
   1. Terbutaline to a client preparing for an external cephalic version
   2. Hydralazine to a client diagnosed with preeclampsia
   3. Methotrexate to a client diagnosed with an ectopic pregnancy
   4. Prochlorperazine to a client diagnosed with hyperemesis gravidarum

8. The nurse is preparing to administer medication in a labor and delivery unit. Which medication should the nurse **question** administering?
   1. Magnesium sulfate to a client diagnosed with preeclampsia
   2. Dinoprostone to a client diagnosed with asthma
   3. Betamethasone to a 27-week pregnant client
   4. Oxytocin to a client diagnosed with an incomplete abortion

9. The nurse is preparing an amnioinfusion for a client experiencing severe variable decelerations of the FHR. Which solution should the nurse expect to administer through the intrauterine pressure catheter? **Select all that apply.**
   1. Normal (0.9%) saline
   2. 5% dextrose in water
   3. Lactated ringer's
   4. Albumin 25% solution
   5. Dextrose in saline

10. The nurse is caring for the pregnant client in labor. The client has had no prenatal care and reports being dependent on opioids throughout her pregnancy. Which interventions for pain control could be provided to this client? **Select all that apply.**
  1. Epidural anesthesia
  2. Butorphanol IV
  3. Morphine IV
  4. Acetaminophen PO
  5. 1% lidocaine locally

11. The nurse is teaching a pregnant client diagnosed with tuberculosis (TB) infection about treatments during pregnancy and effects on her newborn. Which statement indicates the client **understands** the teaching?
  1. "My baby will be born with TB and will be given isoniazid to treat the infection."
  2. "I will not be able to breastfeed, or my newborn could contract TB."
  3. "I should take supplemental pyridoxine during my pregnancy."
  4. "I will not take any medications to treat my TB until I have delivered my baby."

12. The nurse is assisting the certified registered nurse anesthetist (CRNA) in placing an epidural in a laboring client. Which findings would indicate intravascular injection of the local anesthetic? **Select all that apply.**
  1. Tachycardia
  2. Pruritus
  3. Tinnitus
  4. Sedation
  5. Dizziness

13. The nurse prepares to administer topical benzocaine to a client with a fourth-degree episiotomy. Which interventions should the nurse implement? **Rank in order of performance.**
  1. Position the client on their side with the top leg up and forward.
  2. Wash hands and put on nonsterile examination gloves.
  3. Check the client's MAR with the identification band.
  4. Ask the client if she is allergic to any "-caine" drugs.
  5. Apply the benzocaine to the perineal area.

14. The client in labor has an epidural catheter in place for anesthesia. Which intervention is **most important** for the labor and delivery nurse?
  1. Assist the client with breathing exercises during contractions.
  2. Ensure the client's legs are correctly positioned in the stirrups.
  3. Have the significant other wash for the delivery of the baby.
  4. Titrate the epidural medication to ensure an analgesic effect.

15. Which assessment data **warrants immediate** intervention for the client in labor receiving an oxytocin infusion via pump?
  1. The uterus periodically becomes hard and firm.
  2. The client reports an urgency to void.
  3. The client denies the urge to push.
  4. The FHR does not return to baseline.

16. The client diagnosed with preeclampsia and 38 weeks pregnant is admitted to the labor and delivery area. The HCP has prescribed IV magnesium sulfate. Which data indicates the medication is **effective**? **Select all that apply.**
  1. The client has no seizure activity.
  2. The client's urine output is 45 mL/hr.
  3. The client's blood pressure is 148/90.
  4. The client's deep tendon reflexes are 2 to 3+.
  5. The client's apical pulse is 70 beats per minute (bpm).

17. The client is experiencing postpartum hemorrhage and has received methylergonovine. Which intervention is the **priority** when administering this medication?
    1. Check the client's hemoglobin (Hgb) and hematocrit (Hct) levels.
    2. Monitor the client's peripad count frequently.
    3. Assess the client's vital signs every 2 hours.
    4. Determine the client's fundal height.

18. The pregnant client experienced deep venous thrombosis (DVT) with her previous pregnancy. Which medication should the nurse **question** administering to this client? **Select all that apply.**
    1. Unfractionated heparin
    2. Warfarin
    3. Enoxaparin
    4. Rivaroxaban
    5. Dabigatran

19. The labor and delivery nurse is preparing the client for a scheduled cesarean birth. Which interventions should the nurse expect to implement? **Select all that apply.**
    1. Administer famotidine or sodium citrate with citric acid.
    2. Perform an abdominal prep with an antiseptic containing chlorhexidine and alcohol.
    3. Give cephazolin via intravenous piggyback (IVPB).
    4. Administer ondansetron intravenously.
    5. Perform a "time-out" procedure.

20. The pregnant client is diagnosed with preterm labor and the HCP has prescribed nifedipine. Which interventions should the nurse implement? **Select all that apply.**
    1. Teach the client that skin flushing and headaches can occur.
    2. Administer the medication sublingually before meals.
    3. Instruct the client to rise slowly after sitting or lying down.
    4. Discontinue medication if FHR increases 10 bpm over baseline.
    5. Advise the client to avoid grapefruit or grapefruit juice.

21. The nurse is reviewing the laboring client's fetal monitor strip. Which order by the HCP should the nurse **question**?

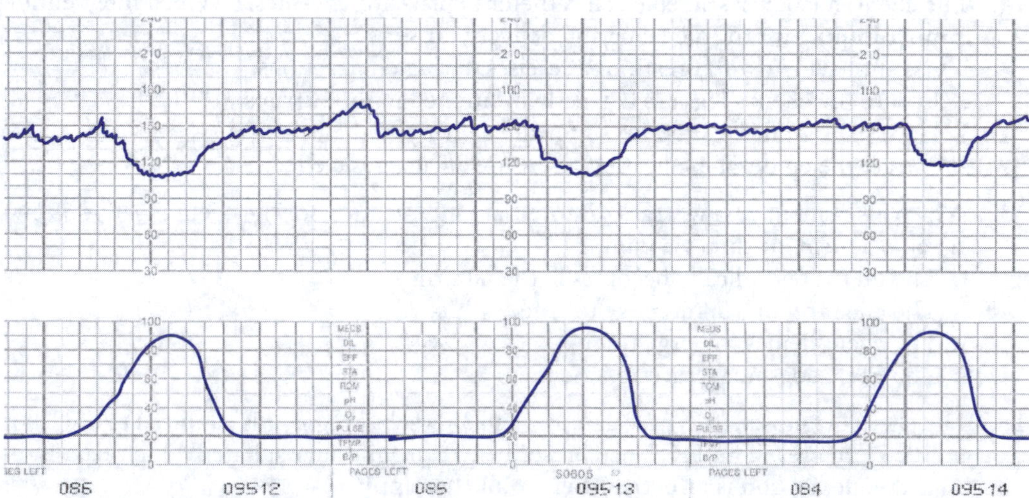

    1. Initiate a saline lock or normal saline IV line.
    2. Administer butorphanol 1 mg IV push (IVP).
    3. Continue oxytocin infusion via IV pump.
    4. Perform a sterile vaginal examination.

22. The nurse is reviewing the laboratory data of a pregnant client in labor at term gestation. Which intervention should the nurse implement?

Laboratory Test	Client Values	Reference Values
White blood cell count (WBC)	11 (10^3 cells/microL)	4.5 to 11.1 × 10^3/cells/microL
Red blood cell count (RBC)	3.9 (10^6 cells/microL)	Men: 4.21 to 5.81 (10^6 cells/microL) Women: 3.61 to 5.11 (10^6 cells/microL)
Hemoglobin (Hgb)	11 g/dL	Men: 14 to 17.3 g/dL Women: 11.7 to 15.5 g/dL
Hematocrit (Hct)	33%	Men: 42% to 52% Women: 36% to 48%
Platelets	300 (10^3/microL)	140 to 400 × 10^3/microL
ABO group	A	
Rh type	Negative (–)	
Culture (vaginal & rectal): Group B streptococcus	Positive	Negative
Rubella	Negative	Positive

1. Administer Rho (D) immune globulin intramuscularly (IM).
2. Administer measles, mumps, rubella (MMR) vaccine subcutaneously.
3. Administer penicillin IVPB.
4. Administer 2 units packed red blood cells (PRBCs) IV.

23. The client diagnosed with preeclampsia is receiving a magnesium sulfate infusion and delivered vaginally. Despite oxytocin and fundal massage, the client is experiencing heavy bleeding. Which medication should the nurse expect to administer?
1. Carboprost tromethamine
2. Methylergonovine
3. Calcium gluconate
4. Ritodrine

24. The nurse is teaching the client about medications and diet during lactation. Which information should the nurse include in the teaching? **Select all that apply.**
1. "Avoid the flu vaccination while breastfeeding as it can expose the baby to influenza."
2. "Do not take over-the-counter (OTC) decongestants such as pseudoephedrine."
3. "Too much caffeine can cause irritability and wakefulness in the newborn."
4. "Low-dose aspirin tablets can be taken as needed for mild pain relief."
5. "Oral contraceptives containing estrogen should be taken daily to prevent pregnancy."

25. The pregnant client diagnosed with bipolar disorder has been taking lamotrigine to control symptoms. The client asks the nurse for information about the medication and pregnancy. Which information should the nurse tell the client? **Select all that apply.**
1. Lamotrigine is the preferred treatment for bipolar disorder in pregnancy.
2. Medication dosage may need to be increased during pregnancy.
3. Serum lamotrigine levels should be obtained every 4 weeks in pregnancy.
4. Breastfeeding is contraindicated with lamotrigine.
5. Lamotrigine causes no significant increase in birth defects.

Transitioning to Extrauterine Life

26. The nurse is caring for a newborn client after an injection of naloxone hydrochloride IM at delivery. The client's vital signs are populated in the following vital sign flowsheet.

Vital Sign Flowsheet	Client Values	Reference Values (term)
Temperature	98.3°F/36.7°C	Axillary: 97 to 100.3°F (36.7 to 37.9°C)
Heart rate	120 bpm	110 to 160 bpm (awake) 80 to 160 bpm (asleep)
Respirations	40 breaths/min	30 to 60 breaths/min
Blood pressure	70/40 mm Hg	65 to 90 mm Hg systolic 45 to 65 mm Hg diastolic

Which assessment data indicates the medication is **effective**?
1. Temperature
2. Heart rate
3. Respiration
4. Blood pressure

27. The nurse is caring for a healthy newborn client. Which vaccination should the nurse expect to administer before the client is discharged? **Select all that apply.**
1. Haemophilus influenzae type b (Hib)
2. Measles, mumps, rubella (MMR)
3. Diphtheria, tetanus, acellular pertussis (DTaP)
4. Hepatitis B (HepB)
5. Inactivated poliovirus (IPV)
6. Pneumococcal conjugate (PCV13)
7. Rotavirus (RV)
8. Influenza (IIV)

28. The nurse is preparing the newborn for circumcision using a Gomco clamp. Which interventions should the nurse implement? **Select all that apply.**
1. Ensure vitamin K was administered at birth.
2. Apply a eutectic mixture of lidocaine and prilocaine.
3. Give 2 ounces of glucose water for pain.
4. Obtain petroleum jelly to place on the penis after the procedure.
5. Administer acetaminophen orally before the procedure.

29. Based on the following assessment of the newborn client, which interventions should the nurse perform? **Select all that apply.**

Assessment	Newborn Finding
Heart rate	110 bpm
Respiration	Slow, weak cry
Muscle tone	Minimal flexion of extremities
Reflex irritability	Grimace with stimulation
Color	Acrocyanosis

1. Suction the mouth and nose.
2. Provide oxygen via a face mask.
3. Administer epinephrine endotracheally.
4. Initiate an IV line of normal saline.
5. Assess for the need to administer naloxone.

30. The client diagnosed with neonatal abstinence syndrome (NAS) is irritable, having difficulty feeding, and sleeping poorly. Which interventions should the nurse expect to implement? **Select all that apply.**
1. Administer morphine orally.
2. Loosely wrap the infant during feedings.
3. Give phenobarbital to control seizures.
4. Collaborate with child protective services.
5. Perform gavage feeding.

31. The premature newborn client is diagnosed with a patent ductus arteriosus (PDA) and is experiencing labored breathing and an increased need for oxygen. Which medication would the nurse anticipate the HCP to order? **Select all that apply.**
1. Indomethacin
2. Ibuprofen
3. Gentamicin
4. Caffeine
5. Captopril

32. The nurse is preparing to administer erythromycin ophthalmic ointment to a newborn client. Which interventions should the nurse implement? **Select all that apply.**
1. Cleanse the client's eyes before application as needed.
2. Apply a thin ribbon of medication to each eye in a single dose.
3. Administer from the inner canthus to the outer canthus.
4. Ensure medication is given within 2 hours of birth.
5. Gently rinse the eye with saline after administration.

Infertility

33. The client diagnosed with infertility tells the clinic nurse about taking St. John's wort for depression. Which statement is the nurse's **best** response?
1. "This herb is useful for depression. I hope it will help."
2. "Did you discuss taking this herb with your psychologist?"
3. "This herb may cause infertility problems."
4. "Is your significant other taking any herbal medication?"

34. The female client is taking clomiphene. Which statement indicates the client **understands** the risk of taking this medication?
 1. "The medication may cause my child to have Down syndrome."
 2. "There are very few risks associated with taking this medication."
 3. "I should stagger the times that I take this medication."
 4. "This medication may increase my chance of having twins."

35. The client diagnosed with infertility and endometriosis is prescribed leuprolide. Which information should the nurse discuss with the client? **Select all that apply.**
 1. Explain that this medication may take 3 to 6 months to work.
 2. Discuss that this medication will help regulate the client's menstrual cycle.
 3. Instruct to take leuprolide every night to help decrease menstrual pain.
 4. Teach that this medication will not affect when the client can have intercourse.
 5. Tell the client not to drink grapefruit juice when taking this medication.

36. The client experiencing infertility is prescribed bromocriptine. The client calls the clinic nurse and reports that she thinks she may be pregnant. Which intervention should the clinic nurse implement **first**?
 1. Schedule the client for a pelvic sonogram.
 2. Instruct the client to quit taking the medication.
 3. Tell the client to make an appointment with the HCP.
 4. Encourage the client to confirm with a home pregnancy test.

37. The client experiencing infertility is receiving menotropin and human chorionic gonadotropin (HCG). Which diagnostic test indicates the medications are **effective**?
 1. A serum HCG level
 2. A serum estrogen level
 3. A negative urine pregnancy test
 4. A hemoglobin A_1c

38. The female client has been taking infertility medications. Which findings indicate ovarian overstimulation syndrome?
 1. Abdominal bloating and vague gastrointestinal discomfort
 2. Bright red vaginal bleeding with golf ball-size clots
 3. A positive fluid wave and lower abdominal wave
 4. Burning and an increased frequency of urinating

39. The nurse administers HCG intramuscularly to the female client diagnosed with infertility. Which instruction should the nurse discuss with the couple regarding this medication? **Select all that apply.**
 1. Explain the need to abstain from sexual intercourse for 14 days after receiving the medication.
 2. Instruct the male partner to wear boxer shorts while his female partner is taking HCG.
 3. Discuss taking the basal metabolic temperature and having sexual intercourse when it becomes elevated 2 degrees.
 4. Advise the couple to have intercourse on the eve of receiving medication and 3 days after receiving medication.
 5. Notify the HCP if you experience swelling of the hands and legs, severe pelvic pain, or shortness of breath.

40. The nurse is preparing a client for in vitro fertilization (IVF). Which statement **best** describes the scientific rationale for administering supplemental progesterone to this client?
 1. To enhance the receptivity of the endometrium to implantation
 2. To provide more hormones to the ovary for egg production
 3. To help regulate the client's monthly menstrual cycle
 4. To decrease galactorrhea in the client if fertilization occurs

41. The male client diagnosed with infertility asks the clinic nurse about methods to improve fertility. Which interventions should the nurse teach the client? **Select all that apply.**
   1. Take a multivitamin daily with zinc.
   2. Consume alcohol and caffeine in moderation.
   3. Testosterone therapy may help increase your sperm count.
   4. Clomiphene taken daily will help increase your fertility.
   5. Avoid smoking and use of nicotine products.

Birth Control

42. The sexually active couple has decided to use a spermicide for birth control. Which information should the nurse discuss with the female partner? **Select all that apply.**
   1. Insert the spermicide before having sexual intercourse.
   2. Douche with vinegar and water immediately after intercourse.
   3. Teach to apply spermicide in the woman's vagina.
   4. Instruct that spermicide is effective up to three times.
   5. Explain this form of birth control will not prevent STIs.

43. Which client should the nurse recommend taking oral contraceptive pills for birth control?
   1. The client smoking two packs of cigarettes a day
   2. The client taking an ACE inhibitor medication
   3. The 65-inch tall client weighing 100 kg
   4. The client with a family history of ovarian cancer

44. Which instructions should the nurse discuss with the client prescribed oral contraceptives for birth control? **Select all that apply.**
   1. "Never take more than one birth control pill a day."
   2. "If breakthrough bleeding occurs, discontinue the pill."
   3. "Take a missed pill as soon as you realize you have missed it."
   4. "Antibiotics will decrease the ovulation suppression effect of the pill."
   5. "Notify the HCP if you experience a severe headache."

45. The sexually active male adolescent tells the school nurse, "I am embarrassed, but I don't know anyone else to tell. Last night when I used a condom with my girlfriend, I got a red itchy rash down there. I don't know what it is or what to do." Which statement is the nurse's **best** response?
   1. "You should abstain from sex until you are older."
   2. "Use a condom made out of a lamb's intestines."
   3. "Do you think your girlfriend gave you an STI?"
   4. "Encourage your girlfriend to use a diaphragm."

46. Which statement indicates to the nurse the client using a vaginal contraceptive ring **understands** the birth control teaching?
   1. "If the ring falls out during intercourse, I should get a new ring."
   2. "I should insert the ring 30 minutes before having intercourse."
   3. "I will remove the ring 3 weeks after I have inserted it."
   4. "I should never use the ring continuously to stop my period."

47. The client is prescribed a 28-day oral contraceptive pack. Which statement **best** describes the scientific rationale for this birth control product?
   1. This causes longer intervals between menses.
   2. A hormone pill daily decreases cramping during menses.
   3. It is not as expensive as other birth control products.
   4. This ensures that the client will take a pill every day.

48. The adolescent client is prescribed the birth control medication depot medroxyprogesterone. Which interventions should the clinic nurse implement? **Select all that apply.**
1. Instruct the client to schedule an appointment every 3 months.
2. Explain that infertility may occur up to 2 years after discontinuing.
3. Demonstrate how to administer the medication subcutaneously in the abdomen.
4. Discuss how to care for the intrauterine device (IUD) inserted in her vagina.
5. Tell the client that she will not have to take a pill every day.

49. The 14-year-old client is prescribed oral contraceptive medication for menstrual irregularity. Which assessment data indicates the medication is **effective**?
1. The client has a period every 28 days.
2. The client has a decrease in abdominal bloating.
3. The client has a negative pregnancy test.
4. The client reports a decrease in facial acne.

Reproductive Hormone Changes

50. Which statement indicates to the nurse that the male client prescribed testosterone pellets for a low testosterone level **understands** the teaching concerning testosterone pellets?
1. "I need to take the pellets every day with food."
2. "I will need to have monthly testosterone levels drawn."
3. "The testosterone pellets will last for 3 to 6 months."
4. "I should notify the HCP if I have more spontaneous erections."

51. The nurse is teaching the early postmenopausal client, prescribed short-term systemic estrogen hormones, about the therapy's benefits. Which information should the nurse include in the teaching? **Select all that apply.**
1. Therapy can reduce hot flashes and night sweats.
2. Therapy can aid in the prevention of osteoporosis.
3. Therapy can reduce vaginal dryness and dyspareunia.
4. Therapy decreases the risk of blood clots and stroke.
5. Therapy decreases memory loss and Alzheimer's disease.

52. The 56-year-old female client tells the nurse that she takes the herb *Angelica sinensis* (dong quai). Which data indicates to the nurse this medication is **effective**?
1. The client has regular menstrual cycles.
2. The client does not have abdominal bloating.
3. The client reports fewer hot flashes.
4. The client has a normal bone density test.

53. The nurse is caring for a client reporting a decreased sexual desire. The HCP has prescribed flibanserin. Which information should the nurse discuss with the client? **Select all that apply.**
1. Alcohol is contraindicated when taking flibanserin.
2. This medication is only for postmenopausal women.
3. This medication can be used to improve sexual performance.
4. Flibanserin should be taken orally, once a day, at bedtime.
5. If you miss a dose, take as soon as you remember, then resume regular schedule.

ANSWERS AND RATIONALES

The correct answer number and rationale are in **boldface blue type.** Rationales for why other answer options are incorrect are also given.

Pregnancy

1. **Correct answers are 4 and 5.**
   1. Category A medications have a remote risk of causing fetal harm and are prescribed for pregnant clients.
   2. Category B medications have a slightly higher risk of causing fetal abnormalities than category A medications, but they are often prescribed for pregnant clients.
   3. Category C medications pose a greater risk than category B medications and are cautiously prescribed for pregnant clients. Medications in this category have either not yet been researched or may show a risk in animal studies.
   4. **Category D medications have a proven risk of fetal harm and are not prescribed for pregnant clients unless the mother's life is in danger.**
   5. **Category X medications have a definite risk of fetal abnormality or abortion.**

2. 1. Iron causes constipation; therefore, the client should increase fluid and fiber to help decrease the possibility of becoming constipated.
   2. Iron causes constipation; therefore, the client is instructed to take a daily stool softener to prevent constipation.
   3. **Ferrous sulfate (Feosol), an iron product, causes the stool to become black and tarry; therefore, the client would not need to notify the obstetrician.**
   4. Iron should be taken between meals, 2 hours after a meal because food decreases absorption of the medication by 50% to 70%.

3. 1. Green leafy vegetables, citrus foods, and nuts such as peanuts and almonds are rich in folic acid.
   2. **Milk, yogurt, and fish are not sources of dietary folic acid.**
   3. A prenatal vitamin with 400 mcg of folic acid is recommended for clients preparing for pregnancy or are pregnant or lactating. Folic acid can prevent neural tube defects, cardiac defects, and cleft lip or palate.
   4. Folic acid can be lost when overcooking foods.

4. **Correct answers are 2, 3, and 5.**
   1. The client should swallow the medication, not crush, chew, or suck on it.
   2. **The medication should be taken on an empty stomach at least 30 minutes before eating.**
   3. **Alcohol can increase central nervous system depressive symptoms (drowsiness, lethargy) of the medication and should be avoided.**
   4. Muscle spasms and rigidity are extrapyramidal side effects and should be reported to the HCP.
   5. **Metoclopramide (Reglan) can cause drowsiness. The client should avoid driving until the medication response is known.**

5. **Correct answers are 1, 2, and 4.**
   1. **ZDV is given orally, as directed, around the clock.**
   2. **The newborn should receive oral zidovudine syrup beginning 8 to 12 hours after birth until 6 weeks old.**
   3. Breastfeeding is not recommended because HIV is present in breast milk.
   4. **The Centers for Disease Control and Prevention (CDC) states that if the client is treated starting in early pregnancy, risk of HIV transmission to the infant can be reduced to 1% or less.**
   5. The choice of delivery method, vaginal or cesarean, is dependent on concentration of the virus in maternal plasma (viral load). Cesarean delivery before onset of labor and rupture of membranes can reduce transmission of the virus that causes HIV; however, the delivery method needs to be individualized for each client.

6. 1. **Terbutaline (Brethine), a beta-adrenergic agonist, causes bronchodilatation. If the client's respiratory rate is greater than 30 or if there is a change in quality of lung sounds (wheezing, rales, or coughing), the HCP should be notified.**
   2. The normal FHR is 110 to 160 bpm; therefore, an FHR of 150 bpm is within normal limits and would not warrant intervention by the nurse.
   3. The client's apical heart rate is just above normal (60 to 100 bpm) and would not warrant intervention by the nurse.
   4. Terbutaline (Brethine) is administered to prevent contractions; therefore, the medication is effective.

7. 1. Terbutaline (Brethine) can be administered to the client preparing for an external version to relax the uterine muscle to manipulate the fetus.
   2. Hydralazine (Apresoline) is commonly used for elevated blood pressure in pregnancy.
   3. Methotrexate, a folic acid antagonist, is used for medical management of an early ectopic pregnancy with an intact fallopian tube.
   4. **Prochlorperazine (Compazine, Stemetil) is contraindicated in pregnancy. Ondansetron (Zofran) and promethazine (Phenergan) are more common medications for nausea and vomiting in pregnancy.**

8. 1. The client diagnosed with preeclampsia would be receiving the anticonvulsant magnesium sulfate to help prevent seizures; therefore, the nurse would not question administering this medication.
   2. **The synthetic prostaglandin dinoprostone (Cervidil) is used cautiously for clients diagnosed with asthma because it can initiate an asthmatic attack; therefore, the nurse should question administering this medication.**
   3. The corticosteroid betamethasone (Celestone) is a medication used to increase surfactant in fetal lungs and would be administered to a client less than 34 weeks pregnant; therefore, the nurse would not question administering this medication.
   4. Oxytocin (Pitocin), a uterine stimulant, would be administered after a client has experienced an incomplete abortion to help the client expel the fetal fragments; therefore, the nurse would not question administering this medication.

9. **Correct answers are 1 and 3.**
   1. **NS is used in amnioinfusions. It can cause slight changes in fetal electrolytes but is an acceptable fluid.**
   2. Dextrose 5% in water is not indicated for amnioinfusions.
   3. **Lactated Ringer's solution is the preferred fluid for amnioinfusions.**
   4. Albumin is a blood product prepared from plasma and is not used for this procedure.
   5. The solution 5% dextrose in normal saline is not indicated for amnioinfusions.

10. **Correct answers are 1, 3, 4, and 5.**
   1. **Epidural anesthesia is not contraindicated in the opioid-dependent client and is an acceptable form of pain management.**
   2. Butorphanol (Stadol) is a narcotic agonist-antagonist and should be avoided in the opioid-dependent client as it can cause acute withdrawal in the mother and in utero withdrawal in the fetus, characterized by fetal tachycardia and fetal death.
   3. **If narcotics can be safely administered, the nurse should not withhold the medication during labor. Giving opioids during acute pain does not enhance an opioid-addicted client's chemical dependence.**
   4. **Acetaminophen administered orally can reduce early labor pain.**
   5. **1% lidocaine can be administered by the HCP before an episiotomy or for perineal repair.**

11. 1. The infant will be tested for congenital TB; however, perinatal transmission is rare.
   2. Breastfeeding is not contraindicated in latent TB.
   3. **Pyridoxine (vitamin B6) is recommended for pregnant clients diagnosed with TB infections to ensure the fetus gets the necessary vitamins.**
   4. Isoniazid, rifampin, and ethambutol are taken daily during pregnancy for TB treatment.

12. **Correct answers are 1, 3, and 5.**
   1. **Tachycardia is a symptom of intravascular injection of a local anesthetic.**
   2. Pruritus or itching is a symptom of an allergic reaction.
   3. **Tinnitus is a symptom of intravascular injection of a local anesthetic.**
   4. Intravascular injection does not cause sedation in the client.
   5. **Dizziness is a symptom of intravascular injection of a local anesthetic.**

13. **Correct order is 3, 4, 2, 1, 5.**
   3. **The nurse must first determine if this is the right client receiving the right medication.**
   4. **The nurse should always check about allergies. With this medication, "-caine" drugs are anesthetics and, if the client is allergic to lidocaine (suturing lacerations) or Novacaine (dental procedures), the client should not receive this medication.**
   2. **Once the nurse determines that this is the right client receiving the right medication and that the client has no allergies, then the nurse must wash their hands and use gloves to administer medication to the perineal area.**

1. This position allows maximum exposure to the area that should be medicated.
5. After completing all previous steps, the nurse can apply the medication.

14. 1. Breathing exercises are important, but protection of the client's lower extremities while under anesthesia should be a priority for the nurse.
2. Because the legs are numb due to the epidural, the nurse must ensure the client's legs are in the stirrups correctly so that the client will not experience neurovascular compromise or any injury to the legs when they are in the stirrups.
3. Preparing the significant other for the delivery is important, but it is not a priority over the safety of the mother's lower extremities.
4. The anesthesiologist or nurse anesthetist would be responsible for administering the anesthesia during delivery.

15. 1. The uterus becoming hard and firm periodically indicates a contraction, which is expected when administering a uterine stimulant.
2. The client wanting to urinate would be expected because the baby's head is pushing against the bladder.
3. Denying the urge to push indicates the client is not in the last stages of labor.
4. During a contraction, FHR will decrease but should return to baseline FHR after the contraction. If this does not occur, it indicates the infant is in distress and warrants immediate intervention. This could also be a clinical manifestation of uterine rupture resulting from uterus overstimulation. The oxytocin (Pitocin) infusion should be stopped immediately.

16. Correct answers are 1 and 4.
1. Magnesium sulfate is administered to prevent seizure activity, so if no seizure activity is occurring, the medication is effective.
2. The client's urine output does not indicate the medication is effective.
3. Magnesium sulfate is not administered to treat the client's blood pressure; therefore, this data cannot be used to evaluate medication effectiveness.
4. Magnesium sulfate is administered to prevent seizure activity and is determined to be effective and in the therapeutic range when the client's deep tendon reflexes are normal, which is 2 to 3+ on a 0 to 4+ scale.
5. The client's apical pulse does not determine effectiveness of magnesium sulfate.

17. 1. The client's Hgb and Hct levels should be monitored, but an ongoing assessment of how much the client is bleeding is the priority.
2. Monitoring the client's peripad count will allow the nurse to directly assess how much the client is bleeding, which will help determine if methylergonovine (Methergine) is effective.
3. Vital signs should be monitored, but an ongoing assessment of how much the client is bleeding is the priority.
4. The client's fundal height should be assessed, but it will not help determine how much blood the client has lost.

18. Correct answers are 2, 4, and 5.
1. Unfractionated heparin does not cross the placenta and is safe to use in pregnancy. A pregnant woman can receive prophylactic anticoagulation therapy until labor begins; then it can be resumed 6 to 12 hours after birth.
2. Warfarin (Coumadin) is contraindicated in pregnancy because of teratogenic effects. It is safe for postpartum use and during lactation.
3. Enoxaparin (Lovenox), a low molecular weight heparin, does not cross the placenta and is safe to use during pregnancy.
4. Rivaroxaban (Xarelto), an oral direct factor Xa inhibitor, is contraindicated in pregnancy because of risk of fetal hemorrhage, malformations, and death.
5. Dabigatran (Pradaxa), a direct thrombin inhibitor, is contraindicated in pregnancy because of teratogenic effects.

19. Correct answers are 1, 2, 3, and 5.
1. Famotidine (Pepcid) or sodium citrate with citric acid (Bicitra) is given before a cesarean section to reduce gastric acid.
2. An abdominal prep is performed using an antiseptic containing chlorhexidine and alcohol (Chloraprep). This antiseptic is effective against methicillin-resistant *staphylococcus aureus* (MRSA), vancomycin-resistant *enterococci* (VRE), and many other viruses and fungi. It needs to dry for 3 minutes to be effective. In an emergency cesarean, a povidone-iodine solution (Betadine) could be used because it requires no drying time.
3. A single prophylactic antibiotic such as cephazolin is recommended to reduce infection risk.
4. Ondansetron (Zofran) may be needed to address nausea and vomiting that can occur

with uterine manipulation during surgery, but this is not given routinely in preparation for a scheduled cesarean.

5. **A "time-out" procedure is performed for client safety to verify the client's identity and surgery to be performed.**

20. Correct answers are 1, 3, and 5.

1. **Skin flushing and headaches are common side effects of nifedipine (Procardia).**
2. The medication is not given sublingually as it may cause serious adverse reactions. It may be administered orally without regard to meals.
3. **Nifedipine is a vasodilator that can cause orthostatic hypotension. The client should be taught to rise slowly after sitting or lying down or call for assistance.**
4. Nifedipine can cause a transient increase in the FHR. An increase in FHR of 10 bpm over baseline should be monitored, but the medication should not be discontinued.
5. **Consuming grapefruit or grapefruit juice with nifedipine can cause an increased amount of medication to be absorbed, causing hypotension or undesirable change in heart rate.**

21. 1. Most laboring clients have a saline lock or IV line. The nurse should not question this order.

2. **The client is experiencing early decelerations, indicative of head compression and possible imminent delivery. The nurse should question administration of butorphanol (Stadol) because if given too close to delivery, it can cause respiratory depression in the newborn.**
3. The contractions are adequately spaced and the fetus is experiencing early decelerations due to head compression. The nurse should not question this order.
4. Performing a sterile vaginal examination can determine the client's cervical dilation. The nurse should not question this order.

22. 1. The decision to administer Rho (D) immune globulin (RhoGAM) depends on the newborn's blood type. This medication is not administered in labor.

2. The client is rubella nonimmune; however, this medication is not administered in labor.
3. **Penicillin (PCN) is administered in labor for clients with a positive group B streptococcus (GBS) culture. If the client is allergic to PCN, then cefazolin, clindamycin, or erythromycin are other options. GBS can be transmitted to the newborn during delivery and can cause sepsis, meningitis, or pneumonia.**
4. The laboratory values for the Hgb and Hct are lower in the pregnant client. At term, however, the Hgb should be at least 11 g/dL and the Hct should be at least 33%. The client's laboratory values are normal; therefore, an infusion of PRBCs is not indicated.

23. 1. **Carboprost tromethamine (Hemabate) is a synthetic prostaglandin that can decrease uterine bleeding postpartum by stimulating contractions.**

2. Methylergonovine (Methergine) is an ergot alkaloid used to stimulate uterine contractions but is contraindicated for clients with hypertension.
3. Calcium gluconate is the antidote for magnesium sulfate toxicity; however, nothing in the stem indicates this is occurring with this client.
4. Ritodrine (Yutopar) is a tocolytic drug used to relax the uterine muscle. Once U.S. Food and Drug Administration (FDA)-approved, it is no longer available in the United States.

24. Correct answers are 2 and 3.

1. The flu shot is not contraindicated in the pregnant or lactating client and can benefit the newborn.
2. **OTC decongestants, such as pseudoephedrine, can decrease milk supply and should not be taken while breastfeeding.**
3. **Excessive caffeine intake by the client can cause irritability and wakefulness in the newborn.**
4. Aspirin should not be taken for mild pain relief because of the association of aspirin and Reye's syndrome in children.
5. Oral contraceptives containing estrogen can decrease milk supply and should be avoided.

25. Correct answers are 1, 2, 3, and 5.

1. **Lamotrigine is the preferred treatment for bipolar disorder in pregnancy.**
2. **Lamotrigine dosage may need to be increased during pregnancy to avoid symptom recurrence. If the dose is increased in pregnancy, the medication should be tapered off in the postpartum period to prepregnancy levels.**

3. **Serum lamotrigine levels should be monitored every 4 weeks during pregnancy. There are no established therapeutic lamotrigine levels, so the dose should be individualized for the client.**
4. The client taking lamotrigine (Lamictal) can breastfeed with pediatric monitoring.
5. **Lamotrigine causes no significant increase in congenital disabilities.**

Transitioning to Extrauterine Life

26. 1. Naloxone is not given to treat temperature instability; therefore, this data does not indicate the medication is effective.
2. The client's heart rate does not determine naloxone's effectiveness.
3. **Naloxone is administered to newborn clients diagnosed with depressed respirations when the mother receives opiates within 4 hours of birth. Naloxone is determined to be effective when the newborn client's respirations are between 30 and 60 breaths per minute. The normal newborn has an irregular breathing pattern. It is important to remember the naloxone dose may need to be repeated if the respiratory effort does not improve or if the opiate has a longer half-life than naloxone.**
4. The client's blood pressure does not determine naloxone's effectiveness.

27. 1. Erythromycin ophthalmic ointment is prophylaxis against *Neisseria gonorrhoeae*, preventing ophthalmia neonatorum in infants of mothers with gonorrhea. It is required by law.
2. Otitis externa is an outer ear canal infection and is unrelated to ophthalmic ointment treatments.
3. Transient strabismus ("crossed eyes") is common in the newborn due to weak eye muscles.
4. Cytomegalovirus can cause infant blindness; however, it cannot be prevented with erythromycin.

28. Correct answers are 1, 2, 4, and 5.
1. **Vitamin K is administered shortly after birth to prevent bleeding. The nurse should confirm this was administered before the circumcision procedure.**
2. **A eutectic mixture of lidocaine and prilocaine (EMLA) cream is applied to the penis before the procedure to anesthetize the area.**
3. The newborn should not be given glucose water or a feeding immediately before the procedure to reduce risk of aspiration.
4. **Petroleum jelly is applied to the penis after the procedure and after each diaper change for 7 days. Petroleum jelly is not needed for a circumcision using a PlastiBell device.**
5. **Acetaminophen given before the procedure and intermittently as needed after the procedure can control pain.**

29. Correct answers are 1, 2, and 5.
1. **The mouth and nose should be suctioned to ensure airway patency.**
2. **The infant is breathing and has a heart rate greater than 100 breaths per minute but is experiencing slow respirations and acrocyanosis, so oxygen should be given via face mask or "blow-by."**
3. Epinephrine treats prolonged bradycardia or asystole in the newborn and is used in codes. This newborn has a normal heart rate, so epinephrine should not be administered now.
4. An IV line is not indicated at this time.
5. **An infant with a normal heart rate and color (acrocyanosis is a normal finding in a newborn) but poor respiratory effort should be assessed for need of naloxone. If the mother received opiates within 4 hours of delivery, naloxone might need to be administered to the infant to counteract respiratory depression.**

30. Correct answers are 1, 3, 4, and 5.
1. **Oral morphine can be given to reduce clinical manifestations of withdrawal.**
2. The newborn should be swaddled during feedings to prevent excessive movements, which can cause increased distress in the client.
3. **Phenobarbital is effective in treatment of opioid withdrawal seizures.**
4. **When a newborn client tests positive for drugs, child protective services becomes involved.**
5. **Gavage feeding may be necessary if the client cannot coordinate sucking and swallowing with breathing. Additionally, it conserves energy in the client.**

31. Correct answers are 1, 2, and 4.
1. **Indomethacin causes the PDA to constrict, which closes the opening. This medication works well in premature infants.**
2. **Ibuprofen works in a similar way to indomethacin and is helpful in closing PDAs in premature infants.**

3. Gentamicin, an aminoglycoside, is commonly given in the neonatal intensive care unit (NICU) to treat enterococcal infections but has a vasodilatory effect on most tissue.
4. **Early caffeine therapy decreases the medical treatment required for a PDA.**
5. Captopril is an ACE inhibitor used to treat hypertension.

32. Correct answers are 1, 2, and 3.
1. **The newborn's eyes should be cleaned as needed before application.**
2. **A thin ribbon of 0.5% erythromycin ointment is applied to each eye. A new ointment tube is used with each newborn to prevent infection spread.**
3. **The ointment is administered in the lower conjunctival sac, beginning at the inner canthus and moving to the outer canthus.**
4. The medication should be given within 1 hour of birth.
5. Excess ointment can be gently wiped off a few minutes after administration; however, the eye should not be washed off with saline.

Infertility

33. 1. This herb is taken to treat depression, but it can cause more infertility problems; therefore, the nurse should discuss this with the client.
2. The client should discuss taking herbs with all HCP, but this is not the nurse's best response.
3. **St. John's wort may cause effects on sperm cells, decreased sperm motility, and decreased viability; therefore, this client should not take this herb.**
4. The significant other taking herbs should not affect the client's fertility; therefore, this is not an appropriate response.

34. 1. There is no increased risk of having a child with Down syndrome when taking this medication.
2. Many risks are associated with taking this fertility medication, including multiple fetuses, pain, visual disturbances, abnormal bleeding, and ovarian failure.
3. This medication should be taken at the same time every day to maintain a therapeutic drug level.
4. **Clomiphene (Clomid), an estrogen antagonist, is an ovarian stimulant that promotes follicle maturation and ovulation. Many follicles can mature simultaneously, resulting in the increased possibility of multiple births.**

35. Correct answers are 1 and 4.
1. **The client should be aware that it may take 3 to 6 months for leuprolide therapy to achieve maximum benefits; therefore, the nurse should discuss the long-term possibility with the client.**
2. Continuous use of this medication may cause amenorrhea or menstrual irregularities.
3. This medication is given intramuscularly once a month or as an implant inserted once every 12 months, but it is not administered daily.
4. **Leuprolide (Lupron), a GnRH medication, does not affect when the client can have intercourse.**
5. This medication is administered intramuscularly. Drinking grapefruit juice does not affect the medication.

36. 1. A pelvic sonogram is used to determine ovarian response to bromocriptine (Parlodel), but because the client thinks she is pregnant, performing a sonogram is not the first intervention.
2. **The client must quit taking bromocriptine (Parlodel) immediately because it can cause fetal miscarriage. Once the client becomes pregnant, the medication is not needed anymore.**
3. The client needs to see the HCP, but it is not the first intervention for the nurse to discuss with the client.
4. The client can perform a home pregnancy test, but it is not the first intervention for the nurse to discuss with the client.

MEDICATION MEMORY JOGGER: The test taker should question administering any medication to a pregnant client. Many medications cross the placental barrier and could affect the fetus.

37. 1. This test determines how much medication has been administered, but it does not indicate that the medication is effective.
2. **The serum estrogen level should increase three to four times the pretreatment baseline if the medications, menotropin (Pergonal), an ovarian stimulant, and HCG are effective. The client may get pregnant.**
3. A negative pregnancy test indicates the medications are not effective.
4. This is the test that determines the 3-month average blood glucose level.

38. 1. Abdominal bloating and vague gastrointestinal discomfort are clinical manifestations of ovarian cancer.
2. This could indicate a miscarriage but does not support an ovarian hyperstimulation syndrome diagnosis.
3. Ovarian hyperstimulation syndrome involves marked ovarian enlargement with fluid exudation into the woman's peritoneal and pleural cavities. This syndrome can result in ovarian cysts that may rupture, causing pain.
4. These are clinical manifestations of urinary tract infections.

39. Correct answers are 4 and 5.
1. HCG acts immediately to promote ovulation; therefore, the couple should not wait to have sexual intercourse.
2. Wearing tight-fitting underwear causes the scrotum to be close to the body, and heat reduces sperm count, which is why boxer shorts are recommended, but this has nothing to do with the HCG medication.
3. Taking the basal metabolic temperature is a first-line intervention for clients experiencing infertility to determine when a woman is ovulating. HCG stimulates ovulation, which should occur within hours to a day or two of medication administration.
4. The couple should have sexual intercourse during this time because this is the probable ovulation period.
5. Hand and leg swelling, severe pelvic pain, and shortness of breath can indicate ovarian hyperstimulation syndrome (OHSS), and the client should notify the HCP.

40. **1. Progesterone enhances receptivity of the endometrium to implantation—progesterone's function in the body—and is the scientific rationale for administering supplemental progesterone to a client preparing for in vitro fertilization (IVF).**
2. Providing more hormones to the ovary for egg production is not the scientific rationale for administering supplemental progesterone to a client preparing to undergo IVF.
3. Menstrual cycle regulation is not the scientific rationale for administering this medication.
4. This is not the scientific rationale for administering this medication.

41. Correct answers are 1, 3, and 5.
1. A multivitamin daily improves nutrition. Zinc has been reported to increase testosterone levels, sperm count, and sperm motility.
2. Alcohol and caffeine should be eliminated from the diet to improve fertility.
3. Testosterone administration will improve hormonal levels, resulting in potential for increased spermatogenesis.
4. Clomiphene (Clomid) is an ovarian stimulant and will not help a male client.
5. Smoking is associated with lower sperm count and motility.

Birth Control

42. Correct answers are 1, 3, and 5.
1. Correct use of spermicide is required for contraceptive efficacy. The spermicide must be in place before intercourse, and the foam is immediately active. If a suppository or tablet is used, it must be inserted 10 to 15 minutes before intercourse to allow time for it to dissolve.
2. Douching is not allowed for at least 6 hours after intercourse; douching will remove the spermicide.
3. Spermicide must be inserted into the female's vagina.
4. Spermicide must be inserted before sexual intercourse. It is only effective for one time.
5. Abstinence or condoms are the only two ways to prevent STIs.

43. 1. The client smoking more than 15 cigarettes a day is at greater risk for cardiovascular complications when taking oral contraceptives.
2. A client taking an ACE inhibitor would have cardiovascular problems. Oral contraceptives elevate blood pressure by increasing both angiotensin and aldosterone; therefore, this client should not take oral contraceptives.
3. A client diagnosed with obesity is at risk for hypertension, hypercholesterolemia, and DVT, and should not take oral contraceptives.
4. Oral contraceptives decrease risk of several disorders, including ovarian and endometrial cancer, pelvic inflammatory disease, premenstrual syndrome, toxic shock, fibrocystic breast disease, ovarian cysts, and anemia. While providing birth control for the client, the client also gets a secondary benefit of decreasing ovarian cancer risk.

44. Correct answers are 3, 4, and 5.
1. The client should be instructed to take any missed pill as soon as the omission is recognized; therefore, the client could and should take more than one pill in a day.

2. Breakthrough bleeding may mean the oral contraceptive dosage is not appropriate, but this is not a reason to discontinue taking the medication. The client should see the HCP.
3. The client should be instructed to take any missed pill as soon as the omission is recognized; therefore, the client could and should take more than one pill in a day. To maintain ovulation suppression, the client must take the medication routinely.
4. Antibiotics decrease effectiveness of some oral contraceptives, and a secondary form of birth control should be used during antibiotic therapy.
5. The client should be instructed to notify the HCP of a severe headache, indicating hypertension and a possible stroke.

45. 1. This statement can be viewed as judgmental. Because the adolescent is already sexually active, it is not going to protect him from fathering a child or getting an STI. The nurse should encourage the sexually active adolescent to use protection.
2. The adolescent's comments should make the school nurse consider an allergic reaction to the condom, most of which are made of latex. Suggesting a type of condom made from lamb's intestines would prevent an allergic reaction.
3. STIs require an incubation period. The red rash area would not occur the following day.
4. A diaphragm is a form of birth control, but most are made of latex, which may cause a reaction for the male adolescent.

46. 1. If the ring is expelled before 3 weeks have passed, it can be washed off in warm water and reinserted. A new one is reinserted only if the expelled ring cannot be used.
2. This statement is appropriate for using a diaphragm, not the ring.
3. The vaginal contraceptive ring works on the same principle that oral contraceptives work. It provides 21 days of hormone suppression, followed by 7 days to allow for menses. The ring slowly releases hormones that penetrate the vaginal mucosa and are absorbed by the blood and distributed throughout the body. The contraception occurs from systemic effects, not local effects in the vagina.
4. It is safe for the client to continuously use the ring by replacing it every 4 weeks. After a period of continuous use, any breakthrough bleeding should disappear.

MEDICATION MEMORY JOGGER: Medications are not usually administered to stop normal body functions; however, the vaginal ring can be used continuously to stop monthly menses.

47. 1. This is not a true statement. The client will have a regular 28-day cycle.
2. Birth control pills will decrease cramping, but 7 days out of the month, the pill the client takes does not contain hormones—it is a placebo.
3. This product is not any more expensive or cheaper than a 21-day product.
4. This 28-day pack contains 21 days of the hormone and 7 days of placebos. The client takes a pill every day. This eliminates the need for the woman to remember which day to restart taking the pill, as she would have to with a 21-day pack, with which the woman takes a pill for 21 days and then no pill for 7 days and then restarts a new pack.

48. Correct answers are 1, 2, and 5.
1. Depot medroxyprogesterone (Depo-Provera) is a safe, effective contraceptive that is effective for 3 months or longer and is administered via intramuscular injection every 3 months to provide continuous protection.
2. When injections are discontinued, an average of 12 months is required for fertility to return. Some women remain infertile for as long as 2 1/2 years.
3. This medication is administered intramuscularly every 3 months.
4. An IUD is not necessary when using this medication. An IUD is inserted by the HCP, not by the client.
5. This medication's advantage is that it is only taken every 3 months, which is why it is recommended for adolescents or women unable to use other methods of birth control reliably.

49. 1. Because the client is receiving the medication for menstrual irregularity, it is effective when the menstrual cycle is regular, which is every 28 days.
2. A decrease in abdominal bloating may occur, but it does not indicate the medication is effective.

3. This should occur, but this is not why the client is taking the medication; therefore, it cannot be used to indicate the medication is effective.
4. Birth control pills positively affect acne, but this is not why the client is taking the medication; therefore, it cannot be used to indicate the medication's effectiveness.

MEDICATION MEMORY JOGGER: The nurse determines medication effectiveness by assessing for the symptoms, or lack thereof, for which the medication was prescribed.

Reproductive Hormone Changes

50. 1. Testosterone pellets are implanted in the upper hip or buttocks, not administered orally.
2. Testosterone levels are drawn 2 to 3 months after beginning therapy, then annually. The normal testosterone range for adult men is 280 to 1,100 ng/dL.
3. Testosterone pellets (Testopel) last 3 to 6 months, then dissolve.
4. Clinical manifestations of low testosterone include a reduced desire for sex, less spontaneous erections, trouble concentrating, weight gain, and loss of muscle mass. A common side effect of testosterone pellets (Testopel) includes more spontaneous erections. The client does not need to notify the HCP.

51. Correct answers are 1, 2, and 3.
1. Short-term systemic estrogen therapy can help reduce hot flashes and night sweats in postmenopausal clients.
2. The FDA approves estrogen therapy for osteoporosis prevention.
3. Estrogen therapy can reduce vaginal dryness and dyspareunia in postmenopausal clients.
4. Estrogen therapy can increase the client's risk of blood clots and stroke.
5. Estrogen therapy does not prevent memory loss or Alzheimer's disease in postmenopausal clients.

52. 1. The nurse would expect that a 56-year-old client should not have normal menstrual cycles.
2. Abdominal bloating is associated with premenstrual syndrome. The nurse would not expect that a 56-year-old client would have normal menstrual cycles.
3. Dong quai is used for menopausal symptoms and premenstrual syndrome. Still, because the client is 56 years old, the nurse should consider the medication effective when there is a lack of menopausal symptoms.
4. This herb does not affect bone density.

53. Correct answers are 1 and 4.
1. Alcohol taken with flibanserin (Addyi) can cause hypotension and syncope. The client should also avoid grapefruit juice as it can change the amount of medication that is absorbed in the body.
2. This medication is approved by the FDA to treat premenopausal women with generalized hypoactive sexual desire disorder.
3. This medication is not intended to improve sexual performance, only to increase sexual desire.
4. Flibanserin (Addyi) is taken orally, once a day, at bedtime. Taking flibanserin any other time increases risk of hypotension, syncope, and accidental injury. The medication can cause drowsiness.
5. If a medication dose is missed, the client should skip the dose. Do not double the medication. Take the medication at the next scheduled time.

REPRODUCTIVE SYSTEM COMPREHENSIVE EXAMINATION

1. The postpartum client, after delivering via cesarean section, is receiving epidural morphine. The unlicensed assistive personnel (UAP) measures the vital signs and enters the findings in the client's electronic health record for the registered nurse (RN) to review. The following flowsheet is populated with the client's vital signs.

Vital Sign Flowsheet	Client Values	Reference Values
Temperature	98°F/36.7°C	Oral: 98°F (36.7°C)
Pulse	84 bpm	60 to 100 bpm
Respirations	10 breaths/min	12 to 20 breaths/min
Blood pressure	98/58 mm Hg	100 to 119 mm Hg systolic 60 to 80 mm Hg diastolic

Which intervention should the nurse implement **first**?
1. Administer naloxone intramuscularly.
2. Assess the client's pain using the numerical (1 to 10) pain scale.
3. Check the client's respiratory rate and pulse oximeter reading.
4. Complete a neurovascular assessment of the client's lower extremities.

2. Which client should the nurse consider at risk for complications when taking sildenafil?
1. A 56-year-old client diagnosed with unstable angina
2. An 87-year-old client diagnosed with glaucoma
3. A 44-year-old client diagnosed with type 2 diabetes
4. A 32-year-old client diagnosed with an L1 spinal cord injury (SCI)

3. The client diagnosed with gestational diabetes asks the nurse, "Why do I have to take shots? Why can't I take a pill?" Which statement is the nurse's **best** response?
1. "The shots will help keep your blood glucose level down better."
2. "Pills may hurt the development of the baby in your womb."
3. "Insulin will help prevent you from having the baby too early."
4. "Pills for diabetes may delay the baby's lung development."

4. The mother diagnosed with preeclampsia has received magnesium sulfate during labor and delivery. Which interventions should the nursery nurse implement for the newborn? **Select all that apply.**
1. Assess the lungs for meconium aspiration.
2. Prepare to administer IV calcium gluconate.
3. Administer 2 ounces of glucose water.
4. Assess the infant's axillary temperature.
5. Stimulate the baby by tapping the feet.

5. The female client tells the nurse that she is taking the herb *Jasminum grandiflorum* (jasmine) to improve her mood and decrease insomnia. Which response by the nurse is **most appropriate**?
1. "You should speak with your HCP about taking this herb."
2. "You should stop taking this herb immediately; it can cause miscarriages."
3. "You should take chasteberry instead to enhance infertility."
4. "No herbal supplements can increase fertility or prevent miscarriages."

6. Which interventions should the nurse implement when the nurse anesthetist is administering spinal anesthesia to a pregnant client in labor? **Select all that apply.**
   1. Administer 500 to 1,000 mL of IV fluid before insertion of the spinal catheter.
   2. Instruct the client to lie on her side in the fetal position during spinal catheter insertion.
   3. Perform a neurovascular assessment on the client's lower extremities.
   4. Monitor the client's blood pressure, pulse, and respirations during spinal anesthesia.
   5. Assist the client with pushing when instructed by the obstetrician.

7. The client, after being raped, is admitted to the emergency department and tells the nurse, "I will kill myself if I get pregnant by this monster." Which statement is the nurse's **best** response?
   1. "Have you ever thought about killing yourself and do you have a plan?"
   2. "There are medications that can be taken within 72 hours to prevent pregnancy."
   3. "A vaginal spermicide can be prescribed that will prevent pregnancy."
   4. "You may have to have an elective abortion if you do become pregnant."

8. The pregnant client asks the nurse, "What does category A mean if the doctor orders that medication for me?" Which statement **best** describes the scientific rationale for the nurse's response?
   1. Category A is the safest medication a client can take when pregnant.
   2. Category A medications are safe as long as the client does not take them during the first trimester.
   3. Research has not determined if these medications are harmful to the fetus.
   4. This category is dangerous to the fetus but could be prescribed in emergencies.

9. The woman with Rh negative blood and a follower of the Jehovah's Witnesses faith delivers an Rh positive baby. The HCP prescribed Rho (D) immune globulin for the mother. Which intervention should the nurse implement **first**?
   1. Administer the Rho (D) immune globulin to the client within 72 hours.
   2. Obtain a signed permit for administering this medication.
   3. Confirm the infant's blood type with the laboratory.
   4. Explain to the client that Rho (D) immune globulin is a blood product.

10. The nurse is caring for the preterm infant in the NICU prescribed aminoglycosides and loop diuretics. Which **adverse** reaction can occur from combining these two types of medications?
    1. Blindness
    2. Intellectual delays
    3. Hearing loss
    4. Skin rash

11. The nurse is caring for the client before inserting prostaglandin E_2 dinoprostone for cervical ripening. Which interventions should the nurse implement? **Select all that apply.**
    1. Ensure the client has signed informed consent for the procedure.
    2. Instruct the client to void before medication insertion.
    3. Have the client maintain a recumbent position for 2 hours after administration.
    4. Prepare to remove the insert in the event of an adverse reaction.
    5. Avoid oxytocin induction for 6 to 12 hours after gel administration.

12. The client has been taking birth control pills for 5 weeks. Which statement from the client **warrants intervention** by the clinic nurse?
    1. "I stay nauseated, and my breasts are very tender."
    2. "I have not had a period since I started the pill."
    3. "I make my boyfriend use a condom even though I am on the pill."
    4. "I took the pills for 3 weeks then stopped for 1 week."

13. The nurse is discussing fertility issues. Which statement indicates the couple is **knowledgeable** of fertility issues?
    1. "My insurance should cover the cost of the medications completely."
    2. "A multifetal pregnancy can result in preterm labor and birth."
    3. "There is an excellent probability we will get pregnant the first time."
    4. "Most of the implanted zygotes will result in a live birth."

14. Which medication for the treatment of postpartum hemorrhage can be administered rectally?
    1. Misoprostol
    2. Carboprost
    3. Oxytocin
    4. Methylergonovine

15. The nurse is caring for the client diagnosed with preeclampsia and receiving magnesium sulfate intravenously. The laboratory reports to the nurse a critically high magnesium level of 6 mg/dL. Which intervention should the nurse implement?
    1. Stop the magnesium infusion immediately.
    2. Notify the HCP to increase the magnesium infusion.
    3. Continue to monitor the client.
    4. Administer calcium gluconate stat.

16. The nurse is caring for a pregnant client who delivered her last baby at 30 weeks gestation. The HCP has prescribed hydroxyprogesterone caproate injections. Which information should the nurse discuss with the client? **Select all that apply.**
    1. "This medication lowers the risk of having another preterm infant."
    2. "Injections are given weekly from 16 to 37 weeks gestation."
    3. "This medication can be used to stop active preterm labor."
    4. "Pain, redness, and swelling can occur at the injection site."
    5. "This medication is intended for clients with multiple gestations."

17. The nurse is providing discharge instructions for the postpartum client concerning birth control methods. Which question is **most important** for the nurse to ask the client?
    1. "Has your doctor discussed when to resume sexual activity?"
    2. "Have you decided if you will be breastfeeding your baby?"
    3. "Are you concerned about how this baby will change your life?"
    4. "Does your partner agree with the type of birth control you will use?"

18. The nurse is caring for a client diagnosed with menopause and prescribed paroxetine mesylate for hot flashes. The client tells the nurse, "I am concerned about taking hormone therapy for my symptoms." Which statement is the nurse's **best** response?
    1. "Hormone therapy is the best way to relieve your hot flashes."
    2. "This medication does not contain any hormones."
    3. "Are you concerned this medication will not help your symptoms?"
    4. "Taking hormones is safe if you only take them for a short time."

REPRODUCTIVE SYSTEM COMPREHENSIVE EXAMINATION ANSWERS AND RATIONALES

1. 1. This is the antidote for morphine overdose, but the nurse would not administer the medication without first assessing the client because these data were provided by the UAP.
2. The client's respiration is less than normal; therefore, the priority should be assessing the respiratory status, not the client's pain level.
3. Because the UAP provided the initial abnormal data, the RN should first assess the client to determine and validate the client's respiratory status.
4. The client's neurovascular status should be assessed because of the epidural analgesia, but the client's respiratory status is the priority.

2. 1. Sildenafil (Viagra), a vasodilator and erectile dysfunction agent, should be used cautiously for clients diagnosed with coronary heart disease. During sexual activity, the client could have a myocardial infarction from the extra demands on the heart. Specifically, clients taking nitroglycerin or any nitrate medication should not take sildenafil (Viagra) because the vasodilatation effect may cause hypotension. A client diagnosed with unstable angina would be taking a nitrate medication.
2. Sildenafil (Viagra) is not contraindicated for clients diagnosed with glaucoma.
3. Sildenafil (Viagra) is not contraindicated for clients diagnosed with type 2 diabetes and may help erectile dysfunction.
4. Sildenafil (Viagra) is not contraindicated for clients diagnosed with an SCI and may help erectile dysfunction.

3. 1. Insulin may better help control the blood glucose level, but that is not the reason why it is used during pregnancy.
2. Oral hypoglycemics are not used during pregnancy because they cross the placental barrier; they stimulate fetal insulin production and may be teratogenic.
3. Insulin has no effect on preterm labor.
4. Oral hypoglycemics do not affect fetal lung development.

4. Correct answers are 2 and 5.
1. There is no data in the stem that indicates that the baby had meconium-stained fluid or is postmature; therefore, the nursery nurse would not assess for meconium aspiration.
2. The antidote for magnesium sulfate toxicity is calcium gluconate; therefore, the nurse should be prepared to administer it.
3. Glucose water is given to infants experiencing hypoglycemia. There is no indication that this infant is experiencing hypoglycemia. The mother does not have diabetes, and hypoglycemia in the infant does not occur due to preeclampsia.
4. The infant's respiratory status should be assessed, not the infant's temperature.
5. The baby is at risk for respiratory or neurological depression; therefore, the nurse should stimulate the baby until the effects of the magnesium sulfate have dissipated.

5. 1. The nurse should advise all clients to discuss herbal supplements with their HCP. Still, this medication can cause a miscarriage, and the client should be instructed to stop the medication immediately.
2. The nurse should instruct the client to stop the herbal supplement *J. grandiflorum* (jasmine) immediately as it can cause miscarriage.
3. Chasteberry is believed to promote ovulation; however, there is a lack of scientific data about herbal supplements. The supplement *J. grandiflorum* (jasmine) should be stopped immediately.
4. This statement cannot be proven as there is a lack of scientific data about herbal supplements.

6. Correct answers are 1, 2, 3, 4, and 5.
1. Spinal anesthesia has been shown to be well tolerated by a healthy fetus when a maternal IV fluid preload of 500 to 1,000 mL precedes the spinal administration.
2. The client can be in the side-lying or fetal position when the spinal anesthesia is being administered.
3. This neurovascular assessment should be performed before and after the spinal anesthesia to determine anesthesia's effectiveness.
4. Baseline vital signs can be obtained 30 minutes to 1 hour before spinal anesthesia; postprocedure vital signs are monitored every 1 to 2 minutes for the first 10 minutes and then every 5 to 10 minutes throughout the delivery.

5. **Spinal anesthesia will cause the pregnant client not to feel the contractions, so the nurse needs to assist the client with pushing.**

7. 1. The client is understandably distressed and is in a crisis. The suicide threat is not imminent in the emergency department, and she would not know if she were pregnant for several weeks.
   2. **There are three emergency contraception options available: (1) Yuzpe regimen, which is a combination of estrogen and progesterone pills administered within 72 hours and a second dose 12 hours later that will initiate the onset of menstrual bleeding within 21 days; (2) the administration of mifepristone (RU 486) plus misoprostol (Cytotec), which will prevent pregnancy; and (3) copper IUD insertion within 5 days of unprotected intercourse, which can prevent pregnancy (99% effective).**
   3. Spermicide after intercourse is not effective in preventing pregnancy.
   4. If the client is adamant about not carrying a baby to term, the nurse should discuss other options to prevent pregnancy.

8. 1. **Category A medications have a remote risk of causing fetal harm and are prescribed for pregnant clients.**
   2. Category B medications are associated with a slightly higher risk than category A medications and are often prescribed for pregnant clients. These medications should not be taken during the first 3 months of pregnancy.
   3. Category C medications pose a greater risk than category B medications and are cautiously prescribed for pregnant clients. Research on medications in this category has not been done or may show risk in animal studies.
   4. Category D medications have a proven risk of fetal harm and are not prescribed for pregnant clients unless the mother's life is in danger. Category X medications have a definite risk of fetal abnormality or abortion.

9. 1. RhoGAM prevents formation of antibodies to the fetus's Rh-positive blood in the mother, but this cannot be done first because the client is a Jehovah's Witness.
   2. The mother must sign a permit when taking this medication, but this is not the nurse's first intervention because the client is a Jehovah's Witness.
   3. The nurse can confirm the newborn's blood type, but this is not the first intervention because the client is a Jehovah's Witness.
   4. **RhoGAM is derived from blood products; therefore, the nurse must explain this to the client whose faith prohibits blood or blood products administration.**

10. 1. Blindness is not associated with the combination of aminoglycosides and loop diuretics.
    2. Intellectual delay is not associated with the combination of aminoglycosides and loop diuretics.
    3. **Ototoxicity can be an adverse reaction to aminoglycosides. Loop diuretics increase risk of ototoxicity. Extent of hearing loss varies and may be irreversible.**
    4. Skin rash can occur from an allergic reaction; however, this can happen with any medication and is not specific to this medication combination.

11. **Correct answers are 1, 2, 3, and 4.**
    1. **The nurse should ensure the client understands the procedure and obtain informed consent.**
    2. **The client should void before medication administration.**
    3. **The client should remain supine with a lateral tilt or in the side-lying position for 2 hours after insert placement to maintain the proper positioning of the insert in the posterior uterine fornix.**
    4. **Prostaglandin E2 dinoprostone insert (Cervidil) is an insert with an attached polyester tape that allows for insert removal if uterine hyperstimulation occurs.**
    5. Prostaglandin potentiates oxytocin's effects; therefore, oxytocin should be avoided for 30 to 60 minutes after removal of the insert.

12. 1. **If clinical manifestations of estrogen excess are apparent (nausea, edema, or breast discomfort), a preparation with lower estrogen content is needed. This statement, therefore, warrants the nurse to intervene.**
    2. Oral contraceptives may decrease or eliminate menstrual flow during initial months of use; therefore, the nurse would not intervene based on this statement.
    3. This statement would warrant praise from the clinic nurse because birth control pills do not protect the client from STIs—only abstinence or condoms can do that.

4. The birth control pill suppresses ovulation for 3 weeks; then, when the pill is not taken, the client has her period. This statement indicates the client understands the teaching and does not warrant intervention.

13. 1. Infertility therapy is costly. Most insurance plans do not cover it at all or may cover only a small portion.
2. Pregnancy with more than twins carries a substantially higher risk to the mother and the fetuses because of preterm labor and birth, placental insufficiency, and increased demand on maternal body systems.
3. There is no guarantee of pregnancy on the first attempt.
4. Most implanted zygotes do not result in live births.

14. 1. Misoprostol (Cytotec) can be administered by mouth, intravaginally, or rectally.
2. Carboprost (Hemabate) is given intramuscularly.
3. Oxytocin (Pitocin) is given IVPB, never by IVP.
4. Methylergonovine (Methergine) is given intramuscularly.

15. 1. A laboratory value of 6 mg/dL is therapeutic; therefore, the nurse should not stop the medication.
2. The magnesium is at a therapeutic level. There is no need to increase the medication.
3. The therapeutic magnesium sulfate level for seizure prevention in preeclampsia is 4 to 8 mg/dL. A normal magnesium level is 1.6 to 2.2 mg/dL. Although a laboratory result of 6 mg/dL is critically high in the normal client, it is a therapeutic value in this client.
4. Calcium gluconate is indicated for magnesium toxicity, resulting in respiratory depression and hyporeflexia. There is no indication that this client is experiencing magnesium toxicity; therefore, the nurse would not administer calcium gluconate.

16. Correct answers are 1, 2, and 4.
1. Hydroxyprogesterone caproate (Makena) is shown to reduce risk of recurrent preterm birth in a client with a history of at least one previous preterm birth and pregnant with a single fetus.
2. Injections are administered intramuscularly every week, beginning at 16 to 20 weeks gestation until 37 weeks gestation.
3. This medication is not intended to treat active preterm labor.
4. Pain, redness, and swelling can occur at the injection site.
5. This medication is only indicated for clients with a single fetus pregnancy, not multiple gestations.

17. 1. This is an appropriate question, but the timing of sexual activity is not an important consideration for a new mother taking her baby home when discussing birth control.
2. This is the most important question because if the mother has decided on breastfeeding, the nurse should discourage use of birth control pills. Birth control pills enter the breast milk and reduce milk production. Breastfeeding may delay ovulation but should not be used as a form of birth control.
3. This is a question that the nurse could ask, but it is not the most important when concerned about birth control.
4. This question could be asked, but the most important issue is protecting the baby if the mother chooses to breastfeed because anything the mother ingests may affect the baby. This includes effects of the type of birth control if the mother chooses to breastfeed.

18. 1. Hormone therapy is helpful for some women in controlling hot flashes; however, this medication does not contain hormones.
2. Paroxetine mesylate (Brisdelle) is a selective serotonin reuptake inhibitor (SSRI) and does not contain any hormones.
3. This is a therapeutic response, and the client is asking for information; therefore, the nurse should provide the facts.
4. Hormone therapy is safe for specific clients on a short-term basis; however, the medication the client is prescribed does not contain hormones.

Musculoskeletal System

It is better to have ten skeletons in your closet, than walk with no bones.

—Anthony Liccione

QUESTIONS

Low Back Pain

1. The client is diagnosed with low back pain and is prescribed cyclobenzaprine. Which instructions should the clinic nurse teach the client? **Select all that apply.**
   1. "Take the medication just before leaving home for work each day."
   2. "Drink a full glass of water with each dose of medication."
   3. "The medication can cause drowsiness that will make driving unsafe."
   4. "Divide the dose of medication between early morning and bedtime."
   5. "Suck on hard candy if you experience a dry mouth."
   6. "Avoid OTC antihistamines while taking this medication."
   7. "Notify the HCP if you experience anxiety, rapid heart rate, or muscle twitching."

2. The orthopedic unit charge nurse is transcribing orders for a client diagnosed with back pain. The health-care provider's (HCP) orders are in the following order sheet.

Client: C.M.	MR# 1234567	Date: Today
Age: 45 years	Allergies: NKDA	Diagnosis: Back pain
PROVIDER ORDERS:		
Bedrest with bathroom privileges		
Physical therapy for hot packs and massage		
Labs: CBC, CMP		
Hydrocodone PRN		
Carisoprodol 250 mg PO t.i.d		
Duloxetine 60 mg PO daily		

Which HCP order(s) should the charge nurse **question**?
1. Bedrest with bathroom privileges
2. Physical therapy for hot packs and massage
3. Labs: CBC, CMP
4. Hydrocodone as needed (PRN)
5. Carisoprodol 250 mg by mouth (PO) t.i.d.
6. Duloxetine 60 mg PO daily

3. The nurse is administering medications to clients on an orthopedic unit. Which medication should the nurse **question**?
   1. Ibuprofen to a client diagnosed with back pain and a history of ulcers
   2. Morphine to a client diagnosed with back pain rated as "6"
   3. Methocarbamol to a client diagnosed with chronic back pain
   4. Acetaminophen with codeine #3 to a client diagnosed with mild back pain

4. The client diagnosed with low back pain is prescribed morphine sulfate. Which interventions should the nurse implement? **Select all that apply.**
   1. Discuss with the HCP starting the client on a stool softener.
   2. Teach the client about rating the pain on a numeric pain scale.
   3. Inform the client to rise quickly from a supine position.
   4. Administer anticonvulsant medications around the clock.
   5. Tell the client to call for assistance when getting out of bed.

5. The client diagnosed with low back pain is scheduled to have a steroid injection in the intrathecal space. Which statement by the client indicates the client **understands** the procedure?
   1. "I will have to curl up like a Halloween cat."
   2. "This procedure will cure my back pain."
   3. "I will have an injection in each of my hips."
   4. "There is no risk with this procedure."

6. The nurse is completing the preoperative checklist for a client diagnosed with a herniated disc. Which information is a **priority** for the nurse to notify the operating room staff?
   1. The client is reporting a headache.
   2. The client is allergic to iodine and aspirin.
   3. The client has not had anything to drink.
   4. The client's hematocrit (Hct) is 43%.

7. The client presents to the outpatient clinic reporting back pain. Which assessment question should the nurse ask **first?**
   1. "What activity did you do to hurt your back?"
   2. "Which over-the-counter (OTC) medications have you taken?"
   3. "Have you used illegal drugs to treat your back pain?"
   4. "Did you miss any work time because of this pain?"

8. The client diagnosed with chronic low back pain has been taking baclofen. Which instruction should the nurse review with the client?
   1. The medication can cause gastric ulcer formation.
   2. The client may consume no more than one glass of wine per day.
   3. The medication must be tapered off when discontinued.
   4. The client should not take the medication before bedtime.

9. The nurse is administering 0900 medications to clients on a medical unit. Which medication should be administered **first**?
   1. Morphine sulfate ER to a client diagnosed with low back pain
   2. Chlorzoxazone to a client on bedrest
   3. Acetaminophen to a client diagnosed with a headache
   4. Diazepam to a client diagnosed with muscle spasms

10. The client is admitted with severe low back pain and prescribed methocarbamol IV piggyback every 8 hours. Which nursing intervention has **priority** when administering this medication?
    1. Ask the client to lie flat for 15 minutes after the IV infusion.
    2. Infuse at a rapid rate of 200 to 250 mL/hr via an infusion pump.
    3. Assess the IV site for extravasation after the infusion is complete.
    4. Monitor liver function laboratory tests daily.

Osteoarthritis

11. The client diagnosed with osteoarthritis is prescribed celecoxib. Which statement(s) by the client **warrants intervention** by the nurse? **Select all that apply.**

1. "I take aspirin daily to help prevent heart disease."
2. "I am allergic to penicillin and aminoglycosides."
3. "I know I am overweight and need to lose 50 pounds."
4. "I walk 30 minutes at least three times a week."
5. "I will take the medication and go right to bed."
6. "I should continue to monitor my blood pressure regularly."

12. The client diagnosed with severe osteoarthritis of the left knee is receiving sodium hyaluronate injected directly into the left knee. Which information should be discussed with the client?

1. Explain that this medication will cause some bleeding into the joint.
2. Instruct the client to avoid any strenuous activity for 48 hours after injection.
3. Discuss that the medication will be injected daily for 7 days.
4. Tell the client that strict bedrest is required for 24 hours after the injection.

13. The nurse is preparing to administer the following medications. Which medication should the nurse **question** administering?

1. Ibuprofen to a client receiving furosemide
2. Nabumetone to a client receiving digoxin
3. Acetylsalicylic acid to a client receiving warfarin
4. Ketorolac intramuscularly to a client on a morphine patient-controlled analgesia (PCA)

14. The client is taking acetylsalicylic acid four to five times a day for severe osteoarthritic pain. Which teaching interventions should the nurse discuss with the client? **Select all that apply.**

1. Do not drink any type of alcoholic beverage.
2. Keep the acetylsalicylic acid bottle out of reach of children.
3. Inform the dentist about taking high doses of acetylsalicylic acid.
4. Maintain a serum salicylate level between 15 and 30 mg/dL.
5. Explain that ringing in the ears is a common side effect.
6. Notify the HCP if you have black or bloody stools.
7. Drink plenty of water while taking acetylsalicylic acid.
8. Teach the client to call the HCP for unrelieved gastrointestinal (GI) discomfort.

15. At 0900, the charge nurse observes the primary nurse crushing an enteric-coated aspirin in the medication room. Which action should the charge nurse implement?

1. Take no action because this is an acceptable standard of practice.
2. Correct the primary nurse's behavior in the medication room.
3. Explain that enteric-coated medication should not be crushed.
4. Complete an adverse occurrence report on the primary nurse.

16. The client diagnosed with osteoarthritis of the hands is prescribed capsaicin cream. Which intervention should the nurse discuss with the client concerning this medication?

1. Wash hands immediately after applying cream.
2. Remove cream immediately if burning of the skin occurs.
3. Apply a heating pad to the affected area after applying cream.
4. After application, do not remove the cream for at least 30 minutes.

17. The client in the hospital is reporting arthritic pain. The prescribed medication for administration is in the following medication administration record (MAR).

Client: W.C.	MR# 1234567	Date: Today
Age: 85 years	Allergies: NKDA	Diagnosis: Arthritis
Medication	**0701–1900**	**1901–0700**
Meloxicam 7.5 mg PO	0900	
Acetylsalicylic acid 81 mg PO	1900	
Acetaminophen 325 mg PO 1 to 2 tablets q 4 to 6 hours, PRN, not to exceed 3,250 mg daily		
Morphine 5 mg IVP every 4 hours PRN severe pain		
Nurse Initials/Credentials	**DN/RN**	**NN/RN**

Which intervention should the nurse implement?
1. Administer meloxicam.
2. Administer acetylsalicylic acid.
3. Administer acetaminophen.
4. Administer morphine IV push (IVP).

18. The client diagnosed with osteoarthritis tells the clinic nurse about taking the herb ginkgo. Which intervention should the nurse implement?
1. Determine what medications the client is currently taking.
2. Praise the client because this herb helps decrease inflammation.
3. Notify the HCP that the client is taking ginkgo.
4. Examine why the client thought they needed to take herbs.

19. The HCP is administering an intraarticular corticosteroid mixed with lidocaine to a client diagnosed with severe osteoarthritis in the right knee. Which statement by the client **warrants intervention** by the nurse?
1. "I have taken off work tomorrow so I can rest my knee."
2. "I am attending physical therapy once a week."
3. "I alternate heat and ice on my knee when I am having pain."
4. "I had one of these just last month, and it helped the pain."

20. The client diagnosed with osteoarthritis who is taking celecoxib calls the clinic and reports having black, tarry stools. Which intervention should the clinic nurse implement?
1. Ask if the client is taking any type of iron preparation.
2. Tell the client not to take any more celecoxib.
3. Instruct the client to bring a stool specimen to the clinic.
4. Explain that this is a side effect of the medication.

Osteoporosis

21. The postmenopausal client is prescribed alendronate to help prevent osteoporosis. Which information should the nurse discuss with the client? **Select all that apply.**
1. "Chew the tablet thoroughly before swallowing."
2. "Eat a meal before taking the medication."
3. "Drink one glass of milk when taking the medication."
4. "Take the medication first thing in the morning."
5. "Remain upright 30 minutes after taking the medication."

22. The client diagnosed with postmenopausal osteoporosis is prescribed calcitonin salmon intranasally. Which instruction should the nurse discuss with the client?
   1. "Notify the HCP if nausea and vomiting occur."
   2. "Decrease calcium and vitamin D intake during drug therapy."
   3. "Remove the nasal spray from the refrigerator immediately before using."
   4. "Expect to experience rhinitis when taking the medication."

23. The client is prescribed raloxifene. Which information should the nurse discuss with the client?
   1. Instruct the client to walk for 10 minutes every hour when traveling in a car.
   2. Encourage the client to decrease smoking cigarettes and drinking alcohol.
   3. Explain that raloxifene will decrease the hot flashes experienced with menopause.
   4. Discuss the importance of performing non weight-bearing activities.

24. The long-term care nurse is preparing to administer calcium gluconate to a client diagnosed with osteoporosis. Which data **warrants** the nurse **questioning** administering this medication?
   1. The client asks the nurse for a walker to ambulate.
   2. The client's oral intake is 850 mL, and urinary output is 1,250 mL.
   3. The client is lethargic, drowsy, and has increasing weakness.
   4. The client has abnormal bleeding when brushing teeth.

25. **Complete the sentence by choosing from the list of options.**

   The HCP has prescribed calcitonin salmon to a client diagnosed with osteoporosis.The nurse knows that the scientific rationale for this medication administration is to ____
   1. Decrease renal excretion of calcium.
   2. Stimulate osteoclast activity.
   3. Decrease bone matrix resorption.
   4. Increase progesterone and estrogen levels.

26. The nurse is discussing ways to prevent osteoporosis with a group of older women. A woman in the audience asks, "Why aren't doctors prescribing hormone replacement therapy (HRT)?" Which statement by the nurse is **most appropriate**?
   1. "There are many other, better ways to treat osteoporosis than HRT."
   2. "HRT treatment is very expensive, and many insurers will not pay."
   3. "There is an increased risk of cancer and deep vein thrombosis associated with HRT."
   4. "Research has shown that HRT is not effective in treating osteoporosis."

27. Which assessment data **best** indicates to the nurse that the medication therapy for a client diagnosed with osteoporosis has been **effective**?
   1. The client's serum calcium level is 7.5 mg/dL.
   2. The client does not experience any pathologic fractures.
   3. The client has adequate urinary output.
   4. The client loses less than 1 inch in height.

28. Which statement indicates the 30-year-old client **understands** the teaching for how to prevent osteoporosis? **Select all that apply.**
   1. "I need to take at least 1,500 mg of calcium daily."
   2. "Milk and dairy products are good sources of vitamin D."
   3. "I must get shots weekly to increase my calcium level."
   4. "I should take steps to prevent osteoporosis now."
   5. "Smoking and alcohol increase my risk of osteoporosis."
   6. "I should continue taking my low-impact aerobics class."

29. Which statement indicates the postmenopausal client diagnosed with osteoporosis **understands** the medication teaching concerning the bisphosphonate alendronate?
1. "I do not use sunscreen when working outside in my yard."
2. "I take the medication with 6 to 8 ounces of tap water."
3. "I drink orange juice when I take the medication at breakfast."
4. "I may experience some heartburn when taking this medication."

Orthopedic Surgery

30. The client who had surgery for a hip fracture is reporting severe pain 45 minutes after the nurse administered morphine IVP. Which intervention should the nurse implement **first**?
1. Administer another dose of morphine.
2. Turn on the television to distract the client.
3. Assess the client's affected leg for alignment.
4. Notify the HCP of the problem.

31. The client postoperative from hip surgery is scheduled to ambulate with the physical therapist. Which intervention should the registered nurse (RN) implement to assure the client's success in **performing** the therapy?
1. Assist the client to the bedside chair with the therapist's help.
2. Administer pain medication 30 minutes before the therapy.
3. Ask the unlicensed assistive personnel (UAP) to brush the client's hair.
4. Allow the client to delay therapy until late in the day.

32. The 84-year-old client diagnosed with a fractured knee cannot rate pain using a numeric pain scale. Which intervention should the nurse implement?
1. Have the client use a pediatric faces scale.
2. Do not try to get the client to rate the pain.
3. The nurse should decide the amount of pain.
4. Check the pulse and blood pressure for elevation.

33. After bilateral knee replacement surgery, the client calls the nurse's desk and reports seeing bruises on both sides of the abdomen while taking a bath. The client's MAR notes an antibiotic, anarcotic analgesic, and enoxaparin. Which statement is the nurse's **best** response to the client?
1. "This is a reaction to the antibiotic you are receiving, and it will need to be changed."
2. "This is caused by straining when trying to have a bowel movement."
3. "This occurs because of your positioning during the surgical procedure."
4. "This happened because of the medication used to prevent complications."

34. After total knee surgery, the client returns to the room with an autotransfusion drainage system (cell saver) device inserted into the wound. Which interventions should the nurse implement? **Select all that apply.**
1. Monitor the drainage in the collection chamber every 30 to 45 minutes.
2. Take the drainage to the blood bank when it reaches 200 mL.
3. Attach a filter to the drainage before administering.
4. Have a second nurse verify the client's identification band.
5. Monitor vital signs every 5 to 15 minutes when transfusing the blood.

35. After hip surgery, the 78-year-old client is to receive a unit of packed red blood cells (PRBCs). The nurse's assessment reveals bilateral crackles in the lungs and 2+ edema of the sacrum. The PRBCs contain 250 mL of cells and 60 mL of preservative solution. At what rate will the nurse set the IV infusion pump after the initial 15 minutes?

____

36. A 10-year-old child sustained a compound fracture of the left forearm and just returned to the unit after open reduction and internal fixation (ORIF). Which interventions should the nurse implement? **Select all that apply.**
   1. Assess the child's ability to rate pain using a pain scale.
   2. Ask the parent to determine when the child needs pain medication.
   3. Apply a heat pack to the cast until the cast is completely dry.
   4. Check the child's fingertips for warmth and color every 15 minutes.
   5. Administer the prophylactic antibiotic as prescribed by the surgeon.

37. The nurse is administering medications at 2100. Which medication should the nurse **question**?
   1. An NSAID to a 24-year-old client recovering from an arthroscopy
   2. An opioid analgesic to a 50-year-old client diagnosed with a fractured femur
   3. A sedative hypnotic to a 65-year-old client after a total knee replacement
   4. A muscarinic antagonist to an 89-year-old male client diagnosed with a hip fracture

38. The client is postoperative from a cervical laminectomy and is prescribed morphine sulfate by PCA pump. Which instruction regarding pain control should the nurse teach the client?
   1. Notify the nurse when needing pain medication.
   2. Press the button on the pump when the client feels pain.
   3. Have the significant other push the button on the pump frequently.
   4. Use the pain medication sparingly to prevent narcotic addiction.

39. The RN and UAP are caring for clients on an orthopedic unit. Which action by the UAP requires **immediate intervention** by the RN?
   1. The UAP obtains a fracture pan for a client with a laminectomy to use.
   2. The UAP attempts to ambulate an elderly client immediately after receiving pain medication.
   3. Before bedtime, the UAP provides a back rub to a client diagnosed with low back pain.
   4. The UAP places moisture barrier cream on a client's perineal area.

ANSWERS AND RATIONALES

The correct answer number and rationale are in **boldface blue type.** Rationales for why other answer options are incorrect are also given.

Low Back Pain

1. **Correct answers are 3, 5, 6, and 7.**
   1. Cyclobenzaprine (Flexeril) is a muscle relaxant. Taking the medication before leaving the house could be a danger to the client and others because this medication can cause drowsiness. The client should not be driving or operating equipment until the client has determined the medication's effect on their body.
   2. Cyclobenzaprine (Flexeril) is a muscle relaxant. There is no need to drink a full glass of water when taking Flexeril.
   3. **Cyclobenzaprine (Flexeril) is a muscle relaxant. The medication acts on the central nervous system and can cause drowsiness. The client should be warned not to drive until the client understands the effects on their body. Driving could be dangerous for the client and others.**
   4. This is prescribing. The HCP will prescribe how frequently the dose should be administered.
   5. **Cyclobenzaprine (Flexeril) is a muscle relaxant. A side effect of Flexeril is a dry mouth, so using hard candy is an appropriate intervention.**
   6. **Cyclobenzaprine (Flexeril) can increase the effects of alcohol and other CNS depressants, such as antihistamines, and should be avoided.**
   7. **Anxiety, restlessness, rapid heart rate, fever, sweating, and muscle twitching could indicate the client is experiencing serotonin syndrome. The client should report these symptoms to the HCP immediately.**

2. **Correct answers are 1 and 4.**
   1. **Bedrest is not recommended for clients with back pain. The inactivity can make the pain even worse and delay the client's recovery. The nurse should question this order.**
   2. Physical therapy for heat and massage is standard therapy for back pain. There is no reason to question this order.
   3. Many medications can affect the kidneys or liver and blood counts. Baseline data should be obtained. There is no reason to question this order.
   4. **Hydrocodone (Vicodin) is an opioid analgesic. This medication order is incomplete. The nurse should contact the HCP for a time limitation.**
   5. Carisoprodol (Soma) is a muscle relaxant used for short-term treatment of back pain, and the HCP's order is complete. There is no reason to question this order.
   6. Duloxetine (Cymbalta), an antidepressant medication, has been shown to reduce lower back pain. The nurse should not question this order (Alev et al., 2017).

MEDICATION MEMORY JOGGER: All medication orders must be complete, and the nurse is responsible for determining all parameters before administering a medication.

3. 1. **Ibuprofen (Motrin) is an NSAID. NSAIDs decrease prostaglandin production in the stomach, increasing the client's risk of developing ulcers. This client has a known risk of peptic ulcer disease (PUD). The nurse should question the medication and discuss this with the HCP.**
   2. Morphine sulfate is an opioid analgesic. Opioid analgesics are administered for pain. The client is in the moderate to severe pain range. The nurse would administer this medication.
   3. Methocarbamol (Robaxin) is a muscle relaxant. Muscle relaxant medications are administered to clients with back pain to relax the muscles and decrease pain. The nurse would administer this medication.
   4. Acetaminophen (Tylenol) is a nonnarcotic analgesic, and when combined with codeine, a narcotic analgesic, the potency of medication for pain relief is increased. The nurse would administer this medication.

4. **Correct answers are 1, 2, and 5.**
   1. **Narcotic pain medications slow peristalsis in the small and large intestines, increasing the risk for constipation and fecal impaction. The nurse should discuss a bowel regimen with the HCP.**
   2. **The nurse should attempt to have the client quantify the pain so that**

intervention effectiveness can be evaluated. The numeric pain scale is one method of objectifying pain.

3. Rising quickly from a flat-on-the-back (supine) position could increase the client's pain. Some medications administered for back pain can cause orthostatic hypotension. The nurse should teach the client to turn on the side and slowly push up on the elbow when getting out of bed.
4. The client may be taking antispasmodic and pain medications, but there is no reason for anticonvulsant medications.
5. **This is a safety issue. The client should call for assistance to prevent falls.**

5. 1. **Intrathecal means into the central nervous system via a lumbar puncture. The client will be positioned with the back arched, like a Halloween cat, for the HCP to insert the needle between the vertebrae.**
2. The procedure provides temporary relief of inflammation of affected nerves.
3. The injections are into the intravertebral space, not into the hips. An injection in the hips indicates an intramuscular injection.
4. There is a risk with any procedure. In this procedure, nerve damage is the most significant risk.

6. 1. The client's report of a headache frequently occurs when clients have not been able to eat or drink, especially caffeine drinks. This is not a priority at this time.
2. **The standard surgical scrub is a povidone-iodine (Betadine) antiseptic skin preparation. The surgical nurse, who prepares the surgical site, should be made aware so that a substitute can be used.**
3. Clients going to surgery should have nothing by mouth for several hours to prevent aspiration during anesthesia.
4. This is a normal Hct level.

7. 1. This is important, but it is not a priority during initial assessment. The nurse should determine how the client has been treating the injury. This would be the second query, not the first.
2. **The priority at this time is to determine what medications have been tried in order to assess the full extent of the injury. This is the first intervention. Adult clients will frequently only seek the HCP's advice and treatment when OTC remedies have failed.**
3. This is an accusatory statement and most likely will make the client mistrust the nurse's objectives. This should not be asked at this time.
4. This is the third query the nurse could ask. Missed work time is important, but to treat the client, the HCP must be aware of attempted treatments.

8. 1. This medication is not known to increase ulcer risk.
2. The client should be warned not to consume any alcohol while taking baclofen. Baclofen is a central nervous system depressant, as is alcohol. The combination of alcohol and baclofen could intensify depressant effects.
3. **Baclofen must be tapered off when being discontinued. Abrupt withdrawal after prolonged use can cause anxiety, agitated behavior, hallucinations, severe tachycardia, acute spasticity, and seizures.**
4. The medication can cause drowsiness, which might assist the client in resting. Administration at bedtime is preferred if this is the case.

MEDICATION MEMORY JOGGER: There is rarely any medication for which the client will be told that concurrent administration with alcohol is appropriate.

9. 1. Morphine sulfate extended release is an opioid analgesic and is a sustained-release tablet. This medication is to provide relief of chronic pain for the day. It does not need to be the first medication administered.
2. Chlorzoxazone (Parafon Forte) is a muscle relaxant. The client prescribed bedrest usually takes a muscle relaxant as a routine medication. It does not need to be administered first.
3. Acetaminophen (Tylenol) is an analgesic. Tylenol (for mild pain) would not be the first medication administration for the nurse treating a client with a headache.
4. **Diazepam (Valium) is a benzodiazepine. A client having muscle spasms is a priority for the nurse. Muscle spasms can be extremely painful. This medication should be administered first.**

10. 1. **Methocarbamol (Robaxin) is a muscle relaxant. The client should be kept recumbent during and for at least 15 minutes after administration of Robaxin IV to reduce orthostatic hypotension risk.**

2. The medication must be administered slowly at a rate of no greater than 300 mg per minute, not by rapid infusion.
3. The IV site should be assessed before initiating medication to prevent complications from extravasation of the medication into the tissues.
4. Robaxin is detoxified by the kidneys, not the liver.

Osteoarthritis

11. Correct answers are 1 and 5.

1. **Celecoxib (Celebrex) is an NSAID. The client should not take aspirin with an NSAID because it can increase risk of gastrointestinal (GI) upset and possible GI bleeding.**
2. Celecoxib (Celebrex) is an NSAID. Allergies to antibiotics are not a contraindication to NSAID use.
3. Celecoxib (Celebrex) is an NSAID. Obesity is not contraindicated in clients taking NSAIDs.
4. Exercising is recommended for clients with osteoarthritis unless it causes pain. This activity is acceptable while taking Celebrex.
5. **The client should not lie down for at least 10 minutes after taking this medication.**
6. Celecoxib (Celebrex) can raise blood pressure, so the client should monitor their blood pressure regularly and tell the HCP if the blood pressure increases.

12. 1. Any bleeding into the joint is a complication. Bleeding into a joint would not be the expected benefit of any type of medication. Sodium hyaluronate (Hyalgan) is a synovial joint lubricant used for relief of osteoarthritis pain.

2. **Sodium hyaluronate (Hyalgan) is a synovial joint lubricant used to relieve osteoarthritis pain unrelieved by NSAIDs. After injection, the client can walk and perform routine daily activities but running, bicycling, or strenuous activity should be avoided. Hyalgan is a preparation of a chemical normally found in high amounts in the synovial fluid. The injection replaces or supplements the body's natural hyaluronic acid that deteriorates due to the inflammation associated with osteoarthritis.**
3. The treatment includes three to five injections, with the client receiving one injection every week.
4. This injection is done in an HCP's office. The client will be able to walk out of the clinic after the injection.

MEDICATION MEMORY JOGGER: The nurse should realize that the joint must have time for the medication to be effective, and daily injections would not allow this. The nurse should recognize that a medication should not cause an abnormal body function, such as bleeding into the joint.

13. 1. Ibuprofen (Motrin) is an NSAID. NSAIDs do not interfere with loop diuretic effectiveness; therefore, the nurse would not question administering Motrin.

2. Nabumetone (Relafen) is a COX-2 inhibitor. COX-2 inhibitors do not interfere with effectiveness of cardiac glycosides; therefore, the nurse would not question administering Relafen.
3. **Acetylsalicylic acid (ASA) is a mild analgesic, but it is also an antiplatelet. Aspirin displaces warfarin from protein-binding sites and will increase the client's bleeding; therefore, the nurse should question administering aspirin.**
4. Ketorolac (Toradol) is an NSAID. Toradol is often administered around the clock to a client in pain, along with a narcotic analgesic. Toradol decreases inflammation to help reduce pain.

14. Correct answers are 1, 2, 3, 4, 6, 7, and 8.

1. **Alcohol displaces warfarin from protein-binding sites and will increase the client's bleeding; therefore, the nurse should instruct the client not to drink alcohol.**
2. **Acetylsalicylic acid (ASA) poisoning can kill children, and all medications, prescription or nonprescription, should be kept out of the reach of children.**
3. **High doses of ASA can cause bleeding; therefore, the dentist should be made aware of the client's medication use.**
4. **Aspirin toxicity can occur when the client takes ASA four to five times a day; therefore, the serum level should be kept within normal limits (15 to 30 mg/dL). Mild toxicity occurs with serum levels above 30 mg/dL, and severe toxicity occurs above 50 mg/dL.**
5. Tinnitus (ringing in the ears) is a sign of aspirin toxicity and should be reported to the HCP.
6. **Black or bloody stools indicate bleeding, and the HCP should be notified.**

7. The client should drink plenty of fluids while taking ASA.
8. Unrelieved GI discomfort should be reported to the HCP.

15. 1. Enteric-coated aspirin should not be crushed.
2. The charge nurse should not correct the primary nurse in front of other staff and, at 0900, there would be other nurses in the medication room.
3. The charge nurse should explain to the primary nurse that enteric-coated ASA should not be crushed because the coating ensures the ASA will dissolve only in the small intestine. The aspirin will be absorbed in the stomach if the coated tablet is crushed.
4. Because the client did not receive the crushed enteric-coated ASA, no adverse occurrence report must be completed. This form is completed if the client's condition has been compromised in some way.

16. 1. Capsaicin (Capsin) is a nonopioid analgesic. This medication is being administered for the hands; therefore, the client should not wash off the medication immediately after application.
2. The client should know that transient burning occurs with the application.
3. Capsaicin (Capsin) is a nonopioid analgesic. The client should not apply heat because this will increase skin burning secondary to the cream application. Burning is increased by heat, sweating, bathing in warm water, humidity, and clothing.
4. Capsaicin (Capsin) is a nonopioid analgesic. The topical cream should be kept in place at least 30 minutes after application because it is being administered for osteoarthritis of the hands. If not being applied to treat the hands, the cream should be washed off immediately.

17. 1. Meloxicam (Mobic) is an NSAID COX-2 inhibitor. These medications are administered around the clock and are not specifically for acute pain.
2. Acetylsalicylic acid (Aspirin, ASA) is a salicylate. Aspirin has side effects, such as GI discomfort, and is not the drug of choice for elderly clients.
3. Acetaminophen (Tylenol) is a nonopioid analgesic. Acetaminophen is generally preferred for use in older clients because it has fewer toxic side effects.
4. Morphine is a narcotic analgesic. It is not used to treat chronic arthritis pain and should be used cautiously in elderly clients.

18. 1. The first intervention the nurse should implement is to determine if the client is taking any medication that will interact with the herb. Ginkgo, along with dong quai, feverfew, and garlic, when taken with NSAIDs, may cause bleeding.
2. Ginkgo is used to treat allergic rhinitis, Alzheimer's disease, anxiety or stress, dementia, tinnitus, vertigo, and poor circulation. It is not known to decrease inflammation.
3. The nurse should determine what medications the client is currently taking and if ginkgo interacts with them before notifying the HCP.
4. The nurse does not need to know why the client thought they needed to take the herb. This is an accusatory intervention. The nurse should support alternative-type medicine if it does not interfere with other medications the client is currently taking.

MEDICATION MEMORY JOGGER: Some herbal preparations are effective, some are not, and a few can be harmful or even deadly. If a client is taking an herbal supplement and a conventional medicine, the nurse should investigate to determine if the combination will cause harm to the client. The nurse should always be the client's advocate.

19. 1. Lidocaine numbs the nerves and the injected steroid will decrease joint inflammation. Resting the knee after injection is an appropriate action for the client. It would not warrant nurse intervention.
2. Physical therapy for range-of-motion exercises is an acceptable conservative treatment for osteoarthritis. The client should inform the physical therapist of the treatment, but this statement does not warrant immediate intervention by the nurse.
3. Alternating ice and heat is an acceptable conservative treatment for easing the pain secondary to osteoarthritis. This statement would not warrant nurse intervention.
4. Lidocaine numbs the nerves, and the steroid injection will decrease joint inflammation. This procedure does provide significant pain relief, but it should not be done more than once every 4 to 6 months because it can hasten the rate of cartilage breakdown. This statement should be reported to the HCP. It is helpful to be aware that clients often go to more than one HCP.

20. 1. Iron preparations can cause black, tarry stool. Still, because the client is taking an NSAID, the nurse should realize tarry stools are a sign of GI distress, a complication of NSAID medications.

2. Celecoxib (Celebrex) is a COX-2 inhibitor NSAID. NSAIDs are notorious for causing GI upset and PUD. Black, tarry stool indicates GI bleeding; therefore, the client should stop taking the medication.

3. A specimen is not sent to the laboratory when the stool is black and tarry. The nurse should know these are findings of GI bleeding.

4. Celecoxib (Celebrex) is a COX-2 inhibitor NSAID. This is not an expected side effect of the medication, and the NSAID should be discontinued immediately.

MEDICATION MEMORY JOGGER: If the client verbalizes a symptom, the nurse assesses data, or if laboratory data indicates that an adverse effect is secondary to a medication, the nurse must intervene. The nurse must implement an independent intervention or notify the HCP because medications can result in severe or life-threatening complications.

Osteoporosis

21. Correct answers are 4 and 5.

1. Alendronate (Fosamax) is a bisphosphonate used to prevent or treat osteoporosis. The client should swallow the medication. The client should not crush, chew, or suck on the medication.

2. Alendronate (Fosamax) is a bisphosphonate used to prevent or treat osteoporosis. The medication should be taken on an empty stomach at least 30 minutes before eating or drinking liquids. Foods and beverages greatly decrease the effect of Fosamax.

3. Alendronate (Fosamax) is a bisphosphonate used to prevent or treat osteoporosis. The medication should be taken on an empty stomach at least 30 minutes before eating or drinking liquids except for water. Never take the medication with tea, coffee, juice, milk, or any liquid other than plain water. Foods and beverages significantly decrease the effect of Fosamax.

4. Alendronate (Fosamax) is a bisphosphonate used to prevent or treat osteoporosis. The medication will irritate the stomach and esophagus if the client lies down; therefore, the medication should be taken when the client can remain upright for at least 30 minutes first thing in the morning.

5. Alendronate (Fosamax) is a bisphosphonate used to prevent or treat osteoporosis. This client must remain upright to facilitate the medication's passage to the stomach and minimize risk of esophageal irritation.

22. 1. Calcitonin salmon (Miacalcin) is a parathyroid calcium regulator used to treat postmenopausal osteoporosis. Nausea and vomiting occur during initial therapy and disappear as treatment continues; therefore, the client does not need to notify the HCP.

2. Calcitonin salmon (Miacalcin) is a parathyroid calcium regulator used to treat postmenopausal osteoporosis. The client should consume an adequate amount of calcium and vitamin D while taking this medication.

3. Calcitonin salmon (Miacalcin) is a parathyroid calcium regulator used to treat postmenopausal osteoporosis. The nasal spray should be at room temperature before use. The nasal spray is not kept in the refrigerator.

4. Calcitonin salmon (Miacalcin) is a parathyroid calcium regulator used to treat postmenopausal osteoporosis. Rhinitis, a runny nose, is the most common side effect with calcitonin nasal spray, but the client should not quit taking the medication if this occurs.

MEDICATION MEMORY JOGGER: Even if the test taker did not know this drug, the method of delivery (intranasal) should have made it easy to choose option 4, "rhinitis."

23. 1. Raloxifene (Evista) is a selective estrogen receptor modulator (SERM). Evista increases venous thrombosis risk; therefore, the client should avoid prolonged immobilization, including driving long distances in a car.

2. Raloxifene (Evista) is a SERM. The client should not just decrease smoking and alcohol. The client needs to stop both activities because they interact with the medication.

3. Raloxifene (Evista) is a SERM. Evista will not reduce hot flashes or flushes associated with estrogen deficiency and may cause hot flashes.

4. Raloxifene (Evista) is a SERM. The nurse should emphasize the importance of regular weight-bearing exercise to help increase bone density.

24. 1. Calcium gluconate (Kalcinate) is an electrolyte replacement. Safety is a priority for clients diagnosed with osteoporosis; therefore, the client requesting a walker would not warrant the nurse's questioning the medication administration.
2. This indicates the client's kidneys are functioning adequately. Calcium gluconate (Kalcinate) is an electrolyte replacement. The nurse would question administering calcium if the client had findings of renal deficiency.
3. Calcium gluconate (Kalcinate) is an electrolyte replacement. The nurse must monitor for clinical manifestations of hypercalcemia, which include drowsiness, lethargy, weakness, headache, anorexia, nausea or vomiting, increased urination, and thirst.
4. Calcium gluconate (Kalcinate) is an electrolyte replacement. Abnormal bleeding is cause for the nurse to investigate but does not warrant questioning this medication because this is not an expected side effect or adverse effect of this medication.

MEDICATION MEMORY JOGGER: The nurse must know accepted standards of practice for medication administration, including which client assessment data and laboratory data should be monitored before administering medication.

25. 1. Calcitonin salmon (Miacalcin) is a parathyroid calcium regulator used to treat postmenopausal osteoporosis. It works to inhibit osteoclasts and increase renal excretion of calcium.
2. Calcitonin salmon (Miacalcin) is a parathyroid calcium regulator used to treat postmenopausal osteoporosis. Inhibiting bone reabsorption by suppressing osteoclast activity is the scientific rationale for administering calcitonin to clients with postmenopausal osteoporosis.
3. Calcitonin salmon (Miacalcin) is a parathyroid calcium regulator used to treat postmenopausal osteoporosis. Miacalcin is a natural product obtained from salmon and is approved for osteoporosis treatment in women who are more than 5 years postmenopause. Calcitonin decreases bone matrix resorption and serum calcium, thus increasing bone density and reducing risk of vertebral fractures.
4. Calcitonin salmon (Miacalcin) is a parathyroid calcium regulator used to treat postmenopausal osteoporosis. The scientific rationale for administering HRT is to increase progesterone and estrogen levels.

26. 1. There are medications to treat and prevent osteoporosis that are safer than HRT and do not cause severe complications that can occur with HRT. HRT is better than some medications in treating osteoporosis, but HRT is not recommended for this purpose because of possible complications.
2. Expense should not be an issue when treating chronic illnesses.
3. Until recently, HRT with estrogen was one of the most common treatments for osteoporosis in postmenopausal women, but research has shown that serious complications can occur from HRT use; therefore, long-term estrogen therapy is no longer recommended.
4. HRT was one of the most common treatments for osteoporosis, but due to complications associated with its use, long-term therapy is no longer recommended.

27. 1. The normal serum calcium level is 8.2 to 10.2 mg/dL. A low calcium level indicates the medication therapy is not effective.
2. As a result of decreased bone density, a client diagnosed with osteoporosis is at risk for pathologic fractures. If the client does not experience these types of fractures, the medication therapy is effective.
3. The client must have a normal renal function to take these medications, but this does not indicate the medication is effective.
4. Any loss of height indicates the medication is not effective. The loss of height occurs as a result of the collapse of vertebral bodies.

MEDICATION MEMORY JOGGER: The nurse determines medication effectiveness by assessing for symptoms, or lack thereof, for which the medication was prescribed.

28. Correct answers are 1, 2, 4, 5, and 6.
1. A woman who does not take estrogen needs about 1,500 mg of calcium daily to minimize risk of developing osteoporosis. The client understands the teaching.
2. The best dietary sources of vitamin D are milk and other dairy products, including yogurt, which indicates the client understands the teaching.

3. Calcium is not available in injections; therefore, the client does not understand the teaching. Dietary treatment, sunshine, or calcium supplements are recommended to maintain adequate serum calcium levels.
4. Osteoporosis is usually diagnosed in older clients, but prevention starts when the client is young. Steps must be taken to maintain bone density and prevent bone demineralization. The client understands this.
5. The client should not smoke because smoking is linked to osteoporosis and decreased bone density. Alcohol should be limited because of the link between heavy alcohol use and bone loss. The client understands the teaching.
6. Regular weight-bearing and muscle-strengthening exercises improve bone strength, balance, and flexibility. The client understands the teaching.

29. 1. Alendronate (Fosamax) is a bisphosphonate. The client should use sunscreen and protective clothing to prevent a photosensitivity reaction caused by this medication.
2. Alendronate (Fosamax) is a bisphosphonate. The medication must be taken with a full glass of water to ensure proper swallowing of the drug and reduce risk of mouth or throat irritation.
3. Alendronate (Fosamax) is a bisphosphonate. The client should not take the medication with orange juice, mineral water, coffee, or other beverages (besides water) because it will significantly decrease medication absorption.
4. Alendronate (Fosamax) is a bisphosphonate. Taking the medication incorrectly may result in mouth or throat irritation or esophageal irritation. Therefore, if the client experiences pain or difficulty swallowing, retrosternal pain, or heartburn, the client should notify the HCP.

Orthopedic Surgery

30. 1. The nurse will be given time limit parameters for the administration of PRN medications, usually a longer time interval than 45 minutes. Because the client has received no relief of pain, the nurse needs to determine the reason for continued pain.
2. Distraction may be needed if the nurse determines that a complication is not occurring.
3. The client is not receiving pain relief from the morphine. At 45 minutes after IVP the client should have better relief than "severe." One cause of unrelieved pain would be dislocation of the affected joint. The nurse should assess the situation to determine further action.
4. The nurse should assess the client before notifying the HCP.

31. 1. The client should be allowed to rest until the therapist is ready to have the client ambulate. Ambulating is not sitting in a bedside chair.
2. The client will be better able to work with the therapist if not experiencing pain. The nurse should anticipate the need for pain control and administer the medication before the therapist arrives to start the therapy.
3. Brushing the client's hair will not assist the therapist in gaining client cooperation with therapy.
4. The client should be encouraged to work with the therapist when therapy is scheduled. The client may be too tired to perform therapy if waiting until late in the day.

32. 1. The nurse should attempt to use another method of rating pain because the client is cognitively unable to use the numeric scale. Young children can point at a face and tell the nurse how they feel. This scale should be presented to the client for use.
2. Pain is a subjective symptom. The nurse should attempt to get the client to describe the pain.
3. Pain is a subjective symptom. The nurse should attempt to get the client to describe the pain. The nurse is not experiencing the pain.
4. Acute pain does cause an elevated pulse and blood pressure, but many other reasons could cause these same elevations. The nurse should attempt to have the client rate their pain.

33. 1. Antibiotics, but not this phenomenon, might cause a rash on the trunk of the body.
2. Straining to have a bowel movement would not cause external abdomen bruising.
3. The client is not positioned on the abdomen for a knee replacement, and great care is taken in the operating room to prevent any client injury. The nurse should never suggest that the client was not positioned correctly.

4. **Enoxaparin (Lovenox) is a low-molecular-weight heparin anticoagulant administered in the "love handles" or upper anterior lateral abdominal walls. Small "bruises" or hematomas in this area suggest a non-life-threatening side effect of this medication's administration.**

34. Correct answers are 1, 3, and 5.

1. **An autotransfusion drainage system collects the client's blood after a particularly bloody surgery. The surgeon is unable to cauterize or suture bones to prevent bleeding. The collections should be monitored frequently, and the blood should be reinfused when the drainage amount is approximately 200 mL. Any blood remaining in the system longer than 4 hours is discarded.**
2. Drainage is not stored for future use. If not used in the immediate postoperative period, it is discarded.
3. **There could be fat globules, tiny bone fragments, and clots in the drainage. A filter must be attached before infusing the product back into the client.**
4. A second nurse is not required to attach the drainage from the client back to the client.
5. **The client should be monitored every 5 to 15 minutes during initial reinfusion as per all blood protocols.**

35. **78 mL per hour. A total of 310 mL of blood product is to be infused (250 mL + 60 mL) over a 4-hour period: 310 mL ÷ 4 = 77.5 mL or 78 mL/hr. Blood cannot hang any longer than 4 hours to prevent infection and contaminated blood. The client has symptoms of congestive heart failure (bilateral crackles and sacrum edema). The nurse should plan to administer blood over the entire 4-hour period to prevent any further fluid volume overload.**

36. Correct answers are 1, 4, and 5.

1. **Children should be included in their care at the level they can understand and participate. A 10-year-old should be able to describe their pain and rate it on a pain scale. The nurse should determine the child's ability and work from there.**
2. The parents may not want the child to receive pain medication because of a fear of narcotics or want the child medicated when the child is not in pain. Pain is a subjective symptom, and the child should request their medication.
3. A heat pack would not be applied to the cast. An ice pack is sometimes ordered to reduce swelling and pain.
4. **The child's neurovascular status should be monitored every 15 minutes when first returning to the floor and then every 2 hours.**
5. **The client will have a prophylactic antibiotic prescribed because this is a surgical procedure.**

37.

1. NSAID medications should relieve pain resulting from an arthroscopy.
2. Opioid analgesics are frequently used to provide pain relief for all types of surgeries.
3. A sedative hypnotic (sleeping pill) would not be questioned for a client after a total knee replacement.
4. **An 89-year-old male client unable to stand while voiding could develop bladder retention when taking muscarinic antagonists. Muscarinic antagonists relax the bladder muscles by blocking involuntary bladder contractions and are used to treat urge incontinence.**

MEDICATION MEMORY JOGGER: The nurse must be knowledgeable of accepted standards of practice for disease processes and conditions. If the nurse administers a medication the HCP has prescribed, and it harms the client, the nurse could be held accountable. Remember, the nurse is a client advocate.

38.

1. The PCA pump was developed to enable clients to control their pain relief. The nurse should assess the amount of relief the client obtains and any complications, but the client does not need to notify the nurse when needing pain medication.
2. **The client can push the button on the PCA pump whenever the client feels pain. There is a 4-hour lockout programmed into the machine to prevent overdose.**
3. No one but the client should push the button for the client to receive medication. The antidote for pain is narcotic medication. If the client is resting and does not have pain, continuous medication administration could result in an overdose.
4. The client should not be concerned with narcotic addiction. The medication should be discontinued before this becomes a problem.

39. 1. A fracture pan is preferred for clients who have back pain or surgeries because the pan has a smaller rim and will displace the back less. The nurse would not need to intervene.

2. The UAP should be instructed not to get the client out of bed immediately after taking pain medication. The client may be drowsy and could fall.

3. A backrub before bedtime would assist the client in resting. The nurse would not need to intervene.

4. UAPs are allowed to apply barrier protectant creams as part of their duties when changing a client who has soiled themselves. The nurse would not need to intervene.

MUSCULOSKELETAL SYSTEM COMPREHENSIVE EXAMINATION

1. The client is 4 hours postamputation. The nurse notes a large amount of bright red blood on the dressing and notifies the surgeon. The client's laboratory values are populated in the chart below.

Laboratory Test	Client Values	Reference Values
Prothrombin time (PT)	22.5	10 to 13 seconds
International Normalized Ratio (INR)	25	0.9 to 1.1 without anticoagulation therapy 2 to 3 with therapy 2.5 to 3.5 if the client has a mechanical heart valve

Which intervention should the nurse implement based on the prothrombin time (PT) and International Normalized Ratio (INR) results?
1. Prepare to administer warfarin.
2. Prepare to administer phytonadione.
3. Apply direct pressure to the residual limb.
4. Prepare to administer protamine sulfate.

2. The day surgery nurse is caring for a client scheduled for an arthrocentesis. Which information **warrants notifying** the surgeon?
1. The client reports a prednisone allergy.
2. The client is allergic to ibuprofen.
3. The client has a historyof peptic ulcer disease (PUD).
4. The client reports getting a rash with soaps.

3. The client is 2 days postoperative right total hip replacement and is receiving enoxaparin subcutaneously. Which laboratory data should the nurse monitor?
1. PT
2. INR
3. There is no laboratory data to monitor.
4. The activated partial thromboplastin time (aPTT)

4. Which medication would the nurse prepare to administer to a client with a right long leg cast and reporting severe itching under the cast?
1. Hydrocortisone acetate topically
2. Pseudoephedrine
3. Diphenhydramine IV
4. Hydroxyzine PO

5. The client diagnosed with a fractured femur has an external fixation device. The nurse assesses reddened, inflamed skin around the insertion site. Which interventions should the nurse implement? **Select all that apply.**
1. Notify the client's HCP.
2. Cleanse the insertion site with alcohol swabs.
3. Put a sterile, nonadhesive dressing on the site.
4. Readjust clamps on the external fixator frame.
5. Apply topical antibiotic ointment.

6. The female client comes to the clinic with an injured right ankle and has an abnormally large amount of ecchymotic tissue. Which question is **most appropriate** for the nurse to ask the client concerning the ecchymotic tissue?
   1. "Is there any chance you could be pregnant?"
   2. "Are you currently taking aspirin routinely?"
   3. "How long did you apply ice to the ankle?"
   4. "Do you take any antihypertensive medications?"

7. The elderly client diagnosed with a fractured hip in Buck's traction has a stage 1 pressure injury on the lateral ankle over the bony prominence. Which intervention should the nurse implement?
   1. Massage the reddened area gently.
   2. Rub moisture barrier cream into the area.
   3. Apply a hydrocolloid dressing to the area.
   4. Put a silver-impregnated dressing on the area.

8. The client diagnosed with osteomyelitis of the right trochanter is receiving vancomycin intravenously. The HCP has ordered a peak and trough on the third dose. Which interventions should the nurse implement when administering the third dose? **Rank in order of performance.**
   1. Administer the medication via an IV pump.
   2. Check the client's identification band.
   3. Have the laboratory draw the trough level.
   4. Request the laboratory to draw the peak level.
   5. Determine the client's trough level.

9. The client diagnosed with low back pain syndrome is prescribed chlorzoxazone. Which statement by the client **warrants intervention** by the nurse?
   1. "I have had this flu since I started taking the medication."
   2. "I am always drowsy after taking this medication."
   3. "I do not drive my car when I take my back pain medicine."
   4. "If I miss a dose, I wait until the next dose time to take a pill."

10. **Complete the sentence by choosing from the list of options.**

    The male client tells the clinic nurse that he takes glucosamine and chondroitin for joint aches. The nurse knows that the scientific rationale for medication administration is to ______________________________
   1. Help reduce inflammation in the joints to decrease pain.
   2. Help prevent joint deformity and improve mobility for the client.
   3. Increase production of synovial fluid in the joint.
   4. Improve tissue function and retard the cartilage breakdown in the joint.

11. **Complete the sentence by choosing from the list of options.**

    The elderly client diagnosed with osteoporosis is prescribed risedronate. The nurse knows the therapeutic goal of this therapy is to ______________________
   1. Help the client regain lost height.
   2. Strengthen the bone and prevent fractures.
   3. Increase calcium absorption by the body.
   4. Improve joint movement.

12. **Complete the sentence by choosing from the list of options.**

    The HCP wants to evaluate efficacy of pharmacologic therapy for the client diagnosed with osteoporosis? The nurse should anticipate the physician to order the __________
   1. Dual-energy x-ray absorptiometry (DEXA)
   2. Serum calcium level
   3. Arthrography exam
   4. Bone scan

13. The client diagnosed with osteoarthritis asks the nurse, "I saw on the television that a medication called celecoxib was good for osteoarthritis. What do you think about it?" Which statement is the nurse's **best** response?
1. "This medication is very good at reducing osteoarthritis pain and stiffness."
2. "This medication does not have the GI side effects of other NSAIDs."
3. "There are some concerns about that medication. You should talk to your doctor."
4. "You should be cautious about the information that you see on the television."

14. The client prescribed the combination medication hydrocodone and acetaminophen calls the clinic, and tells the nurse, "I have not had a bowel movement in more than 3 days." Which statement is the nurse's **best** response?
1. "This medication causes constipation. You need to increase your fluid intake."
2. "Have you been taking the stool softeners I told you to take along with hydrocodone and acetaminophen?"
3. "You should go to the emergency department so that you can see a doctor."
4. "You should take a laxative, and if you do not have a bowel movement within 24 hours, call me."

15. The nurse is preparing to administer medications to clients on an orthopedic floor. Which medication should the nurse **question** administering?
1. NSAID to the client diagnosed with tendonitis and has a history of duodenal ulcer
2. PRN narcotic to a client post-open reduction and internal fixation of the left tibia
3. COX-2 inhibitor to a client diagnosed with osteoarthritis and has joint stiffness
4. Cephalosporin to a client diagnosed with osteomyelitis and an allergy to sulfa drugs

16. The client has a callus on the bony protuberance of the left fifth metatarsal. The client asks the clinic nurse, "My grandmother told me to dissolve an aspirin to put on my corn. Is that all right to use?" Which statement is the nurse's **best** response?
1. "I would recommend using a pumice stone to rub it off, but not the aspirin."
2. "Yes, but make sure you do not get the dissolved aspirin on the surrounding skin."
3. "There are OTC preparations using salicylic acid that will help remove the corn."
4. "This is an old wives' tale, and you should not pay attention to these remedies."

17. The client 4 hours postoperative bunionectomy (hallux valgus removal) is prescribed hydromorphone. The client is reporting pain of 9 on a scale of 1 to 10. Which interventions should the nurse implement? **Select all that apply.**
1. Request the HCP to prescribe a less potent analgesic.
2. Administer the pain medication as prescribed.
3. Encourage the client to use distraction techniques.
4. Assess the client's foot for hemorrhaging findings.
5. Encourage the client to ambulate in the hall.

18. The client diagnosed with Morton's neuroma in the right foot is being injected with bupivacaine along with hydrocortisone. Which discharge instruction should the nurse discuss with the client? **Select all that apply.**
1. Instruct the client to put inner soles in the shoe.
2. Tell the client to soak the foot in warm water.
3. Teach the client to exercise the foot daily.
4. Explain that a moon face may occur after injection.
5. Apply ice and elevate the foot for 24 hours.

19. The nurse is preparing to administer medications to a client diagnosed with intractable pain. The client is reporting a headache and nausea.

Client: H.A.	MR# 1234567	Date: Today
Age: 55 years	Allergies: NKDA	Diagnosis: Intractable pain
Medication	**0701–1900**	**1901–0700**
Regular insulin subcutaneously ac and hs 0 to 60: 1 amp D_{50} 61 to 150: 0 units 151 to 300: 5 units 301 to 450: 10 units >450: Call HCP	0730 BG 175 1130 1630	2100
Levothyroxine 0.75 mcg oral daily	0900	
Buprenorphine buccal 75 mcg every 12 hours IVP	0900	2100
Acetaminophen 650 mg oral every 4 hours PRN		
Ondansetron 4 mg IVP every 6 hours PRN		
Nurse Initials/Credentials	DN/RN	NN/RN

Which medication would the nurse **question**?
1. Regular insulin subcutaneously
2. Buprenorphine buccal
3. Acetaminophen oral
4. Ondansetron IVP

20. The nurse is discussing meloxicam with a client diagnosed with osteoarthritis pain. Which instructions should the nurse teach the client? **Select all that apply.**
1. “Stools may become clay-colored.”
2. “Do not take meloxicam on an empty stomach.”
3. “Notify the HCP if you become weak or dizzy.”
4. “Avoid drinking alcohol.”
5. “Return to the HCP’s office for monthly serum levels of meloxicam.”

MUSCULOSKELETAL SYSTEM COMPREHENSIVE EXAMINATION ANSWERS AND RATIONALES

1. 1. Warfarin (Coumadin) is an anticoagulant that would cause increased bleeding; therefore, the nurse would not prepare to administer this medication.

2. Phytonadione (Vitamin K) increases clotting; therefore, the surgeon would order this medication to decrease prolonged PT. (A normal PT is 12.9 seconds.)

3. Applying direct pressure will help decrease bleeding but will not correct prolonged PT.

4. Protamine sulfate is the antidote for heparin, an anticoagulant. The postoperative client would not be taking heparin.

2. 1. An arthrocentesis is an aspiration of synovial fluid and an injection of pain medication and antiinflammatory medication, such as a steroid. If the client were allergic to the steroid prednisone, the nurse should notify the surgeon.

2. The client would not be receiving any type of NSAID during this procedure; therefore, this information would not warrant notifying the surgeon.

3. A history of PUD would be pertinent if the client was receiving oral steroids, not intraarticular steroids. Therefore, this information would not warrant notifying the surgeon.

4. This information would not be pertinent to this procedure; therefore, this information would not warrant notifying the surgeon.

MEDICATION MEMORY JOGGER: If the client verbalizes a symptom, the nurse assesses data, or if laboratory data indicates that an adverse effect is secondary to a medication, the nurse must intervene. The nurse must implement an independent intervention or notify the HCP because medications can result in serious or life-threatening complications.

3. 1. Enoxaparin (Lovenox) is a low-molecular-weight heparin, an anticoagulant, administered subcutaneously. The PT is monitored when the client is receiving oral anticoagulant therapy.

2. Enoxaparin (Lovenox) is a low-molecular-weight heparin, an anticoagulant, administered subcutaneously. The INR is monitored when the client is receiving oral anticoagulant therapy.

3. Enoxaparin (Lovenox) is a low-molecular-weight heparin, an anticoagulant, administered subcutaneously. This anticoagulant is administered prophylactically to prevent deep vein thrombosis, but it will not achieve a therapeutic value because of its short half-life; therefore, no bleeding studies are monitored.

4. Enoxaparin (Lovenox) is a low-molecular-weight heparin, an anticoagulant, administered subcutaneously. The aPTT is monitored when the client is receiving continuous IV anticoagulant therapy.

MEDICATION MEMORY JOGGER: The nurse must be knowledgeable about diagnostic tests and surgical procedures.

4. 1. Nothing should be put down the cast; therefore, a topical medication would not be appropriate for this client. Hydrocortisone acetate (Caladryl) is an antiitch medication applied to rashes from poison ivy, chicken pox (herpes varicella), etc.

2. Pseudoephedrine (Sudafed) is an antihistamine. This medication is prescribed for allergies or colds and would not be appropriate for this client.

3. Diphenhydramine (Benadryl) is an antihistamine. The IV route for administering an antihistamine is appropriate to prevent or reduce severity of an anaphylactic reaction. It is not used to treat itching.

4. Hydroxyzine (Vistaril) is an antihistamine. Oral hydroxyzine (Vistaril) effectively reduces itching; therefore, this would be an expected order.

5. Correct answers are 1 and 5.

1. An insertion site infection could lead to osteomyelitis; therefore, the HCP should be notified to take further action.

2. Alcohol swabs may cause burning and have a drying effect on the skin; therefore, they are not used to cleanse the area. Instead, a sterile normal saline swab should be used to cleanse the area.

3. Insertion sites are left open to air because of the external fixator frame. A reddened, inflamed area must be treated, not covered up.

4. The nurse never adjusts the clamps. Only the HCP adjusts the clamps.

5. **A topical antibiotic ointment is used to help prevent infection at the insertion sites.**

6. 1. This would be an appropriate question before x-raying the ankle to determine if there is a fracture, but it has nothing to do with the ecchymotic area.
   2. **Ecchymosis (bruising) is secondary to bleeding in the tissue. An abnormal amount of bruising may indicate a bleeding problem. Taking daily aspirin would increase bleeding.**
   3. Applying ice would not increase bruising to the right ankle.
   4. Antihypertensive medication would not affect the ecchymotic area.

7. 1. A stage 1 pressure injury should not be massaged because it may cause further tissue breakdown and damage.
   2. The moisture barrier cream would prevent protective dressing from adhering, and rubbing the area may cause further tissue breakdown and damage.
   3. **A hydrocolloid (Duoderm) dressing provides a barrier and cushion for the reddened area and prevents further breakdown of the reddened area.**
   4. A silver-impregnated dressing is used for pressure injuries that are infected or heavily contaminated and need debridement. A stage I pressure injury is a reddened area that does not require debridement.

8. **Correct order is 3, 5, 2, 1, 4.**

   Vancomycin is an aminoglycoside antibiotic.
   3. **The nurse should first have the trough level drawn to determine how much medication remains in the blood after the drug has been metabolized and excreted.**
   5. **If the facility is capable, the nurse should obtain the trough results before administering medication. This medication is nephrotoxic and ototoxic. If the trough level is above the therapeutic range, the nurse should hold the medication.**
   2. **Before administering any medication, the nurse must determine if it is the right client.**
   1. **After the trough level is drawn and evaluated, and the identification band is checked, then the nurse can administer medication to the client.**
   4. **After the medication has infused over 1 hour, the peak level is drawn 30 minutes to an hour later, depending on hospital policy.**

9. 1. **Chlorzoxazone (Parafon Forte) is a muscle relaxant. This medication causes agranulocytosis. The flulike symptoms are indicative of this reaction and warrant nurse intervention.**
   2. Chlorzoxazone (Parafon Forte) is a muscle relaxant. Drowsiness is an expected side effect of the medication and would not warrant nurse intervention. The nurse should discuss expected drowsiness with the client.
   3. Chlorzoxazone (Parafon Forte) is a muscle relaxant. The client acknowledging not driving the car is an expected comment because this medication causes drowsiness. The statement would not require intervention.
   4. Chlorzoxazone (Parafon Forte) is a muscle relaxant. Missed doses should be taken within 1 hour of the normal dosing schedule time, or the dose should be omitted until the next normal dosing schedule time. Do not double dose. This comment would not warrant intervention.

10. 1. NSAIDs are used to help decrease joint inflammation.
    2. These medications do not treat rheumatoid arthritis (joint deformities), which this client does not have.
    3. These medications do not affect synovial fluid production.
    4. **These OTC medications are recommended to clients with osteoarthritis to help build up and reduce cartilage destruction in the joints.**

11. 1. Risedronate (Actonel) is a bone resorption inhibitor. The height lost in a client diagnosed with osteoporosis results from vertebrae fractures and is permanent.
    2. **Risedronate (Actonel) is a bone resorption inhibitor. This medication inhibits bone resorption and reduces bone turnover. It normalizes serum alkaline phosphatase and reverses osteoporosis progression.**
    3. Risedronate (Actonel) is a bone resorption inhibitor. This medication works by reducing bone loss, not by increasing calcium reabsorption.
    4. Risedronate (Actonel) is a bone resorption inhibitor. This medication improves bone structure, not joint flexibility.

12. 1. **Dual energy x-ray absorptiometry (DEXA) is a painless test that determines bone density at the waist, hip, or spine to estimate the extent of osteoporosis or monitor the client's response to treatment.**
2. A serum calcium level determines how much calcium there is in the blood, not bone strength.
3. An arthrography is used to visualize the joint cavity and identify acute or chronic tears in a joint capsule.
4. A bone scan is performed to detect metastatic or primary bone tumors, osteomyelitis, and aseptic necrosis.

13. 1. Celecoxib (Celebrex) is a COX-2 inhibitor NSAID. This is a true statement, but the nurse should refer the client to the HCP because of the potential adverse effects of the medication.
2. Celecoxib (Celebrex) is a COX-2 inhibitor NSAID. COX-2 inhibitors do not inhibit the isoform of COX that protects the stomach; therefore, there is a lower incidence of gastroduodenal ulcers, but there are potential life-threatening adverse effects associated with COX-2 inhibitors. Therefore, this is not the nurse's best response.
3. **Celecoxib (Celebrex), a COX-2 inhibitor, is used to treat osteoarthritis, but more data is needed to determine how safe the medication is for specific clients. Research shows an increase in heart attacks and strokes, and the drug is contraindicated for clients with liver and renal disease. The nurse should refer the client to the HCP.**
4. Celecoxib (Celebrex) is a COX-2 inhibitor NSAID. The client should be cautious about what is advertised on television regarding medications and ask the nurse or HCP for further clarification before taking the drug.

14. 1. Hydrocodone and acetaminophen is a combination medication that puts a narcotic and nonnarcotic analgesic in the same pill. The client should increase fluid intake because Vicodin slows peristalsis and creates constipation risk, but the client is already constipated so this is not the nurse's best response.
2. Hydrocodone and acetaminophen is a combination medication that puts a narcotic and a nonnarcotic analgesic in the same pill. The client should be taking stool softeners because Vicodin slows peristalsis and creates constipation risk, but the client is already constipated, so this is not the nurse's best response.
3. The client does not need to go to the emergency department yet. The client needs a stimulant laxative to attempt to evacuate the bowel.
4. **Hydrocodone and acetaminophen (Vicodin) is a combination medication that puts a narcotic and a nonnarcotic analgesic in the same pill. The nurse can recommend an OTC stimulant laxative to help evacuate the bowel because the nurse knows that constipation is a side effect of Vicodin. Giving the client a 24-hour deadline for having a bowel movement is a safeguard.**

15. 1. **An NSAID decreases prostaglandin production, a protective mechanism to prevent ulcers. The nurse should question administering this medication to a client with a history of diagnosed ulcers.**
2. A client with an ORIF of the left tibia would be expected to have pain, and the nurse would not question administering a PRN pain medication.
3. A COX-2 inhibitor is prescribed for a client diagnosed with osteoarthritis and joint stiffness; therefore, the nurse would not question administering this medication.
4. Cephalosporins are second- or third-generation penicillins, but they do not have cross-sensitivity to sulfa drugs. The nurse would not question administering this medication.

16. 1. The client cannot use the pumice stone until the callus or corn is softened; this is not the best answer.
2. Dissolved aspirin may help erode the corn over time, but it will also deteriorate good skin. This is not the best answer because it would be very difficult to keep aspirin on the corn only.
3. **Medicated disks impregnated with salicylic acid are available OTC to help dissolve calluses and corns. The salicylic acid softens the callus, which can then be removed with a pumice stone.**
4. Folk remedies often are based on fact and should not be immediately discounted.

17. **Correct answers are 2, 3, and 4.**
1. This surgery causes extreme pain, and potent narcotics are frequently prescribed for this client.

2. **A hallux valgus is a deformity in which the great toe deviates laterally. The surgery to correct this deformity may cause intense throbbing pain at the operative site that requires liberal amounts of potent analgesics.**
3. **This surgery causes intense throbbing pain, and distraction techniques could be used in conjunction with narcotics, but they could not be used alone.**
4. **The nurse should assess the client for any surgical complications before administering the narcotic analgesic.**
5. The client should not be walking on the surgical incision site. The surgery was done on the foot.

18. Correct answer is 5.

1. Bupivacaine (Marcaine) is a local anesthetic. This is considered conservative treatment designed to balance the metatarsal pads, spread the metatarsal heads, and balance foot posture for Morton's neuroma. This does not address the injection procedure.
2. Bupivacaine (Marcaine) is a local anesthetic. Warm water would not do anything for the injection procedure; therefore, the nurse should not recommend this action.
3. Morton's neuroma results in nerve ischemia, and exercise will not help the pathologic changes or the injection procedure.
4. Bupivacaine (Marcaine) is a local anesthetic. Moon face is a sign of prednisone toxicity and occurs with long-term therapy, not a one-time injection of steroids.
5. **Bupivacaine (Marcaine) is a local anesthetic. Morton's neuroma is a plantar digital neuroma of the third branch of the median plantar nerve on the foot resulting in burning pain. The injection relieves the burning and pain, but it does cause edema and pain at the injection site. Elevating the foot and applying ice will address the acute discomfort associated with the injection.**

19.

1. The client's blood glucose is within the parameters stated to receive an insulin dose. The nurse has no reason to discuss medication administration of the insulin with the HCP.
2. **The nurse should discuss this medication with the HCP. The word *buccal* refers to the mouth. The MAR reads to administer the medication IVP. Buprenorphine (Belbuca), an opioid partial agonist, is prescribed for clients with severe long-term pain and requires round-the-clock therapy. It is a film that is applied inside the mouth and absorbed through the buccal mucosa.**
3. The client could have acetaminophen if there is a need for a mild pain reliever.
4. The client could have the ondansetron for nausea.

20. Correct answers are 2, 3, and 4.

1. Meloxicam (Mobic, Vivlodex) is an NSAID that can cause GI bleeding. Stools could become dark and tarry if the client develops an ulcer while taking this drug. Clay-colored stools indicate a bile blockage.
2. **NSAIDs should be taken with food to decrease the risk of gastric erosion and ulcer formation.**
3. **The client could experience bleeding in other parts of the body. Weakness, dizziness, and chest pain could indicate that there is another area of bleeding.**
4. **Alcohol can increase the risk of GI bleeding.**
5. Meloxicam does have required blood level checks. Dosage is determined by the client's report of response to the medication.

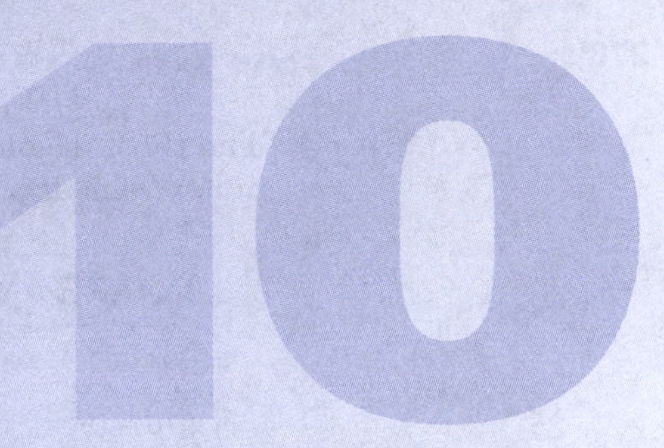

Integumentary System

. . . the foot is more noble than the shoe, and skin more beautiful than the garment . . .

—Michelangelo

QUESTIONS

Burns

1. The client diagnosed with a partial-thickness burn is prescribed mafenide acetate. Which intervention should the nurse implement when applying this medication?
   1. Do not administer if the serum sodium level is decreased.
   2. Assess the client's urine for any increased concentration.
   3. Determine the amount of burned skin using the Rule of Nines.
   4. Premedicate the client before administering the medication.

2. The nurse is discussing the application of silver sulfadiazine cream to a client diagnosed with a partial-thickness burn to the left leg. Which information should the nurse teach the client about how to apply this medication after discharge? **Select all that apply.**
   1. Administer the silver sulfadiazine cream to the burned area twice a day.
   2. A black discoloration can occur on the burned area.
   3. Wear sterile gloves when applying the medication.
   4. Remove the cream at night to allow the wound to dry.
   5. Use roll gauze as a dressing over the cream as needed.

3. The client diagnosed with a full-thickness burn over 40% of the body is admitted to the burn unit 4 hours after the fire. The health-care provider (HCP) writes an order for Ringer's lactate 450 mL/hour. Which interventions should the nurse implement? **Select all that apply.**
   1. Question the HCP's orders.
   2. Administer the IV fluid as prescribed.
   3. Infuse the IV fluid via a pump.
   4. Do not administer more than 200 mL an hour.
   5. Verify the order with another nurse in the burn unit.

4. The client diagnosed with full-thickness burns to the body is receiving fluid resuscitation. Which data indicates the fluid resuscitation is **effective**?

1.

INTAKE AND OUTPUT RECORD				
Day One	**Oral (mL)**	**Intravenous (mL)**	**Urine (mL)**	**Other (Specify) (mL)**
0701–1900	0 mL	3,800 mL	200 mL	Emesis 400 mL
1901–0700	0 mL	1,900 mL	170 mL	
Total	0 mL	5,700 mL	370 mL	400 mL

2.

INTAKE AND OUTPUT RECORD				
Day One	**Oral (mL)**	**Intravenous (mL)**	**Urine (mL)**	**Other (Specify) (mL)**
0701–1900	0 mL	3,800 mL	3 mL	
1901–0700	0 mL	1,900 mL	400 mL	
Total	0 mL	5,700 mL	700 mL	

3.

INTAKE AND OUTPUT RECORD				
Day One	**Oral (mL)**	**Intravenous (mL)**	**Urine (mL)**	**Other (Specify) (mL)**
0701–1900	0 mL	3,800 mL	450 mL	Emesis 400 mL
1901–0700	0 mL	1,900 mL	500 mL	
Total	0 mL	5,700 mL	950 mL	400 mL

4.

INTAKE AND OUTPUT RECORD				
Day One	**Oral (mL)**	**Intravenous (mL)**	**Urine (mL)**	**Other (Specify) (mL)**
0701–1900	0 mL	3,800 mL	2,800 mL	Emesis 400 mL
1901–0700	0 mL	1,900 mL	1,700 mL	
Total	0 mL	5,700 mL	4,500 mL	400 mL

5. The client is admitted to the emergency department (ED) diagnosed with a partial and full-thickness burn to the left hand. Which questions are **most important** for the nurse to ask the client? **Select all that apply.**
1. "When was your last tetanus shot?"
2. "Can you tell me how this burn happened?"
3. "Are you allergic to any medications?"
4. "Have you taken any antibiotics in the last week?"
5. "Are you right- or left-handed?"

6. The client diagnosed with a partial-thickness burn to the entire right leg is being treated with silver sulfadiazine and develops leukopenia. Which medication intervention should the nurse expect the HCP to order?
1. Discontinue the silver sulfadiazine ointment immediately.
2. Continue administering the silver sulfadiazine ointment.
3. Administer aminoglycoside antibiotics intravenously.
4. Administer a hydrocortisone cream to the burned area.

7. Which client should the nurse **use caution** with when applying mafenide acetate to a burned area?
1. A client with laboratory values populated in the chart below

Laboratory Test	Client Values	Reference Values
Blood urea nitrogen (BUN)	15	8 to 21 mg/dL Age ≥90 yr: 10 to 31 mg/dL
Creatinine	0.8	Male: 0.61 to 1.21 mg/dL Female: 0.51 to 1.11 mg/dL
Glomerular filtration rate (GFR)	62	Over 60 mL/min/1.73 m^2
Creatinine clearance (24-hr urine)	100	Male: 85 to 125 mL/min/1.73 m^2 Female: 75 to 115 mL/min/1.73 m^2

2. A client diagnosed with chronic obstructive pulmonary disease
3. A client with vital signs populated in the chart below

Vital Sign Flowsheet	Client Values	Reference Values
Blood Pressure	90/40	100 to 119 mm Hg systolic 60 to 80 mm Hg diastolic
Temperature	98°F	Oral: 98°F (36.7°C)
Pulse	110	60 to 100 bpm
Respirations	24	12 to 20 breaths/min
SpO_2	95%	95% or higher

4. A client diagnosed with type 2 diabetes and taking insulin

8. The client diagnosed with partial- and full-thickness burns to 35% of the body is admitted to the burn department. The HCP has prescribed famotidine. Which statement **best describes** the scientific rationale for administering this medication?
1. Famotidine acts on the cell wall to prevent bacterial growth.
2. Famotidine will help control the client's pain.
3. Famotidine will help decrease the client's nausea and vomiting.
4. Famotidine will help decrease gastric acid production.

9. The HCP prescribed morphine 2 to 5 mg intramuscular (IM) every 2 hours for the client diagnosed with full-thickness burns to the chest and abdominal area. The client reports pain of "10" on a pain scale from 1 to 10. Which intervention should the nurse implement?
1. Administer 5 mg of morphine IM to the client immediately.
2. Contact the HCP to request an increase in the medication.
3. Request a patient-controlled analgesia (PCA) pump for the client.
4. Assess the client for complications and then administer the medication.

10. The client diagnosed with a partial-thickness burn to the back is prescribed silver sulfadiazine. Which information should the nurse discuss with the client concerning this medication?
1. Encourage the client to drink 3,000 mL of water.
2. Discuss the need to eat foods high in protein.
3. Teach the client how to test the urine for ketones.
4. Instruct the client to change the dressing twice a day.

Pressure Ulcers

11. The nurse is using the antimicrobial binding dressing Actisorb Silver 222 for a stage 3 pressure injury on the left hip area. The dressing is a combination of silver and activated charcoal. Which intervention should the nurse implement?
    1. Perform the sterile dressing change twice a day.
    2. Avoid cutting the dressing when applying it to the wound.
    3. Premedicate the client with a narcotic analgesic.
    4. Do not use tape to hold the secondary dressing in place.

12. The client diagnosed with a stage 4 pressure injury on the coccyx area is being treated with an autolytic medication for debridement and an occlusive dressing. The partner of the client asks the nurse, "Why isn't someone doing something about that foul odor my husband has?" Which statement is the nurse's **best** response?
    1. "I will contact your husband's doctor when he makes rounds."
    2. "The odor is secondary to an infection and he is taking antibiotics."
    3. "The odor is an expected reaction to the pressure dressing."
    4. "I am sorry the odor bothers you. We will bathe your husband."

13. The nurse is changing a hydrocolloid antimicrobial barrier dressing with silver for a client diagnosed with a stage 4 pressure injury. Which intervention should the nurse implement **first**?
    1. Rinse the wound with physiologically normal saline.
    2. Remove the old dressing and assess the pressure injury.
    3. Hold the dressing in place for 5 seconds after applying.
    4. Apply sterile gloves when performing the procedure.

14. The nurse is caring for a client diagnosed with a stage 3 pressure injury. The client has a CombiDERM nonadhesive, sterile, hydrocolloidal dressing. Which data indicates the dressing is **ready to be removed**?
    1. The exudate begins to pool on the wound surface.
    2. The drainage color changes from brown to yellow-gray.
    3. The HCP must write an order to remove the dressing.
    4. The softened area is approaching the edge of the dressing.

15. The client diagnosed with a stage 2 pressure injury is prescribed a hydrogel dressing. Which statement indicates the client **understands** the teaching about the hydrogel dressing?
    1. "The hydrogel dressing is soothing and reduces pain."
    2. "It must be used because my pressure injury drains a lot."
    3. "This dressing can only be used if my wound is not infected."
    4. "This dressing is very difficult to apply and remove from the wound."

16. While giving the elderly client a bath, the nurse notices a new, reddened area over the coccyx area, but the skin is intact. Which interventions should the nurse implement? **Select all that apply.**
    1. Notify the wound care nurse to assess the wound.
    2. Apply a bio-occlusive transparent dressing to the area.
    3. Contact the HCP to request a systemic antibiotic.
    4. Turn the client every 2 hours from side to side.
    5. Request a Gel-Overlay mattress for the client's bed.

17. Which client diagnosed with a stage 2 pressure injury should the nurse **question** use of cadexomer iodine gel?
    1. The client diagnosed with an adverse reaction to bovine products
    2. The gel can be used on any client.
    3. The client diagnosed with a pressure injury that is infected
    4. The client with a known sensitivity to iodine

18. The nurse is applying papain-urea topical ointment to a client diagnosed with a stage 3 pressure injury. Which intervention should the nurse implement?
1. Cleanse the wound with a hydrogen peroxide solution.
2. Rub the papain cream directly into the wound.
3. Apply 1/8-inch papain ointment to the pressure injury.
4. Be sure that no medication is applied to viable tissue.

19. The client has been diagnosed with a stage 4 pressure injury with tunneling. Which intervention should the nurse implement when instructed to apply a medicated rope dressing to the wound?
1. Question inserting any medicated dressing into the tunnel.
2. Apply a topical anesthetic to the wound before entering the tunnel.
3. Use a sterile cotton swab and insert the dressing into the tunnel.
4. Insert sterile normal saline into the tunnel after inserting the dressing.

20. The nurse is applying a DermaDress dressing to a client diagnosed with a stage 2 pressure injury on the coccyx. Which interventions should the nurse implement? **Rank in order of performance.**
1. Secure the edges of the dressing with gentle pressure.
2. Remove one side of the backing of the dressing.
3. Clean the wound with DermaKlenz wound cleaner.
4. Place the dressing gently over the wound.
5. Remove the remaining backing to cover the wound.

Skin Disorder

21. The client is prescribed low-dose methotrexate for a psoriasis diagnosis. Which data should the nurse monitor? **Select all that apply.**

Laboratory Test	Client Values	Reference Values
Blood urea nitrogen (BUN)	15	8 to 21 mg/dL Age ≥90 yr: 10 to 31 mg/dL
Creatinine	1.2	Male: 0.61 to 1.21 mg/dL Female: 0.51 to 1.11 mg/dL
Glomerular filtration rate (GFR)	70	Over 60 mL/min/1.73 m^2
Total iron-binding capacity (TIBC)	300	250 to 450 mcg/dL
Platelets	140	140 to 400 × (10^3/microL)
White blood cells (WBC)	10.5	4.5 to 11.1 × (10^3/cells/microL)

1. The glomerular filtration rate (GFR)
2. The blood urea nitrogen (BUN)
3. The creatinine levels
4. The complete blood count (CBC)
5. The iron-binding capacity

22. The client diagnosed with tinea pedis reports intense itching. Which interventions should the nurse discuss with the client? **Select all that apply.**
1. Wash feet with soap and water and dry thoroughly at least twice a day.
2. Soak the feet in vinegar and water twice a day until better.
3. Take the prescribed itraconazole for 1 week a month for 3 months.
4. Wear clean cotton socks and change frequently to keep feet dry.
5. Use over-the-counter (OTC) antifungal powders such as miconazole.

23. The nurse is administering medications. Which intervention or medication should the nurse **question**?
    1. Balneotherapy with medicated tar to a client when the exhaust fan is broken
    2. A colloidal oatmeal bath for a client diagnosed with itching from poison ivy
    3. Sprinkling zinc oxide powder on a client on continuous bedrest
    4. Using zinc oxide topical ointment on a client diagnosed with an excoriated perianal area

24. The nurse is working in a medical unit. Which medication should the nurse administer **first**?
    1. Griseofulvin to a client diagnosed with tinea corporis
    2. Hydroxyzine to a client reporting itching
    3. Acyclovir to a client diagnosed with herpes zoster
    4. Doxycycline to a client diagnosed with acne

25. The HCP ordered lindane lotion to be administered to the client diagnosed with scabies from an extended care facility. Which intervention should the nurse implement?
    1. Apply the ointment by thoroughly massaging it into the scalp.
    2. Bathe the client and then apply the lotion to the client from the neck down.
    3. Scrape the scabies lesions with a sterile needle.
    4. Shampoo the head with lindane and comb with a fine-toothed comb.

26. The nurse is discussing skin care with a teenage client diagnosed with mild acne. Which medication or treatment should the nurse discuss with the client?
    1. Injections of *Clostridium botulinum* into the acne lesions
    2. Applying vitamin E oil directly to the acne pimples to keep them moist
    3. Taking low-dose isotretinoin by mouth daily
    4. Washing the face and neck morning and night with benzoyl peroxide

27. The nurse in a plastic surgeon's office is discharging a client after onabotulinumtoxin A injections. Which discharge instructions should the nurse provide?
    1. The client can expect permanent muscle paralysis.
    2. The client should notify the HCP if edema is noted.
    3. The results will develop slowly over 3 to 10 days.
    4. The only side effect is a localized reaction at the injection site.

28. The client diagnosed with atopic dermatitis (eczema) is prescribed tacrolimus ointment. Which interventions should the nurse implement? **Select all that apply.**
    1. Avoid sunlight getting to the treated areas.
    2. Stop using the medication if redness or itching occurs.
    3. Apply a thin layer to the skin twice a day.
    4. Cover the area with an occlusive dressing.
    5. Take a bath in tepid water before each application.

29. The client calls the clinic to report that she has a painful sunburn. Which information should the nurse discuss with the client? **Select all that apply.**
    1. "Rub the inside of the aloe plant leaves on the sunburn."
    2. "Apply calamine lotion to the most severely burned areas."
    3. "Apply *Echinacea* to the sunburn to take away the pain."
    4. "Use a cool compress of baking soda to help the sunburn heal."
    5. "Add apple cider vinegar to the tub to relieve sunburn pain."
    6. "Soak in an oatmeal bath to help ease pain from the sunburn."
    7. "Warm coconut oil and gently massage on the sunburned area."
    8. "Spread honey on your sunburn to help hydrate the skin."

30. The occupational health nurse is presenting information regarding prevention of skin cancer to a group of workers in an industrial plant. Which information should the nurse include in the program? **Select all that apply.**
    1. Wear sunglasses that wrap around and block UVA and UVB rays.
    2. Many antibiotics lose efficacy if the client is exposed to sunlight.
    3. Use a sunscreen with at least a sun protective factor of 30.
    4. Tanning beds do not have the same damaging rays as the sun.
    5. Check the sunscreen's expiration date before applying it to the skin.

ANSWERS AND RATIONALES

The correct answer number and rationale are in **boldface blue type.** Rationales for why other answer options are incorrect are also given.

Burns

1. 1. The serum sodium level is not affected by mafenide acetate (Sulfamylon), a topical antimicrobial; it is affected when administering silver nitrate, a topical antimicrobial used to treat burns.
2. Urine concentration may be affected by silver sulfadiazine (Silvadene), a topical antimicrobial used to treat burns, but mafenide acetate does not affect urine concentration.
3. This should have been done before the HCP prescribed this medication; therefore, this would not be an appropriate intervention.
4. Mafenide acetate (Sulfamylon) is a topical antimicrobial. The medication causes pain or a burning sensation after its application; therefore, the client should be premedicated.

2. Correct answers are 1, 2, and 5.
1. Silver sulfadiazine (Silvadene) cream is a topical antimicrobial. It is typically applied 1 to 2 times a day.
2. Silver sulfadiazine cream can cause a black or gray discoloration on the skin.
3. Nonsterile gloves are needed to apply the cream, not sterile gloves.
4. The burn should remain covered by the cream at all times.
5. A dressing may be used to cover the wound to prevent the cream from rubbing off.

3. Correct answers are 2 and 3.
1. The nurse should administer this IV fluid as ordered.
2. There are formulas that are used to determine the client's fluid-volume resuscitation. The formulas specify the total amount of fluid that must be infused in 24 hours: 50% in the first 8 hours, followed by the other 50% over the next 16 hours. This is a large amount of fluid, but its administration is not uncommon in clients diagnosed with full-thickness burns over more than 20% of their total body surface.
3. The IV fluids must be infused on a pump to ensure the client receives the correct amount for fluid resuscitation.
4. This is not an unusual amount of fluid to be infused. There is no absolute amount of fluid that a client may require during fluid resuscitation.
5. There is no reason to verify this order with another nurse in the burn unit.

4. 1. A urine output of less than 30 mL/hr would not indicate the fluid resuscitation is effective.
2. A urine output of less than 30 mL/hr would not indicate the fluid resuscitation is effective.
3. The client undergoing fluid resuscitation should have a urine output of 0.5 to 1 mL/kg/hr or approximately 30 to 50 mL/hr for the fluid resuscitation to be effective (Oliver, 2021).
4. An output of greater than 100 mL/hr would indicate the client is losing too much fluid and that the fluid resuscitation is not effective.

5. Correct answers are 1, 2, 3, and 5
1. A tetanus toxoid is administered intramuscularly early in the acute phase of burn care to prevent *Clostridium tetani* infection. If the client has not had a tetanus shot within the last 10 years or if the time is in doubt, a tetanus toxoid booster should be administered.
2. Assessing circumstances surrounding the injury is essential in any burn to identify any related trauma.
3. This is an appropriate question because the client will need medications and burn treatments.
4. This question would not be pertinent to the client's burn and medical care in the ED.
5. This is an appropriate question to determine client needs at discharge. Remember, discharge planning begins upon admission.

6. 1. Silver sulfadiazine (Silvadene) is a sulphonamide antibacterial agent. Leukopenia improves over the treatment course with Silvadene and does not warrant discontinuing the medication.
2. Silver sulfadiazine (Silvadene) is a sulphonamide antibacterial agent. Many clients develop marked leukopenia in response to Silvadene. Leukopenia will improve spontaneously over the

treatment course. Leukopenia does not contraindicate this medication use.

3. Silver sulfadiazine (Silvadene) is a sulphonamide antibacterial agent. Leukopenia secondary to Silvadene therapy does not warrant administration of aminoglycoside antibiotics.
4. Hydrocortisone cream does not treat leukopenia secondary to Silvadene.

7. 1. Mafenide acetate (Sulfamylon) is a topical antimicrobial. Sulfamylon affects the acid-base balance in the body and should not be administered to clients diagnosed with renal disease. A 0.8 mg/dL serum creatinine level is within the normal range for males: 0.61 to 1.21 mg/dL and females: 0.51 to 1.11 mg/dL; therefore, the nurse would not need to use caution with this client.

2. Mafenide acetate (Sulfamylon) is a topical antimicrobial. Sulfamylon impairs the renal mechanism involved in blood buffering, thereby increasing bicarbonate excretion in the urine. When this occurs, the pulmonary system affects a compensatory hyperventilatory status to maintain normal acid-base balance. If this compensation cannot take place as a result of pulmonary disease, the client develops metabolic acidosis.

3. This client has adequate respiratory status; therefore, the nurse would not need to use caution with this client.
4. Mafenide acetate (Sulfamylon) is a topical antimicrobial. There is no reason a client diagnosed with diabetes could not be prescribed mafenide acetate.

8. 1. Silver sulfadiazine (Silvadene), a topical antimicrobial, not famotidine, a histamine$_2$ blocker, acts on the cell membrane and cell wall of susceptible bacteria and binds to cellular DNA.

2. IV opioid medications, not Silvadene, will help decrease the client's pain.
3. Antiemetics, not Silvadene, will help prevent the client's nausea and vomiting.

4. Curling's ulcer (stress ulcer) is an acute ulceration of the stomach or duodenum that forms after a burn injury. Histamine$_2$ antagonists like famotidine (Pepcid) are administered to decrease gastric acid secretion in the acute phase of burn care.

9. 1. The client should receive IV medication, not IM medication.

2. The client should receive IV medication, not IM medication; therefore, the nurse should be a client advocate and notify the HCP for a change in the morphine route.

3. The client should have IV pain medication until hemodynamic stability and unimpaired tissue perfusion return. The PCA pump provides an IV route, and the client can control the amount of medication administered with the PCA, ensuring safe limits of pain medication.

4. The client should receive IV medication, not IM medication; therefore, the nurse should not administer this medication after assessing the client.

10. 1. Silver sulfadiazine (Silvadene) is a sulphonamide antibacterial agent. The client should drink large amounts of fluids to prevent sulfa crystals from forming in the urine.

2. Silver sulfadiazine (Silvadene) is a sulphonamide antibacterial agent. The client should eat foods high in protein for healing purposes, but this does not explicitly concern this medication.
3. Silver sulfadiazine (Silvadene) is a sulphonamide antibacterial agent. Ketones are a byproduct of fat breakdown and would not be specific for teaching about Silvadene.
4. Silver sulfadiazine (Silvadene) is a sulphonamide antibacterial agent. The client should change the dressing twice a day, but this is not part of teaching about the medication Silvadene.

Pressure Ulcers

11. 1. The dressing may be left in place for up to 7 days or may be changed every 24 hours, but it would not be changed twice a day. This does not allow the dressing adequate time to increase wound healing.

2. The nurse should avoid cutting the dressing because particles of activated charcoal may get into the wound and cause discoloration.

3. The dressing change does not warrant administering a narcotic analgesic to the client.
4. Tape should be used to hold the secondary dressing in place or the antimicrobial binding dressing will not remain in the pressure injury.

12. 1. There is no reason to contact the HCP because this is an expected reaction to the pressure dressing.

2. The client may have an infection and is taking antibiotics, but this is not causing the foul odor.

3. This is an expected reaction to the pressure dressing. The foul odor is produced by cellular debris breakdown and does not indicate that the wound is infected.
4. Bathing the husband will not help the odor; therefore, this response is not appropriate.

13. 1. The nurse should rinse the wound with physiologically normal saline, but this is not the first intervention.
2. Removing the old dressing and assessing the pressure injury for healing is the first intervention.
3. This dressing must be held in place for 5 seconds after applying it to the pressure injury.
4. The dressing change is performed with nonsterile gloves using aseptic technique; therefore, this is not an appropriate intervention.

14. 1. This would indicate when an alginate dressing, not a hydrocolloidal dressing, is ready to be removed.
2. The Iodosorb gel, not the CombiDerm dressing, should be changed when the color changes from brown to yellow-gray.
3. The nurse does not need a written order from the HCP to change the dressing.
4. This dressing is an absorbent hydrocolloidal dressing that provides a moist environment, absorbs exudates, and is not damaging to the skin. When the softened area approaches the dressing's edge, it must be removed, and a new one must be applied.

15. 1. Hydrogels help maintain a moist healing environment, granulation, and epithelialization, and they facilitate autolytic debridement. One advantage of a hydrogel dressing is that it is soothing and reduces pain.
2. One disadvantage of hydrogel dressings is that they are not recommended for wounds with heavy exudate.
3. An advantage of using hydrogel dressings is that they can be used when infection is present.
4. An advantage of using hydrogel dressings is that they are easily applied and removed from the wound.

16. Correct answers are 1, 2, 4, and 5.
1. The wound care nurse is usually contacted for a new pressure injury noted in the hospital.
2. Bio-occlusive transparent dressing is a semi-occlusive bacterial and viral barrier that protects skin from exogenous fluid and contaminants. It is used for areas where the skin is intact.
3. A stage 1 pressure injury does not require systemic antibiotic therapy because the skin remains intact.
4. The nurse should turn the client from side to side to remove pressure from the reddened area on the coccyx.
5. A Gel-Overlay mattress uniformly distributes pressure and reduces friction and shear with gel bladders inside a foam core. It is designed to be placed directly on an existing mattress.

17. 1. A Catrix wound dressing, which is a topically applied powder made from bovine tracheal cartilage, not an Iodosorb dressing, would be contraindicated in a client diagnosed with a pressure injury and an adverse reaction to bovine products.
2. The nurse would question Iodosorb use for certain clients because there are some contraindications to its use.
3. Cadexomer iodine gel (Iodosorb), a wound filler, cleanses the wound by absorbing. The nurse would not question use of this gel for the client diagnosed with an infection.
4. Cadexomer iodine gel (Iodosorb) is an iodine-based wound filler. If the client has a known sensitivity to iodine, the nurse should not use this dressing.

MEDICATION MEMORY JOGGER: If the test taker has no idea what the answer to the question is, then the test taker should look at the medication's name. In this question, the medication has "iodo" in the name. This should make the nurse think about iodine and select option 4.

18. 1. Hydrogen peroxide solution should not be used because it may inactivate the papain.
2. Cream should not be rubbed into the wound because it will cause further tissue damage.
3. Papain-urea topical (Accuzyme) ointment is made from the proteolytic enzyme from the fruit of *Carica papaya* and is a debriding product. After cleansing the pressure injury, the nurse should apply 1/8-inch thickness of ointment.
4. Papain-urea topical (Accuzyme) ointment is a potent digestant of nonviable protein matter, but it is harmless to viable tissue.

19. 1. Inserting the medicated dressing is an appropriate intervention; therefore, the nurse should not question this order.

2. Topical anesthetic is not used to dress a stage 4 pressure injury.

3. The nurse must insert the rope dressing into the tunnel to ensure wound healing. Using a sterile cotton swab will allow the dressing to be inserted into the tunnel and will not cause damage to the tissue.

4. The wound should be cleansed with normal saline or some type of sterile solution before dressing the wound, not after dressing the wound.

20. Correct order is 3, 2, 4, 5, 1.

3. The wound needs to be cleaned with some type of solution. Even if the test taker were not familiar with DermaKlenz, they should select this option as the first intervention. DermaKlenz is a mild, rinse-free wound cleanser. DermaKlenz helps loosen and remove debris from wounds for an optimal wound healing environment.

2. DermaDress is a multilayered waterproof sterile dressing, and the nurse must remove one side of the backing before applying it to the wound.

4. After the backing is removed, the nurse should apply the dressing to the wound.

5. The nurse should then remove the remaining back and cover the wound.

1. The nurse should then secure the dressing in place.

Skin Disorder

21. Correct answer is 4.

1. Methotrexate (Rheumatrex) is an antineoplastic agent. The GFR monitors for renal function. Methotrexate is not toxic to the kidneys, so GFR monitoring would not be needed.

2. Methotrexate (Rheumatrex) is an antineoplastic agent. The BUN monitors for renal problems. Methotrexate is not toxic to the kidneys.

3. Methotrexate (Rheumatrex) is an antineoplastic agent. The creatinine monitors for renal problems. Methotrexate is not toxic to the kidneys.

4. Methotrexate (Rheumatrex) is an antineoplastic agent. Methotrexate causes hematopoietic depression. The nurse should monitor for leukopenia, thrombocytopenia, and anemia. The CBC provides information in all these areas.

5. Methotrexate (Rheumatrex) is an antineoplastic agent. Methotrexate does not interfere with iron-binding capacity.

22. Correct answers are 1, 2, 4, and 5.

1. Washing the feet with soap and water and drying thoroughly will keep the area clean so fungus will not grow in this area.

2. Tinea pedis is athlete's foot. The nurse should recommend that the client soak the feet twice a day in a vinegar-and-water solution. If this is not successful in treating the problem, the client should contact the HCP for a prescription of antifungal agent.

3. Itraconazole (Sporanox) is the treatment for tinea unguium, a toenail infection. The HCP would have to prescribe this treatment.

4. Wearing clean cotton socks and changing them frequently prevents the area from being wet, where fungus grows.

5. OTC antifungal powders or creams can help control infection. These generally contain miconazole, clotrimazole, or tolnaftate. Keep using the medicine for 1 to 2 weeks after the infection has cleared to prevent the infection from returning.

23. 1. Balneotherapy involves therapeutic baths with or without medications. Tar baths are recommended for clients diagnosed with severe psoriasis or eczema. Because tars are volatile, the bath area should be well ventilated. The nurse would question this medication at this time.

2. Oatmeal baths (Aveeno) are useful in relieving the itching associated with poison ivy rashes. The nurse would not question this medication.

3. Although the therapeutic duration of relief from powders is brief; powders act as a hygroscopic agent to retain and absorb moisture from the air and reduce friction between skin surfaces and clothing or bedding. The nurse would not question this medication.

4. Zinc oxide (Desitin) ointment is a zinc oxide-based preparation used to treat erythema and excoriated areas of the perineum or around the anus (perianal). The nurse would not question this medication.

24\. 1. Griseofulvin is an antifungal. This client has a diagnosis of fungal infection of the body that is not life-threatening, and the option did not state the client was uncomfortable. The client diagnosed with a comfort problem (itching) should receive the medication first.
2. Hydroxyzine (Atarax) is an antihistamine and is prescribed to relieve itching. Pruritus is an uncomfortable sensation. This client should receive the medication first.
3. Acyclovir (Zovirax) is an antiviral administered several times a day for herpes infections. The viral infection is not life-threatening. The uncomfortable client should receive the medication first.
4. Doxycycline (Vibramycin) is an antibiotic administered orally for acne, but acne is not life-threatening, and the uncomfortable client should receive medication first.

25\. 1. Lindane is an antiparasitic cream. The medication is a cream, not an ointment, and scabies infestations occur on the body, usually between the fingers or toes, wrists, elbows, and waistline. When lindane is used on the scalp, it is used to treat lice, and is shampooed in.
2. Lindane is an antiparasitic cream. All creams, lotions, powders, and the like should be removed before applying a cream to the body, so the client should be bathed before the cream application. The nurse then applies a thin layer of cream over the entire body starting at the neck, avoiding the face and urethral meatus, and including the soles of the feet. The skin is allowed to dry and cool after application. The medication is removed after 8 to 12 hours by a bath or shower.
3. Lindane is an antiparasitic cream. The nurse does not scrape the lesions. Scabies mites burrow under the client's skin, and the medication is applied to the entire body surface area, excluding the face and urethral meatus.
4. Lindane (Kwell) is an antiparasitic cream. This is how to apply Kwell for head lice, not for scabies.

26\. 1. *C. botulinum* is Botox, which is used to decrease appearance of wrinkles, not to treat acne.
2. Clients diagnosed with acne have too much oil production. Applying vitamin E oil would increase the client's problem.
3. Accutane has serious side effects and is used only for those clients diagnosed with severe, disfiguring acne.
4. Benzoyl peroxide is used for mild acne to suppress growth of *Propionibacterium acnes* and promote keratolysis (peeling of the horny layer of the epidermis).

27\. 1. This not a true statement. Paralysis of the facial muscles lasts from 3 to 6 months.
2. Facial edema is expected after the procedure. The nurse should teach the client to apply ice to the site and avoid using alcohol or NSAID products for a week before the procedure.
3. Results of onabotulinumtoxin A (Botox) injections are neither instantaneous nor permanent. Results develop over 3 to 10 days.
4. In addition to mild edema, there can be more side effects to Botox injections. Excessive dosing can cause facial paralysis, and clients can lose the ability to smile, frown, raise the eyebrows, or squint.

28. Correct answers are 1 and 3.
1. Tacrolimus (Protopic) is a topical ointment used for eczema. Tacrolimus increases risk of skin cancer when the client is exposed to ultraviolet (UV) light. The client should be told to avoid direct sunlight or use of tanning beds.
2. Common side effects of Tacrolimus (Protopic) are erythema, pruritus, and a burning sensation at the application site. These reactions lessen as the skin heals. The client should not stop using the medication.
3. This is the regular dosing schedule.
4. The skin should be left uncovered.
5. The client does not have to take a bath before each application. The first application will have absorbed into the skin before the next dose.

29. Correct answers are 1, 2, 3, 4, 5, 6, 7, and 8.
1. The juice from the aloe plant is used topically to treat minor burns, insect bites, and sunburn.
2. Calamine is typically used to decrease itching from poison ivy, oak, or sumac. It can help soothe a sunburn.
3. Echinacea is used topically to treat canker sores or fungal infections, not sunburn.
4. Baking soda paste helps treat insect bites and can soothe a sunburn.
5. Apple cider vinegar is an astringent that can soothe pain and accelerate regeneration of damaged skin from sunburn.

6. **Oatmeal has a soothing effect on the skin and can hydrate areas damaged by the sun.**
7. **Warm coconut oil in a pan and gently massage over the sunburned area to help heal sun-damaged skin.**
8. **Apply a thin layer of honey over the sunburn, leaving it on at least 30 minutes, to hydrate and heal the sunburned skin.**

30. Correct answers are 1, 3, and 5.
    1. **Sunglasses will help prevent eye damage and skin cancer around the eyes.**
    2. Sunlight does not affect efficacy of antibiotics taken internally. Some antibiotics might cause the client to be more susceptible to photosensitivity, but antibiotic effectiveness would not be affected.
    3. **Clients should be told to use a sunscreen of at least SPF 30 when in the sun. The higher the number, the better the blocking of the sun's UV rays.**
    4. Tanning beds use UV rays and may be more damaging than the sun because of the concentrated time clients stay under the tanning bed lamps.
    5. **Sunscreen without an expiration date has a shelf life of no more than 3 years. The shelf life is shorter if the sunscreen is exposed to high temperatures.**

INTEGUMENTARY SYSTEM COMPREHENSIVE EXAMINATION

1. The client diagnosed with stage 4 pressure injury is being treated with an enzymatic debriding agent and occlusive dressing. The nurse notices a foul odor. Which intervention should the nurse implement?
   1. Notify the wound care nurse that there is a foul odor.
   2. Explain to the client that this odor is expected.
   3. Assess the client's oral temperature.
   4. Request an order for an antibiotic from the HCP.

2. The child diagnosed with pediculosis capitis is prescribed lindane. Which information should the nurse discuss with the parents?
   1. "Wash the hair with an antimicrobial shampoo before using lindane."
   2. "Scrub the head and wash the hair for 2 minutes and then remove the lindane."
   3. "Apply the shampoo to dry hair and use a small amount of water to lather."
   4. "Before going to bed, use the lindane shampoo daily for 1 week."

3. Which information should the nurse discuss with the client diagnosed with seborrheic dermatitis of the scalp? **Select all that apply.**
   1. "Use a fine-toothed comb to comb out the hair after shampooing."
   2. "Dry the hair using the high heat setting for at least 5 minutes."
   3. "Apply hydrocortisone 1% to the scalp area twice a day."
   4. "Rotate two or three different types of shampoos daily."
   5. "Use OTC 1% ketoconazole shampoo and gels."

4. The client diagnosed with a verruca vulgaris (wart) on the left ring finger below the knuckle is prescribed salicylic acid colloidal solution. Which information should the nurse discuss with the client? **Select all that apply.**
   1. "Apply the solution to the wart every 12 hours."
   2. "Expect the wart to disappear within 1 week."
   3. "Be careful because the wart may spread easily."
   4. "Do not wear any rings on the left hand."
   5. "Soak the finger in warm water before applying the solution."

5. The nurse is discussing the system to manage Accutane-related teratogenicity (SMART) with a client diagnosed with severe acne. Which statement by the female client would cause the HCP **not** to prescribe isotretinoin?
   1. "The only contraception I use is birth control pills."
   2. "My menstrual cycles have been regular and heavy."
   3. "I hope this works because I am so tired of the acne on my face."
   4. "I will have to come in every month for a pregnancy test."

6. The female client diagnosed with acne is prescribed tetracycline. Which intervention should the nurse include in the medication teaching?
   1. Tell the client to take the medication with milk or milk products.
   2. Explain that this medication may cause discolored teeth.
   3. Tell the client to use sunscreen and protective clothing when outside.
   4. Advise the client to take birth control pills.

7. The child is diagnosed with impetigo on the hands. The HCP prescribes topical mupirocin. Which intervention should the nurse demonstrate to the parents when discussing this medication?
   1. Apply the ointment with sterile gloves.
   2. Scrape the lesions before applying the ointment.
   3. Soak the hands in soapy water.
   4. Cleanse the impetigo with hydrogen peroxide.

8. The client diagnosed with cellulitis of the left arm is seen in the clinic. Which interventions should the nurse expect the HCP to prescribe when discharging the client home? **Select all that apply.**
   1. Apply topical corticosteroid ointment to the affected area.
   2. Take a 7- to 10-day regimen of systemic antibiotics.
   3. Apply moist compresses to the reddened, inflamed skin.
   4. Continue activity as needed with no specific restrictions.
   5. Elevate the left arm on two pillows.

9. Which procedure should the nurse teach the client scheduled for a chemical face peel?
   1. "Do not wear any type of makeup for 1 week before the scheduled procedure."
   2. "Apply a heat lamp to the face for 10 minutes three times a day."
   3. "Take all the prescribed antibiotics for 5 days before the procedure."
   4. "Clean the face and hair with hexachlorophene for 3 days before the procedure."

10. The client has a diagnosis of second- and third-degree burns to 40% of the body. The HCP writes an order for 9,000 mL of fluid to be infused over the next 24 hours. The order reads that one-half of the total amount should be administered in the first 8 hours, with the other one-half being infused over the remaining 16 hours. What rate would the nurse set the IV pump for during the first 8 hours?

    ____

11. The client diagnosed with acute herpes zoster is prescribed oral acyclovir. Which statement by the client indicates the client **needs more** medication teaching?
    1. "I am so glad this medication will cure my shingles."
    2. "I will have to take the pill five times a day."
    3. "I should take this medication for 7 to 10 days."
    4. "If the shingles get near my eyes, I will call my HCP."

12. The client diagnosed with male pattern baldness is prescribed finasteride. When should the nurse evaluate the **medication's effectiveness**?
    1. After the client has been taking the medication for 1 month
    2. When the client states there are no hair strands in the comb
    3. At the time the client's hair changes texture and color
    4. One year after taking the hair growth stimulant medication daily

13. The registered nurse (RN) and the unlicensed assistive personnel (UAP) are caring for a client experiencing pruritus. Which tasks should the nurse delegate to the UAP? **Select all that apply.**
    1. Help the client turn, cough, and deep breathe every 2 hours.
    2. Place mittens on both of the client's hands.
    3. Administer diphenhydramine orally.
    4. Remove all caffeine-containing products from the room.
    5. Apply a moisturizing lotion to the client's skin.

14. The client has been applying a topical hydrocortisone cream to rough, dry skin for more than 2 years. Which data should the nurse assess in the client?
    1. Check for clinical manifestations of adrenal insufficiency.
    2. Assess for a buffalo hump and a moon face.
    3. Assess for thin, fragile skin in the area near the dry, rough skin.
    4. Monitor the client's serum blood glucose level.

15. The parents of a 2-year-old child diagnosed with measles call the pediatric clinic and tell the nurse the child is very uncomfortable, irritable, and fretful. Which recommendation should the nurse discuss with the parents?
    1. Alternate ibuprofen with children's aspirin every 4 hours.
    2. Apply diphenhydramine cream to the rash.
    3. Administer acetaminophen elixir to the child.
    4. Tell the parents that there is no medication for the child.

16. The client reports inability to sleep because of pruritus secondary to skin irritation on the lower extremities. Which information should the nurse discuss with the client? **Select all that apply.**
    1. Take hydroxyzine at bedtime.
    2. Apply antibacterial ointment to the skin irritation.
    3. Soak the lower extremities in warm, soapy water.
    4. Place an occlusive dressing over the irritated skin.
    5. Dress in warm, woolen clothing for bedtime.

17. Which statement describes the **advantage** of taking valacyclovir over acyclovir for the client diagnosed with acute herpes infection?
    1. Valacyclovir does not cost as much as acyclovir.
    2. Valacyclovir only requires taking medication three times a day.
    3. Acyclovir has to be taken for a longer period of time.
    4. Acyclovir must be taken on an empty stomach.

18. The client diagnosed with psoriasis has been prescribed secukinumab to treat the plaque. Which clinical manifestations **would alert** the nurse to a potential adverse reaction to the medication?
    1. The client reports symptoms of sinusitis, and there are round red welts on the skin.
    2. The client reports weakness and dizziness upon rising from a chair.
    3. The client reports constipation requiring frequent stimulant laxatives.
    4. The client reports left calf tenderness, and the calf is 2 inches larger than the right.

19. The nurse is teaching the parents of a child diagnosed with eczema about crisaborole ointment. Which should the nurse teach the parents when administering the medication?
    1. Apply sterile gauze after administration.
    2. Limit the child's intake of green vegetables.
    3. Wash hands before and after applying the ointment.
    4. Monitor the child's stools for a change in bowel pattern.

INTEGUMENTARY SYSTEM COMPREHENSIVE EXAMINATION ANSWERS AND RATIONALES

1. 1. This odor does not indicate that the wound is infected; therefore, the nurse should not notify the wound care nurse usually responsible for treating a stage 4 pressure injury.
   2. **When an enzymatic debriding agent is used under an occlusive dressing, a foul odor is produced by cellular debris breakdown. The nurse should explain to the client that the odor is expected.**
   3. This odor does not indicate that the wound is infected; therefore, the nurse would not need to assess the client's temperature to determine if there is an elevation.
   4. This odor does not indicate that the wound is infected; therefore, the client would not need to be receiving antibiotic therapy.

2. 1. Lindane (Kwell) is an antiparasitic shampoo. The hair does not need to be shampooed with an antimicrobial solution before applying lindane.
   2. Lindane (Kwell) is an antiparasitic shampoo. The head must be scrubbed for 4 minutes before rinsing the shampoo.
   3. **Lindane (Kwell) is an antiparasitic shampoo. This child has head lice and the treatment of choice is shampooing the hair with Kwell. It should be applied to dry hair with a small amount of water so that the medication is not washed off the hair but is rubbed into the hair to kill the lice.**
   4. Lindane (Kwell) is an antiparasitic shampoo. The Kwell shampoo may be repeated in a week to kill newly hatched lice, but it should not be used daily nor does it matter what time of day the shampoo is used. Daily shampooing with Kwell may cause central nervous system toxicity, especially in children.

3. **Correct answers are 4 and 5.**
   1. A fine-toothed comb is used to remove nits for clients diagnosed with head lice; it is not used to treat seborrheic dermatitis (dandruff).
   2. Using the hairdryer on the high heat setting will further dry out the scalp and increase dandruff production.
   3. Corticosteroids help symptoms by reducing inflammation, itching, and discomfort and are generally recommended for short-term use for the skin, not the scalp.
   4. **Two or three different types of shampoos should be used in rotation to prevent seborrhea from becoming resistant to a specific shampoo. This treatment for dandruff is used initially; then, as the condition improves, treatment can be less frequent.**
   5. **Antifungal agents such as ketoconazole work by reducing the amount of *Malassezia* yeast in affected areas of the body.**

4. **Correct answers are 1, 4, and 5.**
   1. **Acid therapy (16% salicylic acid and 16% lactic acid) is a common way to remove warts. It should be applied every 12 to 24 hours for up to 12 weeks.**
   2. The wart should disappear in 2 to 3 weeks.
   3. Warts are only slightly contagious but the acid therapy will not cause the wart to spread.
   4. **The wart can spread by removing and putting on rings so it would be encouraged to avoid wearing rings on the affected hand.**
   5. **Soaking the wart in warm water will soften the thickened skin of the wart and help with solution absorption.**

5. 1. **Isotretinoin (Accutane), an acne treatment, has been associated with birth defects. If the client is placed on Accutane the client must participate in the iPledge program, pledging to take precautions against becoming pregnant while taking the medication. The client must use two forms of birth control when taking Accutane because Accutane is extremely damaging to the fetus. The SMART protocol has been instituted to ensure that no female clients are or become pregnant while taking this medication.**
   2. Accutane is extremely damaging to the fetus, and because the client is having regular and heavy menses, the HCP could prescribe this medication knowing that the client is not pregnant.
   3. Accutane is prescribed for acne; therefore, this statement would not cause the HCP not to prescribe Accutane.
   4. One requirement of the SMART protocol is a pregnancy test monthly because Accutane is extremely damaging to the fetus.

6. 1. Tetracycline, an antibiotic, should not be taken with milk or milk products because those products prevent medication absorption in the stomach.
2. Tetracycline may cause discoloration or a yellow-brown color of the teeth in children younger than 8 years old or in the fetus of a pregnant client. This client is not pregnant and is an adult; therefore, this intervention is not appropriate.
3. Photosensitivity (sun reaction) may occur in persons taking tetracycline; therefore, the client should be taught to use safety precautions when in the sunlight.
4. The female client should use a nonhormonal method of contraception because birth control pills interact with the tetracycline and the client will be unprotected from pregnancy.

7. 1. The parents should wash their hands before administering the medication and can use nonsterile gloves or a tongue depressor when applying medication. They do not need to use sterile gloves, but they should not touch the affected area.
2. Scraping the lesions would hurt the child and cause bleeding, which results in a scab, which, in turn, must be removed before applying ointment. Do not scrape the lesions.
3. The soapy water will help to remove the central site of bacterial growth, giving the topical antibiotic the opportunity to reach the infected site.
4. Hydrogen peroxide is not used to cleanse impetigo. A 1:20 Burow's solution may be used to put compresses on the impetigo.

8. Correct answers are 2, 3, and 5.
1. Cellulitis is not a topical infection and is not treated with topical ointments.
2. Systemic antibiotic therapy is the treatment of choice for cellulitis, an inflammation of skin and subcutaneous tissue.
3. Apply warm or cool moist compresses to the area to help decrease pain and redness.
4. The HCP would prescribe rest with extremity immobilization.
5. Elevating the arm will help decrease edema.

9. 1. There is no reason the client cannot wear makeup before the procedure, especially for 1 week. Makeup is not allowed for a few weeks after the procedure.
2. Heat lamp use is not prescribed before having a chemical face peel.
3. A chemical face peel does not necessitate antibiotic therapy before the procedure, but the client may be prescribed antibiotics after the procedure.
4. Cleaning the face and hair with hexachlorophene will decrease risk of infection during and after the procedure.

10. **563/hr. Because one-half of the total dose of 9,000 mL should be administered in the first 8 hours, the nurse should determine how many milliliters should be given in the first 8 hours: 9,000 mL ÷ 2 = 4,500 mL. Then, the 4,500 must be divided by 8 to determine the rate per hour: 4,500 ÷ 8 = 562.5, or rounded up to 563. There are formulas that are used to determine the client's fluid-volume resuscitation. The formulas specify the total amount of fluid that must be infused in 24 hours, 50% in the first 8 hours followed by the other 50% over the next 16 hours. This is a large amount of fluid, but it is not uncommon in clients diagnosed with full-thickness burns covering more than 20% of the total body surface area.**

11. 1. Acyclovir (Zovirax) is an antiviral medication. The client must understand that no medication will cure a herpes viral infection. Zovirax shortens the symptom time and speeds healing, but it does not cure the shingles. The client needs more medication teaching.
2. Acyclovir (Zovirax) is an antiviral medication. This medication is prescribed for five times a day dosing because of the short half-life of the medication.
3. Acyclovir (Zovirax) is an antiviral medication. The medication is prescribed for 7 to 10 days when the client has an acute exacerbation of a herpes virus.
4. Acyclovir (Zovirax) is an antiviral medication. If the herpes zoster occurs near or in the eyes it could cause blindness and is considered an ophthalmic emergency.

12. 1. Finasteride (Propecia) is a hair growth stimulant. The medication must be taken for at least 1 year before determining adequate response to the medication.
2. Finasteride (Propecia) is a hair growth stimulant. Not finding any hair in the comb does not indicate the medication is stimulating hair growth.
3. Finasteride (Propecia) is a hair growth stimulant. Hair texture and color have nothing to do with determining medication effectiveness.

4. Finasteride (Propecia) is a hair growth stimulant. Approximately 50% of clients regrow hair, and it may require up to 1 year of daily treatment to determine if the medication is effective.

13. Correct answers are 2 and 5.

1. Turning, coughing, and encouraging the client to turn, cough, and deep breathe is a task that can be delegated, but will not address pruritis.
2. **The UAP can place mittens on the client's hands to discourage the client from scratching.**
3. The nurse cannot delegate medication administration.
4. Caffeine will keep the client awake and should be discouraged, but will not address pruritis.
5. **The UAP can put moisturizing lotion on the client. This is not considered a medication.**

14. 1. The client would not experience clinical manifestations of systemic withdrawal because of a steroid being applied topically.

2. The client would not experience clinical manifestations of prednisone toxicity because topical steroids are used.
3. **After prolonged use of topical steroids, the dermis and epidermis will atrophy, resulting in thinning of the skin, striae, and purpura; therefore, the nurse should assess for this data.**
4. The client would not have elevated blood glucose levels because the medication is a topical cream.

15. 1. Ibuprofen is an NSAID. Aspirin is also an NSAID, but a child should not take aspirin because it may cause Reye's syndrome.

2. Diphenhydramine (Benadryl), an antihistamine ointment, should not be applied to the rash area.
3. **Acetaminophen (Tylenol) elixir is the drug of choice for children to decrease irritability and any discomfort.**
4. There is no treatment for the measles. It must run its course. A mild nonnarcotic analgesic such as Tylenol can decrease irritability and discomfort.

16. Correct answer is 1.

1. **Hydroxyzine (Atarax) is an antihistamine medication that decreases itching and is also prescribed as a sedative at bedtime because it is effective in producing a restful and comfortable sleep.**
2. Antibacterial ointment will not help the client sleep; therefore, it is not information the nurse should discuss with the client.
3. Warm, soapy water will not help decrease itching and may increase skin irritation.
4. An occlusive dressing will not help decrease the client's itching issue.
5. Wool and other rough fabrics can overheat the child and increase skin irritation.

17. 1. Valacyclovir (Valtrex) is an antiviral. Valtrex costs more than acyclovir; therefore, the cost is not an advantage.

2. **Acyclovir (Zovirax) requires the client to take medication five times a day and Valtrex is taken only three times a day. Fewer dosing times increase compliance with the medication and are an advantage of Valtrex. Valacyclovir (Valtrex) is an antiviral, as is acyclovir (Zovirax).**
3. Both antiviral medications are taken for the same period of time; therefore, there is not an advantage to taking Valtrex.
4. Both medications can be taken with or without food; therefore, this is not an advantage to taking Valtrex.

18. 1. Secukinumab (Cosentyx) is an interleukin-17 antagonist that reduces inflammation by targeting cells involved in the inflammatory process. Adverse effects include sinusitis, upper respiratory infections, oral candida infections, oral herpes infection, exacerbations of inflammatory bowel diseases (IBDs) (Crohn's disease, ulcerative colitis), nasopharyngitis, and urticaria. It is administered subcutaneously once a week for 4 weeks and then once a month. Clients are taught to self-administer the medication.

2. Weakness and dizziness are not associated with Cosentyx.
3. The drug can cause diarrhea associated with exacerbations of IBD.
4. Blood clots are not associated with this medication.

19. 1. Crisaborole (Eucrisa) is a phosphodiesterase 4 inhibitor approved for use in psoriasis in children and adults. The ointment should be applied and rubbed into a plaque, but not covered with a sterile dressing.

2. There are no food restrictions.
3. **The parent should apply the ointment after washing hands. Using unsterile gloves, apply the ointment, rub it in, then remove the gloves and wash hands.**
4. Eucrisa does not affect bowel patterns.

Immune Inflammatory System

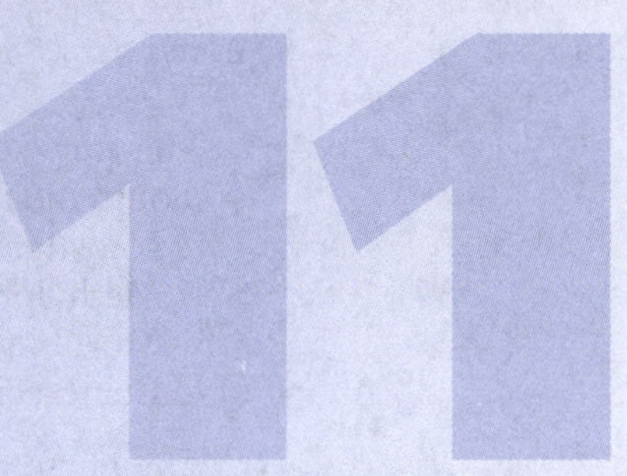

Whatever you do, always give 100%. Unless you're donating blood.

—Bill Murray

QUESTIONS

Autoimmune Disease

1. The nurse is administering medications to the clients on a medical unit. Which medication should the nurse **question** administering?
   1. Atropine to a client diagnosed with myasthenia gravis (MG)
   2. Chloroquine to a client diagnosed with a butterfly rash
   3. Prednisone to a client diagnosed with polymyalgia rheumatica
   4. Pyridostigmine to a client in a cholinergic crisis

2. The female client diagnosed with systemic lupus erythematosus (SLE) reports to the nurse that she has pain, has stiffness when getting up in the morning, and takes ibuprofen to help ease the pain and stiffness. Which question is **most important** for the nurse to ask the client?
   1. "How often do you have to take ibuprofen?"
   2. "Do you take the medication on an empty stomach?"
   3. "Does the medication help with menstrual cramping too?"
   4. "Have you noticed an improvement in the pain and stiffness?"

3. The client diagnosed with multiple sclerosis (MS) is prescribed IV hydrocortisone. The client has a saline lock. Which procedures should the nurse follow when administering the medication? **Rank in order of performance.**
   1. Administer the diluted medication intravenously over 1 to 2 minutes.
   2. Aspirate the syringe to obtain a blood return.
   3. Flush the saline lock with 2 mL of sterile normal saline.
   4. Flush the saline lock again with 2 mL of normal saline.
   5. Check the client's identification bands against the MAR.

4. The client diagnosed with MS is prescribed baclofen. Which data should the nurse assess? **Select all that apply.**
   1. The client's serum baclofen levels
   2. The client's report of urinary urgency
   3. The client's muscle rigidity
   4. The client's range of motion
   5. The client's blood urea nitrogen
   6. The client's creatinine levels
   7. The client's muscle spasticity
   8. The client's pain level

5. The nurse is administering 0800 medications on a medical floor. Which medication should the nurse administer **first**?
1. Neostigmine bromide to a client diagnosed with myasthenia gravis (MG)
2. Methylprednisolone to a client diagnosed with lupus erythematosus
3. Morphine to a client diagnosed with Guillain-Barré (GB) syndrome
4. Etanercept to a client diagnosed with rheumatoid arthritis (RA)

6. The nurse administered edrophonium to a client diagnosed with rule-out MG. Which response by the client indicates the client has MG?
1. The client loses the ability to breathe without mechanical support.
2. The client's strength improves briefly without findings of fasciculations.
3. The client cannot gaze at the ceiling for 2 minutes without fatigue.
4. The client's paroxysmal atrial tachycardia converts to normal sinus rhythm.

7. The client diagnosed with an acute gout attack is prescribed allopurinol. The client's laboratory values are populated in the chart below.

Laboratory Test	Client Values	Reference Values
Serum creatinine	0.9 mg/dL	Male: 0.61 to 1.21 mg/dL Female: 0.51 to 1.11 mg/dL
Serum uric acid	4.2 mg/dL	Men: 4 to 8 mg/dL Women: 2.7 to 7 mg/dL
White blood cells (WBC)	9 (10^3/cells/microL)	4.5 to 11.1 (10^3/cells/microL)
Total iron-binding capacity	325 mcg/dL	250 to 450 mcg/dL
Glucose	98 mg/dL	Fasting <100 mg/dL Random <200 mg/dL

Which laboratory data indicates the medication is **effective**? **Select all that apply.**
1. Serum creatinine
2. Serum uric acid
3. White blood cells (WBC)
4. Total iron-binding capacity (TIBC)
5. Glucose

8. The client diagnosed with MG reports that the anticholinesterase medication makes them nauseous. Which information should the nurse teach the client?
1. Decrease the dose of the medication.
2. Hold the medication and notify the health-care provider (HCP).
3. Take the medication with milk or crackers.
4. Take an over-the-counter (OTC) proton-pump inhibitor.

9. The client diagnosed with paranoid schizophrenia has been taking chlorpromazine. The client tells the psychiatric clinic nurse that they have frequent joint pain and stiffness and get a rash when in the sun. Which statement is the nurse's **best** response?
1. "This is part of your illness and will go away if you ignore it."
2. "What have your voices said about the aches, pains, and rash?"
3. "Don't take your medication today and come in to see the HCP."
4. "This is a reaction to medications and you can no longer take medications."

HIV and AIDS

10. The clinic nurse is discussing medication compliance with a client diagnosed with AIDS. Which information should the nurse discuss with the client? **Select all that apply.**
1. Availability of insurance to pay for medications
2. Whether the client wants to try to manage the disease without medications
3. Including OTC herbs in the medication regimen
4. Importance of taking multiple vitamins at least twice a day
5. Ability to change the medication regimen if side effects are not tolerable

11. The nurse received a needle stick with a contaminated needle from a client diagnosed with AIDS. Which medications should the nurse begin within hours of the needle stick?
1. A combination of antiviral and antifungal medications with an antibiotic
2. A combination of an integrase inhibitor and nucleoside reverse transcriptase inhibitors
3. Single-agent therapy with a nonnucleoside transcriptase inhibitor
4. No medications are recommended to prevent conversion to HIV-positive

12. The pregnant client's HIV test is positive. Which medication should the client be given during labor to **prevent** transmission of the virus to the fetus?
1. Efavirenz
2. Lopinavir
3. Zidovudine
4. Ganciclovir

13. The nurse is caring for clients diagnosed with AIDS. Which actions by the unlicensed assistive personnel (UAP) **warrant immediate** action by the registered nurse (RN)? **Select all that apply.**
1. The UAP uses nonsterile gloves to empty the client's urinal.
2. The UAP takes a glass of grapefruit juice to the client.
3. The UAP dons gloves to remove the client's meal tray.
4. The UAP provides a tube of moisture barrier cream to the client.
5. The UAP fills the client's water pitcher with ice and water.

14. The home health-care nurse is caring for a client diagnosed with HIV infection. The client's laboratory values are populated in the chart below.

Laboratory Test	Client Values	Reference Values
HIV viral load	positive	negative
White blood cell count (WBC)	5 (10^3/microL)	4.5 to 11.1 × 10^3/microL
Erythrocyte sedimentation rate (ESR)	13 mm/hr	Adult less than 50 years: 0 to 15 mm/hr Adult 50 years and older: 0 to 20 mm/hr
CD4 count	299 cells/microL	332 to 1,642 cells/microL

Which laboratory data suggests the **need** for prophylaxis with trimethoprim sulfa?
1. HIV viral load
2. WBC count
3. Erythrocyte sedimentation rate
4. CD4 count

15. The client diagnosed with AIDS is to receive an initial dose of amphotericin B. Which intervention should the nurse implement **first**?
   1. Administer IV piggyback (IVPB) in 500 mL of D_5W over 6 hours.
   2. Administer meperidine 25 mg IV push (IVP) over 5 minutes.
   3. Administer a test dose of 1 mg over 20 minutes.
   4. Administer acetaminophen 650 mg orally.

16. The client diagnosed with AIDS and cytomegalovirus retinitis is prescribed ganciclovir. The client has a single lumen implanted port. Which information about the medication should the home health-care nurse discuss with the client? **Select all that apply.**
   1. The client will have to take the medication for the rest of their life.
   2. The client will take the medication for 1 week each month.
   3. The medication should infuse over 1 hour via infusion pump.
   4. The medication can run simultaneously with the client's total parenteral nutrition (TPN).
   5. The medication is administered twice daily for the first few weeks of treatment.

17. The client diagnosed with HIV has a positive skin test for tuberculosis (TB). Which medication order should the nurse anticipate? **Select all that apply.**
   1. Isoniazid
   2. Ethambutol
   3. Pyrazinamide
   4. Enfuvirtide
   5. Rifampin

18. The intensive care nurse is preparing to administer trimetrexate to a client diagnosed with AIDS and *Pneumocystis jiroveci* pneumonia (PJP). Which interventions should the nurse implement? **Select all that apply.**
   1. Administer IV via gravity infusion.
   2. Administer concurrently with leucovorin.
   3. Monitor the client's complete blood count (CBC).
   4. Monitor the client's liver enzymes.
   5. Maintain nothing by mouth during drug administration.

Allergies

19. The client diagnosed with allergies is prescribed diphenhydramine. Which statement indicates the client **understands** the teaching concerning this medication?
   1. "If I get any ringing in my ears, I should notify my HCP."
   2. "I will probably get drowsy when I take this medication."
   3. "It is not uncommon to get a buffalo hump or moon face."
   4. "I will have to taper off the medications when I quit taking them."

20. The client has a severe anaphylactic reaction to insect bites. Which **priority** discharge intervention should the nurse discuss with the client?
   1. "Wear an insect repellent on exposed skin."
   2. "Keep prescribed antihistamines with you."
   3. "Have an epinephrine auto-injector available at all times."
   4. "Wear a medication alert identification bracelet."

21. The client diagnosed with seasonal allergic rhinitis is prescribed fluticasone. Which interventions should the nurse implement? **Select all that apply.**
   1. Instruct the client not to eat licorice.
   2. Explain that this is for short-term use.
   3. Instruct the client not to use this with other nasal decongestants.
   4. Have the client notify the HCP if nasal bleeding occurs.
   5. Tell the client to stop the spray if nasal stinging occurs upon first use.

22. Which client should the nurse **question** administering fexofenadine? **Select all that apply.**
1. The client smoking two packs of cigarettes daily
2. The client running 2 miles every day
3. The client diagnosed with an antibiotic allergy
4. The client experiencing nasal congestion and sneezing
5. The client diagnosed with asthma

23. The client is prescribed clemastine prophylactically for allergies. Which statement indicates the client **needs more** teaching concerning this medication?
1. "I will suck on hard candy if I have a dry mouth."
2. "I will notify my HCP if I take an OTC medication."
3. "I will experience some blurred vision when taking clemastine."
4. "I need to maintain adequate fluid intake when taking this medication."

24. The clinic nurse is discussing OTC oxymetazoline nasal spray with a client experiencing nasal congestion. Which information should the nurse discuss with the client? **Select all that apply.**
1. "Do not use the oxymetazoline nasal spray for more than 3 to 5 days."
2. "Spray the medication into the open nostril while inhaling deeply."
3. "Clear the nose immediately after using the nasal spray."
4. "Immediately swallow the postnasal medication residue."
5. "Take additional nasal sprays if congestion is not relieved."

25. The client taking a nasal glucocorticoid spray calls the clinic nurse and reports that the medication is not helping their condition. Which question should the nurse ask the client **first**?
1. "Are you sure you are taking the spray correctly?"
2. "Did you shake the bottle before taking the spray?"
3. "What time of the day are you taking the medication?"
4. "How long have you been using the spray?"

26. Which interventions should the nurse implement for the elderly client receiving antihistamine therapy? **Select all that apply.**
1. Auscultate the client's breath sounds.
2. Assess the client's level of consciousness.
3. Evaluate the client's intake and output.
4. Encourage the client to ambulate.
5. Provide an acid-ash diet for the client.

27. The nurse is administering a dose of an IV antibiotic to the client. Twenty minutes into the infusion the client reports shortness of breath, itching, and difficulty swallowing. Which intervention should the nurse implement **first**?
1. Prepare to administer subcutaneous epinephrine.
2. Discontinue the client's IV antibiotic.
3. Assess the client's apical pulse and blood pressure.
4. Administer 10 L of oxygen via nasal cannula.

Rheumatoid Arthritis

28. The client diagnosed with rheumatoid arthritis (RA) is prescribed hydroxychloroquine sulfate. Which statements indicate the client **needs more** teaching concerning the medication? **Select all that apply.**
1. "I will get my eyes checked every 6 months."
2. "I should not drink alcohol while taking this drug."
3. "It is important to take this medication with milk."
4. "I will call my HCP if the pain is not relieved in 2 weeks."
5. "Loss of balance is common while taking hydroxychloroquine sulfate."

29. The client diagnosed with RA is taking leflunomide. Which comment by the client **warrants** intervention by the nurse?
   1. "I have noticed that I am starting to lose my hair."
   2. "I sometimes get dizzy and drowsy."
   3. "My spouse and I are trying to start a family."
   4. "I will not get any vaccines while taking this medication."

30. Which instruction should the nurse discuss with the client diagnosed with RA and prescribed methotrexate? **Select all that apply.**
   1. "Use a soft-bristled toothbrush when brushing teeth."
   2. "Wear warm clothes when it is less than 40°F."
   3. "Gargle with mouthwash at least four times a day."
   4. "Use sunscreen with an SPF 15 or lower when outside."
   5. "Take NSAIDs only as ordered by the HCP while taking this medication."

31. The client diagnosed with RA is taking phenylbutazone. Which statement requires the nurse to **question** administering this medication?
   1. "I have had a sore throat and fever the last few days."
   2. "I have not had a bowel movement in more than 3 days."
   3. "I can't believe I have gained 3 pounds in the last month."
   4. "I have been having trouble sleeping at night."

32. The client diagnosed with RA has been taking methotrexate for 2 weeks. The client's laboratory values are populated in the chart below.

Laboratory Test	Client Values	Reference Values
Serum creatinine	0.9 mg/dL	Male: 0.61 to 1.21 mg/dL Female: 0.51 to 1.11 mg/dL
Red blood cells (RBC)	2.5 (10^6 cells/microL)	Men: 4.21 to 5.81 (10^6 cells/microL) Women: 3.61 to 5.11 (10^6 cells/microL)
White blood cells (WBC)	9 (10^3/cells/microL)	4.5 to 11.1 (10^3/cells/microL)
Hemoglobin (Hgb)	14.5 g/dL	Men: 14 to 17.3 g/dL Women: 11.7 to 15.5 g/dL
Hematocrit (Hct)	43%	Men: 42% to 52% Women: 36% to 48%

Which laboratory data **warrants** intervention by the nurse?
   1. Serum creatinine
   2. Red blood cell (RBC)
   3. White blood cell (WBC)
   4. Hemoglobin (Hgb)
   5. Hematocrit (Hct)

33. Which assessment data should the nurse expect for the client diagnosed with RA and taking sulfasalazine?
   1. Orange or yellowish discoloration of the urine
   2. Ulcers and irritation of the mouth
   3. Ecchymosis of the lower extremities
   4. A red, raised skin rash over the back

34. The client recently diagnosed with RA is prescribed 4 grams of aspirin daily. Which statement indicates the client **needs more** teaching concerning the medication?
1. "I will decrease my dose for a few days if my ears start ringing."
2. "I should take my aspirin with meals, food, milk, or antacids."
3. "I need to take the entire aspirin dose at night before going to bed."
4. "If I have any stomach upset, I will take enteric-coated aspirin."

35. The client diagnosed with RA is prescribed prednisone for an acute episode of pain. The client asks the nurse, "Because it helps the pain so much, why can't I be on this forever?" Which statement is the nurse's **best** response?
1. "The medication will cause you to have a buffalo hump or moon face."
2. "The medication has long-term side effects, such as osteoporosis."
3. "If you continue taking the medication, it may cause an Addisonian crisis."
4. "There are other medications that can be prescribed to help the pain."

36. The client diagnosed with RA is prescribed capsaicin. Which information should the nurse discuss with the client? **Select all that apply.**
1. Apply the cream as needed for severe arthritic pain.
2. Notify the HCP if skin burning occurs after application.
3. It may take up to 3 months for the medication to become effective.
4. Rub the cream into the skin until no cream remains on the surface.
5. Wash hands with vinegar or soap after application of the cream.

37. The client diagnosed with RA is taking etodolac. The client is reporting a headache. Which intervention should the nurse implement?
1. Administer two aspirins.
2. Administer an additional dose of etodolac.
3. Administer one oral narcotic analgesic.
4. Administer two acetaminophen tablets.

Immunizations

38. The nurse in the pediatrician's office is recording a child's immunizations. Which information is the nurse **required** to document? **Select all that apply.**
1. The vaccinations the client should have received
2. Adverse events reported by the client, even if unrelated to the vaccine
3. Vaccine information statement (VIS) edition and date given to the client
4. The vaccination type, manufacturer, and lot number
5. The date the next required vaccination should be administered
6. The name and title of the person administering the vaccine
7. The address of the location where the vaccine was given

39. The mother of a child scheduled to receive the measles, mumps, and rubella vaccination asks the nurse, "What could happen to my child if I don't let you give the vaccination?" Which statement is the nurse's **best** response?
1. "If your child gets one of the diseases, it could lead to serious complications."
2. "Your child will not be allowed to attend any public school in the country."
3. "Nothing can happen to you or the child if your child doesn't get the vaccination."
4. "You sound worried. Have you heard of problems associated with the shot?"

40. A 4-year old child received an immunization for varicella earlier in the day. The parent calls the clinic and tells the nurse that the child now has chickenpox because the child has a fever of 101°F (38.3°C). The client's vital signs are populated in the following vital sign flowsheet.

Vital Sign Flowsheet	Client Values	Reference Values
Temperature	101°F/38.3°C	Oral: 98°F (36.7°C)
Pulse	120 bpm	80 to 150 bpm
Respirations	24 breaths/min	20 to 40 breaths/min
Blood pressure	98/64 mm Hg	89 to 112 mm Hg systolic 46 to 72 mm Hg diastolic

Which statement is the nurse's **best** response?
1. "You signed a permit knowing this might happen as a result."
2. "You need to take the child to the emergency department now."
3. "Has the child been exposed to any illness recently?"
4. "This is a reaction to the injection, but it is not chickenpox."

41. Which clients should the nurse **question** administering a live virus vaccine? **Select all that apply.**
1. The child with fear of needles and health-care personnel
2. The child living with a grandparent undergoing chemotherapy
3. The child who has not received an immunization previously
4. The child with Jehovah's Witnesses as parents
5. The immunosuppressed child on prednisone
6. The child diagnosed with otitis media
7. The child with a low-grade fever

42. The nurse is preparing to administer measles, mumps, and rubella vaccinations to a 15-month-old child. Which is the correct administration procedure?
1. Inject the medication into the dorsogluteal muscle.
2. Use the deltoid muscle for the injection.
3. Administer the medication into the vastus lateralis muscle.
4. Give subcutaneously in the abdomen.

43. The 14-year-old adolescent has not received the varicella vaccine, and the HCP cannot determine that the teen has ever had chickenpox. Which statement indicates the correct administration procedure?
1. Administer the single-dose injection as soon as possible.
2. Administer two injections at least 4 weeks apart.
3. Administer a series of three injections over 6 months.
4. Do not administer the vaccine because by age 13 the client is immune to varicella.

44. The parent of a child about to receive the intramuscular inactivated poliovirus vaccine (IPV) asks the nurse, "Why can't my child get the oral vaccine like I took when I was a child?" Which statement by the nurse is the **best** explanation to give the client?
1. "I don't know why, but the manufacturer has stopped making the oral drug."
2. "There were some cases of polio that developed from the oral vaccine."
3. "I will check with your HCP and see about changing the order."
4. "The intramuscular route is more effective in preventing polio than the oral route."

45. The clinic nurse has administered several recommended vaccinations to a 2-month-old infant. Which discharge instructions should the nurse give to the parents? **Select all that apply.**

1. Notify the HCP if the infant has a high-pitched cry.
2. Use a humidifier in the infant's room to reduce congestion.
3. Give the infant the prescribed amount of acetaminophen for comfort.
4. Keep the infant in the parents' room at night for a few days.
5. Explain that research does not support immunizations cause autism.

ANSWERS AND RATIONALES

The correct answer number and rationale are in **boldface blue type.** Rationales for why other answer options are incorrect are also given.

Autoimmune Disease

1. 1. Atropine, an antimuscarinic, works opposite of the cholinesterase inhibitors administered to treat MG. Still, atropine, in small doses, is prescribed to reduce the gastrointestinal (GI) side effects of the cholinesterase inhibitor. The nurse would not question this medication.
2. The antimalarial medication, chloroquine, is prescribed to treat cutaneous lupus erythematosus. The nurse would not question this medication.
3. The client diagnosed with polymyalgia rheumatica must take the prescribed corticosteroid medication, prednisone, or the client can become blind. The nurse would not question this medication.
4. Pyridostigmine (Mestinon), a cholinesterase inhibitor, is prescribed to increase the available amount of acetylcholine for muscle movement. A client in a cholinergic crisis has too much medication on board. The nurse would question administering this medication until the crisis is resolved.

2. 1. This may be asked, but it is not the most important question.
2. This is the most important question. The client reports pain and stiffness upon awakening in the morning. Taking NSAIDs then places the client at risk for developing peptic ulcer disease. The client should be taught to take these medications with food.
3. NSAID medications are frequently taken by female clients to relieve menstrual cramps. This is not the most important question.
4. This is the reason the client is taking the medication. NSAIDs are used to treat pain and stiffness, but they are also helpful in decreasing the inflammation associated with SLE and allow a reduction in the steroid dosage.

3. Correct order is 5, 2, 3, 1, 4.
5. The nurse must determine that the "right" medication is being administered to the "right" client. This is the first step.
2. The nurse should assess the IV catheter placement before administering medication. If there is a blood return, the catheter is in the vein.
3. The nurse should flush the saline lock with 2 mL of sterile saline before administering the medication to ensure that previously administered medication is flushed from the line and to avoid inadvertent mixing of medications.
1. Glucocorticoid hydrocortisone (Solu-Cortef) can be administered safely over 1 to 2 minutes.
4. The final step is to flush the saline lock to ensure the client receives all prescribed medication.

4. Correct answers are 2, 3, 4, 7, and 8.
1. There is no serum baclofen level.
2. Antispasmodic baclofen (Lioresal) can cause urinary urgency, so this should be assessed.
3. Antispasmodic baclofen (Lioresal) is administered to treat spasticity associated with MS. The nurse should assess for muscle spasticity, rigidity, movement, and pain to determine medication effectiveness.
4. The nurse should assess for muscle spasticity, rigidity, movement, and pain to determine baclofen's effectiveness.
5. The medication can affect the liver, but it does not damage the kidneys.
6. The medication can affect the liver, but it does not damage the kidneys.
7. Antispasmodic baclofen (Lioresal) is administered to treat spasticity associated with MS. The nurse should assess for muscle spasticity, rigidity, movement, and pain to determine medication effectiveness.
8. The nurse should assess for muscle spasticity, rigidity, movement, and pain to determine medication effectiveness.

5. **1. Cholinesterase inhibitor neostigmine bromide (Prostigmin) must be administered precisely on time to maintain muscle movement and ability to swallow for clients diagnosed with MG. This is the priority medication.**
2. Methylprednisolone (Solu-Medrol), a glucocorticoid, can be administered within the 30-minute acceptable time frame.

3. Morphine, a narcotic analgesic pain medication, is a priority, but not over the prevention of aspiration and maintaining the client's ability to use the respiration muscles.
4. Biologic response modifier etanercept (Enbrel) can be administered within the 30-minute acceptable time frame.

6. 1. Edrophonium (Tensilon), a cholinesterase inhibitor, is used to help diagnose MG and to determine if a client diagnosed with MG is in a cholinergic versus myasthenic crisis. A client losing the ability to breathe without mechanical support when given Tensilon is in a cholinergic crisis in which too much medication is in the body.
2. This response is the response that is diagnostic of MG.
3. This is a nonpharmacologic test that can be performed to assess for MG. This is a positive finding, but it does not apply to edrophonium (Tensilon), a cholinesterase inhibitor.
4. An unlabeled use for edrophonium (Tensilon), a cholinesterase inhibitor, is to terminate paroxysmal atrial tachycardia, but this does not diagnose MG.

7. Correct answer is 2.
1. Serum creatinine levels may be decreased if allopurinol levels are increased; however, the value is normal. Serum creatinine does not determine if allopurinol (Zyloprim) is effective for gout treatment.
2. The main problem with gout is hyperuricemia. A normal value indicates suppression of uric acid production by the body and that the medication, allopurinol (Zyloprim), is effective.
3. Allopurinol can cause decreased CBC and platelet counts; however, a change in WBCs does not indicate the medication is effective.
4. Total iron-binding capacity is not affected by allopurinol (Zyloprim).
5. Allopurinol (Zyloprim) can cause hypoglycemia but does not indicate effectiveness in treating gout.

MEDICATION MEMORY JOGGER: The nurse determines medication effectiveness by assessing for the symptoms or laboratory values, for which the medication was prescribed.

8. 1. The nurse should not tell the client to decrease the medication dose. Achieving the correct dose is extremely difficult and may require frequent modification, especially when the client is under stress or has an illness. Only the HCP should advise the client about the correct dose.
2. Holding the medication could result in respiratory compromise. The nurse should teach the client how to minimize medication side effects.
3. The nurse should teach the client how to minimize medication side effects. Taking the medication with milk or crackers will reduce GI effects. The HCP can prescribe small doses of atropine to counteract the side effects if this suggestion is unsuccessful, but the client must take the medication.
4. The client does not need an OTC medication to counteract the side effect of nausea.

9. 1. These symptoms are not part of schizophrenia and should be investigated.
2. The hallucinations the client has are not part of actual physical symptoms. Further investigation is needed to determine if the client is having a reaction to the antipsychotic medication chlorpromazine (Thorazine).
3. This is the best response by the nurse. These are symptoms of drug-induced SLE. The nurse should make sure the HCP sees the client.
4. The nurse should not tell the client that they would no longer be able to take medications to control symptoms of schizophrenia. The antipsychotic medication, chlorpromazine (Thorazine), may need to be changed to a different medication. Medication compliance in clients diagnosed with psychiatric illnesses can be poor. This statement would give the client a reason not to take any medication.

HIV and AIDS

10. Correct answers are 1 and 5.
1. If the client does not have insurance to help pay for the medications, the client may have trouble complying with the regimen. The current regimens include four or more daily medications costing more than $6,000 per drug per year.
2. Currently, AIDS cannot be managed without medications. With the medications, it is possible to reduce the viral load to undetectable in serum samples.
3. Many OTC medications and herbs interact with the medications used to treat AIDS. The nurse should assess each OTC preparation taken by the client but should not encourage their use.

4. One multiple vitamin is usually sufficient. The body excretes any water-soluble vitamin that is not needed.
5. **Many antiretroviral therapies have side effects that can be effectively treated; however, if the client cannot tolerate the side effects, the medication regimen can be altered.**

MEDICATION MEMORY JOGGER: Some herbal preparations are effective, some are not, and a few can be harmful or even deadly. If a client is taking an herbal supplement and a conventional medicine, the nurse should investigate to determine if the combination will cause harm to the client. The nurse should always be the client's advocate.

11. 1. These medications treat actual infections and are sometimes administered prophylactically, but they will not prevent conversion to HIV-positive status.
2. **The combination of specific medications depends on the health-care facility's protocol, but most include a combination of two nucleoside reverse transcriptase inhibitors and an integrase inhibitor. The Centers for Disease Control and Prevention (CDC) has a hotline that can provide specific recommendations at 800-458-5231 or www.cdc.gov.**
3. Single-agent therapy is not recommended because of the speed at which the virus can mutate.
4. There are medications that can possibly prevent conversion to HIV-positive status.

12. 1. Efavirenz (Sustiva), a nonnucleoside reverse transcriptase inhibitor, is not approved for prevention of transmission of HIV in pregnant women.
2. Lopinavir (Kaletra), a protease inhibitor, is not approved to prevent transmission of HIV to the fetus.
3. **Although zidovudine (AZT), a nucleoside reverse transcriptase inhibitor, is a pregnancy category C drug, research has proved that taking the drug during pregnancy reduces risk of maternal-to-fetal transmission of the HIV virus by almost 70%. This is the only medication approved for this purpose.**
4. Ganciclovir (Cytovene), an antiviral, is not approved for prevention of transmission of HIV to the fetus.

13. Correct answers are 2 and 3.
1. This is a standard precaution and does not require nurse intervention.
2. **Many protease inhibitors used to treat AIDS can interact with grapefruit juice. The nurse should stop the UAP until the nurse can determine if the client is receiving a medication that would interact with grapefruit juice.**
3. **The client's meal tray does not have body fluids that can transmit the HIV virus to the UAP; therefore, this action warrants nurse intervention. The UAP needs to understand how the HIV virus is transmitted.**
4. The client can apply their own moisture barrier protection cream. This does not warrant immediate intervention by the nurse.
5. This is a comfort measure and does not warrant nurse intervention.

MEDICATION MEMORY JOGGER: Grapefruit juice can inhibit metabolism of certain medications. Specifically, grapefruit juice inhibits cytochrome P450-3A4 found in the liver and the intestinal wall. The nurse should investigate any medications the client is taking if the client drinks grapefruit juice.

14. 1. The client diagnosed HIV positive could be expected to have a positive viral load. This is not a reason to begin trimethoprim sulfa (Bactrim).
2. This is a normal WBC count and is not a reason to start a prophylactic antibiotic.
3. The erythrocyte sedimentation rate assists in diagnosing acute inflammation, but this is a normal rate and does not indicate the need for trimethoprim sulfa (Bactrim).
4. **The client with a CD4 count of less than 300 (Normal is 332 to 1,642 cells/microL) is at risk for developing *Pneumocystis jiroveci* pneumonia (PJP). Trimethoprim sulfa (Bactrim) is a prophylaxis for PJP.**

15. 1. The medication should be administered daily over 6 hours, but not before the nurse knows the client will not have a reaction to the medication. Amphotericin B (Fungizone), an antifungal agent, is compatible only with D_5W.
2. Meperidine (Demerol) is used as a premedication to prevent an extrapyramidal reaction.
3. **The first action by the nurse is to administer a small test dose of amphotericin B (Fungizone), an antifungal agent, to assess the client's potential response.**
4. This is done to prevent a febrile reaction to the medication.

16. Correct answers are 3 and 5.
1. Before highly active antiretroviral therapy (HAART), the client would have had to continue taking the antiviral agent ganciclovir (Cytovene) for the rest of their life to prevent blindness. With HAART, the CD4 counts can rebound, and the client usually only needs to take the medication for 3 to 6 months.
2. This is not the regimen for the antiviral agent ganciclovir (Cytovene).
3. **Initial therapy is IV, and care must be taken not to infuse the medication too rapidly. The infusion should be administered on a pump for over 1 hour.**
4. The medication is incompatible with TPN.
5. **Ganciclovir (Cytovene) is administered twice a day during the first few weeks of treatment, then once a day 5 to 7 times a week.**

MEDICATION MEMORY JOGGER: Nothing should run in the same line as TPN. This is an infection-control issue.

17. Correct answers are 1, 2, 3, and 5.
1. **Isoniazid (INH) is the first-line therapy for active TB in combination with other medications.**
2. **Ethambutol (Myambutol), an antiinfective, is a treatment for TB.**
3. **Pyrazinamide (Tebrazid) is the first-line therapy of active TB in combination with other medications.**
4. Enfuvirtide (Fuzeon), an HIV fusion inhibitor, is the newest classification of drugs used to treat HIV viral infections, but it is effective against viruses, not bacteria.
5. **Rifampin is the first-line therapy of active TB in combination with other medications.**

18. Correct answers are 2, 3, and 4.
1. The medication should infuse over 60 to 90 minutes and, for best control, the infusion should be placed on an infusion pump.
2. **Leucovorin is the "rescue factor" to prevent an adverse reaction to trimetrexate (Neutrexin). The nurse should have both medications infusing simultaneously.**
3. **The medication trimetrexate (Neutrexin) can cause myelosuppression; therefore, the CBC should be monitored by the nurse.**
4. **The medication trimetrexate (Neutrexin) can cause a transient elevation in the client's liver enzymes; therefore, the nurse should monitor this laboratory result.**
5. The client does not have to be NPO while receiving this medication.

Allergies

19.
1. Tinnitus (ringing in the ears) is not a side effect of diphenhydramine (Benadryl), an antihistamine; tinnitus usually occurs with aspirin toxicity.
2. **Antihistamines such as diphenhydramine (Benadryl) cause drowsiness; therefore, the client should avoid driving or engaging in hazardous activities.**
3. A buffalo hump and moon face are side effects of glucocorticoids, not of antihistamines.
4. Diphenhydramine (Benadryl), an antihistamine, does not require tapering when discontinuing the medication.

20.
1. Wearing insect repellent is an appropriate intervention, but if the client has an insect bite, the repellent will not help prevent anaphylaxis; therefore, this is not the priority intervention.
2. Antihistamines are used for clients with anaphylaxis. Still, it takes at least 30 minutes for the medication to work, and if the client has an insect bite, it is not the priority medication.
3. **Clients with documented severe anaphylaxis should carry an epinephrine auto-injector (EpiPen), a prescribed injectable device containing epinephrine that the client can administer to themselves in case of an insect bite. This will save the client's life; therefore, this is the priority intervention.**
4. The client should wear a medication alert (MedicAlert) identification bracelet stating the allergy, but it will not help the client if they are bitten by an insect; therefore, it is not the priority intervention.

21. Correct answers are 1, 2, 3, and 4.
1. **Glucocorticoid intranasal spray, such as fluticasone (Flonase), should be used with caution for clients taking herbal supplements such as licorice, which can potentiate the glucocorticoid effects.**
2. **Therapy usually begins with two sprays in each nostril twice a day and then decreases to one dose per day for a specific period.**

3. **Concomitant use of a local nasal decongestant spray may increase risk of nasal irritation or bleeding. Both sprays may be used together for a client diagnosed with chronic rhinitis but not for seasonal allergies.**
4. **Nasal bleeding indicates broken mucous membranes that can allow direct access to the bloodstream, increasing the likelihood of systemic effects of the drug. The HCP should be notified if nose bleeds occur.**
5. Temporary nasal stinging may occur at the beginning of therapy. Discontinuing the medication is not necessary.

MEDICATION MEMORY JOGGER: Some herbal preparations are effective, some are not, and a few can be harmful or even deadly. If a client is taking an herbal supplement and a conventional medicine, the nurse should investigate to determine if the combination will cause harm to the client. The nurse should always be the client's advocate.

22. Correct answers are 1 and 5.
1. **H_1 receptor antagonist fexofenadine (Allegra) is contraindicated for clients diagnosed with asthma and clients using nicotine because of its anticholinergic effects on the respiratory system.**
2. There are no contraindications for use of H_1 receptor antagonists for clients running daily; therefore, the nurse would not question administering this medication.
3. There are no contraindications for H_1 receptor antagonists for clients with antibiotic allergies; therefore, the nurse would not question administering this medication.
4. H_1 receptor antagonist fexofenadine (Allegra) is prescribed prophylactically for clients with nasal sneezing and tearing of the eye; therefore, the nurse would not question administering this medication.
5. **Fexofenadine (Allegra) and other antihistamines are contraindicated for clients diagnosed with asthma because they dry the upper and lower respiratory tract secretions and cause an asthma exacerbation.**

23.
1. This medication has anticholinergic effects; therefore, a dry mouth is an expected side effect. Sucking on hard candy will help relieve the dry mouth. This statement indicates the client understands the teaching.
2. The client is at risk for an anticholinergic crisis and should notify the HCP or pharmacist of taking clemastine (Tavist), an H_1 receptor antagonist. This statement indicates the client understands the teaching.
3. **The client should be aware of clinical manifestations with an anticholinergic crisis such as blurred vision, confusion, difficulty swallowing, and fever or flushing. This statement indicates the client needs more teaching about the medication, clemastine (Tavist), an H_1 receptor antagonist.**
4. This medication has anticholinergic effects. The client should maintain adequate fluid intake to help prevent dehydration. This statement indicates the client understands the teaching.

24. Correct answers are 1 and 2.
1. **Prolonged use of oxymetazoline (Afrin 12-Hour Nasal Spray), a sympathomimetic, causes hypersecretion of mucous and nasal congestion to worsen once the drug effects wear off. This sometimes leads to a cycle of increased drug use as the condition worsens. This rebound congestion is why it should not be used for more than 3 to 5 days.**
2. **The client should use a finger to close the nostril not receiving the medication. The spray tip should be inserted into the open nostril. When spraying, the client should inhale deeply through the nose.**
3. The client should avoid clearing the nose immediately after spraying so that the medication can stay in the nares.
4. The postnasal medication should be spat out, not swallowed.
5. The medication should be administered exactly as prescribed. Additional dosing will not speed relief of nasal congestion.

25.
1. This is an appropriate question, but it is not the first question the nurse should ask the client.
2. The nasal glucocorticoid spray bottle should be shaken thoroughly, but this is not the first question the nurse should ask the client.
3. The client should take the medication as prescribed, but this is not the first question the nurse should ask the client.
4. **The nasal glucocorticoid spray medication may take 2 to 4 weeks to be effective; therefore, the nurse should first determine how long the client has been taking the medication.**

26. Correct answers are 1, 2, and 3.
1. **Anticholinergic effects of antihistamine therapy may trigger bronchospasms; therefore, the nurse should assess for wheezing or difficulty breathing.**
2. **Elderly clients are at an increased risk of increased sedation and other anticholinergic effects; therefore, the nurse should assess the consciousness level.**
3. **Antihistamines promote urinary retention, and the nurse should ensure adequate intake and output.**
4. Antihistamines cause drowsiness; therefore, the nurse should institute safety and fall precautions and not encourage the client to ambulate without assistance.
5. There are no dietary precautions for clients taking antihistamines.

27. 1. The drug of choice for an anaphylactic reaction is epinephrine (Adrenalin) administered subcutaneously, but it is not the first intervention.
2. **The nurse should realize that the client is having an allergic reaction to the IV antibiotic and immediately discontinue the medication. This is the nurse's first intervention.**
3. The nurse should not take time to assess the client when it is apparent the client is having an allergic reaction to the IV antibiotic.
4. Oxygen should be applied, but it is not the nurse's first intervention in this situation. The antibiotic that is causing the anaphylactic reaction should be discontinued first.

Rheumatoid Arthritis

28. Correct answers are 4 and 5.
1. Hydroxychloroquine sulfate (Plaquenil), a disease-modifying antirheumatic drug (DMARD), can cause pigmentary retinitis and vision loss, so the client should have a thorough vision examination every 6 months. The client does not need more teaching.
2. Hydroxychloroquine sulfate (Plaquenil), a DMARD, may increase liver toxicity risk when administered with hepatotoxic drugs; therefore, alcohol use should be eliminated during therapy. The client does not need more teaching.
3. The medication should be taken with milk to decrease GI upset. The client does not need more teaching.
4. **The medication hydroxychloroquine sulfate (Plaquenil), a DMARD, takes 3 to 6 months to achieve the desired response. Many clients do not experience significant benefits. The client needs more teaching.**
5. **Loss of balance and coordination is an adverse effect of hydroxychloroquine sulfate (Plaquenil), a DMARD. The client needs more teaching and should notify the HCP.**

MEDICATION MEMORY JOGGER: Drinking alcohol is always discouraged when taking any prescribed or OTC medication because of potential adverse interactions. The nurse should encourage the client not to drink alcoholic beverages.

29. 1. Alopecia is a common side effect of the DMARD leflunomide (Arava). This should be discussed with the client before starting the medication, and methods of coping with hair loss should be explored. This comment would not warrant intervention by the nurse.
2. This medication causes dizziness; therefore, this comment would not warrant intervention by the nurse.
3. **The DMARD leflunomide (Arava) is teratogenic. Women must undergo the drug-elimination procedure, and men must take 8 grams of cholestyramine three times daily for 11 days to minimize any possible risk of harm to the fetus their partner is carrying.**
4. The client should avoid vaccinations with live vaccines during and after therapy; therefore, this comment does not require nursing intervention.

30. Correct answers are 1 and 5.
1. **Methotrexate, a DMARD, causes bone marrow depression, which may lead to abnormal bleeding; therefore, the client should use a soft-bristled toothbrush.**
2. Methotrexate does not affect the client's response to cold weather.
3. The client is at risk for mouth ulcers and should not use any commercially available mouthwash. The client should rinse the mouth with water after eating and drinking.
4. Methotrexate, a DMARD, may increase sensitivity of the skin to sunlight. The client should use a sunscreen of SPF 30 or higher and wear protective clothing when sun exposure is unavoidable.

5. NSAIDs and salicylates taken with methotrexate can cause elevated levels of methotrexate in the blood, leading to toxicity. Careful monitoring of methotrexate levels is required.

31. 1. The most dangerous adverse reaction to phenylbutazone (Butazolidin), a pyrazoline NSAID, is blood dyscrasias, which are manifested in the client by flu-like symptoms.

2. Constipation is not a side effect of phenylbutazone (Butazolidin), a pyrazoline NSAID. The nurse would not question administering the medication.
3. Weight gain is not a side effect of phenylbutazone (Butazolidin), a pyrazoline NSAID. The nurse would not question administering the medication.
4. Insomnia is not a side effect of phenylbutazone (Butazolidin), a pyrazoline NSAID. The nurse would not question administering the medication.

MEDICATION MEMORY JOGGER: Usually, if a client is prescribed a new medication and has flu-like symptoms within 24 hours of taking the first dose, the client should contact the HCP. These are clinical manifestations of agranulocytosis, which indicate the medication has caused a sudden drop in the WBC count, leaving the body defenseless against bacterial invasion.

32. 1. The serum creatinine is within the normal range of 0.61 to 1.21 mg/dL for men and 0.51 to 1.11 mg/dL for women.

2. This RBC count indicates anemia (low RBC count and Hgb/Hct resulting from low RBCs), which would warrant intervention by the nurse. The normal RBC is 4.21 to 5.81 (10^6 cells/microL) for men and 3.61 to 5.11 (10^6 cells/microL) for women.

3. The WBC count is within the normal range of 4.5 to 11.1 × 10^3/microL.
4. The hemoglobin (Hgb) is within the normal range of 14 to 17.3 g/dL for men and 11.1 to 15.5 g/dL for women.
5. The hematocrit (Hct) is within the normal range of 42% to 52% for men and 36% to 48% for women.

33. 1. Sulfasalazine (Azulfidine), an antirheumatic, may cause an orange or yellowish discoloration of urine and the skin. This is expected and is not significant.

2. Stomatitis is not an expected side effect of sulfasalazine (Azulfidine), an antirheumatic medication. The HCP should be notified.
3. Ecchymosis (unexplained bleeding) is not an expected side effect of sulfasalazine (Azulfidine), an antirheumatic. The HCP should be notified.
4. A rash is not an expected side effect. The HCP should be notified.

34. 1. This aspirin dose is just less than the toxic dose that produces tinnitus and hearing loss, but this is the dose needed to treat RA. The client should reduce the dose by two to three tablets per day until the tinnitus resolves. This statement indicates the client does not need more teaching.

2. GI side effects are common with aspirin therapy; therefore, the client should take aspirin with food. This statement indicates the client does not need more teaching.

3. The aspirin should be taken in divided doses (three to four 325-mg tablets four times a day). This statement indicates the client needs more teaching.

4. Enteric-coated aspirin produces less gastric distress than plain, buffered aspirin. The client's statement does not need more teaching.

35. 1. A buffalo hump and moon face are expected side effects, are not life-threatening, and would not be a problem if the client took the medication forever. These side effects affect body image, but most individuals in severe pain would rather have body-image problems than pain.

2. Prednisone, a glucocorticoid, has serious long-term side effects that can lead to possible life-threatening complications; therefore, the client cannot take prednisone forever.

3. An Addisonian crisis (adrenal insufficiency) is a complication that may occur when the client abruptly stops prednisone, a glucocorticoid medication, but not if it is tapered off.
4. This response does not answer the client's question; therefore, it is not the best response.

36. Correct answers are 4 and 5.

1. Pain relief lasts only as long as the topical analgesic, capsaicin (Zostrix), is applied regularly, not as needed (PRN).
2. Transient burning may occur with the application if applied fewer than three to four times daily. Burning usually disappears after a few days but may continue for 2 to 4 weeks or longer.
3. If the pain persists longer than 1 month, the client should discontinue the cream and notify the HCP.

4. **The cream capsaicin (Zostrix), a topical analgesic, should be rubbed into the skin until little or no cream is left on the skin's surface.**
5. **Hands should be washed immediately after cream is applied to the skin with soap or vinegar so the client does not accidentally spread capsaicin (Zostrix) to the eyes, nose, or mouth.**

37. 1. The client should not take aspirin, an NSAID, while taking etodolac (Lodine), another NSAID.
2. The client should not receive an additional dose of a routine medication being administered for treatment of RA.
3. The nurse should administer a nonnarcotic analgesic for a headache, not a narcotic.
4. **Acetaminophen, a nonnarcotic analgesic, would be the most appropriate medication for the client experiencing a headache and taking etodolac (Lodine), an NSAID.**

Immunizations

38. Correct answers are 2, 3, 4, 6, and 7.
1. This may be important information to give to the parent, but it is not the legal requirement for immunization documentation.
2. **The CDC and Federal Drug Administration (FDA) require all HCPs to report any adverse events reported by the client, using the Vaccine Adverse Events Reporting System (VAERS), even if the HCP believes the event is unrelated to the immunization.**
3. **Vaccine information statements (VISs) are developed by the CDC. The HCP is required to give a copy to the client and allow the client to read the statement before administering the vaccination.**
4. **The National Childhood Vaccine Act of 1986 requires that a permanent record of the vaccinations a child receives be maintained. The required information includes: date of vaccination; route and site of vaccination; vaccine type, manufacturer, lot number, and expiration date; and name, address, and title of the person administering the vaccination.**
5. This may be important information to give to the parent, but it is not the legal requirement for immunization documentation.
6. **The name and title of the person administering the vaccination is required documentation.**
7. **The office or clinic address where the vaccine was given is required documentation. Providers can add the contact information to an existing VIS but cannot make any substantive changes to the document.**

39. 1. Potential complications of measles include blindness and deafness. Potential complications of mumps include aseptic meningitis. For adolescent and adult males, orchitis is another complication. Potential complications for rubella include arthritis in women and congenital disabilities or miscarriage for pregnant women.
2. The public school system encourages all children to be immunized according to CDC prevention guidelines, but there are exceptions. The nurse should know the requirements for the state where the nurse is practicing.
3. Immunizations prevent many illnesses.
4. This parent is asking for information, not a therapeutic conversation.

MEDICATION MEMORY JOGGER: The nurse must be knowledgeable of accepted standards of practice for disease processes and conditions. If the nurse administers a medication that the HCP has prescribed, and the medication harms the client, the nurse could be held accountable. The nurse is a client advocate and should provide truthful information to the client.

40. 1. The parent may have allowed the immunization to occur, but specific signed permission is not needed.
2. The nurse should teach the parent how to care for the child, not send the child to the emergency department.
3. The problem is probably related to the immunization, not a secondary infection.
4. **The varicella vaccine can cause a fever spike to 102°F (38.8°C), a mild rash with a few lesions, and pain and redness at the injection site. The nurse should tell the parents how to care for the child.**

41. Correct answers are 2 and 5.
1. Most children are afraid of being hurt by the injections, but this is not a reason to question administering the injection.

2. **The child will shed the vaccine in the urine and feces. The grandparent is immunocompromised as a result of the chemotherapy and could become ill. This child should receive an inactivated vaccine. The nurse should question this vaccine.**
3. This is a reason to give the vaccine, not question it.
4. Jehovah's Witnesses do not refuse vaccinations because of religious beliefs.
5. **This child is immunocompromised, could become ill, and should receive an inactivated vaccine.**
6. According to the CDC, a child can be vaccinated even if they have an ear infection (otitis media).
7. According to the CDC, a child can still be vaccinated if they have a low-grade fever, cold, or mild diarrhea.

42. 1. This is not a safe administration site for a 15-month-old child.
2. This is not the best site for a toddler.
3. **Infants and toddlers should receive intramuscular injections in the vastus lateralis muscle, the large muscle of the thigh. This muscle is large and away from any nerves that could be damaged by the injection.**
4. The immunizations are given intramuscularly, not subcutaneously.

43. 1. The child has a chronic disease, and it is very important for the child to receive all immunizations.
2. The child is at greater risk of complications of the illnesses the immunizations prevent because of diabetes. The child should receive all recommended immunizations.
3. The child does not "get used" to the needles, and the child likely will mind the injections.
4. **Children diagnosed with chronic illnesses are encouraged to receive a yearly flu vaccine.**

44. 1. The injection should be administered, but a single injection is not sufficient for the age of this child.
2. **The correct procedure for a child age 13 or older is to administer two injections at least 4 weeks apart.**
3. Two injections are recommended. Three injections are the recommended schedule for hepatitis B.
4. Adults can become ill with varicella.

45. Correct answers are 1, 3, and 5.
1. **The parent should notify the HCP if the infant has a high-pitched cry, because it is a clinical manifestation of the infant having an adverse immunization effect.**
2. Vaccinations should not cause congestion; therefore, a humidifier is not needed.
3. **Acetaminophen is the treatment used to manage side effects of sore injection sites and fever.**
4. The parents do not have to keep the infant in their room.
5. **Research in various countries has found no link between vaccines and autism spectrum disorders (see www.vaccines.com).**

IMMUNE INFLAMMATORY SYSTEM COMPREHENSIVE EXAMINATION

1. The client presents to the clinic reporting that his girlfriend was diagnosed with hepatitis B yesterday. The client asks the nurse, "Can you give me something so that I won't get hepatitis?" Which statement is the nurse's **best** response?
   1. "You should take 500 mg of OTC vitamin C every day."
   2. "You need to have hepatitis B vaccine injections starting today."
   3. "At this time, there is no treatment to ensure you don't get hepatitis."
   4. "You need to receive an injection of gamma globulin IM today."

2. The 4-year-old is prescribed prednisolone for juvenile arthritis. Which statement by the child's mother **warrants immediate** intervention?
   1. "My child is current with all the required immunizations."
   2. "I can crush the tablet and put it in some of their favorite pudding."
   3. "My 2-year-old child is at home with chickenpox."
   4. "I need to notify my HCP if my child's temperature is higher than 100°F."

3. The client diagnosed with AIDS is receiving IV acyclovir. Which intervention should the home health-care nurse implement when administering this medication?
   1. Restrict all visitors when administering this medication.
   2. Arrange for IV tubing and bag to be incinerated.
   3. Store reconstituted solutions at room temperature.
   4. Have the pharmacy mix the medication for 1 week at a time.

4. The client diagnosed with AIDS has a pruritic rash with pinkish-red macules. Which medication should the nurse suspect is causing the rash?
   1. Trimethoprim-sulfamethoxazole
   2. Nelfinavir
   3. Efavirenz
   4. Zidovudine

5. The home health-care nurse is reviewing the list of daily medications prescribed to the client diagnosed with AIDS. Which medication **needs** further clarification by the nurse?
   1. Prednisone
   2. Fluoxetine
   3. Saquinavir
   4. Nevirapine

6. The client diagnosed with Guillain-Barré (GB) syndrome is reporting pain. The client has an order for morphine 2 mg IVP. Which interventions should the nurse implement? **Rank in order of performance.**
   1. Administer the morphine over 5 minutes.
   2. Assess the client's respiratory status.
   3. Check the two identifiers against the MAR.
   4. Sign out the medication per hospital policy.
   5. Check the last time the morphine was administered.

7. The spouse of the client diagnosed with GB syndrome asks the nurse, "Don't you have something that will cure this disease?" Which statement is the nurse's **best** response?
   1. "Long-term steroid therapy will help reverse paralysis."
   2. "High doses of IV antibiotics may help cure GB syndrome."
   3. "There is no medication known that will cure this disease."
   4. "Alefacept has side effects, but it can cure GB syndrome."

8. The client diagnosed with MS is being treated with interferon beta-1a. Which diagnostic test should the nurse monitor to determine the medication **effectiveness**?
   1. The cerebrospinal fluid WBC count
   2. The magnetic resonance imaging (MRI) scan
   3. An electromyogram (EMG)
   4. An electroencephalogram (EEG)

9. The client diagnosed with MS tells the nurse, "I have problems having regular bowel movements." Which statement indicates the client **needs more** medication teaching?
   1. "I am taking a stimulant laxative tablet every day."
   2. "I am taking a fiber laxative daily."
   3. "I take a stool softener at bedtime."
   4. "I keep a glass of water with me at all times."

10. The client diagnosed with systemic lupus erythematosus (SLE) is prescribed azathioprine. Which teaching should the nurse discuss with the client? **Select all that apply.**
    1. Instruct the client on how to use a glucometer.
    2. Tell the client to come to the office for laboratory tests.
    3. Explain that low-grade fevers are expected initially.
    4. Discuss the need for recording an accurate urinary output.
    5. Teach the use of sunscreen and protective clothing outdoors.
    6. Emphasize how the medication will cure SLE in 12 weeks.
    7. Advise female clients to avoid pregnancy during drug therapy.
    8. Tell the client to avoid concurrent use of salicylates or NSAIDs.

11. The clinic nurse is caring for a client requesting to be up to date on their vaccinations. Which interventions should the nurse implement? **Rank in order of performance.**
    1. Educate the client about the vaccines.
    2. Screen for contraindications and precautions.
    3. Document the vaccinations.
    4. Prepare the vaccinations.
    5. Review immunization history.
    6. Assess the needed immunizations.
    7. Administer the vaccines.

12. The client diagnosed with RA is undergoing long-term therapy with hydroxychloroquine. Which actions by the client indicate compliance with the medication teaching? **Select all that apply.**
    1. The client takes the medication with food.
    2. The client does not drink any alcoholic beverages.
    3. The client drinks at least 3,000 mL of water daily.
    4. The client has not had any unexplained weight loss.
    5. The client sees the ophthalmologist every 6 months.

13. The nurse is preparing to administer a COVID-19 vaccination. Which vaccination schedule is correct? **Select three correct answers.**
    1. Administer BNT162b2, manufactured by Pfizer-BioNTech, as two injections, 21 days apart.
    2. Administer BNT162b2, manufactured by Pfizer-BioNTech, as one injection.
    3. Administer mRNA-1273, manufactured by Moderna, as two injections, 28 days apart.
    4. Administer mRNA-1273, manufactured by Moderna, as one injection.
    5. Administer JNJ-78436735, manufactured by Johnson & Johnson, as two injections, 21 days apart
    6. Administer JNJ-78436735, manufactured by Johnson & Johnson as one injection.

14. The hospital nurse has developed a latex allergy. Which **action** should the hospital nurse implement?
1. Investigate working for a home health-care agency.
2. Wash hands thoroughly instead of wearing gloves.
3. Request a box of nonlatex gloves from the hospital.
4. File workers' compensation with the employee health nurse.

15. The nurse is caring for an 8-year-old child diagnosed with poison ivy. The child's parent is concerned about the child attending school and experiencing itching. Which medication should the nurse recommend to help **decrease** pruritus while in school?
1. An oatmeal bath
2. A calamine and diphenhydramine lotion
3. Oral diphenhydramine
4. Polymyxin

16. The nurse is preparing to administer morning medications to a client. The prescribed medication for administration is in the following medication administration record (MAR).

Client: A.C.	MR# 1234567	Date: Today
Age: 65 years	Allergies: NKDA	Diagnosis: 1-day postoperative total knee replacement
Medication	**0701–1900**	**1901–0700**
Ceftriaxone 150 mg IV q 12 hours	0900	2100
Enoxaparin 40 mg SQ daily	0900	
Cyclosporine 300 mg b.i.d.	0900	2100
Morphine 2 mg IV q 2 hours PRN pain		
Nurse Initials/Credentials	**DN/RN**	**NN/RN**

Which medication should the nurse **question** administering?
1. Ceftriaxone
2. Enoxaparin
3. Cyclosporine
4. Morphine

17. The nurse is preparing to administer morning medications. Which medication should the nurse administer **first**?
1. Hydrocodone to the client with pain rated a 7 on a pain scale of 1 to 10
2. Furosemide IVP to a client with 2+ pitting edema
3. Metformin by mouth to a client diagnosed with type 2 diabetes
4. Neostigmine orally to the client diagnosed with myasthenia gravis

IMMUNE INFLAMMATORY SYSTEM COMPREHENSIVE EXAMINATION ANSWERS AND RATIONALES

1. 1. Vitamin C will increase immune system efficiency but will not prevent the client from getting hepatitis B.
2. Vaccines provide immunity when administered before exposure to hepatitis B, but they are ineffective in preventing hepatitis B after exposure.
3. This is a false statement because there is a treatment available.
4. Gamma globulin may be administered to a client exposed to hepatitis B within 24 hours to 7 days of exposure to the virus. This will provide passive immunity to the client.

2. 1. While the child is receiving prednisolone (Pediapred), a glucocorticoid, immunizations should not be administered. If a child is immunocompromised, then only attenuated vaccines can be administered.
2. This medication can be crushed because it is not a sustained-release formulation or enteric coated.
3. Children taking prednisolone (Pediapred), a glucocorticoid, are more prone to infection and should avoid exposure to measles or chickenpox while taking prednisolone.
4. Steroid medication suppresses the immune system; therefore, an elevated temperature should be reported to the HCP.

3. 1. There is no reason to restrict visitors during medication administration. The client is immunocompromised, which may require restriction of visitors with known infections.
2. Ganciclovir and acyclovir (Cytogenesis), an antiviral medication, are teratogenic and carcinogenic; therefore, they must be disposed of in a manner that protects the environment. They should be burned at a high temperature to prevent the chemical from reaching the environment.
3. The reconstituted solutions must be stored in the refrigerator to protect their efficacy.
4. The medication acyclovir (Cytogenesis), an antiviral medication, is only viable for 24 hours after mixing the solution; therefore, the pharmacy cannot mix a week at a time.

4. 1. An antibiotic trimethoprim-sulfamethoxazole (Bactrim) sulfa allergy with this type of rash develops in up to 60% of clients diagnosed with AIDS.
2. Common side effects of antiretroviral medication nelfinavir (Viracept) are hyperglycemia and diarrhea, but not allergic rashes.
3. Common side effects of nonnucleoside reverse transcriptase inhibitor efavirenz (Sustiva) are central nervous system symptoms but not allergic rashes.
4. GI intolerance and bone marrow suppression are common side effects of a nucleoside analog reverse transcriptase inhibitor AZT or (Invirase), but allergic rashes are not.

MEDICATION MEMORY JOGGER: When a client develops a rash and is receiving an antibiotic, the nurse should suspect that the antibiotic is the cause of the rash.

5. 1. The nurse would need further clarification for glucocorticoid prednisone (Deltasone) steroid because the client is already immunosuppressed, and this medication would further suppress the immune system.
2. The nurse must realize that depression is common in clients diagnosed with chronic illnesses; therefore, a prescription for selective serotonin reuptake inhibitor fluoxetine (Prozac) would not need further clarification.
3. Antiviral medications such as antiretroviral medication saquinavir (Invirase) are commonly prescribed for clients diagnosed with AIDS to suppress replication of the AIDS virus.
4. Nonnucleoside reverse transcriptase inhibitors such as nevirapine (Viramune) are commonly prescribed for clients diagnosed with AIDS to suppress replication of the AIDS virus.

6. Correct order is 5, 4, 2, 3, 1.
5. One of the medication Rights is the right time, and the nurse must check PRN medications to make sure they are within the prescribed time frame.
4. Narcotics are locked up and must be signed out and accounted for before administering.
2. If the client's respiratory rate is less than 12 breaths a minute, the morphine medication should be questioned.
3. The Joint Commission has mandated that the nurse identify the client with two identifiers before administering medication.

1. The nurse should administer morphine over 5 minutes to avoid respiratory depression, hypotension, or circulatory collapse.

7. 1. There is no medication that can cure GB.
2. There is no medication that can cure GB.
3. At this time, the medical treatment for Guillain-Barré (GB) is supportive until the GB resolves on its own.
4. Alefacept (Amevive) is a medication used to treat psoriasis.

8. 1. WBCs in the cerebrospinal fluid indicate an infection such as meningitis, not MS.
2. Biologic response modifier interferon beta-1a (Avonex) can reduce frequency of relapse by 30% and decrease appearance of new lesions on the MRI by 80%. The decrease in the appearance of new lesions indicates the medication is effective.
3. The EMG would not help determine if the medication was effective because the results will be skewed from previous damage.
4. The EEG would not help determine if the medication was effective because it measures the brain activity, not appearance of plaque.

MEDICATION MEMORY JOGGER: The nurse must be knowledgeable about accepted standards of practice for medication administration, including which of the client's assessment data, laboratory data, or diagnostic tests should be monitored to determine medication effectiveness.

9. 1. Bisacodyl (Dulcolax) is a stimulant laxative and should not be taken every day because it will cause a decrease in bowel tone. The client diagnosed with MS already has difficulty with bowel tone.
2. The client diagnosed with MS is at risk for constipation, fecal incontinence, and fecal impaction because of decreased bowel tone. A fiber laxative increases the stool's bulk and helps prevent constipation; therefore, the medication teaching is effective.
3. The client diagnosed with MS is at risk for constipation, fecal incontinence, and fecal impaction because of decreased bowel tone. A stool softener (Colace) will help prevent constipation and can be taken at any time of day; therefore, the medication teaching is effective.
4. Increasing the fluid intake will help the bulk laxative to work and will help soften the stool; therefore, the client understands the medication teaching.

10. Correct answers are 2, 5, and 7.
1. The client's blood glucose level is not affected by azathioprine (Imuran); therefore, there is no need to monitor the glucose level.
2. Bone marrow depression may occur when taking azathioprine (Imuran). The client must have a CBC and platelet count every week for the first month of therapy, then bimonthly for 2 to 3 months, and monthly after that.
3. Low-grade fever is not expected and is a clinical manifestation of infection. This must be reported to the HCP.
4. Kidney function is monitored through laboratory tests, not the client's urine output.
5. Azathioprine can increase skin cancer risk. The client should be taught to wear sunscreen and protective clothing outdoors and to avoid tanning booths.
6. Azathioprine is used to slow or stop the disease process; it is not a cure.
7. Female clients should avoid pregnancy during therapy and for at least 4 months after medication therapy is complete. Breastfeeding should be avoided.
8. The client may continue to take salicylates, NSAIDs, and steroids while taking azathioprine.

11. Correct order is 5, 6, 2, 1, 4, 7, 3.
5. The nurse should first review the client's immunization history to determine what vaccines are needed.
6. The nurse should use the current Advisory Committee on Immunization Practices schedule to determine what vaccines are needed based on the client's immunization history.
2. The next step is to screen for vaccine contraindications and precautions to avoid adverse events after vaccinations.
1. The nurse should educate the client about the vaccines and provided written documentation.
4. The nurse should prepare the vaccines properly.
7. The nurse should administer the vaccines by following recommended routes and sites.
3. The final step is to document the vaccinations with the appropriate information in the client's medical record (CDC, 2021).

12. Correct answers are 1, 2, and 5.
1. The client should take the hydroxychloroquine (Plaquenil) medication with meals or milk to reduce GI distress.

2. Alcohol should be avoided because it will increase the possibility of liver toxicity.
3. Constipation is not a side effect of hydroxychloroquine (Plaquenil); therefore, the client does not need to increase fluid intake. Diarrhea is a side effect.
4. Weight gain or loss would not be an indicator of hydroxychloroquine (Plaquenil) medication compliance.
5. Hydroxychloroquine (Plaquenil) can cause retinopathy, blurred vision, and difficulty focusing; therefore, the client should have periodic eye examinations.

13. Correct answers are 1, 3, and 6.
1. The COVID vaccine manufactured by Pfizer-BioTech is given as two injections, 21 days apart.
2. The COVID vaccine manufactured by Pfizer-BioTech is given as two injections, 21 days apart.
3. The COVID vaccine manufactured by Moderna is given as two injections, 28 days apart.
4. The COVID vaccine manufactured by Moderna is given as two injections, 28 days apart.
5. The COVID vaccine, manufactured by Johnson & Johnson, is one injection.
6. The COVID vaccine, manufactured by Johnson & Johnson, is one injection.

14. 1. All nurses must wear gloves when exposed to blood and body fluids, regardless of the work setting.
2. According to Standard Precautions, the nurse must wear gloves when exposed to blood and body fluids.
3. The hospital must provide nonlatex gloves, and the nurse must keep them available for use when the nurse may be exposed to blood and body fluids.
4. This is not a workers' compensation issue. The nurse has not been injured.

15. Correct answers are 2 and 5.
1. Baths cannot be given at school.
2. Caladryl, a topical antihistamine, is calamine lotion and diphenhydramine (Benadryl) combined. The lotion dries the lesions, and the topical (Benadryl) decreases itching. This medication can be administered at school.
3. Oral diphenhydramine (Benadryl), an H_1 antagonist, could have the systemic effect of drowsiness, which would interfere with the child's ability to function.
4. Polymyxin, an antibiotic ointment, is a combination antibiotic, but it is not administered for a topical dermatitis.

16. 1. The nurse would not question administering ceftriaxone (Rocephin), a broad-spectrum antibiotic. The client has had surgery, and antibiotics are prescribed prophylactically.
2. Enoxaparin (Lovenox), a low-molecular-weight heparin, is prescribed to prevent deep vein thrombosis, and the nurse would not question administering this medication.
3. Cyclosporine (Neoral), an immunosuppressant, is not an expected medication to be prescribed for a client recovering from total knee replacement. The nurse should determine why the client is receiving this medication. The client taking cyclosporine has had some type of organ transplant. This is important information to include in discussions with others caring for the client.
4. The nurse would expect the postoperative client to receive a narcotic analgesic pain medication.

17. 1. Pain medication such as hydrocodone (Vicodin), a narcotic analgesic, is a priority, but not over a medication that will prevent a potentially life-threatening event.
2. Furosemide (Lasix), a loop diuretic, would be administered to treat the edema, but it is not a priority for someone with 2+ edema.
3. Metformin (Glucophage), a biguanide, is not given for a life-threatening condition; therefore, it can be administered after the Prostigmin.
4. A client diagnosed with MG must take medications on time to ensure muscle function while eating or performing activities of daily living. Neostigmine (Prostigmin), an anticholinesterase, is one of the few medications that must be administered exactly on time.

12 Cancer Treatments

When you have exhausted all possibilities, remember this: You haven't.

—Thomas Edison

QUESTIONS

Chemotherapy

1. The client has received chemotherapy 2 days a week every 3 weeks for the past 8 months. The client's current laboratory values are populated in the chart below.

Laboratory Test	Client Values	Reference Values
Platelets	89 (10^3/microL)	140 to 400 × 10^3/microL
Neutrophils	50%	40% to 75%
White blood cells (WBC)	5.2 (10^3/cells/microL)	4.5–11.1 (10^3/cells/microL)
Hemoglobin (Hgb)	10.3 (g/dL)	Men: 14–17.3 g/dL Women: 11.7–15.5 g/dL
Hematocrit (Hct)	31%	Men: 42% to 52% Women: 36% to 48%

Which information should the nurse teach the client? **Select all that apply.**
1. "Use an electric razor when shaving."
2. "Avoid individuals with colds or other infections."
3. "Be careful when using sharp objects such as scissors."
4. "Plan for periods of rest to prevent fatigue."
5. "Use a soft-bristled toothbrush when brushing teeth."

2. The nurse is preparing to administer 0900 medications on an oncology floor. Which medication should the nurse administer **first**?
1. An analgesic to a client with a headache of "3" on the pain scale
2. An antiemetic to a client who might become nauseated
3. A mucosal barrier agent to a client diagnosed with peptic ulcer disease (PUD)
4. A biologic response modifier to a client with low red blood cell (RBC) counts

3. The client receiving mitotic inhibitors (plant alkaloids) for cancer reports to the clinic nurse being "so clumsy lately that I can't even pick up a dime." Which statement is the nurse's **best response**?
   1. "This is normal and will resolve when your therapy is complete."
   2. "There is no reason to worry about a minor side effect of the drugs."
   3. "Have you also noticed a difference in your bowel movements?"
   4. "Are you also weak and dizzy when you try to stand up?"

4. The client has received the second dose of chemotherapy and is ready for discharge. Which information should the nurse teach the client?
   1. Tell the client to notify the HCP of a temperature of 100°F (37.7°C).
   2. Have the client drink dietary supplements three times a day.
   3. Encourage the client to stay away from all people outside of the home.
   4. Apply a continuous ice pack to the IV site.

5. The nurse is reviewing laboratory data of a male client receiving chemotherapy. Which intervention should the nurse implement?

Client: C.D.	MR# 123456	Date: Today
Laboratory Test	**Client Values**	**Reference Values**
White blood cells (WBC)	2.4	4.5–11.1 (10^3/cells/microL)
Red blood cells (RBC)	4.0	Men: 4.21–5.81 (10^6 cells/microL) Women: 3.61–5.11 (10^6 cells/microL)
Hemoglobin (Hgb)	11.6	Men: 14–17.3 g/dL Women: 11.7–15.5 g/dL
Hematocrit (Hct)	34.2	Men: 42%–52% Women: 36%–48%
Mean corpuscular volume (MCV)	83	Men: 77–97 fl Women: 78–98 fl
Mean corpuscular hemoglobin concentration (MCHC)	31	33–36 g/dL
Coefficient of variation in RBC distribution width index (RDWCV)	12	11.6–14.8
Platelets	110	140 to 400 × 10^3/microL
DIFFERENTIAL		
Neutrophils	40	40%–75% (2.7–6.5 × 10^3/microL)
Lymphocytes	50	12%–44% (1.5–3.7 × 10^3/microL)
Monocytes	2	4%–9% (0.2-0.4 × 10^3/microL)
Eosinophils	6	0%–5.5% (0.05–0.5 × 10^3/microL)
Basophils	20	0%–1% (0–0.1 × 10^3/microL)

   1. Assess for an infection.
   2. Assess for bleeding.
   3. Assess for shortness of breath.
   4. Assess for pallor.

6. At 1000, the client diagnosed with cancer and receiving chemotherapy is reporting unrelieved nausea. Which intervention should the nurse implement?

Client: W.S.	MR# 1234567	Date: Today
Age: 60 years	Allergies: NKDA	Diagnosis: Cancer
Medication	**0701–1900**	**1901–0700**
Ondansetron 4 mg IVP every 4 hours PRN	0900 DN/RN	0100 NN/RN 0500 NN/RN
Morphine 2 mg IVP every 2–3 hours PRN		0315 NN/RN
Prochlorperazine 5 mg PO t.i.d. PRN		0639 NN/RN
Nurse Initials/Credentials	**DN/RN**	**NN/RN**

1. Administer another prochlorperazine.
2. Discuss the nausea medications with the HCP.
3. Teach the client how to control nausea at home.
4. Turn the client on their side to prevent aspiration.

7. The client diagnosed with cancer has developed diarrhea after the third round of chemotherapy. Which intervention should the clinic nurse implement?
1. Have the client take up to 12 loperamide 2-mg tablets per day.
2. Place the client on a clear liquid diet.
3. Medicate the client with promethazine suppositories.
4. Discuss adding a fiber supplement to the client's diet.

8. The client has received five treatments of combination chemotherapy for a diagnosis of lung cancer. Which data indicates the medications **are effective**?
1. The client's hair has begun to grow back in again.
2. The client only has nausea during the treatments.
3. The client reports being able to ambulate around the block.
4. The client's lung sounds are clear.

9. Which statement by the client receiving adjunct chemotherapy for a breast cancer diagnosis **warrants immediate** intervention by the nurse?
1. The client reports numbness and tingling in her feet.
2. The client reports that she feels unattractive without hair.
3. The client says she is unable to eat for 2 days after treatment.
4. The client tells the nurse she has lost 2 pounds since the last treatment.

10. The client receiving IV chemotherapy was nauseated and vomited twice the day before. Which intervention should the nurse implement?
1. Ask the dietary department to provide full liquids.
2. Hold all meal trays until the client is not nauseated.
3. Premedicate the client before each meal.
4. Have the client suck on ice chips frequently.

Biologic Response Modifier

11. Which instruction(s) should the nurse teach the client receiving oprelvekin? **Select all that apply.**
    1. Report any edema of arms, legs, or both.
    2. Take the pill with food to prevent gastric distress.
    3. Monitor the blood glucose levels daily.
    4. Inform the HCP if vision becomes blurred.
    5. Store the medication in the refrigerator.

12. The client diagnosed with chronic kidney disease is prescribed erythropoietin. Which intervention should the nurse implement? **Select all that apply.**
    1. Administer it intramuscularly in the deltoid.
    2. Have the client take acetaminophen for pain.
    3. Monitor the client's CBC.
    4. Teach the client to pace activities.
    5. Inform the client not to drive for 90 days.

13. **Complete the sentence by choosing from the list of options.**

    The health-care provider (HCP) prescribed interferon alfa-2b to a client diagnosed with hepatitis C. The nurse knows that the scientific rationale for this medication administration is to ______________________
    1. Suppress cell proliferation in proliferative diseases.
    2. Decrease production of cytotoxic macrophages.
    3. Increase production of suppressor genes.
    4. Reprogram virus-infected cells to inhibit virus replication.

14. The client diagnosed with cancer has received several treatments of combination chemotherapy. The client's current laboratory values are populated in the chart below.

Laboratory Test	Client Values	Reference Values
Neutrophils	79%	40% to 75%
White blood cells (WBC)	2.2 (10^3/cells/microL)	4.5–11.1 (10^3/cells/microL)

    Which hematopoietic growth factor should the nurse administer?
    1. Darbepoetin
    2. Oprelvekin
    3. Filgrastim
    4. Erythropoietin

15. The nurse on an oncology floor is administering morning medications. Which medication should the nurse **question**?
    1. Vitamin B_{12} to a client diagnosed with pernicious anemia
    2. Erythropoietin to a client diagnosed with chronic lymphocytic leukemia
    3. Filgrastim to a client diagnosed with a solid tissue tumor
    4. Heparin intravenously to a client diagnosed with disseminated intravascular coagulation (DIC)

16. The nurse is preparing to administer pegfilgrastim. Which interventions should the nurse implement when administering this medication? **Select all that apply.**
    1. Use a 1-mL 5/8-inch syringe needle and administer it in the deltoid muscle.
    2. Mix the powder with sterile normal saline and administer it within 1 hour.
    3. Assess the client's blood pressure and pulse before administration.
    4. Hold the medication 24 hours before or after chemotherapy.
    5. Monitor the client's WBC count and the absolute neutrophil count.

17. The client, after receiving darbepoetin, calls the clinic nurse and reports aching in the back and legs. Which statement is the nurse's **best response**?
 1. "This is unrelated to the medication. You may be getting the flu."
 2. "You should come to the clinic immediately to see the HCP."
 3. "This is an expected side effect of the medication and can be treated."
 4. "Have you taken your blood pressure medication today?"

18. Which client should the nurse **question** receiving epoetin alfa?

1.

Client: J.S.	MR# 345555	Date: Today
Age: 74 years	Allergies: Penicillin	Diagnosis: End-stage renal disease
Sex: Female	Height: 64 inches	Weight: 50 kg

2.

Client: M.A.	MR# 875334	Date: Today
Age: 44 years	Allergies: NKDA	Diagnosis: Essential hypertension
Sex: Male	Height: 72 inches	Weight: 113 kg

3.

Client: J.S.	MR# 345555	Date: Today
Age: 60 years	Allergies: Sulfa drugs	Diagnosis: Lung cancer and metastasis
Sex: Female	Height: 66 inches	Weight: 60 kg

4.

Client: W.D.S.	MR# 3290809	Date: Today
Age: 14 years	Allergies: NKDA	Diagnosis: Anemia and leukopenia
Sex: Male	Height: 63 inches	Weight: 47 kg

19. The client on the medical unit diagnosed with anemia is a Jehovah's Witness and the HCP orders erythropoietin. Which intervention should the nurse implement?
 1. Question the order on religious grounds.
 2. Have the client sign an informed consent.
 3. Ask the laboratory to confirm the RBC count.
 4. Administer the medication subcutaneously.

20. The client is scheduled to receive anakinra. Which data should make the nurse **question** administering the medication?
 1. The client has joint deformities of the hands.
 2. The client has a temperature of 100.4°F (38°C).
 3. The client received a dose 2 days ago at the same time.
 4. The client took acetaminophen for a headache 2 hours ago.

Hormone Therapy

21. The 45-year-old female client with a family history of breast cancer asks the nurse, "Is there anything I can do to improve my chances of not getting breast cancer like my sister and mother?" Which statement is the nurse's **best** response?
 1. "There are medications and lifestyle changes to reduce the risk."
 2. "No. Clients that have a strong family history just have to hope they don't get it."
 3. "You sound worried. Would you like to talk about how you feel?"
 4. "Do any other relatives have breast or other female cancers?"

22. **Complete the sentence by choosing from the list of options.**

The HCP has prescribed hormone suppression therapy to the client diagnosed with prostate cancer. The nurse knows that the scientific rationale for this medication administration is to ______________________________
1. Increase the client's libido and ability to maintain an erection.
2. Shrink the prostate tissue by destroying tumor cells during replication.
3. Produce menopausal-like symptoms.
4. Decrease cellular growth.

23. The male client diagnosed with prostate cancer is receiving a leuprolide implant. Which procedure is the **correct** method of administration?
1. Use a tuberculin syringe and administer it subcutaneously.
2. Insert the 16-gauge needle at a 30-degree angle into the abdomen.
3. Place the medication into the rectal vault using a nonsterile glove.
4. Administer with an antacid to prevent peptic ulcer disease.

24. The postmenopausal client diagnosed with breast cancer is placed on anastrozole. Which data indicates the medication is **effective**?
1. The client reports a positive body image.
2. The client can discuss her feelings openly.
3. The client's bone and lung scans are negative.
4. The client's DNA ploidy tests show diploid cells.

25. The client diagnosed with AIDS is prescribed megestrol. Which data indicates the medication is **effective**?
1. The Kaposi's lesions have become light brown.
2. The client ate 90% of the meals served.
3. The client experiences a decrease in nausea.
4. The client can complete activities of daily living (ADLs).

26. The client diagnosed with a brain tumor is prescribed dexamethasone. Which instructions should the nurse teach? **Select all that apply.**
1. "Take the medication with food."
2. "The medication may increase appetite."
3. "Do not abruptly stop taking the medication."
4. "Decadron may cause a headache and nystagmus (involuntary eye movements)."
5. "Let me show you how to perform a subcutaneous injection."

27. The female client had a left breast biopsy that revealed breast carcinoma. The following laboratory data reports estrogen and progesterone influence on the tumor. Which medications should the nurse discuss with the client?

Client: J.D.	MR# 567890	Date: Yesterday
Cytochemical Report		
Estrogen receptor assay: Greater than 45% of the cell nuclei stained Progesterone receptor assay: Greater than 20% of the cell nuclei stained		

1. Supplemental estrogen and progesterone hormone
2. Glucocorticoid and mineral corticoid hormones
3. Gonadotropin-releasing hormone (GnRH) agonists
4. Antiestrogen and progesterone hormone medications

28. The 60-year-old female client has taken hormone replacement therapy (HRT) to control menopausal symptoms for the last 9 years. Which statement by the nurse indicates the client's **risk** for developing breast cancer?
1. "The risk of getting cancer decreases each year that the client takes hormones."
2. "The risk is the same as for women not taking HRT."
3. "The risk increases each year the client is taking HRT."
4. "The risk is only slightly greater while taking HRT."

29. The 39-year-old female client diagnosed with breast cancer is prescribed tamoxifen. Which information is **most important** for the nurse to teach the client?
1. The medication will cause menopause symptoms.
2. Tamoxifen may cause vaginal discharge and nausea.
3. Tamoxifen will slow the growth of estrogen-positive tumors.
4. It is essential to see the gynecologist regularly.

Investigational Protocol

30. The client is scheduled to receive an investigational medication for cancer treatment. Which is the nurse's **first** intervention?
1. Explain the risks and benefits of the medication to the client.
2. Administer the medication per the protocol.
3. Contact the pharmacy to deliver the medication to the unit.
4. Find information on administration procedures and side effects.

31. Which statement is the **primary** reason to enroll a client in an investigational protocol for cancer treatment?
1. The HCP feels that the investigational drug has the best chance of a cure.
2. The client has failed conventional treatment, and there is a poor prognosis.
3. The HCP can provide care at a reduced rate because of subsidies.
4. The client does not like the standard treatment regimen for their disease.

32. The registered nurse (RN) is caring for clients on an oncology unit. Which task is an **appropriate** delegation or assignment by the nurse? **Select all that apply.**
1. Have the licensed practical nurse (LPN) administer the IV investigational medication.
2. Request the unlicensed assistive personnel (UAP) to measure and record the client output.
3. Assign a new graduate nurse to care for a client receiving PRBCs.
4. Delegate care of a seriously ill client taking an investigational drug to a RN.
5. Ask the UAP to reposition the client receiving an investigational drug.

33. The nurse is working in a clinic that uses investigational protocols to determine the effectiveness of new medications. Which information regarding use of placebo medications should the nurse teach the clients?
1. Placebos are not used in investigational protocols because of ethical considerations.
2. The placebo will contain the active ingredient under study in the protocol.
3. Clients in the control group will receive a medication that does not help the disease.
4. Clients should insist on not being placed in the group that gets the placebo pill.

34. The nurse working in an outpatient clinic is screening clients for inclusion in an investigational medication protocol for rheumatoid arthritis (RA). Which screening questions should the nurse include? **Select all that apply.**
1. Which medications has the client been prescribed for arthritis?
2. Which herbs and over-the-counter (OTC) medications have the client taken?
3. Is the client allergic to any soaps or clothing dyes?
4. Does the client have any other immune system disease?
5. Does the client have insurance to pay for the medication?

35. The client participating in an investigational protocol calls the clinic and tells the nurse that the medications have made them "sick to my stomach all night." Which statement is the nurse's **best response**?
1. "You should consider whether or not you want to be in the study."
2. "This must be uncomfortable for you. Let's talk about your feelings."
3. "Come to the clinic to see the HCP. You may be reacting to the drug."
4. "This is a temporary problem and will go away with future doses."

36. The client receiving an investigational medication protocol must be hydrated with at least 1,000 mL of IV fluid in the 4 hours immediately before infusion of the investigational medication. At which rate would the nurse set the pump?

____

37. The nurse is administering medications on a medical unit. Which medication should the nurse administer **first**?
1. The investigational medication to a client wanting to go home now
2. The investigational medication to the client who has not signed a permit
3. The investigational medication that must be administered at a specific time
4. The investigational medication that must infuse over 24 hours

38. The nurse on an oncology unit is administering morning investigational protocol medications. To which client stating the following should the nurse **question** administering medications?
1. "I am sure I am getting better every day."
2. "I'm not sure I want to continue this treatment."
3. "The doctor told me there were no guarantees."
4. "Can you explain the side effects of the medication?"

Surgery for Cancer

39. The client has had an implanted port placed to receive chemotherapy. When the nurse attempts to access the device, there is no backflow of blood, and the nurse meets resistance when flushing. Which intervention should the nurse take to access the implanted port?
1. Forcefully insert 3 mL of heparin into the port.
2. Flush the implanted port with 5 to 10 mL of normal saline.
3. Instill a prescribed amount of urokinase into the port.
4. Schedule the client for a newly implanted port placement.

40. The nurse is accessing a newly implanted port IV line. Which interventions should the nurse implement? **Rank in order of performance.**
1. Set up the sterile field and don sterile gloves.
2. Cleanse the skin with antiseptic skin prep.
3. Palpate the port rim with two fingers.
4. Insert a noncoring needle between the fingers.
5. Explain the procedure to the client and wash hands.

41. The client diagnosed with cancer of the head of the pancreas has had a Whipple procedure (pancreatoduodenectomy). Which discharge instructions should the nurse teach the client?
1. "Administer insulin subcutaneously."
2. "Take acetaminophen for an elevated temperature."
3. "Change the surgical dressing weekly."
4. "Increase the calories and protein in the diet."

42. The nurse assesses excoriated, contaminated skin surrounding the colostomy stoma of a client diagnosed with colon cancer. Which intervention should the nurse implement **first**?
1. Request a consult from a wound ostomy continence nurse.
2. Apply a skin barrier protectant paste around the stoma.
3. Gently cleanse the area with mild soap and water.
4. Replace the pouch with one that is 1/3 inch larger than the stoma.

43. The client diagnosed with prostate cancer has had prostate surgery using spinal anesthesia. Which safety precaution should the postanesthesia care nurse use?
1. Cover the client with a heating device to avoid hypothermia.
2. Keep the head of the bed elevated until feeling returns to the legs.
3. Medicate the client with IV narcotic analgesics for pain.
4. Hold pressure on the epidural insertion site for at least 5 minutes.

44. The client with an implanted port has completed the chemotherapy medications and is ready for discharge. Which intervention should the nurse take to prepare the client for discharge?
1. Teach the client how to manage the port at home.
2. Insert a sterile, noncoring needle into the port.
3. Flush the port with saline followed by heparin.
4. Scrub the port access with povidone-iodine.

45. The client diagnosed with ovarian cancer had an extensive bowel resection and is receiving total parenteral nutrition (TPN). Which laboratory data should the nurse monitor daily?
1. Blood urea nitrogen and creatinine levels
2. Sodium, potassium, and glucose levels
3. Urine and serum osmolality levels
4. CA-125 and carcinoembryonic antigen (CEA)

46. The client had a right upper lobectomy for a lung cancer diagnosis and returns to the intensive care unit with a patient-controlled analgesia (PCA) pump for pain control. Which intervention should the nurse implement **first**?
1. Show the client how to use the PCA pump.
2. Obtain a new cartridge of medication.
3. Determine the level of pain relief obtained.
4. Check the HCP orders against the settings.

47. The client had a Whipple resection (pancreatoduodenectomy) for pancreatic cancer and has arterial blood gas values populated in the chart below.

Arterial Blood Gas		Adult Reference Values
pH	7.29	7.35 to 7.45
Pco_2	40	35 to 45 mm Hg
Hco_3	18	22 to 26 mmol/L
Po_2	100	80 to 95 mm Hg

Which medication should the nurse prepare to administer?
1. IV normal saline at a keep-open rate
2. IV insulin by continuous infusion
3. Sodium bicarbonate intravenously
4. Sliding-scale insulin isophane subcutaneous

Chronic Pain

48. The client diagnosed with terminal cancer is experiencing significant pain. Which information is **most important** for the hospice nurse to teach the client and significant other?
1. If the pain medications are not working, try to divert the client's attention.
2. Take pain medications at the onset of pain before it becomes severe.
3. Do not allow family or friends to visit when the client is in pain.
4. Too much narcotic pain medication will cause the client to become addicted.

49. The client calls the nursing station and requests pain medication. When the nurse enters the room with the narcotic medication, the nurse finds the client laughing and talking with visitors. Which intervention should the nurse implement?
1. Administer the client's prescribed pain medication.
2. Confront the client's narcotic-seeking behavior.
3. Wait until the visitors leave to administer any medication.
4. Check the MAR to see if there is a nonnarcotic medication ordered.

50. Which discharge instructions should the nurse provide for the client diagnosed with cancer taking hydrocodone with acetaminophen as needed (PRN) for pain?
1. Take the medication only when the pain is severe.
2. Use acetaminophen for any pain unrelieved by the medication.
3. Notify the HCP if the medication relieves the pain.
4. Increase the fluid intake and roughage in the diet.

51. The client diagnosed with cancer notifies the nurse of pain that is "11" on the pain scale but cannot localize it to a specific area or describe when it began. Which intervention should the nurse implement?
1. Discuss the importance of knowing where the pain is located.
2. Prepare to administer the prescribed narcotic pain medication.
3. Refer the client to a chaplain or social worker for counseling.
4. Ask the client to use the Faces Pain Scale to rate the pain.

52. The terminally ill client reports that the pain is getting progressively worse despite hourly IV narcotic pain medication administered in increasingly higher doses. Which intervention should the nurse implement?
1. Request an increase in medication dosage from the HCP.
2. Ask the significant other to try to distract the client.
3. Use therapeutic communication to discuss the client's concerns.
4. Teach the client nonpharmacologic pain control measures.

53. The client diagnosed with cancer tells the nurse that they hate feeling "doped up" during the day but need pain medication to rest at night. Which statement is the nurse's **best response**?
1. "Sometimes it is necessary to take as much medication as you can to get to sleep. Ask the HCP for stronger medications."
2. "I am sure that this must be uncomfortable for you. You need to talk about how you are feeling."
3. "We could try to balance your pain medications with sleeping medications to help you get comfortable at night."
4. "Too much pain medication will cause you to have many other complications and should be avoided."

54. The nurse administered narcotic pain medication to a client diagnosed with cancer then assessed the client 30 minutes later. Which data indicates the medication was **effective**?
1. The client keeps their eyes closed, and the drapes are drawn.
2. The client uses guided imagery to help with pain control.
3. The client states that the pain has gone down 5 points on the scale.
4. The client is lying as still as possible in the bed.

55. The client admitted with intractable pain from an osteosarcoma diagnosis is being discharged. Which information should the nurse emphasize with the client?
   1. The client will need to accept some pain as part of the disease process.
   2. Most pharmacies will be able to fill the medication whenever it is needed.
   3. The client should plan to have an adequate medication supply on weekends and holidays.
   4. The client should return to the hospital if the pain returns.

56. The nurse is caring for a client diagnosed with cancer. At 1000 the client is reporting pain and nausea. Based on the medication administration record (MAR), which intervention should the nurse implement?

Client: M.F.	MR# 1234567	Date: Today
Age: 55 years	Allergies: NKDA	Diagnosis: Cancer
Medication	**0701–1900**	**1901–0700**
Ondansetron 4 mg IVP every 4 hours PRN	0900 DN/RN	
Morphine sulfate 2 mg IVP every 2–3 hours PRN	0800 DN/RN	0575 NN/RN
Liquid morphine sulfate 10 mg PO every hour PRN		0100 NN/RN
Prochlorperazine 5 mg PO t.i.d. PRN	0730 DN/RN	
Prochlorperazine 5–10 mg IVP every 2 hours PRN		
Nurse Initials/Credentials	**DN/RN**	**NN/RN**

   1. Administer liquid morphine 10 mg orally and hold any antiemetic medication.
   2. Administer prochlorperazine and morphine, but use separate syringes.
   3. Administer liquid morphine now and ondansetron in 3 hours.
   4. Administer 2 mg of morphine combined with 10 mg of prochlorperazine IV.

57. The client diagnosed with chronic pain is prescribed morphine sulfate controlled release and liquid morphine. Which statement **best describes** how to administer the medications?
   1. Administer the controlled release morphine at prescribed intervals and the liquid morphine PRN.
   2. Administer both morphine medications PRN for the client's chronic pain.
   3. Administer the liquid morphine every 4 hours and the controlled release morphine PRN pain.
   4. Administer the morphine sulfate controlled release for breakthrough pain and hold the liquid morphine.

ANSWERS AND RATIONALES

The correct answer number and rationale are in **boldface blue type.** Rationales for why other answer options are incorrect are also given.

Chemotherapy

1. Correct answers are 1, 3, and 5.

1. A platelet count of less than 100,000 is the definition of thrombocytopenia. The nurse should teach measures to prevent bleeding, such as using an electric razor.

2. This is good information to teach, but it is not based on the laboratory values. The client's white blood cells (WBC) and absolute neutrophil counts are within the normal range.

3. A platelet count of less than 100,000 is the definition of thrombocytopenia. If the client sustains a cut, the blood will not clot.

4. This is good information to teach, but it is not based on the laboratory values. Fatigue related to cancer and its treatment is real and should be addressed, and Hgb and Hct levels of around 8 and 24 could cause fatigue, but the client's levels do not indicate this.

5. A platelet count of less than 100,000 is the definition of thrombocytopenia. The nurse should teach measures to prevent bleeding, such as using a soft-bristled toothbrush.

2. 1. A "3" is considered mild pain and could wait until the more emergent client is medicated.

2. Anticipatory nausea and vomiting are very difficult to control. The nurse needs to medicate the client to prevent nausea. This client should be medicated first.

3. At 0900 the breakfast tray meal should have already been consumed. Administering a mucosal barrier agent after a meal places medication in the stomach that will coat the food, not the stomach lining. This medication should be retimed for 0730 and not administered until later in the morning after the breakfast meal has had a chance to leave the stomach for this dose.

4. This medication stimulates bone marrow to produce RBCs. The medication's full effect will not be seen for 30 to 90 days. It could be administered after the antiemetic and analgesic.

3. 1. This is not normal and could indicate that the client is developing neuropathy from the medications. The danger is that the innervation to the small bowel may be compromised as well. It will not go away when the therapy is complete.

2. This is not a minor side effect of the medication; it may indicate that the client must be changed to a different antineoplastic agent.

3. This may indicate a potential life-altering complication of chemotherapy. The client may have nerve damage caused by the mitotic inhibitors or plant alkaloid medications. The intestinal nerves may also be compromised, causing decreased peristalsis. The nurse should assess the situation and notify the HCP (American Cancer Society, 2021).

4. Plant alkaloid medications do not cause orthostatic hypotension.

4. 1. The client should be given information regarding potential complications of therapy and when to notify the HCP. A temperature of 100°F (37.7°C) or more should be immediately discussed with the HCP. The client could be developing an infection and must be treated as soon as possible.

2. The client may or may not need dietary supplements at this time. The client should be referred to a dietitian for a consultation regarding nutritional status, but dietary supplements three times a day would not allow the client to enjoy normal foods. This would be recommended if the client were not tolerating any normal dietary intake.

3. Clients should not isolate themselves from enjoying the extended family. They should be told to avoid clients diagnosed with a known contagious illness.

4. If the client has a tender vein that has been assessed by the HCP and found not to be extravasation of the medication, the client can apply intermittent warm packs. Ice packs restrict blood flow to the area.

MEDICATION MEMORY JOGGER: Usual discharge instructions include teaching the client to notify the HCP in case of a fever. The test taker might choose this option based on standard procedure.

5\. 1. **The client has a low WBC count, which is 2.4 times 10^3, or 2,400 actual WBCs counted. Of this amount, only 40% are mature neutrophils capable of fighting a bacterial invasion. Multiply 2,400 times 40% (0.4) and determine that the absolute neutrophil count is 960. This count, far below the normal count, puts the client at risk for infection. The nurse should assess the client for infection.**
2. The client's platelet count is less than normal (140,000–400,000), but it is still greater than 100,000. Less than 100,000 is thrombocytopenia. Critical values begin at 50,000.
3. The client's Hgb level is less than normal, but not critically low. This client might fatigue easily because of oxygen demands on the body, but should not be short of breath with this Hgb level.
4. The Hgb and Hct levels are below normal in values, but not enough for the client to become pale as a result.

MEDICATION MEMORY JOGGER: The nurse must be aware of which laboratory values should be monitored for specific medication administration.

6\. 1. Prochlorperazine (Compazine Spansules) is used before meals to control nausea so the client can eat. This did not control nausea, so the nurse should discuss the situation with the HCP.
2. **The client is having unrelieved nausea, and the night nurse has already tried to control the nausea with all medication that the HCP has ordered. It is time to notify the HCP to discuss alternative medications or increase the dosage of ondansetron (Zofran).**
3. Clients experiencing discomfort are not ready to be taught anything. This client needs to know that controlling nausea is possible in the hospital before being ready to learn how to control it at home.
4. The stem of the question did not say the client was sedated. There is no reason to position the client on the side.

7\. 1. The maximum dose of loperamide (Imodium), an antidiarrheal, per day is 16 mg. This would exceed the recommended dose per day.
2. Clear liquids will not provide the needed bulk to the stools and will not provide sufficient calories to prevent malnutrition.
3. Promethazine (Phenergan) is an antiemetic, not an antidiarrheal, and any medication administered by the rectal route would probably be expelled before absorbing into the client's system.
4. **Clients experiencing diarrhea need to add bulk to the diet in the form of fiber supplements or dietary intake to decrease the liquid nature of the stools.**

8\. 1. The client's hair will grow when treatments are discontinued and sometimes during the treatments, but this does not indicate the medications are killing cancer cells.
2. Nausea during or after treatments is not a measure of cell kill.
3. **The client being able to tolerate activity indicates the client has adequate lung capacity. This indicates the lung cancer has not enveloped the entire lung field and that medications are effective. Lung cancer has a poor prognosis, and the treatment goal is to improve or maintain quality of life.**
4. The client's lung fields being clear does not indicate the quality of life or cell kill.

9\. 1. **This client may have metastasis to the spinal column, and this information should be immediately reported to the HCP for emergency evaluation. The client could become paralyzed.**
2. Body image suffers when a client has alopecia (hair loss) from antineoplastic agents, but it is not life-threatening or permanent.
3. Being able to resume nutritional intake after 2 days is not a cause for immediate intervention by the nurse.
4. Treatments are scheduled every 3 to 4 weeks, and a 2-pound weight loss is not significant in this time period.

10\. 1. The client should receive whatever the client wishes to eat within the prescribed diet. The nurse should not autocratically decide the client should consume full liquids.
2. The client may wish to attempt to eat. The nurse should not autocratically decide the client should not eat.
3. **The client may tolerate meals after receiving an antiemetic medication 30 minutes before each meal. The nurse can administer a PRN medication before each meal or request a routine medication order from the HCP.**
4. The client will not become dehydrated while receiving IV fluids with antineoplastic medications. Ice chips will not prevent nausea.

Biologic Response Modifier

11. Correct answers are 1, 4, and 5.

1. **Oprelvekin (Neumega) is a biologic response modifier that acts on the bone marrow to increase platelet production. It can also cause cardiovascular stimulation, tachycardia, vasodilation, palpitations, dysrhythmias, and edema. The client should report any of these clinical manifestations as well as shortness of breath or blurred vision immediately.**
2. Oprelvekin (Neumega), a biologic response modifier, is administered by subcutaneous injection.
3. Oprelvekin (Neumega), a biologic response modifier, does not affect blood glucose levels.
4. **The client should notify the HCP of blurred vision immediately so the medication can be discontinued. Blurred vision could indicate papilledema (optic nerve swelling) (University of Pennsylvania, 2021).**
5. **Oprelvekin (Neumega) should be stored in the refrigerator.**

12. Correct answers are 2, 3, 4, and 5.

1. Erythropoietin (Procrit or Epogen) is a biologic response modifier that stimulates the body to produce RBC. The medication is administered subcutaneously.
2. **Erythropoietin (Procrit or Epogen) is a biologic response modifier that stimulates the bone marrow to produce RBCs. Bone marrow is located inside the bones. The client may experience aches and pains in the bony areas as a result. Tylenol usually will remedy this side effect.**
3. **Epogen stimulates RBC production, and the CBC should be monitored at regular intervals.**
4. **This should be done for any client diagnosed with anemia to prevent fatigue. The medication is ordered to treat anemia.**
5. **Because the potential for seizures exists during periods of rapid Hct increase, the client should be warned not to drive or operate any heavy equipment for 90 days until the Hct has stabilized.**

13. 1. Interferon alfa-2b (Intron A), a biologic response modifier, is useful for several disease processes because of its different mechanisms of action. Suppression of cell proliferation is the desired action in clients diagnosed with leukemia.

2. Interferon alfa-2b (Intron A) does not affect macrophages.
3. Intron A does not increase tumor suppressor genes.
4. **Interferon alfa-2b (Intron A) reprograms virus-infected cells to inhibit viral replication. This is the reason that it is useful in treating hepatitis.**

14. 1. Darbepoetin (Aranesp) is a hematopoietin growth factor that stimulates RBC production. The question does not give the client's RBC count. (The advantage of Aranesp over Procrit or Epogen, which also stimulates RBC production, is that it is administered once a week instead of daily.)

2. Prelvekin (Neumega) is a hematopoietin growth factor that stimulates platelet production. The question does not refer to the client's platelet count.
3. **Filgrastrim (Neupogen) is a hematopoietic growth factor that stimulates WBC production. This client has a low WBC count and thus is at risk for an infection. The client's absolute neutrophil count is only 1,738 (2.2 multiplied by 1,000 equals 2,200, then multiply this number by 0.79 to get 1,738). Clients with an absolute neutrophil count below 2,500 are at risk for infection.**
4. Erythropoietin (Epogen or Procrit) is a hematopoietic growth factor that stimulates RBC production.

15. 1. Vitamin B_{12} (Cyanocobalamin), a vitamin replacement, is the treatment for pernicious anemia. The nurse would not question administering this medication.

2. **Erythropoietin (Epogen or Procrit) is a biologic response modifier that stimulates the bone marrow to produce more cells. Stimulation of bone marrow is questioned when the cancer is in the bone marrow.**
3. Filgrastim is a biologic response modifier that stimulates WBC production. Stimulation of the bone marrow is not questioned in clients diagnosed with solid tissue tumors. The nurse would not question administering this medication.
4. Heparin is part of the standard treatment regimen for disseminated intravascular coagulation.

16. **Correct answers are 1, 4, and 5.**
 1. **Pegfilgrastim (Neulasta) is a hematopoietic growth factor that stimulates WBC production over an extended period. The medication is administered subcutaneously with a 1-mL, 5/8-inch needle, and the deltoid muscle is an appropriate area to administer the medication.**
 2. The medication comes in a vial of 10 mg per mL already prepared. If mixed for an IV infusion, dextrose 5% in water is used.
 3. The client receiving an RBC stimulant (Epogen, Procrit, Aranesp) should have their blood pressure monitored because rapid increases in Hct will also increase blood pressure. This does not happen with Neulasta, which stimulates WBC production.
 4. **Pegfilgrastim (Neulasta) is a hematopoietic growth factor that stimulates WBC production over an extended period. Cytotoxic chemotherapy acts on the bone marrow to decrease WBC production, an opposite response. The nurse should hold the medication and resume it 24 hours after chemotherapy administration.**
 5. **The nurse should monitor WBC and absolute neutrophil count to determine if Neulasta is effective.**

17. 1. Darbepoetin (Aranesp) is an extended-release formulation of a biologic response modifier that stimulates RBC production. Aching in the back and legs is probably caused by bone marrow hyperstimulation to produce RBCs, not by the flu.
 2. Darbepoetin (Aranesp) is an extended-release formulation of a biologic response modifier that stimulates RBC production. The HCP does not need to see the client immediately. Acetaminophen (Tylenol) will usually treat the problem. The HCP only needs to see the client if OTC analgesic medications do not relieve the pain.
 3. **Darbepoetin (Aranesp) is an extended release formulation of a biologic response modifier that stimulates RBC production. Bone marrow Hyperstimulation is the probable cause of the aches and should be treated with OTC pain medications.**
 4. Darbepoetin (Aranesp) is an extended release formulation of a biologic response modifier that stimulates RBC production. The client's blood pressure should be monitored during administration of medications that increase Hct, but not taking blood pressure medication would not cause aches in the bones.

MEDICATION MEMORY JOGGER: The nurse must be aware of safety precautions when administering medications.

18. 1. Epoetin alfa (Epogen or Procrit) is a biologic response modifier that stimulates RBC production. Epogen is frequently administered to clients diagnosed with end-stage kidney disease to stimulate their bodies to produce RBCs. The kidneys naturally produce erythropoietin to stimulate RBC production, but clients with renal disease may not be able to produce the cytokine, erythropoietin. It is not contraindicated in elderly clients.
 2. **Epoetin alfa (Epogen or Procrit) is a biologic response modifier that stimulates RBC production. A rapid increase in Hct level, which may occur with Epogen, can result in uncontrolled hypertension. The client must have hypertension well controlled for Epogen to be administered safely. The nurse would question this medication for this client.**
 3. Epoetin alfa (Epogen or Procrit) is a biologic response modifier that stimulates RBC production. The client diagnosed with lung cancer and metastasis would be a candidate for Epogen. The nurse would not question this medication.
 4. Epoetin alfa (Epogen or Procrit) is a biologic response modifier that stimulates RBC production. Epogen is given to clients diagnosed with anemia. Leukopenia will not be increased or decreased by the medication. Epoetin alpha can be given to pediatric clients over one month of age.

19. 1. Members of the Jehovah's Witnesses church refuse to allow transfusion of blood and blood products. Procrit is not a blood product; it is the client's own body making RBCs. There is no reason to question the medication on religious grounds.
 2. The client in the hospital signs a permit to treat when admitted. There is no need for another consent form.
 3. The laboratory does not need to confirm the data.
 4. **The nurse should administer the medication. Erythropoietin (Procrit) is administered subcutaneously.**

20. 1. Anakinra (Kineret) is an immune modulator. Hand deformities indicate RA. Anakinra (Interleukin 1) is used to treat RA in clients having failed other treatments.

2. Anakinra (Kineret) is an immune modulator. This medication suppresses the immune system and should not be administered to anyone with an infection. A temperature greater than 100°F (37.7°C) indicates an infection.

3. The normal dosing schedule is every 2 days at the same time.

4. Acetaminophen (Tylenol) does not interfere with Anakinra, and a headache would not indicate an infection.

Hormone Therapy

21. 1. Tamoxifen (Tamofen) and raloxifene (Evista), anti-estrogen medications, have been researched in the STAR trial and have proven efficacy in reducing risk of breast cancer in women having primary relatives with breast cancer. Lifestyle modifications such as consuming a low-fat diet and avoiding obesity are also recommended to reduce risk of breast cancer.

2. There are lifestyle modifications and hormone-suppressing medications that can reduce the risk of developing breast cancer.

3. The client is asking for information and the nurse should provide factual information.

4. This statement does not address the client's question.

22. 1. Hormone suppression therapy in a male client would decrease the client's libido and decrease the ability to sustain an erection.

2. Hormone suppression therapy does not destroy cancer cells; it works by changing the hormonal environment of the host and depriving cancer of the hormones that stimulate its growth.

3. This is a true statement, but it is not the rationale for how the medications work in the body.

4. Gender-specific cancers may replicate better in the presence of hormones specific to that sex. Suppressing the androgens produced in the testes results in a reduction in the tumor growth rate.

23. 1. Leuprolide (Lupron) is a luteinizing hormone-releasing hormone (LHRH) agonist. The medication is an implant that slowly dissolves. The drug is formulated in a pellet that is dispensed through a 16-gauge needle.

2. Leuprolide (Lupron) is a LHRH agonist. Lupron is an implant that slowly dissolves over 1 month to 6 months depending on the dosage. The drug is formulated in a pellet that is dispensed through a 16-gauge needle under the skin on the abdomen (American Cancer Society, 2021b).

3. Leuprolide acetate (Lupron) is a LHRH agonist. This is not a suppository.

4. Leuprolide acetate (Lupron) is a LHRH agonist. The medication does not cause PUD and is not administered orally.

24. 1. Anastrozole (Armidex) is an aromatase inhibitor. Aromatase inhibitors block estrogen production and androgen precursors, but they do not have any positive effect on body image. The client may experience a negative effect on body image if she develops facial hair (hirsutism).

2. Anastrozole (Armidex) is an aromatase inhibitor. Aromatase inhibitors are not antidepressants and would not affect the client's ability to express her feelings.

3. Anastrozole (Armidex) is an aromatase inhibitor. Aromatase inhibitors are used to treat postmenopausal breast cancer. Two prime metastasis sites for breast cancer are the lungs and bones. Negative findings in these areas indicate the medication is effective.

4. DNA ploidy tests are conducted on tumor cells at the beginning of treatment to determine disease prognosis. The test is not used to monitor therapy progress.

25. 1. Megestrol (Megace) is an antineoplastic medication. Kaposi's lesions are normally light brown to a purple color, so this does not indicate medication effectiveness.

2. Megestrol (Megace) is an antineoplastic medication. Megace is an antineoplastic hormone used to treat metastatic cancer of the breast and endometrium. A medication side effect is an increased appetite. It is prescribed in unlabeled use for improving the appetite in clients diagnosed with AIDS under the name of Appetrol.

3. Megestrol (Megace) is an antineoplastic medication. Megace does not treat nausea.

4. Megestrol (Megace) is an antineoplastic medication. Megace would not affect the ability to perform ADLs, except indirectly by increasing the client's nutritional intake.

MEDICATION MEMORY JOGGER: The nurse must be aware that some medications are used for other than the original purpose. Megace is one such medication.

26. **Correct answers are 1, 2, and 3.**
   1. **Dexamethasone (Decadron) is a glucocorticoid. All steroids can cause gastric upset, so the client should take the medication with food.**
   2. **Dexamethasone (Decadron) is a glucocorticoid. Steroids usually increase appetite, contributing to the client's weight gain.**
   3. **Dexamethasone (Decadron) is a glucocorticoid. Decadron is a steroid, and when discontinuing a steroid, the client should be informed about tapering the medication. Decadron is the steroid of choice for disease processes occurring in the skull.**
   4. Dexamethasone (Decadron) is a glucocorticoid. The client may have a headache because of increased intracranial pressure from the tumor growth. Decadron decreases edema surrounding the tumor and would help to prevent a headache.
   5. Dexamethasone (Decadron) is a glucocorticoid. Decadron is administered orally or IV, not subcutaneously.

27. 1. This laboratory data indicates that the client's tumors grow best in the presence of estrogen and progesterone. Supplemental estrogen and progesterone would encourage tumor growth.
   2. The adrenal hormones are not indicated by this laboratory data.
   3. GnRH medications are used to suppress male androgens in clients diagnosed with prostate cancer.
   4. **Estrogen and progesterone receptor assays are interpreted as follows: greater than 20% is favorable to tumor growth, 11% to 20% is borderline, and less than 10% is unfavorable. A favorable finding indicates that the client's tumor responds well to the presence of estrogen and progesterone. Suppressing or removing the ability to produce these hormones slows tumor growth. Anti-estrogen and progesterone hormone medications would accomplish this.**

28. 1. This is a false statement. The risk increases with prolonged use.
   2. This is a false statement. Evidence indicates that the risk increases for women taking HRT.
   3. **Risk of developing breast cancer increases each year the client takes HRT. Current research also implicates HRT in the development of cardiovascular disease.**
   4. This is a false statement. The risk increases with prolonged use.

29. 1. Tamoxifen (Nolvadex or Tamofen) is an anti-estrogen. Nolvadex will cause menopausal symptoms, but this is not the most important consideration to teach the client.
   2. Tamoxifen (Nolvadex or Tamofen) is an anti-estrogen. Nolvadex may cause vaginal discharge and nausea, but this is not the most important consideration to teach the client.
   3. Tamoxifen (Nolvadex or Tamofen) is an anti-estrogen. The fact that Nolvadex slows growth of estrogen-positive tumors is the scientific rationale for administering this medication, but it is not the most important consideration to teach the client.
   4. **Tamoxifen (Nolvadex or Tamofen) is an anti-estrogen. Tamoxifen increases the client's risk of developing endometrial cancer. Tamoxifen acts as an estrogen agonist on receptors in the uterus, causing proliferation of endometrial tissue that may result in endometrial cancer. For this reason, the client must see the gynecologist regularly. This is the most important information to teach the client.**

Investigational Protocol

30. 1. Explaining the medication's risks and benefits to the client is the HCP's responsibility, not the nurse's.
   2. The nurse should administer the medication per protocol, but not until the nurse knows the mechanism of action and potential side effects.
   3. The nurse cannot administer the medication until it is available, but this is not the first action.
   4. **The nurse must know what the drug is, how it works in the body, and the potential side effects to assess before administering any medication, especially an investigational medication.**

MEDICATION MEMORY JOGGER: If the test taker placed the options in order of performance, then the test taker could eliminate options 2 and 3.

31. 1. The HCP will enroll clients that fit the protocol requirements. An investigational protocol is being tried to determine treatment efficacy, weighing risks and benefits to the client. The investigation part is to determine what the risks and benefits are. It is not necessarily the best chance for a cure.
2. Ethically, oncology clients will not be enrolled in a protocol if standard therapy regimens have a good chance of providing an extension of life or quality of life for the client. If the client has received conventional therapy and has not responded well, the HCP may suggest an investigational protocol. Usually, this means the client has a poor prognosis before an investigational protocol is discussed.
3. Investigational protocol medication- and treatment-related expenses are provided at no cost to the client, but this is not the primary reason to place the client in a study.
4. This may be a reason the client chooses to participate in a study, but it is not the primary reason for enrolling the client in an investigational study.

32. Correct answers are 2, 3, 4, and 5.
1. An experienced oncology nurse familiar with the investigational protocol should care for this client; an LPN should not.
2. Measuring and recording client output is an appropriate delegation.
3. A new graduate nurse can care for a client receiving PRBCs. This is an appropriate assignment.
4. Care of a seriously ill client taking an investigational drug can be assigned to a RN.
5. The UAP can reposition the client receiving an investigational drug.

33. 1. Placebos are not unethical as long as the clients have been informed of the possibility of receiving a placebo and of being randomly placed in a control group.
2. A placebo is an inactive substance resembling a medication that may be given experimentally or for its psychological effect.
3. Clients in investigational studies are informed that there are control groups that receive an inert medication for comparison to the medication group to determine the medication's statistical effectiveness in treating the disease being studied.
4. Clients are not allowed to request this, as no client wants to "not be treated." In a true investigational protocol, the clients are randomly selected for the medication group and the control group.

34. Correct answers are 1, 2, and 4.
1. The nurse should ask what has been prescribed for the client and how the client responded to the medications.
2. Herbs and OTC medications may affect the client's response to the proposed medication; therefore, this is an appropriate question to ask the client.
3. Soaps and clothing dyes should not affect administration of a systemic medication for arthritis.
4. The client's response to the investigational medication for an immune system disease (RA) could be affected by a comorbid immune system disease. The nurse should assess this.
5. Medications, required laboratory tests, and HCP visits are free to the client in an investigational protocol. The ability to pay for the medication is not an issue.

35. 1. This is not for the nurse to determine. The HCP should assess the client to decide if the side effect of nausea can be controlled.
2. The client has a real physiological problem, not a psychological one that requires a therapeutic conversation.
3. The HCP should assess the client to determine if the side effect of nausea can be controlled. In any event, the side effects experienced by the client must be documented by the HCP. This is the nurse's best response.
4. This is a misleading and possibly false statement.

36. 250 mL. IV infusion pumps are set at an hourly rate. The nurse is to infuse 1,000 mL in 4 hours. 1,000 divided by 4 equals 250 mL/hour.

37. 1. The client may want to leave "now," but this does not make the client the priority to receive their medication.
2. The nurse cannot administer the medication until the client has signed the protocol permits. This is not the first client to receive the medication.
3. Any medication that requires specific timing should be administered at the time required. This medication has priority.
4. A medication that is to be infused over 24 hours could wait to be administered until after the timed medication.

38. **1. The client is expressing a hope in the treatment. This is not a reason to question administering the medication.**
2. This client is having doubts about continuing the treatment. Until the client decides they wish to continue the treatment, the nurse should hold the medication and have the HCP discuss the client's concerns. The nurse should question administering this medication. The client has the right to withdraw from a protocol at any time.
3. The HCP should never guarantee a positive response for any treatment. The nurse would not question administering the medication.
4. The nurse should explain the medication's side effects to the client. Unless the client has concerns after the nurse teaches the client about the side effects, the nurse should administer the medication.

Surgery for Cancer

39. 1. Forcefully instilling anything into the port will push a clot into the client's body. Heparin is an anticoagulant, not a thrombolytic. It will not dissolve a clot. Anticoagulants prevent clot formation.
2. Flushing anything will infuse a clot into the client's body, possibly resulting in a stroke, pulmonary embolus, or myocardial infarction.
3. Urokinase is a thrombolytic. Instilling a small amount into the lumen of the implanted port and allowing the medication to sit in the catheter may dissolve the clot. The procedure may need to be repeated more than once to dissolve the entire clot (Chang et al., 2017).
4. The HCP determines if a new port should be placed and then schedules the procedure with the surgical staff.

MEDICATION MEMORY JOGGER: The nurse should learn medication by specific classifications. Anticoagulants do not dissolve clots; only thrombolytics dissolve clots. The "ase" ending in urokinase should clue the test taker to choose this option because thrombolytics are enzymes, and enzymes usually end in "ase."

40. **Correct order is 5, 1, 2, 3, 4.**
5. The nurse should always inform the client of procedures before attempting to complete the task. The nurse should wash hands on entering the room.
1. The next step is to prepare the equipment and sterile field for the procedure to begin. Central line dressing kits contain sterile gloves for the nurse to use when performing the procedure.
2. Central line dressing kits include antiseptic solutions to be used to cleanse the skin. The nurse should know and follow the facility's procedure for accessing central line IV catheters.
3. Implanted ports can be palpated through the skin to determine where the port diaphragm is. The nurse then places a finger on each side of the diaphragm to maintain the correct placement target.
4. The diaphragm of the implanted port is designed to be punctured repeatedly over months to years. A noncoring needle (Huber) is used to prevent damage to the diaphragm. The nurse places the needle between the fingers and inserts it until the needle strikes the back of the reservoir.

41. **1. The Whipple procedure removes the islet cells of the pancreas, thus creating diabetes. The client must be knowledgeable about how to treat diabetes and administer insulin.**
2. The client should be instructed to notify the HCP of an elevated temperature, not mask the symptoms of an infection.
3. The client should be taught to change the dressing daily. Waiting until once a week to change the dressing could result in the client having an undiscovered wound infection.
4. The client will now have the diabetes diagnosis and should follow a calorie-controlled diet.

42. 1. This should be done, but the nurse cannot wait until the wound care nurse arrives to implement skin protection for the client.
2. The nurse should apply a skin barrier paste to protect the skin around the stoma after cleansing the stoma and surrounding skin with mild soap and water.
3. The skin barrier paste will not adhere to fecal-contaminated skin. The nurse should first gently cleanse the skin. Mild soap acts as an abrasive to remove feces and old barrier paste.
4. The pouch is replaced after the skin has been cleaned and protected.

43. 1. The client may need a warmed blanket in the postanesthesia care unit (PACU) but not a heating device.

2. If the anesthetic agent reaches the upper thoracic and cervical spinal cord, the client's respiratory muscles may be temporarily paralyzed. Keeping the head of the bed slightly elevated will prevent paralysis from occurring.

3. This would not be a safety measure; it is a pain control measure.

4. The anesthesiologist or nurse anesthetist, not the PACU nurse, is responsible for removing the catheter.

44. 1. The advantage of implanted ports is that the client does not have to care for the port at home. The port should be flushed monthly at the time of the therapy sessions. The skin forms a natural barrier to infection.

2. This is done when the client is being prepared to receive the chemotherapy, not when the client is being discharged.

3. The nurse should ensure that all chemotherapy is infused into the client by flushing the port with normal saline. Instilling heparin into the port, reservoir, and catheter will help prevent clot formation in the catheter.

4. This is done when the client is being prepared to receive the chemotherapy, not when the client is being discharged.

45. 1. These laboratory tests monitor kidney function and are not needed to monitor TPN.

2. TPN solution contains high concentrations of glucose, proteins, lipids, and electrolytes. The nurse should monitor this laboratory data.

3. Urine and serum osmolality levels are monitored for diabetes insipidus, not TPN.

4. CA-125 and CEA levels may be monitored to follow the progress of the disease, but they are not daily tests and are not used for TPN.

46. 1. This should be done before the nurse leaves the client with the nurse call light access button, but it is not the first action.

2. This is done when a new cartridge is needed. The client should have a new cartridge in the pump because the pump came with the client from the operating room.

3. Determining the level of pain relief obtained is necessary, but not until the nurse determines that the medication is being administered correctly.

4. The nurse is still responsible for determining that the client is receiving the right dose of the right medication at the right time. The nurse should compare the settings to the HCP orders before the other steps.

47. 1. This blood gas indicates metabolic acidosis. Normal saline at a keep-open rate would not treat metabolic acidosis.

2. Clients after islet cell removal are at risk for diabetes mellitus complications. The blood gas results indicate metabolic ketoacidosis, and the treatment is continuous infusion of regular insulin.

3. Bicarbonate infusion to correct acidosis is avoided because it can precipitate a sudden (and potentially fatal) decrease in serum potassium.

4. Humulin N insulin is not administered by sliding scale, and for acidosis, the treatment is the more rapid-acting Humulin R insulin.

Chronic Pain

48. 1. The nurse should tell the client to notify hospice staff if the client is not receiving adequate pain relief.

2. The nurse should teach the client to take the pain medications as soon as the client begins to feel uncomfortable. Waiting to take the medication can make it difficult to get the pain under control.

3. This would isolate the client unnecessarily. The client may always need medications to control the pain. Visitors should be sensitive to the client, and if the client becomes drowsy from the medication, then they should sit quietly near the client.

4. The client is terminally ill. Addiction is not an issue.

49. 1. Chronic pain is difficult to describe to persons not experiencing pain. It is demoralizing and can result in clinical depression. Clients have to adjust to living with pain and try to be as normal as possible. This is a classic picture of chronic pain. Pain is whatever the client says it is and occurs whenever the client says it does. The nurse should not judge the client; the nurse should administer pain medication.

2. The nurse should not confront the client's behavior. If the nurse is concerned that the client is exhibiting narcotic-seeking behavior, the nurse should discuss this with the HCP.

3. The client is in pain now; the nurse should not wait to administer the medication.
4. The nurse should administer the pain medication, not substitute a different medication.

MEDICATION MEMORY JOGGER: The nurse should remember basic tenets of nursing, for example, that pain is whatever the client says it is. Then, the answer to this question is obvious.

50. 1. The nurse should teach the client to take the pain medications as soon as the client begins to feel uncomfortable. Waiting to take the medication can make it difficult to get the pain under control.
2. The nurse should instruct the client to avoid using other forms of acetaminophen (Tylenol), a nonnarcotic analgesic. The maximum daily adult dose is 4 grams. Each hydrocodone with acetaminophen (Vicodin) tablet contains 500 mg of Tylenol, and Vicodin HP contains 660 mg.
3. The client needs to notify the HCP only if the pain is unrelieved.
4. Hydrocodone slows peristalsis. The client should increase fluids and roughage in the diet to prevent constipation.

51. 1. The client in chronic pain often cannot localize pain and may describe it as "all over" or "taking over my whole body." This is not important.
2. The nurse should administer pain medication without further delay.
3. The client does not need a referral based on the information given.
4. There is no need to use a different scale. The client has rated the pain for the nurse.

52. 1. The client is receiving increasing amounts of narcotics without relief. The nurse should determine if there is some spiritual distress affecting the client's perception of the pain. An increased dose schedule has been tried without success.
2. Distraction techniques would not be successful with this level of pain.
3. The nurse should determine if some spiritual distress affects the client's perception of pain. Increasing the client's pain medications has been tried without success. Therapeutic communication techniques are designed to allow the client to verbalize feelings.
4. The client will not be willing or able to cooperate with any teaching until pain has been controlled.

53. 1. Stronger medications would only make the client feel drowsier. The nurse should discuss ways of helping the client get the rest needed at night.
2. The client is not discussing feelings. The client is talking about not getting rest at night.
3. Sleep medications (sedatives or hypnotics) are better options to induce sleep that the client needs at night. A combination of pain relief and sleep medication might be needed to allow the client to rest.
4. The nurse should not discourage the client from taking the medication needed to improve the quality of life. The nurse should teach the client how to cope with the side effects of all medications.

MEDICATION MEMORY JOGGER: The test taker should know the medications by specific classifications. Medications in the same classification usually share the same side effects and adverse effects, and the same interventions are needed to administer the medications safely.

54. 1. Keeping the eyes closed and drapes drawn would not indicate the pain medication is effective. These actions may be the client's way of dealing with pain.
2. Using guided imagery is an excellent method to assist with pain control, but it does not indicate medication effectiveness.
3. Because pain is whatever the client says it is and occurs whenever the client says it does, a client's report of reduced pain indicates the medication is effective.
4. This action may be the client's way of dealing with pain, but it does not indicate the medication is effective.

55. 1. The client should be told that there are many different methods of relieving pain, and all available methods would have to have failed for this to be true.
2. This is not true, but it is what many clients believe to be true. Neighborhood pharmacies are usually willing to provide the medications their clientele require. Still, they may need advanced notice to obtain the amount of narcotics required to fill a prescription for a client diagnosed with cancer.
3. Narcotic prescriptions need to be issued electronically in most situations. The client should try to anticipate when the medication needs to be refilled, or they may run out over a weekend or holiday. Hospice will arrange to obtain any medication at any time for clients receiving their service.

4. The client's pain has not been cured; it has only been controlled. The client will have pain if they do not take the medications as prescribed. The client should only notify the HCP if the pain becomes uncontrollable again on the prescribed pain control regimen.

56. 1. The client is nauseated. Liquid morphine (Roxanol), a narcotic analgesic, can be taken orally or sublingually, but this could increase nausea and cause vomiting. Morphine can be combined with an antiemetic to provide pain and nausea relief.

2. Prochlorperazine (Compazine) and morphine are compatible in the same syringe. Using two syringes is not cost-effective and would take more time to administer medications.

3. The ondansetron (Zofran) has not relieved the client's nausea. The nurse should try IV prochlorperazine (Compazine). The client is nauseated. Liquid morphine (Roxanol) can be taken orally or sublingually, but this could increase nausea and cause vomiting.

4. Prochlorperazine (Compazine) and morphine are compatible in the same syringe. Morphine (for the pain) should be administered over 5 minutes; Compazine (for nausea) should be administered at a rate of 5 mg per minute. The nurse could administer both medications in one syringe over 5 minutes safely.

57. 1. Morphine sulfate controlled release is a sustained-release formulation and is administered routinely every 6 to 8 hours to control chronic pain. Roxanol is administered sublingually to treat breakthrough pain. This is the correct administration procedure.

2. Morphine sulfate controlled release is not a PRN medication for pain.

3. Morphine sulfate controlled release is not a PRN medication for pain. Roxanol is absorbed very quickly through the veins under the tongue. The dosing for liquid morphine (Roxanol) is more frequent than every 4 hours.

4. Morphine sulfate controlled-release will not control breakthrough pain because of its sustained-release formulation. The liquid morphine (Roxanol) should not be held.

CANCER TREATMENTS COMPREHENSIVE EXAMINATION

1. The postchemotherapy client calls the clinic nurse and reports having mouth ulcers that make it difficult to eat. Which statement is the nurse's **best response**?
   1. "It is fine if you are not able to eat for a while. Just be sure to drink."
   2. "Try swishing a teaspoon of antacid in your mouth before meals."
   3. "You must force yourself to get some nourishment, even if it hurts."
   4. "This is expected and will go away in a week to 10 days."

2. The client about to receive chemotherapy is reporting nausea and nervousness. Based on the MAR, which of the PRN medications should the nurse administer?

Client: P.R.	MR# 345678	Date: Today
Age: 42 years	Allergies: NKDA	Diagnosis: Cancer
Medication	**0701–1900**	**1901–0700**
Ondansetron 4 mg IVP every 4 hours PRN		
Morphine sulfate 2 mg IVP every 2–3 hours PRN		
Lorazepam 2 mg IVP every 2 hours PRN		
Prochlorperazine 5 mg PO t.i.d. PRN		
Prochlorperazine 5–10 mg IVP every 2 hours PRN		
Nurse Initials/Credentials	**DN/RN**	**NN/RN**

   1. Ondansetron IVP
   2. Morphine IVP
   3. Lorazepam IVP
   4. Prochlorperazine IVP

3. The client is participating in a clinical trial for a new antineoplastic agent. Which statement is the purpose of Phase I of the clinical trial?
   1. Determine optimum dosing, scheduling, and toxicity of the medication.
   2. Determine effectiveness against specific tumor types.
   3. Compare the new medication with the standard treatment procedures.
   4. Investigate further to determine if the medication may have other uses.

4. The client diagnosed with cancer reports frequent nausea. Which information is **most important** for the nurse to discuss with the client?
   1. Teach the client to take an antiemetic 30 minutes before meals.
   2. Have the client keep a record of nausea to discuss with the HCP.
   3. Notify the HCP if the client becomes dehydrated.
   4. The significant other should provide the client with their favorite foods.

5. The nurse is reviewing the laboratory report of a client diagnosed with cancer. Which biologic response modifier medication should the nurse **question?**

Client: K.S.	MR# 123456	Date: Today
Laboratory Test	**Client Values**	**Reference Values**
WBC	10.2	4.5–11.1 (10^3/cells/microL)
RBC	3.56	Men: 4.21–5.81 (10^6 cells/microL) Women: 3.61–5.11 (10^6 cells/microL)
Hgb	8.4	Men: 14–17.3 g/dL Women: 11.7–15.5 g/dL
Hct	25.1	Men: 42%–52% Women: 36%–48%
Mean corpuscular volume (MCV)	72	Men: 77–97 fl Women: 78–98 fl
Mean corpuscular hemoglobin concentration (MCHC)	26	33–36 g/dL
Coefficient of variation in RBC distribution width index (RDWCV)	9.2	11.6–14.8
Platelets	79	140 to 400 × 10^3/microL
DIFFERENTIAL		
Neutrophils	83	40%–75% (2.7–6.5 × 10^3/microL)
Lymphocytes	17	12%–44% (1.5–3.7 × 10^3/microL)
Monocytes	0	4%–9% (0.2–0.4 × 10^3/microL)
Eosinophils	0	0%–5.5% (0.05–0.5 × 10^3/microL)
Basophils	0	0%–1% (0–0.1 × 10^3/microL)

1. Erythropoietin
2. Oprelvekin
3. Interferon
4. Filgrastim

6. The client diagnosed with a solid tissue tumor is scheduled to receive chemotherapy. The client's current laboratory values are populated in the chart below.

Laboratory Test	Client Values	Reference Values
Neutrophils	12%	40% to 75%
White blood cells (WBC)	5.9 (10^3/cells/microL)	4.5–11.1 (10^3/cells/microL)

Which intervention should the nurse implement **first**?
1. Administer the chemotherapy as ordered.
2. Assess the client's temperature and lung sounds.
3. Provide the client with a soft-bristled toothbrush.
4. Premedicate the client with an aminoglycoside antibiotic.

7. The nurse is preparing to administer a **vesicant** antineoplastic medication through a peripheral IV catheter. Which intervention is the **priority intervention**?
   1. Have the medication mixed in a large volume of IV fluid.
   2. Tell the client to let the nurse know if the IV site becomes red.
   3. Place the infusion on an IV infusion pump.
   4. Start new IV access before starting administration.

8. The client receiving chemotherapy for a diagnosis of non-Hodgkin's lymphoma asks the nurse, "Why do I need to take steroids? I've heard they can cause problems." Which statement is the nurse's **best response**?
   1. "Steroids suppress replication of lymphoid tissue and cause cell death."
   2. "Steroids will decrease inflammation caused by the tumor cells."
   3. "The problems caused by the steroids are nothing compared to cancer."
   4. "It is possible to have the HCP order different medications for cancer."

9. The client receiving doxorubicin for breast cancer has developed alopecia. Which information is **most helpful** for the nurse to provide the client?
   1. Have the client shave her entire head as a comfort measure.
   2. Encourage the client to purchase a wig that matches her hair.
   3. Try to get the client to discuss her feelings about alopecia.
   4. Discuss measures to prevent scalp sunburn.

10. The client taking chemotherapy has developed a white, patchy area on the tongue and buccal mucosa. Which medication is the **best treatment** for this condition?
    1. Ketoconazole to swish and swallow
    2. Metronidazole by mouth
    3. Miconazole topically
    4. Doxycycline orally

11. Today's laboratory report values for a client receiving chemotherapy are populated in the chart below.

Laboratory Test	Client Values	Reference Values
Platelets	13 (10^3/microL)	140 to 400 × 10^3/microL
Neutrophils	72%	40% to 75%
White blood cells (WBC)	4.8 (10^3/cells/microL)	4.5–11.1 (10^3/cells/microL)
Hemoglobin (Hgb)	11.2 (g/dL)	Men: 14–17.3 g/dL Women: 11.7–15.5 g/dL
Hematocrit (Hct)	34%	Men: 42% to 52% Women: 36% to 48%

    Which intervention should the nurse implement?
    1. Have the laboratory draw a type and cross-match.
    2. Request an order for antibiotics from the HCP.
    3. Prepare to transfuse 10 units of platelets.
    4. Place the client on neutropenic precautions.

12. The nurse is assessing the client **before** initiating the seventh round of chemotherapy. Which question is **most important** for the nurse to ask the client before beginning treatment?
    1. "Has your insurance company precertified you to receive more than six treatments?"
    2. "How have you dealt with the fatigue that occurs with cancer treatments?"
    3. "Did you take all of the prescription for antinausea medications?"
    4. "Have you experienced any difficulty swallowing or had a temperature?"

13. The client diagnosed with cancer tells the clinic nurse, "I am so afraid that I will die a horribly painful death." Which statement is the nurse's **best response**?
 1. "That is a concern. Let's sit down and discuss your concerns. I am here to talk if you need to."
 2. "Pain does not occur for everyone, but if it does, your HCP can prescribe medications to control it."
 3. "This does happen sometimes, and it is a valid concern. I hope this does not happen to you."
 4. "There are medications that can be prescribed to control the pain, but they can cause you to become addicted."

14. The nurse is caring for clients on an oncology unit. Which medication should the nurse administer **first**?
 1. The scheduled dose of leucovorin
 2. The narcotic pain medication for a client with pain of 10 on the pain scale
 3. The antiemetic to a client reporting nausea and emesis of 200 mL
 4. The third dose of an aminoglycoside antibiotic to a client with a fever

15. The HCP has ordered two units of packed red blood cells (PRBC) for the client diagnosed with cancer and anemia. Which interventions should the nurse implement? **Rank in order of performance.**
 1. Initiate the transfusion at 10 mL per hour.
 2. Assess the client's lung sounds.
 3. Place the blood on an infusion pump.
 4. Run the transfusion at a 4-hour rate.
 5. Check the blood with another nurse.

16. The client diagnosed with a solid tissue tumor is prescribed darbepoetin. Which data should the nurse monitor?
 1. The WBC counts
 2. The client's lung capacity
 3. The client's blood pressure
 4. The platelet counts

17. The client diagnosed with cancer is being prepared for surgery. Which information should the outpatient surgery nurse convey to the surgeon **immediately**?
 1. The client takes digoxin for heart problems.
 2. The client stopped taking acetylsalicylic acid last week.
 3. The client has been taking clopidogrel every day.
 4. The client becomes nauseated after receiving anesthesia.

18. The nurse is preparing a client for discharge with intractable pain and a home infusion pump with narcotic medication. Which information should the nurse include? **Select all that apply.**
 1. Teach the client about phlebitis or infection findings.
 2. Have the client sign out the medication.
 3. Remind the client to document pain for the HCP.
 4. Refer the client to a home health agency.
 5. Discuss infusion pump use.

19. The client receiving chemotherapy has developed stomatitis. Which referral should the nurse implement?
 1. Refer to a social worker.
 2. Refer to a dietician.
 3. Refer to a hospice nurse.
 4. Refer to a physical therapist.

20. The nurse working on a medical unit is caring for a client diagnosed with metastatic breast cancer and is receiving capecitabine. Which intervention should the nurse implement? **Select all that apply.**
    1. Administer the medication orally 30 minutes after breakfast.
    2. Have the client chew the tablet before swallowing.
    3. Assess the soles of the feet and palms of the hands for blistering.
    4. Monitor the client's white blood cells.
    5. Administer the IV medication through a central line.

21. The nurse on a medical unit is caring for a client diagnosed with advanced HER2-negative breast cancer and prescribed everolimus. Which should the nurse teach the client?
    1. Teach the client to notify the HCP if developing lung problems or wheezing.
    2. Instruct the client to alternate taking the medication between days and nights.
    3. Have the client take the medication before rising from bed and remain NPO for 2 hours.
    4. Remind the client to check blood pressure and radial pulse before taking medication.

22. The client diagnosed with cancer reports anorexia. Which medication might the nurse discuss with the HCP that might **increase** the client's appetite?
    1. Folinic acid
    2. Cyanocobalamin
    3. Megestrol acetate
    4. Pantoprazole

CANCER TREATMENTS COMPREHENSIVE EXAMINATION ANSWERS AND RATIONALES

1. 1. It is unacceptable for the client to be unable to eat. The client needs a positive nitrogen balance if the client is to respond well to the treatment.

2. This is a suggestion to alleviate pain caused by mouth ulcerations resulting from chemotherapy. The antacid coats the tender mucosal lining. If this does not work, there are numbing medications that the HCP can prescribe.

3. This will cause pain and result in the client dreading mealtime. Some interventions can help the client with the problem.

4. This may be expected as a result of chemotherapy, and it will go away when the client's immune system has time to recover from the insult caused by chemotherapy, but it is not the best response. The nurse should try to help the client deal with the mouth ulcers.

2. 1. Ondansetron (Zofran), a 5-HT_3 receptor agonist, will help nausea, but it will not affect the client's nervousness.

2. Morphine, an opioid analgesic, can produce analgesia and has bronchodilating effects, but it will not treat nausea or nervousness.

3. Lorazepam (Ativan), a benzodiazepine, is a sedative-hypnotic with antiemetic and antianxiety properties. The nurse should administer this medication to treat both of the client's reported symptoms.

4. Prochlorperazine (Compazine) is an antiemetic that will treat nausea but not nervousness. This is not the best medication for the nurse to administer.

MEDICATION MEMORY JOGGER: The test taker should know medications by the specific classifications. Medications in the same classification usually share the same side effects and adverse effects, and the same interventions are needed to administer medications safely.

3. 1. Determining optimum dosing, scheduling, and toxicity of a medication is the purpose of a Phase I clinical trial. Clients participating in Phase I and II trials are not placed in the trials unless their cancers have failed to respond to standard treatment procedures.

2. Determining the effectiveness of a medication against specific tumor types is the purpose of a Phase II clinical trial.

3. Comparing a new medication with the standard treatment procedures is the purpose of a Phase III clinical trial.

4. Further investigation to determine if a medication may have other uses is the purpose of a Phase IV clinical trial (American Cancer Society, 2021c).

4. 1. To prevent nausea, the client should take an antiemetic 30 minutes before attempting to eat. Maintaining the client's nutritional status is the most important information for the nurse to discuss.

2. There is no reason for the client to keep a record of nausea. If the nausea is not controlled, the client should report it to the HCP.

3. Reporting to the HCP that a client has become dehydrated is important, but if the nurse can assist with interventions to maintain the client's nutritional status, the client will also be able to maintain their hydration status.

4. The client should not try to eat favorite foods when nauseated. Doing so may create an aversion to these foods, and then the favorite foods will not be helpful if dealing with anorexia.

5. 1. Erythropoietin (Procrit) is a biologic response modifier that is administered to increase RBC production. The client's levels are below normal. The nurse would not question administering this medication.

2. Oprelvekin (Neumega) is a biologic modifier administered to increase platelet production. The client's levels are below normal. The nurse would not question administering this medication.

3. Interferon (Intron A) is a biologic modifier that would not be questioned based on information provided by a CBC.

4. Filgrastim (Neupogen), a biologic response modifier, is administered to increase WBC production. It is discontinued when the WBC is 10,200 or 10.2×10^3. The nurse should hold this medication and notify the HCP of the client's laboratory values.

6. 1. The client is neutropenic despite the number of WBCs. The absolute neutrophil count is only 708 (5,900 × 0.12 = 708); normal is greater than 2,500. This client is at great risk of developing an infection. The nurse would hold the chemotherapy and discuss the absolute neutrophil count with the HCP.

2. This client's laboratory data indicates a significant risk for infection. The nurse should assess the client for any clinical manifestations of an infection.

3. This is an intervention for thrombocytopenia, not neutropenia.

4. The client may need to be prescribed antibiotic therapy, but aminoglycoside antibiotics are used mainly for methicillin-resistant *Staphylococcus aureus* infections (MRSA).

7. 1. The medication is usually mixed in small volumes of fluid because the nurse should not leave the client during administration of a vesicant.

2. The nurse should not leave the client. The nurse can observe this complication directly.

3. Infusion pumps are controversial because the pump could force the vesicant medication into the client's tissue and cause more extensive damage.

4. When administering a vesicant medication into a peripheral IV line, the nurse must know that the vein is patent and that there is little likelihood of extravasation occurring. This phenomenon involves the leaking of minute amounts of medication into the tissue because the catheter has been in the vein too long, and an insertion site enlargement has occurred. The nurse should start a new IV site.

8. 1. Steroid medications are particularly useful in treating lymphomas because they exert direct toxicity on lymphoid tissue by suppressing cancer cell mitosis and lymphocyte dissolution.

2. Steroids do suppress inflammation, but this is not the reason to administer these medications to clients diagnosed with lymphoma.

3. This is a derogatory statement and does not address the client's concerns.

4. Other prescribed medications have side effects also. The nurse should not undermine the HCP by suggesting this.

9. 1. Doxorubicin (Adriamycin) is an antineoplastic agent. Shaving the entire head would not create comfort. Hair keeps heat in the body and is aesthetic.

2. Doxorubicin (Adriamycin) is an antineoplastic agent that can cause alopecia. Wearing a wig that matches the client's hair color and style will allow the client to appear in public without others making comments about her hair loss.

3. This is assuming that the client wants to discuss feelings about her body image.

4. The nurse should warn the client about being in the sun without covering her head, but it is not the most helpful information.

10. 1. Ketoconazole (Nizoral) is an anti-infective medication that treats yeast infections. White, patchy areas in the mouth indicate oral candidiasis, a yeast infection. The correct administration procedure is to have the client swish the medication around in the mouth and then swallow the medication to treat esophageal areas.

2. Metronidazole (Flagyl) is a gastrointestinal antiinfective that treats intestinal amoebae, vaginal trichomonas, and anaerobic bacteria, not yeast infections.

3. Miconazole (Monistat) is an antifungal used to treat yeast infections, but applying a topical cream to the oral mucosa would cause pain, and it would not adhere to mucosal lining.

4. Doxycycline (Vibramycin) is an antibiotic that would further destroy the good bacteria needed to keep yeast in check. This would increase the client's problem.

11. 1. Clients are not transfused unless Hgb is less than 8 and Hct is less than 24. There is no reason to type and cross-match the client.

2. The client's absolute neutrophil count (3,456) is higher than 2,500, indicating that the client has adequate circulating neutrophils to protect against infection.

3. Thrombocytopenia is defined as a platelet count of less than 100,000. If it is less than 50,000, the client is at risk for bleeding; if it is less than 20,000, the client is at great risk for hemorrhage. This client's platelet count is 13,000. The nurse should prepare to infuse platelets to prevent hemorrhage.

4. The client's absolute neutrophil count is higher than 2,500, so the client has adequate circulating neutrophils to protect against infection. The client does not need to be placed in reverse isolation (neutropenic precautions).

12. 1. This may be an important question for the business manager to ask, but this is not the nurse's responsibility. The nurse should be concerned with administering medications safely.
2. How the client deals with fatigue is not important when deciding if it is safe to administer chemotherapy.
3. Using up a prescription is not the most important question when assessing the client for side effects or adverse effects of chemotherapy.
4. The medications' full effect will not occur until between treatments. Nadir counts of WBCs and other clinical manifestations relating to the chemotherapy should be assessed. The nurse should assess for stomatitis, infections, and nutritional status. A fever would indicate infection, and difficulty swallowing could indicate mouth inflammation (stomatitis) or ulcerations.

13. 1. The nurse should address the client's concern with information. The client did say, "I am afraid," but accurate information can alleviate fear. This is not the best response.
2. The nurse should inform the client about pain control options. After the client has accurate information, the nurse can address the fear, if it still exists.
3. This does not give the client the information the client is seeking.
4. Addiction should not be a concern of the client. Although it is a remote possibility, usually, the client will taper the medication dose if it is too high. This client is worried about dying in pain. Addiction need not be a concern for a terminally ill client.

14. **1. Leucovorin (folinic acid), a rescue factor, is used as a rescue medication for certain drugs. Rescue medications are precisely timed to prevent life-threatening complications. The nurse should administer this medication first.**
2. Pain is a priority, but it is not life-threatening if the client has to wait for a few minutes to receive pain medication.
3. An antiemetic medication is a priority, but it is not life-threatening if the client has to wait to receive antiemetic medication.
4. The client has already had two doses of the medication. This is not the priority medication to administer.

MEDICATION MEMORY JOGGER: The classification of "rescue factor" should provide the test taker with a clue about priority.

15. **Correct order is 2, 5, 3, 1, 4.**
2. The first step should be to assess the client for clinical manifestations of fluid volume overload. Lung crackles would indicate to the nurse to infuse the PRBCs as slowly as possible.
5. Blood products require two nurses to verify that the correct product is being administered. This is the second step.
3. Administering infusions is safer when the nurse uses a pump. Infusion devices prevent inadvertent rapid fluid administration, and pumps also prevent the transfusion from slowing down (blood is very thick) and not infusing within the time period.
1. Blood should initially be transfused at a very slow rate. The most common time for a life-threatening complication to occur is within the first 15 minutes of the transfusion. The nurse should not leave the client being given the transfusion for 15 minutes and should perform vital signs every 5 minutes. If, at the end of the 15 minutes, the client has not experienced any difficulty with the blood product, then the nurse should adjust the infusion rate to transfuse PRBCs within 4 hours.
4. Setting the transfusion to infuse within the time period is the final step before the nurse leaves the client's room.

16. 1. Darbepoetin (Aranesp) is a hematopoietic growth factor that stimulates RBC production. Monitoring WBC count would be appropriate for clients receiving Neupogen and Neulasta, both of which stimulate WBC production.
2. Darbepoetin (Aranesp) is a hematopoietic growth factor that stimulates RBC production. Darbepoetin will not affect the client's lung capacity.
3. Darbepoetin (Aranesp) is a hematopoietic growth factor that stimulates RBC production. When the Hct level rises, it can increase blood pressure. The nurse should monitor the client's blood pressure.
4. Darbepoetin (Aranesp) is a hematopoietic growth factor that stimulates RBC production. Monitoring platelet counts would be appropriate for a client receiving oprelvekin (Neumega), which stimulates platelet production.

17. 1. Many clients take digoxin and do fine during surgery. The HCP should be aware of the client's cardiac status when they

performed the history and physical. The nurse does not have to notify the surgeon about this medication.

2. The client stopped taking aspirin last week. The nurse does not have to notify the surgeon about this medication.
3. **Clopidogrel (Plavix) is an antiplatelet medication the client has been taking. It should be discontinued at least 7 days before surgery. The nurse should notify the surgeon because the surgery will need to be rescheduled.**
4. Many clients become nauseated after anesthesia. The nurse would not have to notify the surgeon.

18. Correct answers are 1, 4, and 5.

1. **Because this client will be monitoring the IV injection site, the nurse should teach the client about clinical manifestations of phlebitis (for a peripheral IV) or infection and what to do if they occur.**
2. The client will not receive the medication from the hospital pharmacy. The client will obtain the medication from a neighborhood pharmacy or from a home health-care agency pharmacy.
3. There is no need for the client to self-document the pain.
4. **Arrangements for follow-up care should be made with a home care agency.**
5. **The medications will be administered using a pump designed for this purpose. The nurse should make sure the client is able to operate the pump.**

19. 1. Stomatitis is a buccal mucosa inflammation. A social worker would not be able to help this client.

2. **Stomatitis is a buccal mucosa inflammation. A dietitian can help the client by providing foods the client can swallow without too much chewing and simultaneously receive adequate nutrition. The nurse should refer the client to the dietitian.**
3. Stomatitis is not a terminal process. Hospice nurses care for the terminally ill.
4. Stomatitis is a buccal mucosa inflammation. A physical therapist would not be able to help with this client.

MEDICATION MEMORY JOGGER: The test taker must know medical terminology.

20. Correct answers are 1, 3, and 4.

1. **Capecitabine (Xeloda) is an oral antineoplastic agent used to treat advanced breast cancer and colon and rectum cancer. It is not a first-line medication. Because it is an oral medication, the nurse on a medical unit may be required to administer the medication, depending on the facility's policy. Regardless, the nurse must be fully aware of these medications' actions, side effects, and adverse reactions. The medication should be administered 30 minutes after a meal, whole, and with a full glass of water.**
2. The pill must be swallowed whole.
3. **An adverse reaction can be pain, tenderness, swelling, or blistering of the soles of the feet and palms of the hands with peeling. The client should immediately notify the HCP if noticing problems in these areas.**
4. **The medication can lower the client's white blood cell (WBC) count and increase infection risk.**
5. The medication is taken orally.

21. 1. **The oral antineoplastic medication everolimus (Afinitor) can result in severe lung issues for the client. The nurse should report any finding of breathing difficulties to the HCP immediately.**

2. The medication should be taken at the same time daily.
3. The medication should be taken after a meal with a full glass of water.
4. There is no reason to take the pulse and blood pressure before taking this medication.

22. 1. Folinic acid is a vitamin that can assist the nurse when working with cancer clients to improve nutritional status or act as a rescue factor to prevent permanent damage from some antineoplastic agents. It is not administered to increase appetite.

2. Cyanocobalamin (vitamin B_{12}) is needed by the body to produce red blood cells and prevent nutritional imbalances, but it is not administered to increase appetite.
3. **Megestrol acetate (Megace, Appetrol) is an antineoplastic agent found to have appetite-increasing properties in some clients. It is given in an oral suspension.**
4. Pantoprazole (Protonix) is a proton-pump inhibitor used to decrease stomach acid production and is helpful in the prevention and treatment of gastric ulcers, but it does not increase appetite.

Mental Health Disorders

Mental health problems don't define who you are. They are something you experience. You walk in the rain and you feel the rain, but, importantly, YOU ARE NOT THE RAIN.

—Matt Haig

QUESTIONS

Major Depressive Disorder

1. The client diagnosed with a major depressive disorder and taking fluoxetine reports feeling confused and restless. The client's vital signs are populated in the following vital sign flowsheet.

Vital Sign Flowsheet	Client Values	Reference Values
Temperature	101°F/38.3°C	Oral: 98°F (36.7°C)
Pulse	110 bpm	60 to 100 bpm
Respirations	24 breaths/min	12 to 20 breaths/min
Blood pressure	158/100 mm Hg	100 to 119 mm Hg systolic 60 to 80 mm Hg diastolic

Which intervention should the clinic psychiatric nurse implement?
1. Determine if the client has flu-like symptoms.
2. Instruct the client to stop taking fluoxetine.
3. Recommend the client take the medication at night.
4. Explain that these are expected side effects (ESEs).

2. The client diagnosed with a major depressive disorder asks the nurse, "Why did my psychiatrist prescribe a selective serotonin reuptake inhibitor (SSRI) medication rather than another type of antidepressant?" Which statement by the nurse is **most appropriate**?
1. "Probably it is the medication that your insurance will cover."
2. "You should ask your psychiatrist why the SSRI was ordered."
3. "SSRIs have fewer side effects than other classifications."
4. "The SSRI medications work faster than other medications."

3. The client diagnosed with pneumonia is admitted to the medical unit. The nurse notes the client is taking an antidepressant medication. Which data **best indicates** that the antidepressant therapy is **effective**?
   1. The client reports a "2" on a 1 to 10 scale, with "10" being very depressed.
   2. The client reports not feeling very depressed today.
   3. The client gets out of bed and completes activities of daily living (ADLs).
   4. The client eats 90% of all meals that are served during the shift.

4. The client diagnosed with depression is prescribed phenelzine. Which statement by the client indicates to the nurse the medication teaching is **effective**?
   1. "I am taking the herb ginseng to help my attention span."
   2. "I drink extra fluids, especially coffee and iced tea."
   3. "I am eating three well-balanced meals a day."
   4. "At a family cookout, I had chicken instead of a hot dog."

5. The client diagnosed with a major depressive disorder is prescribed brexpiprazole in addition to their antidepressant. Which information should the nurse teach? **Select all that apply.**
   1. Inform the client that weight gain can occur.
   2. Teach the client to report urges to gamble, impulse shop, or binge eat.
   3. Instruct the client to avoid all over-the-counter (OTC) medications.
   4. Advise the client to avoid saunas or hot tubs.
   5. Explain to the client the need to rise slowly from a sitting position.

6. The client diagnosed with a major depressive disorder has been taking amitriptyline for more than 1 year and tells the psychiatric clinic nurse about wanting to stop taking the antidepressant. Which intervention is **most important** for the nurse to discuss with the client?
   1. Ask questions to determine if the client is still depressed.
   2. Ask why the client wants to stop taking the medication.
   3. Tell the client to notify the HCP before stopping the medication.
   4. Explain the importance of tapering off the medication.

7. The client diagnosed with a major depressive disorder is prescribed duloxetine. The client tells the nurse, "I am going to take my medication at night instead of in the morning." Which statement is the nurse's **best** response?
   1. "You really should take the medication in the morning for the best results."
   2. "It is all right to take the medication at night. It may help you sleep."
   3. "The medication should be taken with food, so you should not take it at night."
   4. "Have you discussed taking the medication at night with your psychiatrist?"

8. The client admitted to the psychiatric unit for a diagnosis of major depressive disorder and attempted suicide is prescribed an antidepressant medication. Which interventions should the psychiatric nurse implement? **Select all that apply.**
   1. Assess the client's apical pulse and blood pressure.
   2. Check the client's serum antidepressant level.
   3. Monitor the client's liver function status.
   4. Provide for and ensure the client's safety.
   5. Evaluate the effectiveness of the medication.

9. After an attempted suicide and then diagnosed with major depression, the client is being discharged from the psychiatric facility after a 2-week stay. Which discharge intervention is **most important** for the nurse to implement?
   1. Provide the family with the phone number to call if the client needs assistance.
   2. Encourage the client to keep all follow-up appointments with the psychiatric clinic.
   3. Ensure the client has no more than a 7-day supply of antidepressants.
   4. Instruct the client not to take any OTC medications without consulting with the HCP.

10. The client prescribed an antidepressant 1 week ago tells the psychiatric clinic nurse, "I really don't think this medication is helping me." Which statement by the psychiatric nurse is **most appropriate**?
1. "Why do you think the medication is not helping you?"
2. "You should talk to the HCP about your concern."
3. "You need to come to the clinic so we can discuss this."
4. "It takes about 3 weeks for your medication to work."

Bipolar Disorder

11. Which statements indicate the client diagnosed with bipolar disorder and taking lithium **understands** the medication teaching? **Select all that apply.**
1. "I must monitor my daily lithium level."
2. "I will make sure I do not get dehydrated."
3. "I need to taper the dose if I quit taking it."
4. "I should take the medication with food."
5. "I will not eat foods high in tyramine."

12. The nurse is preparing to administer lithium to a client diagnosed with bipolar disorder. The client's laboratory values are populated in the chart below.

Drug Levels	Client Values	Reference Values
Lithium	1.2 mg/dL	0.6 to 1.2 mEq/L

Which intervention should the nurse implement?
1. Administer the medication.
2. Hold the medication.
3. Notify the HCP.
4. Verify the lithium level.

13. To which client should the nurse **question** administering lithium?
1. The 54-year-old client on a 4-g sodium diet
2. The 23-year-old client taking an antidepressant medication
3. The 42-year-old client taking a loop diuretic
4. The 30-year-old client with a urine output of 40 mL/hour

14. The 24-year-old female client diagnosed with bipolar disorder is prescribed valproic acid. Which question should the nurse ask the client?
1. "Have you ever had a migraine headache?"
2. "Are you taking any type of birth control?"
3. "When was the last time you had a seizure?"
4. "How long since you have had a manic episode?"

15. The client diagnosed with bipolar disorder is taking lithium. Which statement by the client **warrants further clarification** by the nurse?
1. "I will limit the amount of caffeine I drink."
2. "I really enjoy playing soccer on weekends."
3. "I will drink at least 2,000 mL of water a day."
4. "I need to call my HCP if I develop diarrhea."

16. The client diagnosed with bipolar disorder is taking lithium medication. The client's laboratory values are populated in the chart below.

Drug Levels	Client Values	Reference Values
Lithium	3.1 mg/dL	0.6 to 1.2 mEq/L

Which treatments should the nurse expect the health-care provider (HCP) to prescribe? **Select all that apply.**
1. No treatment, this is within the therapeutic range.
2. Initiate IV therapy with isotonic sodium chloride.
3. Prepare the client for immediate hemodialysis.
4. Administer the antidote for lithium toxicity.
5. Monitor the client's cardiac status on telemetry.

17. The client diagnosed with bipolar disorder is prescribed carbamazepine. Which data indicates the medication is **effective**?
1. The client is able to control extremes between mania and depression.
2. The client's serum carbamazepine level is within the therapeutic range.
3. The client reports a "3" on a depression scale of 1 to 10; "10" indicates severely depressed.
4. The client has a decrease in delusional thoughts and hallucinations.

18. The client diagnosed with bipolar disorder is prescribed lithium and later admitted to the psychiatric unit in an acute manic state. Which intervention should the nurse implement **first**?
1. Determine the client's serum lithium level.
2. Assess why the client quit taking the lithium.
3. Implement care for the client's physiological needs.
4. Administer a stat dose of lithium to the client.

19. Which information should the nurse discuss with the client diagnosed with bipolar disorder and taking carbamazepine? **Select all that apply.**
1. Instruct the client to use a soft-bristled toothbrush.
2. Encourage the client to get ophthalmic examinations annually.
3. Teach the client to monitor blood pressure daily.
4. Tell the client to avoid hazardous activities.
5. Teach the client to wear sunscreen when outdoors.

20. The client diagnosed with bipolar disorder is prescribed cariprazone. Which interventions should the nurse discuss with the client? **Select all that apply.**
1. Instruct the client to monitor therapeutic serum levels.
2. Tell the client to maintain adequate fluid intake.
3. Encourage the client to avoid alcohol.
4. Stop medication if the radial pulse is less than 60 beats per minute (bpm).
5. Explain ways to prevent orthostatic hypotension.

Schizophrenia

21. The client admitted to the psychiatric unit diagnosed with schizophrenia is prescribed clozapine. Which laboratory data should the nurse evaluate?

Arterial Blood Gas	Client Values	Reference Values
pH	7.35	7.35 to 7.45
Pco_2	36 mm Hg	35 to 45 mm Hg
Hco_3	22 mmol/L	22 to 26 mmol/L
Po_2	90 mm Hg	80 to 95 mm Hg

Blood Count	Client Values	Reference Values
Red blood cell count (RBC)	4.8 (10^6 cells/microL)	Male: 4.21 to 5.81 (10^6 cells/microL) Female: 3.61 to 5.11 (10^6 cells/microL)
White blood cell count (WBC)	10.5 × 10^3/microL	4.5 to 11.1 × 10^3/microL
Platelets	150 × 10^3/microL	140 to 400 × 10^3/microL

Drug Levels	Client Values	Reference Values
International normalized ratio (INR)	0.9	0.9 to 1.1 without anticoagulation therapy 2 to 3 with therapy 2.5 to 3.5 if the client has a mechanical heart valve

1. The client's international normalized ratio (INR)
2. The client's white blood cell (WBC) count
3. The client's red blood cell (RBC) count
4. The client's arterial blood gases (ABGs)

22. The client admitted to the psychiatric unit experiencing hallucinations and delusions is prescribed risperidone. Which intervention should the nurse implement?
1. Provide the client with a low tyramine diet.
2. Assess the client's respiration for 1 full minute.
3. Instruct the client to change positions slowly.
4. Monitor the client's intake and output.

23. The male client diagnosed with schizophrenia is prescribed ziprasidone. Which statement to the nurse indicates the client **understands** the medication teaching?
1. "I need to keep taking this medication even if I become impotent."
2. "I should not go out in the sun without wearing protective clothing."
3. "This medication may cause my breast size to increase."
4. "I may have trouble sleeping when I take this medication."

24. The client diagnosed with schizophrenia is prescribed clozapine. Which information should the nurse discuss with the client concerning this medication? **Select all that apply.**
   1. Discuss the need for regular exercise.
   2. Instruct the client to monitor for weight gain.
   3. Tell the client to take the medication with food.
   4. Explain to the client the need to stop taking aspirin.
   5. Encourage the client to quit smoking cigarettes.

25. The client diagnosed with paranoid schizophrenia is prescribed aripiprazole. Which statement **best** describes the scientific rationale for administering this medication?
   1. It decreases anxiety associated with hallucinations and delusions.
   2. It increases dopamine secretion in the brain tissue to improve speech.
   3. It reduces positive symptoms of schizophrenia and improves negative symptoms.
   4. It blocks cholinergic receptor sites in the diseased brain tissue.

26. Which information should the nurse discuss with the client diagnosed with schizophrenia and prescribed an atypical antipsychotic medication? **Select all that apply.**
   1. Drink decaffeinated coffee and tea.
   2. Decrease the dietary salt intake.
   3. Eat six small, high-protein meals a day.
   4. Report muscle spasms and rigidity.
   5. Monitor glucose levels and lipid levels.

27. The nurse is discussing the prescribed antipsychotic medication with a family member of a client diagnosed with schizophrenia. Which information should the nurse discuss with the family member?
   1. Explain the need for the family member to give the client the medication.
   2. Encourage the family member to learn cardiopulmonary resuscitation (CPR).
   3. Discuss the need for the client to participate in a community support group.
   4. Teach the family member what to do in case the client has a seizure.

28. Which assessment data indicates quetiapine is **effective** for the client diagnosed with paranoid schizophrenia?
   1. The client does not exhibit any tremors or rigidity.
   2. The client reports a "2" on an anxiety scale of 1 to 10.
   3. The family reports the client is sleeping all night.
   4. The client denies having auditory hallucinations.

29. The client diagnosed with paranoid schizophrenia has been taking haloperidol for several years. Which statement indicates the client **needs additional teaching** concerning this medication?
   1. "I know that if I have any rigidity or tremors, I must call my HCP."
   2. "I eat high-fiber foods and drink extra water during the day."
   3. "I am more susceptible to colds and the flu when taking this medication."
   4. "This medication will make my hallucinations and delusions go away."

30. The 43-year-old female client diagnosed with schizophrenia has been taking chlorpromazine for 20 years. Which assessment data **warrants discontinuing** the medication?
   1. The client has had menstrual irregularities for the past year.
   2. The client has to get up very slowly from a sitting position.
   3. The client reports having a dry mouth and blurred vision.
   4. The client has fine, worm-like movements of the tongue.

Anxiety Disorder

31. The client diagnosed with a general anxiety disorder is prescribed alprazolam. Which information should the clinic nurse discuss with the client? **Select all that apply.**
1. Explain to the client this medication is for short-term use.
2. Inform the client that rage and excitement are expected side effects.
3. Tell the client to avoid foods that are high in vitamin K.
4. Discuss the importance of not driving due to drowsiness.
5. Instruct the client to take the medication with at least 8 ounces of water.

32. The female client taking lorazepam for panic attacks tells the clinic nurse that she is trying to get pregnant. Which intervention should the nurse implement **first**?
1. Tell the client to inform the obstetrician she is taking lorazepam.
2. Instruct the client to quit taking the medication.
3. Determine how long the client has been taking the medication.
4. Encourage the client to stop taking lorazepam before getting pregnant.

33. The nurse is preparing to administer alprazolam to a client diagnosed with a generalized anxiety disorder. Which intervention should the nurse implement **before** administering the medication?
1. Assess the client's apical pulse.
2. Assess the client's serum potassium level.
3. Assess the client's anxiety level.
4. Assess the client's blood pressure.

34. The client diagnosed with obsessive-compulsive disorder (OCD) is prescribed sertraline. Which statement indicates the client **understands** the medication teaching?
1. "If I experience sexual dysfunction, I will not notify my HCP."
2. "It will take a couple of months before I see a change in my behavior."
3. "I need to be careful because SSRIs may cause physical addiction."
4. "I am glad I do not need to go to my psychologist's appointments."

35. After returning from the war 1 month ago, the client is diagnosed with post-traumatic stress disorder (PTSD) and prescribed paroxetine. The client asks the nurse, "Will this medication really help me? I don't like feeling this way." Which statement is the nurse's **best** response?
1. "The medication will make you feel better within a couple of days."
2. "Why do you think the medication won't help you feel better?"
3. "Nothing really helps PTSD unless you go to counseling weekly."
4. "Because the traumatic event was within 1 month, the paroxetine should be helpful."

36. The elderly client diagnosed with a panic attack disorder is in the busy day room of a long-term care facility and appears anxious. The client is starting to hyperventilate, tremble, and sweat. Which intervention should the nurse implement **first**?
1. Administer alprazolam.
2. Assess the client's vital signs.
3. Remove the client from the day room.
4. Administer sertraline.

37. The client diagnosed with an anxiety disorder is prescribed alprazolam. The client calls the clinic and reports a dizzy, weak feeling when getting out of the chair. Which intervention should the nurse implement?
1. Instruct the client to quit taking the medication.
2. Make an appointment for the client to come to the clinic.
3. Determine if the client is drinking enough fluids.
4. Discuss ways to prevent orthostatic hypotension.

38. The conscious client was admitted to the emergency department after an overdose of alprazolam. Which intervention should the nurse implement? **Select all that apply.**
   1. Prepare to administer an emetic with activated charcoal.
   2. Prepare the client for hemodialysis.
   3. Prepare to administer the antidote flumazenil IV.
   4. Prepare to administer a whole bowel irrigation.
   5. Prepare supplies for endotracheal intubation.

39. The client is having a computed tomography scan and starts having a severe anxiety attack. The HCP prescribed diazepam, IV push (IVP). Which intervention should the nurse implement?
   1. Dilute the diazepam with normal saline and administer IVP.
   2. Do not dilute diazepam and inject in a port closest to the client.
   3. Inject the diazepam into a 50-mL normal saline bag and infuse.
   4. Question the order because diazepam should not be administered IV.

Attention Deficit-Hyperactivity Disorder

40. The 10-year-old child diagnosed with attention deficit-hyperactivity disorder (ADHD) is taking methylphenidate. Which assessment data **warrants intervention** from the pediatric clinic nurse?
   1. The child has gained 3 kg in the last month.
   2. The child's pulse is 98 and blood pressure is 100/70.
   3. The child has multiple bruises on the arm.
   4. The child sits quietly in the examination room.

41. The 7-year-old child newly diagnosed with ADHD is prescribed methylphenidate as a sustained-release tablet. Which information should the nurse discuss with the parents? **Select all that apply.**
   1. "Have your child take the medication with food."
   2. "Weigh your child weekly in the morning."
   3. "Administer the medication at night."
   4. "Keep a behavior diary on your child."
   5. "Protect the child from direct sunlight."

42. The 6-year-old child diagnosed with ADHD is admitted to the pediatric department after having an emergency appendectomy. Which intervention should the nurse implement when administering methylphenidate to the child?
   1. Check the child's glucose level.
   2. Administer with a full glass of water.
   3. Monitor the child's vital signs.
   4. Assess the child's incisional wound.

43. The 14-year-old adolescent diagnosed with ADHD is taking lisdexamfetamine. Which statement indicates to the nurse that the adolescent **understands** the medication teaching?
   1. "I can carry my medication in a personal pill container with me at school."
   2. "I hate that I have to go to the school nurse to take my medication."
   3. "I just take my medication on days that I have important tests."
   4. "A friend of mine has ADHD, and I gave him one of my pills."

44. The mother of a male child diagnosed with ADHD tells the school nurse she does not want her son to take methylphenidate and wants to know about other medications her son could take. Which statement is the nurse's **best** response?
   1. "There are no other medications that work as well as methylphenidate."
   2. "Why are you worried about your child taking methylphenidate?"
   3. "There is a nonstimulant medication called atomoxetine that your child could take."
   4. "I think that is something you should discuss with your child's doctor."

45. The mother of a 7-year-old child taking methylphenidate for an ADHD diagnosis calls the pediatric clinic and tells the nurse her daughter has lost 4 pounds in the past 2 weeks. Which action should the nurse implement?
   1. Make an appointment for the child to see the HCP.
   2. Instruct the mother to discontinue methylphenidate.
   3. Explain that this is a normal response to the medication.
   4. Tell the mother to increase the child's caloric intake.

46. Which assessment data indicates lisdexamfetamine has been **effective** for the 8-year-old child diagnosed with ADHD?
   1. The child has two notes from the school for inappropriate behavior in 1 week.
   2. The child sleeps 8 hours a night and falls asleep during the day.
   3. The child can sit and play a game for 30 minutes with a friend.
   4. The child has difficulty following verbal instructions from the teacher.

47. Which diagnostic test should the nurse expect the HCP to monitor for the child diagnosed with ADHD and prescribed methylphenidate?
   1. Complete blood count (CBC)
   2. Serum potassium and sodium levels
   3. An annual bone density test
   4. Serum methylphenidate level

Sleep Disorder

48. The male client diagnosed with chronic obstructive pulmonary disease (COPD) is admitted to the medical unit. During the admission process, the client tells the nurse about the inability to sleep without diazepam every night. Which intervention should the nurse implement?
   1. Inform the client that clients diagnosed with COPD should not take diazepam.
   2. Ask the client when the last seizure activity occurred.
   3. Determine what effect the diazepam has on the client after taking it.
   4. Ask the HCP for an order for diazepam.

49. The elderly client being prepped for major abdominal surgery describes taking alprazolam as needed (PRN) many years now for nerves. Which information should the nurse discuss with the HCP?
   1. Discuss prescribing another benzodiazepine medication postoperatively.
   2. Make sure that the alprazolam is ordered after surgery.
   3. Taper the medication to prevent complications.
   4. Change the alprazolam to a medication for sleep.

50. The client diagnosed with insomnia is scheduled for sleep studies. The client provides the nurse with their medication list.

Medication and Dose	Scheduled Time
Captopril 50 mg	With breakfast, at lunch, and bedtime
Diphenhydramine 25 mg	Bedtime
Furosemide 40 mg	With breakfast
Levothyroxine 50 mcg	With breakfast

Which medication should the nurse instruct the client to avoid taking before the sleep study?
1. Captopril
2. Diphenhydramine
3. Furosemide
4. Levothyroxine

51. The HCP has prescribed lorazepam for a female client receiving chemotherapy reporting an inability to sleep. Which information should the nurse teach the client?
1. "Do not attempt to become pregnant while taking lorazepam."
2. "Avoid consuming too much alcohol while taking lorazepam."
3. "Exercise before going to bed to help sleep restfully."
4. "Addiction and dependence is not a problem with this medication."

52. The day shift nurse finds an elderly client difficult to arouse during the initial morning shift assessment. The nurse reviews the client's medication record for the last 24 hours.

Client: J.S.	MR# 345555	Date: Yesterday
Age: 74 years	Allergies: Penicillin	Diagnosis:
Sex: Female	Height: 64 inches	Weight: 50 kg
Medication	0701–1900	1901–0700
Furosemide 40 mg PO daily	0900 DN K+ 3.8	
Digoxin 0.125 mg PO daily	0900 DN AP 93 Dig level 1.4	
Acetaminophen 650 mg PO Q 4–6 hours PRN		2115 NN
Promethazine 12.5 mg IVP Q 3–4 hours PRN nausea		0425 NN
Temazepam 15 mg PO Q HS PRN		2115 NN
Nurse Initials/Credentials	DN/RN	NN/RN

Which intervention should the nurse implement **first**?
1. Notify the HCP of the client's current status.
2. Make sure the client has a call light within reach.
3. Call a code and initiate CPR.
4. Reassess the client's neurological status in 1 hour.

53. The client being admitted to the medical unit gives the nurse a list of medications taken at home.

J.D. Medication List

Medication	Time Taken
Levothyroxine 0.75 mcg	Before breakfast
Omeprazole OTC	Before breakfast
Captopril	Before breakfast
Melatonin	At night

Which question should the nurse ask the client?
1. "Why do you take the levothyroxine?"
2. "Does your emesis have red or dark-brown flecks in it?"
3. "What was your blood pressure before starting captopril?"
4. "Do you have difficulty sleeping at night?"

54. The male client is diagnosed with narcolepsy. Which OTC preparations should the nurse teach the client about?
1. Caffeinated beverages and diphenhydramine
2. Flavored water and beta carotene
3. Milk with added vitamin D and saw palmetto
4. Carbonated sodas and black cohosh

55. The 10-year-old client has begun to sleepwalk, a parasomnia disorder. Which information should the nurse provide the parents of the child? **Select all that apply.**
1. "Give the child a mild sedative 2 hours before bedtime."
2. "Place a lock on the outer door beyond the child's reach."
3. "Guide the child back to bed and let them remain asleep."
4. "Have the child practice guided imagery before bedtime."
5. "Administer atomoxetine every morning."

56. The client diagnosed with obstructive sleep apnea reports falling asleep at inappropriate times. The HCP has prescribed solriamfetol. Which instructions should the nurse give the client about the medication? **Select all that apply.**
1. Take a maximum-strength caffeine tablet twice a day.
2. Do not use the medication if you use a CPAP machine.
3. Monitor your blood pressure daily.
4. Notify your HCP of violent or abnormal behaviors.
5. Take the medication as needed for daytime sleepiness.

Substance Abuse Issues

57. The client diagnosed with chronic alcoholism is admitted to the medical unit for pneumonia. Which medication should the nurse expect the HCP to prescribe to **prevent** delirium tremens?
1. Chlordiazepoxide
2. Thiamine
3. Disulfiram
4. Fluoxetine

58. Which client should the nurse expect the HCP to prescribe methadone?
1. A client addicted to cocaine
2. A client addicted to heroin
3. A client addicted to amphetamines
4. A client addicted to hallucinogens

59. The client is discussing wanting to quit smoking cigarettes with the clinic nurse. Which intervention is **most successful** in helping the client to quit smoking cigarettes?
1. Encourage the client to attend a smoking cessation support group.
2. Discuss tapering the number of cigarettes smoked daily.
3. Instruct the client to use nicotine replacement therapy, such as a patch.
4. Explain that clonidine can be taken daily to help decrease withdrawal symptoms.

60. The client is prescribed methadone. Which intervention should the nurse discuss with the client?
1. Take the medication on an empty stomach.
2. Decrease the fiber in the diet while taking the medication.
3. Do not take methadone if the radial pulse is less than 60 bpm.
4. Learn how to prevent orthostatic hypotension.

61. The client has taken alprazolam daily for the past 2 years. Which clinical manifestations would **warrant intervention** by the nurse?
1. Nausea, vomiting, and agitation
2. Yawning, rhinorrhea, and cramps
3. Disorientation, lethargy, and craving
4. Ataxia, hyperpyrexia, and respiratory distress

62. Which client would be **most appropriate** to prescribe disulfiram?
1. A client diagnosed with chronic alcoholism admitted to the medical unit
2. A highly motivated client wanting to quit drinking alcohol
3. A client taking amphetamines for more than 1 year
4. A highly motivated client wanting to quit taking heroin

63. A client in the medical unit has been having nothing by mouth (NPO) for 3 days and is reporting a headache. What should the nurse ask the client to determine the cause of the headache?
1. "Do you eat a diet high in glucose?"
2. "How often do you drink alcohol?"
3. "Do you take sleeping pills regularly?"
4. "How often do you drink caffeinated beverages?"

64. The client diagnosed with chronic alcoholism comes to the emergency department (ED) reporting no alcoholic drinks in more than 1 week. Which intervention should the ED nurse implement **first**?
1. Implement seizure precautions according to hospital policy.
2. Rehydrate the client with large amounts of IV fluids.
3. Discuss withdrawal treatment in a hospital environment.
4. Administer thiamine through an IV route.

65. The client with a history of substance abuse is brought to the ED by a friend. The client has a staggering gait and reports feeling short of breath. The client's vital signs are populated in the following vital sign flowsheet.

Vital Sign Flowsheet	Client Values	Reference Values
Temperature	104°F/40°C	Oral: 98°F (36.7°C)
Pulse	106 bpm	60 to 100 bpm
Respirations	24 breaths/min	12 to 20 breaths/min
Blood pressure	128/90 mm Hg	100 to 119 mm Hg systolic 60 to 80 mm Hg diastolic

Which question should the nurse ask the client's friend?
1. "How many alcoholic drinks has your friend had today?"
2. "When was the last time your friend took amphetamines?"
3. "Has your friend been inhaling any type of paint thinner?"
4. "Through which route and at what time did your friend take cocaine?"

66. Which pharmacologic intervention should the nurse discuss with the client requesting help to quit smoking marijuana?
1. Explain that there is no specific pharmacologic intervention.
2. Instruct the client to use a nicotine patch or chew nicotine gum.
3. Encourage the client to have the HCP prescribe an antianxiety medication.
4. Discuss tapering dronabinol over a 2-week period.

67. The client is prescribed fluoxetine for a diagnosis of clinical depression after the client's spouse died. Which question should the nurse ask the client when discussing this medication?
1. "How do you feel about taking this medication?"
2. "Do you have insurance to pay for the medications?"
3. "Does your diet include a lot of aged cheese and wine?"
4. "Are you currently taking any angiotensin-converting enzyme (ACE) inhibitors?"

ANSWERS AND RATIONALES

The correct answer number and rationale are in **boldface blue type.** Rationales for why other answer options are incorrect are also given.

Major Depressive Disorder

1. 1. Confusion and restlessness would not indicate the flu. The elevated temperature should make the nurse suspect a possible serious complication of the SSRI fluoxetine (Prozac).
   2. Serotonin syndrome is a serious complication of SSRIs. Fluoxetine (Prozac) produces mental changes (confusion, anxiety, and restlessness), hypertension, tremors, sweating, hyperpyrexia (elevated temperature), and ataxia. Conservative treatment includes stopping the SSRI and supportive therapy. If untreated, expected side effects can lead to death.
   3. Taking the SSRI fluoxetine (Prozac) medication at night will not treat serotonin syndrome.
   4. These are not ESEs. They require nursing intervention.

2. 1. Medication cost or insurance type should not be a reason one medication is prescribed over another.
   2. This is passing the buck, and the psychiatric nurse should be knowledgeable about medications.
   3. SSRIs have the same efficacy as monoamine oxidase inhibitors (MAOs) and tricyclics, but SSRIs are safer because they do not have the sympathomimetic effects (tachycardia and hypertension) and anticholinergic effects (dry mouth, blurred vision, urinary retention, and constipation) of the MAOs and tricyclics.
   4. All antidepressant medications take at least 14 to 21 days to become effective.

3. 1. Depression is subjective; therefore, asking the client to rate the depression on a scale of 1 to 10 best indicates medication effectiveness. Subjective data can be put on a scale to make it objective.
   2. This is a very vague statement; therefore, it is not the best indicator of medication effectiveness.
   3. Completing ADLs indicates the client is not severely depressed, but it does not objectively support that the client's antidepressant medication is effective.
   4. Consuming 90% of the food may indicate the client is not depressed, but the nurse does not know how the client eats when severely depressed; therefore, it is not the best indicator of the medication's effectiveness.

MEDICATION MEMORY JOGGER: The nurse determines medication effectiveness by assessing for the symptoms, or lack thereof, for which the medication was prescribed.

4. 1. The client should use herbs cautiously because ginseng causes headaches, tremors, mania, insomnia, irritability, and visual hallucinations.
   2. The client should refrain from drinking too many beverages containing caffeine.
   3. Eating three balanced meals a day is not information that the nurse would teach about MAOs.
   4. Taking phenelzine (Nardil), a monoamine oxidase (MAO) inhibitor, requires adherence to strict dietary restrictions concerning tyramine-containing foods, such as processed meat (hot dogs, bologna, and salami), yeast products, beer, and red wines. Eating these foods can cause a life-threatening hypertensive crisis.

MEDICATION MEMORY JOGGER: Some herbal preparations are effective, some are not, and a few can be harmful or even deadly. If a client is taking an herbal supplement and a conventional medicine, the nurse should investigate to determine if the combination will cause harm to the client. The nurse should always be the client's advocate.

5. Correct answers are 1, 2, 4, and 5.
   1. The nurse should inform the client that weight gain is a common side effect of brexpiprazole (Rexulti) and to notify the HCP of significant weight increases.
   2. Impulse control disorders, such as binge eating, gambling, shopping or similar, can occur or be enhanced with brexpiprazole (Rexulti), and the client should notify the HCP.

3. The client should discuss any OTC medications or herbal products with their HCP before taking them, but *all* OTC medications are not avoided.
4. The nurse should teach the client to avoid extremes in temperature because brexpiprazole (Rexulti) can impair body temperature regulation.
5. Orthostatic hypotension can occur in clients taking brexpiprazole (Rexulti). The nurse should teach clients to change positions slowly to avoid falls.

6. 1. The nurse should discuss what behavior led to the client being prescribed antidepressants and determine if the client is still depressed, but the most important thing to discuss with the client is that the amitriptyline (Elavil), a tricyclic antidepressant, should not be discontinued abruptly.
2. The nurse should discuss why the client wants to stop taking the medication, but the most important intervention is to teach the client that medication must be tapered. The client could quit taking the medication without telling an HCP; therefore, teaching safety is a priority.
3. The client should notify the HCP before stopping the medication, but the most important intervention is to keep the client safe and inform the client to taper off medication.
4. The client must first know the importance of needing to taper off medication because rebound dysphoria, irritability, or sleepiness may occur if amitriptyline (Elavil), a tricyclic antidepressant, is discontinued abruptly. Then the client should see the HCP to determine what action should be taken because the client doesn't want to take the medication.

7. 1. Duloxetine (Cymbalta), an atypical antidepressant, does not need to be taken in the morning to be more effective.
2. Antidepressants may cause central nervous system (CNS) depression, which causes drowsiness; therefore, taking duloxetine (Cymbalta), an atypical antidepressant, at night may help the client sleep at night and relieve daytime sedation. This is the nurse's best response.
3. Antidepressants do not need to be taken with food because they do not cause gastrointestinal distress.
4. The nurse can provide factual information to the client without contacting the HCP. Taking antidepressants at night is not contraindicated; therefore, the nurse can share this information with the client.

8. Correct answers are 1, 3, and 4.
1. Antidepressant medications may cause orthostatic hypotension. The nurse should question administering the medication if the blood pressure is less than 90/60.
2. Antidepressant medications do not have a therapeutic blood level. Medication effectiveness and side effects are determined by the client's behavior.
3. Many antidepressants may cause hepatotoxicity; therefore, the nurse should monitor the client's liver function tests.
4. The nurse should ensure the client's safety. Many antidepressants may cause orthostatic hypotension and increase risk for dizziness, falls, and injuries.
5. Antidepressant medications take at least 3 weeks to become effective; therefore, when the client is first admitted to the psychiatric department and prescribed an antidepressant, evaluating for medication effectiveness is not an appropriate intervention.

9. 1. Providing phone numbers for the client and family is an intervention that the nurse could implement, but it is not a priority over the psychological and physical safety of the client.
2. Follow-up appointments are essential for the client after being discharged from a psychiatric facility, but the appointments are not a priority over the psychological and physical safety of the client.
3. Ensuring the psychological and physical safety of the client is a priority. As antidepressant medications become more effective (after at least 3 weeks), the client is at a higher risk for suicide; therefore, the nurse should ensure that the client cannot take a medication overdose.
4. This is an appropriate intervention. Effects of OTC medications are important, but are not a priority over the psychological and physical safety of the client.

10. 1. The nurse should realize this medication takes at least 3 weeks to work; therefore, this question is not helpful to the client.
2. The nurse should not refer the client to the HCP. The client needs factual information about the medication, and the nurse should be prepared to provide that information.

3. The nurse should realize this medication takes at least 3 weeks to become effective and the client does not need to come into the clinic to be told that fact.
4. **The client probably was told this information but may have forgotten it, or the client may not have been told. The most appropriate response is to provide information so that the client realizes it takes 3 weeks for the medication to work and the client may not feel better until that time has elapsed.**

Bipolar Disorder

11. **Correct answers are 2 and 4.**
    1. The lithium level is monitored by a venipuncture serum level, which must be done by a laboratory. It is not a test to be done at home.
    2. **Lithium (Eskalith), an antimania medication, acts like sodium in the body so dehydration can cause lithium toxicity; therefore, the client should not become dehydrated.**
    3. Lithium should not be stopped because bipolar disorder is a chemical imbalance and the client must continue taking this medication or manic behavior will return.
    4. **The client should take lithium, an antimania medication, with food to decrease gastrointestinal upset.**
    5. Foods high in tyramine should be avoided when taking MAO inhibitors, an antidepressant.
12. 1. **The therapeutic serum level is 0.6 to 1.2 mEq/L. Because the lithium level is within the parameters, the nurse should administer lithium, an antimania medication.**
    2. This is within therapeutic range; therefore, the nurse should not hold the medication but should administer it.
    3. This is within therapeutic range; therefore, the nurse should administer the medication.
    4. There is no reason to verify the lithium level; therefore, the nurse should administer the medication.

MEDICATION MEMORY JOGGER: The nurse must be knowledgeable about accepted standards of practice for medication administration, including which client assessment data and laboratory data should be monitored before administering medication.

13. 1. The client taking lithium, an antimania medication, should have adequate sodium intake because a salt-free diet reduces lithium excretion and can lead to lithium toxicity. The nurse would not question administering the medication to this client.
    2. Many clients diagnosed with bipolar disorder are prescribed an antidepressant medication and an antimania drug to treat bipolar disorder; therefore, the nurse would not question administering this medication.
    3. **Diuretics increase lithium excretion from the kidneys; therefore, the nurse would question administering lithium (Eskalith), an antimania medication, to this client.**
    4. The nurse would not question administering lithium to a client with an adequate urine output.
14. 1. Valproic acid (Depakote), an anticonvulsant medication, may be used to help prevent migraine headaches, but this is not an appropriate question to ask this client.
    2. **Valproic acid (Depakote), an anticonvulsant medication, is a category D drug, which means it will cause harm to the fetus and should not be prescribed to a female of childbearing age not using reliable birth control methods.**
    3. Often, a medication classification can be prescribed for another disease process. The nurse must know what the drug is prescribed for, as stated in the stem of the question.
    4. Depakote takes 2 to 3 weeks to become therapeutic; therefore, this question is not pertinent.

MEDICATION MEMORY JOGGER: Any time a female client of childbearing age is prescribed a routine medication, the nurse should think about a possible pregnancy.

15. 1. Caffeine has a diuretic effect that can cause lithium sparing by the kidneys, which may cause lithium toxicity. This statement indicates the client understands the lithium (Eskalith) medication teaching.
    2. **Playing soccer or any sport that includes running can lead to dehydration. The nurse must make sure the client understands the need to stay well hydrated during the activity; therefore, this comment indicates the need for further clarification for the client taking lithium (Eskalith), an antimania medication, by the nurse.**

3. The client needs to maintain adequate fluid intake to prevent dehydration. This statement indicates the client understands the medication teaching.
4. Diarrhea is a sign of lithium toxicity and the client should notify the HCP so that a serum lithium level can be evaluated. This statement indicates the client understands the medication teaching.

16. Correct answers are 2, 3, and 5.

1. This is an extremely high toxic level that requires immediate treatment. The therapeutic range for the client taking lithium (Eskalith), an antimania medication, is 0.6 to 1.5 mEq/L.
2. **This is an extremely high toxic level that requires IV therapy.**
3. **Extremely high toxic levels of lithium require hemodialysis and supportive care.**
4. There is no known antidote for lithium toxicity.
5. **The nurse must monitor cardiac function to assess rhythm disturbances.**

17.

1. **Carbamazepine (Tegretol), an anticonvulsant medication, is prescribed as a mood stabilizer. Mood stabilizers are prescribed because they can moderate extreme shifts in emotions between mania and depression; therefore, this data indicates the medication is effective.**
2. Serum drug levels determine if the medication is at a toxic level, but they do not indicate that the client's mania is controlled; therefore, this does not indicate the drug is effective.
3. Carbamazepine is prescribed to treat mania in bipolar disorder, not depression; therefore, a depression scale does not indicate anything about the medication's effectiveness.
4. A client diagnosed with bipolar disorder experiences a mood disorder, not a thought disorder such as schizophrenia; therefore, this data does not indicate carbamazepine, an anticonvulsant medication, is effective in treating bipolar disorder.

MEDICATION MEMORY JOGGER: The nurse determines medication effectiveness by assessing for the symptoms, or lack thereof, for which the medication was prescribed.

18.

1. This would be an appropriate intervention, but the client's physiological needs are a priority.
2. The nurse must assess why the client is not compliant with lithium (Eskalith), an antimania medication, but in an acute manic state, the client cannot answer this question; therefore, it is not the first intervention.
3. **This is the first intervention because the client is in an acute manic state and the client's physiological need is the priority.**
4. Lithium (Eskalith), an antimania medication, takes 2 to 3 weeks to become therapeutic; therefore, a stat dose of lithium orally will not help the manic state. Lithium is not available in the intramuscular (IM) or IV route.

19. Correct answers are 4 and 5.

1. Recommending use of a soft-bristled toothbrush is specific for clients taking phenytoin (Dilantin), another anticonvulsant medication, but not for Tegretol.
2. Anticonvulsant carbamazepine (Tegretol) does not affect visual acuity; therefore, there is no reason to recommend this health promotion activity for this client.
3. Tegretol does not affect the blood pressure; therefore, there is no reason to recommend this health promotion activity for this client.
4. **The client should avoid driving and other hazardous activities until the effects of the anticonvulsant carbamazepine (Tegretol) are known because this medication may cause sedation and drowsiness.**
5. **The client should wear protective clothing and sunscreen (SPF 45 or higher) when outdoors, as carbamazepine (Tegretol) can make the client more susceptible to sunburn.**

20. Correct answers are 2, 3, and 5.

1. Cariprazine (Vraylar) does not have a therapeutic serum level. The medication is evaluated by decreased occurrence and severity of manic episodes.
2. **The nurse should teach the client to drink plenty of water to avoid dehydration that can increase side effects of cariprazine (Vraylar).**
3. **The nurse should teach the client that using alcohol together with cariprazine (Vraylar) can cause dizziness, drowsiness, and confusion. The client should avoid alcohol while on the medication.**

4. The radial pulse is not evaluated before taking cariprazine, and the client should take the medication even if the pulse is less than 60 bpm.
5. **Cariprazine can cause orthostatic hypotension; therefore, the nurse needs to discuss ways to prevent it.**

Schizophrenia

21. 1. International normalized ratio (INR) is used to monitor effectiveness of the anticoagulant warfarin, not for clozapine.
2. **Weekly WBCs are taken because the client is at risk for fatal agranulocytosis. Initially, the clozapine (Clozaril), an atypical antipsychotic medication, will not be administered if the WBC count is not available.**
3. The client's RBC count is not affected by clozapine.
4. The respiratory system is not affected by clozapine (Clozaril), an atypical antipsychotic; therefore, ABGs do not have to be evaluated when taking this medication.

MEDICATION MEMORY JOGGER: Usually, if a client is prescribed a new medication and has flu-like symptoms within 24 hours of taking the first dose, the client should contact the HCP. These are signs of agranulocytosis, which indicates the medication has caused a sudden drop in WBC count, leaving the body defenseless against bacterial invasion.

22. 1. Atypical antipsychotics do not have any food interactions. A low-tyramine diet is prescribed for clients taking an MAOI, an antidepressant.
2. Respirations are not assessed to determine medication effectiveness, nor are they used to determine when to question the medication; therefore, this is not an appropriate intervention for risperidone (Risperdal), an atypical antipsychotic.
3. **A side effect of all types of antipsychotics is orthostatic hypotension (lightheadedness, dizziness), which can be minimized by moving slowly when assuming an erect posture.**
4. The client's renal system is not affected by risperidone (Risperdal), an atypical antipsychotic; therefore, it does not need to be monitored while taking this medication.

23. 1. Atypical antipsychotic medications have a lower risk of sexual dysfunction than conventional antipsychotic medications; therefore, if the client experiences impotency, the client should call his HCP. This statement does not indicate the client understands the medication teaching.
2. Atypical antipsychotic medications do not cause photosensitivity (unlike conventional antipsychotic drugs). This statement does not indicate the client understands the medication teaching.
3. Atypical antipsychotic medications do not cause gynecomastia (unlike conventional antipsychotic drugs). This statement indicates that the client does not understand the medication teaching.
4. **Ziprasidone (Geodon), an atypical antipsychotic, is well-tolerated, but the most common side effect is difficulty sleeping, perhaps because of the histamine antagonist blockade effect of the drug. This comment indicates the client understands the teaching.**

24. Correct answers are 1, 2, and 5.
1. **Clozapine (Clozaril), an atypical antipsychotic, can promote significant weight gain; therefore, the client should exercise regularly, monitor weight, and reduce caloric intake.**
2. **Clozaril promotes weight gain.**
3. Clozaril does not cause gastrointestinal distress and can be taken with food or an empty stomach.
4. Aspirins do not affect taking this medication.
5. **Cigarette smoking may decrease effectiveness of clozapine (Clozaril), an atypical antipsychotic.**

25. 1. Clients diagnosed with schizophrenia do not have an anxiety disorder and this medication does not help decrease anxiety.
2. Aripiprazole (Abilify), a dopamine system stabilizer (DDS), affects receptor sites for dopamine and does not increase dopamine secretion.
3. **Like other antipsychotics, aripiprazole (Abilify), a DDS, treats positive and negative symptoms of schizophrenia, but it does so with fewer side effects than other antipsychotics. This medication does not cause significant weight gain, hypotension, or prolactin release, and it poses no risk of anticholinergic effects or dysrhythmias.**
4. This medication does not block cholinergic receptors.

26. Correct answers are 1, 4, and 5.

1. **Caffeine-containing substances will negate antipsychotic medication effects; therefore, the client should drink caffeine-free beverages such as decaffeinated coffee and tea and caffeine-free colas.**
2. Salt intake does not affect antipsychotic medication, nor does it affect schizophrenia; therefore, dietary intake of salt does not need to be decreased.
3. Small meals and protein do not affect antipsychotic medications, nor will they affect schizophrenia; therefore, the client does not have to eat high-protein meals.
4. **Long-term use of typical antipsychotic medications may lead to a condition called tardive dyskinesia (TD), exhibited by muscle spasms and rigidity.**
5. **Atypical antipsychotics may increase the client's risk of developing diabetes and high cholesterol; therefore, the client's weight, glucose levels, and lipid levels should be monitored regularly.**

27.

1. The client should be responsible for taking their medication and not relying on the family member to administer it. The nurse should encourage the family member to promote the client's independence.
2. There is no reason for the family member to learn CPR because antipsychotic medications do not cause death.
3. The nurse should encourage the family member to attend a support group for families of people diagnosed with schizophrenia. If there are any groups available for people diagnosed with schizophrenia, then the client should attend one. The nurse should encourage the family member to let the client take care of their mental illness.
4. **Antipsychotic medications lower the seizure threshold, even if the client does not have a seizure disorder; therefore, the nurse should discuss what to do if the client has a seizure.**

28.

1. Tremors or rigidity indicate the client is having extrapyramidal side effects of antipsychotic medications. Such activity does not indicate the medication is effective.
2. Antipsychotic medications are not prescribed for anxiety; therefore, anxiety cannot be evaluated to determine if the drug is effective.
3. Sleeping all night is a good sign for the client, but it does not determine if the medication is effective.
4. **Antipsychotic medications are prescribed to decrease clinical manifestations of schizophrenia. If the client denies auditory hallucinations, then the atypical antipsychotic quetiapine (Seroquel) medication is effective.**

MEDICATION MEMORY JOGGER: The nurse determines medication effectiveness by assessing for the symptoms, or lack thereof, for which the medication was prescribed.

29.

1. Rigidity and tremors are signs of extrapyramidal side effects and should be reported to the HCP. The client does not need additional teaching.
2. Haloperidol (Haldol), a conventional antipsychotic, has anticholinergic effects, including constipation. Increasing fiber and fluid intake will help prevent constipation. This statement does not indicate that the client needs additional teaching.
3. **Haloperidol (Haldol), a conventional antipsychotic, can cause agranulocytosis, diminishing the client's ability to fight infection, but the medication (if the client does not develop the adverse effect of agranulocytosis) does not cause the client to have increased susceptibility to colds and the flu. If the client has a fever or sore throat, the HCP should be notified, and if the WBC count is elevated, the medication will be discontinued.**
4. This statement indicates the client understands why the haloperidol (Haldol), a conventional antipsychotic, is being taken. This indicates the medication teaching is effective.

MEDICATION MEMORY JOGGER: Usually, if a client is prescribed a new medication and has flu-like symptoms within 24 hours of taking the first dose, the client should contact the HCP. These are signs of agranulocytosis, which indicates the medication has caused a sudden drop in the WBC count, leaving the body defenseless against bacterial invasion.

30.

1. Menstrual irregularity is a common side effect of conventional antipsychotic medications like chlorpromazine (Thorazine) and would not warrant discontinuing the medication.
2. Orthostatic hypotension is a common side effect of conventional antipsychotic medications and would not warrant discontinuing the medication.

3. Anticholinergic effects are common side effects of conventional antipsychotic medications and would not warrant discontinuing the medication.
4. **Exhibiting fine, worm-like movements of the tongue is a symptom of tardive dyskinesia, which is an adverse effect that may develop after months or years of continuous therapy with a conventional antipsychotic medication. The conventional antipsychotic medication chlorpromazine (Thorazine) should be discontinued and a benzodiazepine should be administered.**

MEDICATION MEMORY JOGGER: The test taker should question administering any medication to a pregnant client or a client trying to become pregnant. Many medications cross the placental barrier and could affect the fetus.

Anxiety Disorder

31. Correct answers are 1 and 4.
1. **Alprazolam (Xanax), a benzodiazepine, has the potential for dependency, but that potential can be minimized by using the lowest effective dosage for the shortest time necessary.**
2. Rage, excitement, and heightened anxiety are signs of paradoxical reactions and should be reported to the HCP. The medication will be discontinued.
3. There is no contraindication to eating foods high in vitamin K and taking Xanax.
4. **Alprazolam (Xanax), a benzodiazepine, can initially cause drowsiness, so the client should not drive automobiles or use machinery.**
5. There is no reason for the client to take the medication with 8 ounces of water.

32. 1. The client should inform the obstetrician of the panic attacks and the lorazepam (Ativan) therapy, but this is not the nurse's first intervention.
2. The client must quit taking the medication because it can harm a fetus. Still, if the client has been on long-term therapy, the medication should be discontinued gradually to prevent withdrawal symptoms.
3. **The nurse should first determine how long the client has been taking lorazepam (Ativan), a benzodiazepine, and what dosage (or how many pills) to determine if the medication can be discontinued abruptly or if it must be gradually decreased.**
4. The nurse should encourage the client to stop taking the Ativan before getting pregnant, but the first intervention is to assess the client to determine how long she has been taking the medication.

33. 1. The client's apical pulse would not be monitored before the nurse administering the benzodiazepine alprazolam (Xanax).
2. The client's potassium level would not be monitored before the nurse administering the Xanax.
3. **The nurse must assess the client's anxiety level on a scale of 1 to 10, with 10 being the most anxious, before administering the benzodiazepine alprazolam (Xanax). If the nurse does not do this, there is no way to evaluate medication effectiveness later.**
4. The client's blood pressure would not be monitored before the nurse administers the Xanax.

34. 1. Common side effects of SSRIs include nausea, headache, insomnia, and sexual dysfunction. If these side effects develop, the client would need to notify the HCP or might be inclined to stop taking the medication due to the side effect. The client does not understand the medication teaching.
2. **The beneficial effects of SSRIs develop slowly, taking several months to become maximal when treating OCD. The client understands this.**
3. SSRIs are antidepressants used to treat OCD. They do not have addictive properties. The client does not understand the medication teaching.
4. The client should continue to go to a counselor or psychologist to determine the cause of the anxiety so that the client can eventually discontinue the SSRI sertraline (Zoloft). The client does not understand the medication teaching.

35. 1. This is not an accurate statement. Initial responses can be seen within 2 weeks, but may take up to 2 to 3 months for maximal response.
2. The nurse should not ask the client "Why?" It is a confrontational question and does not answer the client's question.
3. The client should continue with cognitive therapy, but this is a very negative statement and is not the nurse's best response.
4. **SSRIs reduce the three core symptoms of PTSD: re-experiencing, avoidance or emotional numbing, and hyperarousal.**

The paroxetine (Paxil), an SSRI medication, is most effective if taken within 3 months of the traumatic event and may take up to 2 or 3 months for maximal response.

36\. 1. The benzodiazepine alprazolam (Xanax) is an appropriate medication for an anxiety attack, but it will take at least 15 to 30 minutes for the medication to treat the physiological clinical manifestations.
2. The client is in distress. The nurse should not assess the client; the nurse needs to help the client.
3. This is the most appropriate intervention. The nurse should remove the client from the busy day room to help decrease the anxiety attack.
4. SSRIs can be used to treat panic attacks, but the SSRI sertraline (Zoloft) takes weeks to work; therefore, it would not be helpful in an acute panic attack.

MEDICATION MEMORY JOGGER: Remember that when a client is in distress, medication usually takes too long to work to help the client immediately. The nurse should always treat the client directly.

37\. 1. Feeling dizzy and weak when getting out of a chair indicates orthostatic hypotension, which is a common side effect of antianxiety medications and is not a reason to quit taking the anxiolytic alprazolam (Xanax).
2. Feeling dizzy and weak when getting out of a chair indicates orthostatic hypotension, which is a common side effect of antianxiety medications and is not a reason for the client to come to the clinic.
3. Feeling dizzy and weak when getting out of a chair indicates orthostatic hypotension, which is a common side effect of antianxiety medications, and fluid intake would not affect the client's behavior.
4. Feeling dizzy and weak when getting out of a chair indicates orthostatic hypotension, which is a common side effect of antianxiety medications, such as the anxiolytic alprazolam (Xanax). The nurse should instruct the client to rise slowly from the sitting to the standing position to avoid dizziness.

38\. **Correct answers are 3 and 5.**
1. The use of an emetic with activated charcoal is not used for benzodiazepine toxicity (Kang et al., 2020).
2. Hemodialysis is not used for benzodiazepine toxicity.
3. The antidote, flumazenil (Romazicon), can be given to reduce benzodiazepine-induced sedation, although it is not routine.
4. A whole bowel irrigation performed with large volumes of macrogol solutions (GoLYTELY) is not prescribed for alprazolam overdose (Kang et al., 2020).
5. The treatment for benzodiazepine toxicity is supportive care. The nurse should ensure the supplies for endotracheal intubation are at the bedside.

39\. 1. The anxiolytic diazepam (Valium) is oil based and should not be diluted with normal saline.
2. The nurse should administer the anxiolytic diazepam (Valium) undiluted for at least 1 minute for each 5 mg of medication in the IV port closest to the client's hand so the medication can get to the client's bloodstream faster.
3. Valium should be administered as an IVP, not as an IV piggyback (IVPB).
4. Valium can be administered safely via the IV route and is recommended for acute, severe anxiety attacks because it will be effective within 1 to 5 minutes.

Attention Deficit-Hyperactivity Disorder

40\. 1. Weight gain would not warrant intervention; weight loss would be of concern to the nurse.
2. These vital signs are within normal limits for a 10-year-old child.
3. The nurse should further investigate the cause of the bruises because this could be an adverse effect of methylphenidate (Ritalin), a CNS stimulant, caused by leukopenia, anemia, or both. It could also be the result of child abuse. Either way, it warrants intervention by the nurse.
4. Sitting quietly in the examination room would indicate methylphenidate (Ritalin), a CNS stimulant, is effective and would not warrant nurse intervention.

MEDICATION MEMORY JOGGER: If the client verbalizes a symptom, if the nurse assesses data, or if laboratory data indicates an adverse effect secondary to a medication, the nurse must intervene. The nurse must implement an independent intervention or notify the HCP because medications can result in serious or even life-threatening complications.

41. Correct answer is 4.

1. Methylphenidate (Ritalin), a CNS stimulant, should be taken on an empty stomach (30 to 45 minutes before a meal).
2. The child's weight should be taken two to three times weekly, and any significant weight loss should be reported.
3. The medication should be administered in the morning, and the last medication should be given no later than 1600 so that the child can sleep. This medication is a CNS stimulant.
4. **A behavior diary should be kept to chronicle the response and symptoms to methylphenidate (Ritalin), a CNS stimulant. This diary should be brought to all follow-up visits with the HCP.**
5. The medication is not affected by sunlight; therefore, this is not correct information.

42.

1. Methylphenidate (Ritalin), a CNS stimulant, does not affect glucose level; therefore, the nurse would not need to check this level.
2. The medication should be administered with food to decrease gastrointestinal upset, but it does not need to be given with a full glass of water.
3. **CNS stimulation induces catecholamine release with a subsequent increase in heart rate and blood pressure; therefore, the nurse should assess the child's vital signs.**
4. The nurse should assess the child's surgical wound, but it is not pertinent when administering methylphenidate (Ritalin), a CNS stimulant. The nurse must administer the Ritalin no matter what the wound looks like.

43.

1. Most schools have a "zero drug tolerance" policy and do not allow students to carry personal medication. The adolescent must keep the medication in the original prescription container. This statement indicates the student does not understand the medication teaching.
2. **Lisdexamfetamine (Vyvanse), a CNS stimulant, has high abuse potential and is not allowed to be carried by students in the school. This statement indicates the adolescent understands the medication teaching, specifically, that the medication will be kept by the school nurse.**
3. Lisdexamfetamine (Vyvanse), a CNS stimulant, must be taken daily, usually twice a day. It is not a PRN medication. The student does not understand the medication teaching.
4. The adolescent should not be giving prescription medication to another child. This statement does not support that the adolescent understands the medication teaching.

44.

1. This is a false statement. There are other medications that can be taken for ADHD.
2. The word "why" is considered argumentative, and the nurse should try to provide information to the mother.
3. **Atomoxetine (Strattera) is a medication that has the same efficacy as methylphenidate (Ritalin), a CNS stimulant, and is not a scheduled drug. Parents hesitant to administer stimulants to their children now have a reasonable alternative. The nurse should provide factual information.**
4. The nurse can discuss medications with the mother. The mother would have to obtain a drug prescription, but the school nurse must know about medications.

45.

1. **Growth rate may stall in response to nutritional deficiency caused by anorexia. A 4-pound weight loss in 2 weeks is cause for investigation. The child needs to be seen by the HCP.**
2. Methylphenidate (Ritalin), a CNS stimulant, should not be discontinued abruptly because rebound hyperactivity or withdrawal symptoms can occur.
3. This is not a normal response to methylphenidate (Ritalin), a CNS stimulant, and the child should be seen by the HCP.
4. This may need to be done, but the child needs to see the HCP to determine why the child has lost 4 pounds in 2 weeks. This is not normal for a 7-year-old child.

46.

1. Inappropriate behavior at school would not indicate the child's medication is effective.
2. The CNS stimulant lisdexamfetamine (Vyvanse) is not administered to help the child sleep all the time; therefore, this medication is not effective, and the child is receiving too much medicine.
3. **The child's ability to focus on a specific activity indicates the CNS stimulant lisdexamfetamine (Vyvanse) is effective. Inability to focus on one task at a time and jumping from one activity to another are ADHD signs.**
4. Difficulty in following verbal instruction is an ADHD symptom. This indicates the medication is not effective.

MEDICATION MEMORY JOGGER: The nurse determines medication effectiveness by assessing for the symptoms, or lack thereof, for which the medication was prescribed.

47. **1. The CNS stimulant methylphenidate (Ritalin) is metabolized in the liver and excreted by the kidneys. Impaired organ function can increase serum drug levels. The medication may cause leukopenia, anemia, or both. The HCP would order a CBC, differential, and platelet count.**
2. Potassium and sodium levels are not monitored for methylphenidate (Ritalin).
3. The growth rate may slow as a result of nutritional deficiency caused by anorexia, but the child's bone density is not affected; therefore, this diagnostic test is not monitored.
4. There is no serum drug level for methylphenidate (Ritalin).

MEDICATION MEMORY JOGGER: The nurse must know accepted standards of practice for medication administration, including which client assessment data and laboratory data should be monitored while a client is taking long-term medication.

Sleep Disorder

48. 1. Diazepam (Valium), a benzodiazepine, can depress respirations, but this client has already been taking the medication.
2. Diazepam (Valium), a benzodiazepine, is administered to clients during a seizure to treat a seizure, but this client has informed the nurse that it is being taken for sleep.
3. The client has already told the nurse that the Valium is used to induce sleep.
4. Benzodiazepines should be tapered off when the client is trying to stop taking them. The nurse should request an order for the diazepam (Valium).

49. **1. The client is having abdominal surgery, so the client will be NPO for a while. Alprazolam (Xanax), a benzodiazepine, is only manufactured as an oral medication; therefore, the client will need a similar medication postoperatively. The nurse should discuss this with the HCP.**
2. The client will be NPO after a major abdominal surgery. Xanax only comes in an oral preparation.
3. If the client plans to stop taking Xanax, it should be tapered, but the stem does not indicate a need to discontinue medication.
4. Alprazolam (Xanax), a benzodiazepine, is being taken PRN, not just for sleep but also for anxiety.

50. 1. Angiotensin-converting enzyme (ACE) inhibitors such as captopril are administered to treat hypertension or for prophylaxis in clients diagnosed with diabetes and would not interfere with a sleep study.
2. Antihistamines such as diphenhydramine (Benadryl) can cause drowsiness in many clients. The client should not take any medication that would interfere with the test being interpreted correctly.
3. Loop diuretics such as furosemide are administered early in the day to prevent nocturia and effects should have worn off before the sleep study begins. Sleep studies are conducted during the night.
4. Normal routine doses of thyroid medication such as levothyroxine would not interfere with a sleep study.

51. **1. The nurse should teach the client not to attempt to get pregnant while receiving chemotherapy or taking lorazepam (Ativan), a benzodiazepine. Ativan is a pregnancy category D drug. Ativan is very useful in controlling chemotherapy-induced nausea and vomiting, so the HCP is attempting to achieve a dual use for the medication—improved sleep and relief of chemotherapy-induced nausea.**
2. Lorazepam (Ativan), a benzodiazepine, can interact with alcohol, increasing CNS depression. The client should not consume alcohol at all.
3. Exercise immediately before bedtime can increase the client's inability to sleep. Exercising a few hours before bedtime is suggested.
4. Clients taking benzodiazepines may become dependent on medications and they are at high risk for addiction. The medications are tapered off if they are being discontinued.

52. 1. This situation requires further evaluation by the nurse before notifying the HCP.
2. Safety is a priority. The client received a sedative medication and an antinausea medication within the past 10 hours. Elderly clients frequently require longer periods of time to clear medications from their systems.
3. The client is not in a code situation. The client is lethargic, probably from the medications.

4. The nurse should reevaluate the client in 30 to 60 minutes, but in the meantime safety is the first intervention.

53. 1. There is only one reason to take levothyroxine (Synthroid) as a thyroid replacement. The nurse should know this.
2. There is no indication that the client is vomiting. Omeprazole (Prilosec) is frequently taken for gastroesophageal reflux disease (GERD).
3. The blood pressure before beginning captopril (Capoten) is not essential. The current blood pressure and amount of control the client achieves while taking Capoten are important.
4. Melatonin is an OTC hormone that many people take to prevent jet lag or induce sleep.

54. 1. Caffeine may help the client achieve some measure of alertness, whereas products containing diphenhydramine (Benadryl) can increase the client's problem because this medication is used in OTC sleep aids. The client should be taught about both.
2. Flavored water will not have any effect on narcolepsy. Beta carotene is a precursor to vitamin A and is often taken to treat degenerative eye diseases.
3. Milk with vitamin D is useful for clients diagnosed with osteoporosis and saw palmetto is used to treat benign prostatic hypertrophy. The question does not state that the client has either of these conditions.
4. Carbonated drinks should be avoided by clients with a GERD diagnosis. Black cohosh is used for menstrual irregularities, menopausal symptoms, and as an antispasmodic. The question does not state that the client has either of these problems.

55. Correct answers are 2 and 3.
1. A mild sedative would increase the child's inability to awaken during the night if needed. No medication is useful to treat sleepwalking.
2. This is a safety measure to keep the child from exiting the house during the night.
3. It is difficult to arouse a sleepwalker. The child should be guided back to bed and allowed to remain asleep.
4. Guided imagery will not stop sleepwalking.
5. Atomoxetine (Strattera) is administered for ADHD, not for sleepwalking.

56. Correct answers are 3 and 4.
1. The client should avoid caffeine and other OTC medications while using solriamfetol (Sunosi) unless directed by the HCP.
2. The client should continue to use their continuous positive airway pressure (CPAP) machine while on this medication.
3. Solriamfetol (Sunosi) can cause an increase in blood pressure, especially in patients with a hypertension diagnosis. The nurse should teach the client to monitor their blood pressure and call the HCP if it becomes elevated.
4. Solriamfetol (Sunosi) can cause agitation, irritability, and other abnormal behaviors. The nurse should teach the client to report any feelings of recklessness or violence immediately.
5. Solriamfetol (Sunosi) is taken regularly to treat daytime sleepiness from narcolepsy or obstructive sleep apnea. The medication is not taken PRN.

Substance Abuse Issues

57. 1. Chlordiazepoxide (Librium), a benzodiazepine, diminishes anxiety and has anticonvulsant qualities to provide safe withdrawal from alcohol. It may be ordered every 4 hours or PRN to manage adverse effects from withdrawal, after which the dose is tapered to zero.
2. Thiamine (vitamin B_1), a vitamin, is prescribed for clients diagnosed with chronic alcoholism. It is prescribed to prevent Wernicke's encephalopathy, not to prevent delirium tremens.
3. Disulfiram (Antabuse), an abstinence medication, is used when a client wishes to quit drinking alcohol. It prevents the breakdown of alcohol and causes the client to vomit when alcohol is consumed.
4. Fluoxetine (Prozac) is an antidepressant. Antidepressants are not used to prevent delirium tremens.

MEDICATION MEMORY JOGGER: The nurse must be knowledgeable about accepted standards of practice for disease processes and conditions. If the nurse administers a medication the HCP has prescribed and it harms the client, the nurse could be held accountable. Remember, the nurse is a client advocate.

58. 1. Methadone, an abstinence medication, would not help a client addicted to cocaine.
2. Methadone, an abstinence medication, blocks the craving for heroin.

3. Methadone would not help a client addicted to amphetamines.
4. Methadone would not help a client addicted to hallucinogens, such as lysergic acid diethylamide (LSD).

59. 1. A smoking cessation support group may be helpful, but nicotine withdrawal is a physical withdrawal, and medication should be used to help with withdrawal symptoms.
2. Tapering the number of cigarettes daily is not the most successful method to quit smoking cigarettes.
3. Using a nicotine patch or chewing nicotine gum is the most successful way to help with nicotine withdrawal symptoms.
4. Clonidine is used to help prevent delirium tremens in a client diagnosed with alcohol dependence.

60. 1. Methadone, an opiate agonist, causes gastrointestinal distress, which can be minimized by taking medication with food.
2. Methadone causes constipation; therefore, the client should increase fiber intake to help prevent constipation.
3. Methadone does not affect the pulse; therefore, the pulse does not need to be monitored before taking the medication.
4. Methadone, an opiate agonist, causes drowsiness, lightheadedness, dizziness, and a transient drop in blood pressure; therefore, the nurse should discuss how to prevent orthostatic hypotension. Methadone is used to treat heroin withdrawal.

61. 1. Nausea, vomiting, and agitation, along with tachycardia, diaphoresis, tremors, and marked insomnia, are adverse effects of CNS depressants, such as alprazolam (Xanax), a benzodiazepine.
2. Yawning, rhinorrhea, and cramps are signs of withdrawal from opiates, such as heroin, meperidine, morphine, and methadone.
3. Disorientation, lethargy, and craving are signs of withdrawal from a stimulant, such as crack cocaine and amphetamines.
4. Ataxia, hyperpyrexia, and respiratory distress are signs of a stimulant overdose, such as crack cocaine and amphetamines.

62. 1. The client must want to quit drinking alcohol. Nothing in the question indicates this, so it would not be appropriate to prescribe disulfiram for this client.
2. Disulfiram (Antabuse), an abstinence medication, is only effective in highly motivated clients because the success of pharmacotherapy is entirely dependent on client compliance. This client is highly motivated to quit drinking alcohol.
3. Disulfiram (Antabuse), an abstinence medication, inhibits acetaldehyde dehydrogenase, the enzyme that metabolizes alcohol. It is not used for amphetamine abuse.
4. Disulfiram inhibits acetaldehyde dehydrogenase, the enzyme that metabolizes alcohol. It is not used for heroin abuse.

63. 1. The fact that the client has not had any food in 3 days may be a cause for the headache. The nurse does not need to ask the client the time of the last meal because the nurse is aware of this information. The type of diet the client ate before being NPO for 3 days would not be an appropriate question in determining the cause of the client's headache.
2. Alcohol withdrawal does not cause a headache.
3. Regularly taking sleeping pills would not cause a headache.
4. A hallmark symptom of caffeine withdrawal is a headache, along with fatigue, depression, and impaired performance of daily activities. This question would be most appropriate for the nurse to ask the client.

64. 1. The nurse should implement seizure precautions, but it is not the first intervention.
2. Immediately on arrival at a hospital, the client should be rehydrated with large amounts of IV physiologic fluids. This is the first intervention.
3. After treating delirium tremens, the client must undergo a course of withdrawal treatment in a therapeutic milieu, but it is not the first intervention in the emergency department.
4. Malnutrition is a severe complication of chronic alcoholism, especially thiamine (vitamin B_1) deficiency, which can result in neurologic impairments; therefore, thiamine must be administered intravenously. This is not the first intervention.

65. 1. The nurse would not suspect alcohol overdose with these clinical manifestations.
2. The nurse would not suspect amphetamine overdose with these clinical manifestations.
3. The nurse would not suspect the client was inhaling paint thinner with these clinical manifestations.

4. **Respiratory distress, ataxia, hyperpyrexia, convulsions, coma, or stroke are clinical manifestations of cocaine overdose. This question would be most appropriate for the nurse to ask based on the client's clinical manifestations.**

66. 1. Marijuana use disorder is similar to other substance abuse disorders, but the FDA currently approves no medication for treatment. Behavioral therapy can be a helpful treatment to stop smoking marijuana (National Institute on Drug Abuse, 2020).

2. Nicotine replacement therapy is used by clients trying to quit smoking cigarettes, not marijuana.
3. Antianxiety medications are not used to treat clients wanting to quit smoking marijuana.
4. Dronabinol (Marinol) is a synthetic derivative of tetrahydrocannabinol (THC), the principal constituent of marijuana. It is prescribed to clients receiving chemotherapy to help treat nausea and vomiting.

67. 1. Many people do not acknowledge mental illness as a problem and may not believe in taking antidepressant medications. The client may see taking medications as a weakness or feel as if the medication will change them somehow. The nurse must determine if the client will take fluoxetine (Prozac), a selective serotonin reuptake inhibitor (SSRI), and provide information necessary to allow the client to make an informed choice.

2. Clients with difficulty in procuring medications will usually inform the nurse. It is not a question the nurse should ask.
3. Aged cheese and wine contain tyramine, which should be avoided when taking an MAO inhibitor, not a SSRI.
4. Some beta blockers may interact with an SSRI, but ACE inhibitors do not.

MENTAL HEALTH DISORDERS COMPREHENSIVE EXAMINATION

1. The nurse is leading a medication group in a psychiatric unit. Which information should the nurse discuss with the client concerning antipsychotic medications after discharge? **Select all that apply.**
   1. Instruct the client to chew sugarless gum to help dry mouth.
   2. Teach the client about orthostatic hypotension.
   3. Explain that the medication may cause drowsiness.
   4. Discuss that these medications may cause sexual dysfunction.
   5. Instruct the client to call the HCP if flu-like symptoms occur.

2. The female client diagnosed with anorexia nervosa is in the inpatient psychiatric unit receiving olanzapine and therapy. Which data suggests the medications are **effective**?
   1. The client eats at least 90% of the meal.
   2. The client has a weight gain of 1 kg.
   3. The client has no symptoms of hay fever.
   4. The client states she will eat all her meals.

3. The clinic nurse is assessing a client 3 weeks after a suicide attempt. The client was prescribed sertraline. Which behavior indicates the medication is **effective**?
   1. The client sleeps 14 to 16 hours a day.
   2. The client has lost 3 pounds.
   3. The client regrets the suicide attempt.
   4. The client has started a new job.

4. The client diagnosed with panic disorder is taking a phenelzine. Which statement by the client **warrants immediate** intervention?
   1. "I am very careful about what I eat."
   2. "I have been taking dextromethorphan for my cough."
   3. "I took two acetaminophen for my headache."
   4. "I only drink one cup of coffee a day."

5. Which task is **most appropriate** for the registered nurse (RN) to assign to the licensed practical nurse (LPN) working in the psychiatric department?
   1. Administer alprazolam to a client diagnosed with a panic disorder.
   2. Administer haloperidol to a client experiencing tardive dyskinesia.
   3. Administer lithium medication to a client diagnosed with bipolar disease and a lithium level of 2.0 mEq/L.
   4. Administer oral thiamine to a client diagnosed with chronic alcoholism experiencing delirium tremens.

6. Which statement is the scientific rationale for prescribing atomoxetine for a child diagnosed with ADHD?
   1. It increases acetylcholine levels and the brain's cholinergic function.
   2. This medication normalizes reuptake of certain neurotransmitters.
   3. This medication is a nonstimulant, nonnarcotic that regulates impulse control.
   4. It results in mild CNS stimulation to control the child's behavior.

7. The client diagnosed with insomnia asks the nurse, "Why did my HCP prescribe zolpidem and tell me to quit taking acetaminophen and diphenhydramine?" Which response by the nurse is **most appropriate**?
   1. "Over-the-counter medications are not as good as prescriptions."
   2. "Acetaminophen and diphenhydramine are addicting. You should not take it nightly."
   3. "You are concerned that your HCP gave you a prescription drug."
   4. "Zolpidem will help you get to sleep and stay asleep through the night."

8. The nurse on the substance abuse unit is administering medications. Which medication should the nurse **question** administering?
   1. Chlordiazepoxide to a client admitted for alcohol detoxification
   2. Haloperidol to a client diagnosed with phencyclidine psychosis
   3. Clonidine to client with a blood pressure of 88/60
   4. Thiamine intravenously to a client diagnosed with Wernicke-Korsakoff syndrome

9. The client is brought to the ED by a friend. The client is hypervigilant, has not slept in 3 days, has dilated pupils, has an apical pulse of 118 bpm, and has a runny nose. Which substance should the nurse suspect the client is abusing?
   1. Cannabis
   2. Heroin
   3. Cocaine
   4. Alcohol

10. The client diagnosed with anorexia nervosa is admitted to the medical department for total parenteral nutrition (TPN) because of her emaciated condition. Which task can be delegated to the unlicensed assistive personnel (UAP)? **Select all that apply.**
    1. Evaluate the client's intake and output.
    2. Obtain the client's daily weight.
    3. Change the TPN tubing during the bath.
    4. Escort the client to the hospital cafeteria.
    5. Perform a glucometer check every 6 hours.

11. Which statement **best** supports the scientific rationale for pharmacologic treatment in clients diagnosed with substance abuse?
    1. Medications allow the clients to take a medication legally for their problem.
    2. Medications permit safe withdrawal and help prevent relapse.
    3. Medications will prevent all side effects of substance abuse withdrawal.
    4. Medications allow the clients to have a psychological reason to quit the substance abuse.

12. The client wants to quit smoking cigarettes. The client has been to a smoking cessation support group and has used nicotine patches but has not been successful. Which recommendation should the nurse give the client?
    1. "Chew nicotine gum instead of using the patch."
    2. "Try an OTC medication to help quit smoking."
    3. "Take 500 mg of vitamin C twice a day."
    4. "Ask your HCP for a prescription for bupropion."

13. The client diagnosed with schizophrenia is hallucinating and attacking other clients in the psychiatric unit. The client has a PRN order for 50 mg of chlorpromazine IM. The medication comes in a vial with 100 mg per mL. How many milliliters should the nurse administer?

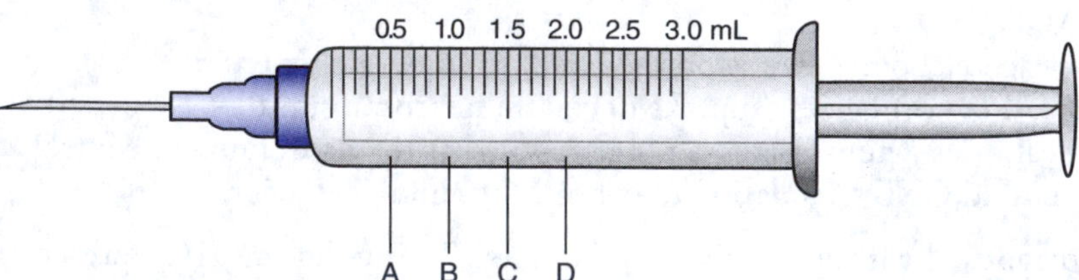

Designate the spot on the syringe.
1. A
2. B
3. C
4. D

14. The client diagnosed with chronic alcoholism is prescribed multivitamins via IV route because of malnutrition. The IV solution turns yellow after injecting the multivitamin. Which intervention should the nurse implement?
1. Notify the pharmacist about the discoloration of the IV.
2. Cover the IV bag and tubing with light-resistant material.
3. Administer the medication as prescribed and take no action.
4. Discard the IV bag and obtain another vial of medication.

15. The client diagnosed with schizophrenia is admitted to the medical department for pneumonia and is exhibiting involuntary movements of the tongue and lips.

Client:	MR# 123456	Date: Today
Age:	Allergies: NKDA	Diagnosis:
Sex:	Height: 69 inches	Weight: 165 pounds
Medication	**0701–1900**	**1901–0700**
Chlorpromazine 50 mg PO b.i.d.	0900 1800	
Lorazepam 2 mg PO daily		2100
Cefuroxime 750 mg IVPB every 6 hours	1200 1800	2400 0600 NN
Maalox 30 mL PRN	1200	
Nurse Initials/Credentials	**DN/RN**	**NN/RN**

Which medication should the nurse **question** administering?
1. Chlorpromazine
2. Lorazepam
3. Cefuroxime
4. The nurse should not question administering any of these medications.

16. The nurse is administering medications on a psychiatric unit. Which client should the nurse discuss with the HCP?
1. The 17-year-old client diagnosed with bipolar disorder and is receiving risperidone
2. The client diagnosed with schizophrenia and is receiving cimetidine
3. The client diagnosed with a heroin dependency and is receiving rifampin
4. The 16-year-old client diagnosed with anorexia nervosa and is receiving amitriptyline

17. The 17-year-old adolescent female diagnosed with anorexia is prescribed desipramine. Which data indicates the medication is **not effective**?
1. The client's mood has improved.
2. The client does not fight with her parents.
3. The client is verbalizing wanting to go to college.
4. The client is preoccupied with shape and weight.

MENTAL HEALTH DISORDERS COMPREHENSIVE EXAMINATION ANSWERS AND RATIONALES

1. **Correct answers are 1, 2, 4, and 5.**
   1. **Antipsychotic drugs produce varying degrees of muscarinic cholinergic blockade, including dry mouth, blurred vision, and photophobia. Chewing sugarless gum may help dry mouth.**
   2. **Antipsychotic medications promote orthostatic hypotension by blocking alpha-adrenergic receptors on blood vessels; therefore, the nurse should teach the client about orthostatic hypotension.**
   3. The sedative effects of antipsychotic medications should have subsided by the time the client is discharged; therefore, this is not an appropriate teaching for discharge. Sedation is common during the early days of treatment, but it subsides within a week or so.
   4. **Antipsychotics can cause sexual dysfunction in women and men, so this should be discussed by the nurse.**
   5. **Flu-like symptoms are a sign of agranulocytosis, a rare but serious reaction to antipsychotic medications. In agranulocytosis, the body loses its ability to fight infection.**

2. 1. The client eating 90% of the meal does not indicate the client has gained weight.
   2. **Therapy and administration of the antipsychotic olanzapine (Zyprexa) are effective if the client gains weight. The 2.2 pounds is excellent weight gain for a client diagnosed with anorexia.**
   3. The antipsychotic olanzapine (Zyprexa) does not impact clinical manifestations of hay fever.
   4. The client can say anything, but weight gain indicates the medication is effective.

MEDICATION MEMORY JOGGER: The nurse determines medication effectiveness by assessing for the symptoms, or lack thereof, for which the medication was prescribed.

3. 1. Sleeping most of the day does not indicate sertraline (Zoloft), an SSRI, is effective. This may indicate the client is very depressed or is taking too much medication.
   2. Weight loss or gain may indicate the client is depressed.
   3. Verbalizing remorse does not indicate the medication is effective.
   4. **Setting new goals and priorities, such as getting a job, indicates the client may no longer be depressed, and sertraline (Zoloft), an SSRI, is effective.**

4. 1. Clients taking phenelzine (Nardil), an MAOI, must not eat foods high in tyramine because this causes a life-threatening complication. This statement does not warrant intervention.
   2. **Dextromethorphan (Robitussin) interacts with MAOIs to produce hypertension, fever, and coma. This statement warrants intervention.**
   3. Acetaminophen (Tylenol) does not interact with MAOIs; therefore, this statement does not warrant intervention.
   4. Caffeine should be limited when taking MAOIs, but it may be consumed in moderation. This statement does not warrant intervention.

MEDICATION MEMORY JOGGER: Some classes of medications are notorious for adverse reactions and MAO inhibitors, which are prescribed rarely for depression, are among the worst.

5. 1. **This client is stable and has a diagnosis of panic attacks. Administering alprazolam (Xanax), a benzodiazepine, would be an appropriate task to assign to an LPN.**
   2. Tardive dyskinesia is a life-threatening complication of antipsychotic medications such as haloperidol (Haldol), and the nurse should not delegate the care of an unstable client.
   3. This lithium level is toxic, and the client should not receive any lithium (Lithobid).
   4. The client should receive IV, not oral, thiamine (B_1), a vitamin. The client is not stable, and the nurse should not delegate this medication administration.

6. 1. This is the scientific rationale for administering donepezil (Aricept) to a client diagnosed with Alzheimer's disease.
   2. This is the scientific rationale for administering lithium to a client diagnosed with bipolar disorder.

3. **Atomoxetine (Strattera), a norepinephrine reuptake inhibitor, is prescribed for ADHD because it is not a CNS stimulant or controlled substance. It acts to increase norepinephrine and regulate impulse control, organizes thoughts, and focuses attention. It does not decrease appetite, and the child does not need to take drug holidays.**
4. This is the scientific rationale for administering methylphenidate (Ritalin) to children diagnosed with ADHD.

7. 1. Some OTC medications are as effective as prescription medications; therefore, this is a false statement.
2. Tylenol PM combines acetaminophen and diphenhydramine (Benadryl), and it is not addictive.
3. The client did not verbalize this concern. The client needs factual information, not a therapeutic response.
4. **Zolpidem (Ambien CR) allows the client to fall asleep and stay asleep, which is why it is prescribed for clients diagnosed with insomnia. Short-term use does not result in an addiction to this medication.**

8. 1. Chlordiazepoxide (Librium), a benzodiazepine, is used to prevent delirium tremens; therefore, the nurse would not question this medication.
2. Haloperidol (Haldol), an antipsychotic, is prescribed for psychosis; therefore, the nurse would not question this medication.
3. **Clonidine (Catapres), an alpha-adrenergic agonist, is administered primarily to treat hypertension, but it is also used to reduce withdrawal symptoms from opioids, nicotine, and alcohol. The nurse would question administering this medication because of the client's low blood pressure, no matter why it is being prescribed.**
4. Thiamine (B_1), a vitamin, is used to diminish Wernicke-Korsakoff encephalopathy, characterized by confusion, memory loss, and loss of cranial nerve function resulting from chronic alcohol abuse.

9. 1. Cannabis is marijuana and results in a lack of sense of time, apathy, and increased appetite, not the clinical manifestations the client is experiencing.
2. Heroin abuse results in slurred speech, sedated appearance, apathy, and decreased emotional pain, not hypervigilance nor insomnia.
3. **Hypervigilance, insomnia, dilated pupils, and a runny nose are clinical manifestations of cocaine abuse.**
4. Alcohol abuse results in lack of control, hostility, rationalization, grandiosity, confusion, and blackouts, not the clinical manifestations this client has.

MEDICATION MEMORY JOGGER: Many illegal substances that are abused by clients may produce the same symptoms, so the test taker must focus on symptoms that are different, such as "runny nose" for cocaine.

10. Correct answers are 2 and 5.
1. The nurse cannot delegate evaluation of assessment data. The UAP can obtain the intake and output but not evaluate it.
2. **The UAP can obtain the client's weight. This does not require judgment.**
3. The UAP should not be manipulating the IV, IV pump, or IV tubing. TPN is a medication, and the nurse cannot delegate medication administration.
4. The client is anorexic, and any food intake should be evaluated by the nurse. Having the UAP go to the cafeteria removes the employee from the unit for an extended period; therefore, this is not an appropriate task to delegate.
5. **TPN is high in glucose, and the client's glucose level should be monitored every 6 hours. The UAP can perform this skill.**

11. 1. Substance abuse, whether involving legal or illegal substances, is still abuse, and the client needs psychological intervention to help with the abuse. The pharmacologic intervention helps with the physiologic withdrawal, with the scientific rationale being to help the client not take any type of medication, legal or illegal.
2. **The two primary purposes for prescribing medication for clients addicted to alcohol, sedatives or hypnotics, and benzodiazepines are to permit safe withdrawal from the substance and to prevent relapse into addiction again.**
3. No medications used in substance abuse detoxification can prevent all side effects.
4. This statement is not true.

12. 1. The nicotine patch and nicotine gum are nicotine replacement products; if one doesn't work, neither will the other one.
2. The nicotine patch is an OTC medication, so this recommendation is not helpful to the client.

3. Nicotine lowers vitamin C levels in the body, so it will not help the client with withdrawal symptoms from nicotine.
4. Bupropion (Wellbutrin) is an antidepressant that has been proved to be an adjunct to smoking cessation.

13. 1. This is the correct amount of chlorpromazine (Thorazine) to administer to the client. 100 divided by 50 is 0.5 mL.
2. This would be a medication error and would be administering 100 mg of medication, or twice the dose prescribed.
3. This would be a medication error and would be administering 150 mg of medication, or three times the dose prescribed.
4. This would be a medication error and would be administering 200 mg of medication, or four times the dose prescribed.

MEDICATION MEMORY JOGGER: Most pharmaceutical companies package medication in amounts that are usually prescribed by the HCP. If the nurse uses more than one vial to administer a medication, then the nurse should seek clarification of the prescription.

14. 1. Multivitamins in the IV solution cause the IV solution to be yellow; therefore, there is no reason to notify the HCP.
2. This IV does not need to be protected from light. The yellow color is normal for this IV therapy.
3. This IV therapy is commonly known as a "banana bag" because of the yellow color of the IV solution. The nurse should administer the medication as prescribed.
4. This is not cost-effective because the yellow color is normal for this medication.

15. 1. Involuntary movements of the tongue and lips are clinical manifestations of tardive dyskinesia, an adverse reaction to first-generation antipsychotic medications such as chlorpromazine (Thorazine).
2. Antianxiety medications, such as lorazepam (Ativan), do not cause tardive dyskinesia.
3. Antibiotics, such as cefuroxime (Zinacef), do not cause tardive dyskinesia.
4. The client has clinical manifestations of tardive dyskinesia, which is an adverse reaction to a first-generation antipsychotic medication such as chlorpromazine (Thorazine). The nurse must intervene when assessing these clinical manifestations.

16. 1. Risperidone (Risperdal), an antipsychotic, is the drug of choice for an adolescent diagnosed with bipolar disorder.
2. Cimetidine (Tagamet), a histamine blocker, may reduce effects of antipsychotic medications and lead to medication failure. The client diagnosed with schizophrenia would be taking an antipsychotic medication, so the nurse should discuss an alternate medication to decrease the client's gastric acidity.
3. The client receiving rifampin (Rifadin), an antituberculin, must receive it to prevent resistant strains of tuberculosis and protect the community.
4. Amitriptyline (Elavil), a tricyclic antidepressant, has shown efficacy in promoting weight gain in clients diagnosed with anorexia nervosa; therefore, the nurse would not need to discuss this medication with the HCP.

17. 1. Desipramine (Norpramin), a tricyclic antidepressant, is administered to improve mood; therefore, this indicates the medication is effective.
2. Arguing with the parents will not determine medication effectiveness.
3. Verbalizing future goals will not determine medication effectiveness.
4. Being preoccupied with shape and weight is a symptom of anorexia and indicates desipramine (Norpramin), a tricyclic antidepressant, is not effective.

MEDICATION MEMORY JOGGER: The nurse determines medication effectiveness by assessing for the symptoms, or lack thereof, for which the medication was prescribed.

14

Sensory Deficits

Memories establish the past; Senses perceive the present; Imaginations shape the future.

—Toba Beta

QUESTIONS

Eye Disorder

1. The client diagnosed with open-angle glaucoma is prescribed ophthalmic drops. The client is demonstrating instilling the medication. Which action by the client **warrants intervention**?
   1. The client washes their hands before instilling the medication.
   2. The client squeezes the bridge of the nose after administering the medication.
   3. The client keeps the eyes open immediately after administering the medication.
   4. The client does not touch the dropper to the eye when instilling the medication.

2. The client diagnosed with glaucoma is prescribed latanoprostene bunod ophthalmic medication. Which information should the nurse discuss with the client? **Select all that apply.**
   1. Place the ophthalmic medication in the lower conjunctival sac.
   2. Apply the ophthalmic drops at the same time as other ophthalmic medications.
   3. Remove contact lenses for medication administration.
   4. Notify the health-care provider (HCP) if changes in eyelash length or color occur.
   5. Store the unopened ophthalmic medication in the refrigerator.
   6. Notify the HCP if you notice a brownish color of the iris of the eye or eyelid.

3. The client diagnosed with glaucoma is prescribed epinephrine ophthalmic drops. Which statement indicates the client **understands** the teaching?
   1. "I will call my HCP if I start experiencing any eye pain."
   2. "This medication does not interfere with any OTC medication."
   3. "I will probably experience anxiety, nervousness, and muscle tremors."
   4. "After putting the medication in my eyes, I must lie down for 1 hour."

4. The client is undergoing eye surgery and the nurse is administering cycloplegic ophthalmic medication. Which intervention should the nurse implement?
   1. Don sterile gloves before administering medication.
   2. Tape the client's eyelids shut with nonadhesive tape.
   3. Place an eye catheter at the outer canthus to insert medication.
   4. Explain that the eyes will be paralyzed for 24 to 48 hours.

5. The client diagnosed with bilateral conjunctivitis is prescribed antibiotic ophthalmic ointment. Which interventions should the nurse implement when discussing the medication with the client? **Select all that apply.**
   1. Apply a thin line of ointment evenly along the inner edge of the lower lid margin.
   2. Press the nasolacrimal duct after applying the antibiotic ointment.
   3. Don nonsterile gloves before administering the medication.
   4. Apply antibiotic ointment from the outer canthus to the inner canthus.
   5. Instruct the client to sit with the head slightly tilted back or lie supine.

6. The client reports having dry and irritated eyes to the clinic nurse. Which intervention should the nurse implement **first**?
   1. Recommend the client use artificial tears in both eyes.
   2. Assess the eyes for any redness or discharge.
   3. Check the client's eyes using the ophthalmoscope.
   4. Evaluate the client's cardinal fields of vision.

7. The client called the emergency department (ED) and told the nurse that bleach had splashed into both eyes. Which action should the nurse tell the client to perform **first**?
   1. Come to the ED immediately.
   2. Determine if the client has a normal saline flush.
   3. Apply antibiotic ointment and patch the eyes bilaterally.
   4. Cleanse the eye continuously with tap water.

8. To which client should the nurse **question** administering betaxolol ophthalmic drops?
   1. The client diagnosed with open-angle glaucoma
   2. The client diagnosed with end-stage liver failure
   3. The client diagnosed with allergies to sulfa
   4. The client diagnosed with chronic obstructive pulmonary disease (COPD)

9. Which statement **best** describes the scientific rationale for administering mydriatic ophthalmic medication to a client diagnosed with glaucoma?
   1. It constricts the pupil, causing the pupil to dilate in low light.
   2. It dilates the pupil to reduce aqueous humor production.
   3. It decreases aqueous humor production but does not affect the eye.
   4. It is used as adjunctive therapy primarily to reduce intraocular pressure.

10. The nurse is preparing to administer ophthalmic medication to the client. To which area should the nurse administer the medication?

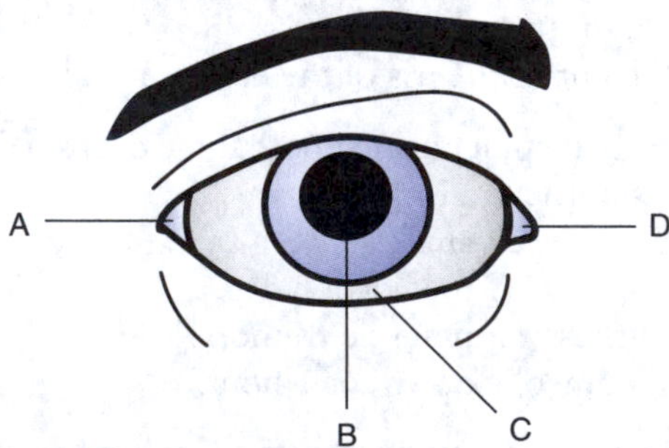

   1. A
   2. B
   3. C
   4. D

Ear Infection

11. The nurse is teaching parents how to instill antibiotic otic drops in their 6-year-old child diagnosed with otitis media. Which instruction should the nurse discuss with the parents? **Select all that apply.**
1. Insert the otic medication in the affected ear after pulling the earlobe upward and back.
2. After instilling medication, gently massage the area immediately anterior to the ear.
3. Gently pull the pinna downward and straight back when inserting ear drops.
4. Allow the child to lie quietly on the side after instilling ear drops into the affected ear.
5. Insert the dropper with prescribed medication deep into the ear canal and instill drops.

12. Which statement indicates that the parent **understands** the procedure for administering otic drops to the child diagnosed with otitis media?
1. "I should clean my child's ear canal very gently with cotton swabs."
2. "I will warm the drops to room temperature before instilling them."
3. "I can place a heating pad over my child's ear after putting in the drops."
4. "I need to place the dropper gently into my child's ear canal."

13. The 4-year-old child diagnosed with otitis media with effusion is not prescribed systemic antibiotics. The parent asks the nurse, "Why didn't the doctor order antibiotics for my child?" Which statement is the nurse's **best** response?
1. "Your child is too young to receive antibiotics."
2. "You should discuss this with your child's HCP."
3. "Because your child did not have a fever, the doctor did not order antibiotics."
4. "Most HCPs prescribe ear drops instead of antibiotics."

14. The parent of a 5-year-old child diagnosed with five ear infections in the past 6 months asks the nurse, "What can be done because my child keeps having ear infections?" Which response by the nurse is **most appropriate**?
1. "There are many different types of antibiotics, and one will work."
2. "You are concerned your child keeps having ear infections?"
3. "Does your child dunk his head underwater during bath time?"
4. "Your child may need tubes inserted into both ears."

15. The parent of a 23-month-old child diagnosed with acute otitis media calls the clinic and tells the nurse their child is crying and pulling at her ears. Which action should the nurse implement?
1. Instruct the parent to give acetaminophen elixir as prescribed on the bottle.
2. Determine when the parent gave the last dose of the prescribed antibiotic.
3. Tell the parent to administer two chewable low-dose aspirins every 6 hours.
4. Encourage the parent to hold the child and rock her until she falls asleep.

16. The nurse is administering otic drops to a 5-year-old child diagnosed with acute otitis media. How should the nurse implement the interventions? **Rank in order of performance.**
1. Brace the administering hand against the child's head above the ear.
2. Insert the required number of drops and gently massage the tragus.
3. Explain the procedure to the child in developmentally appropriate terms.
4. Gently pull the top of the child's ear up and back.
5. Keep the child on the unaffected side for several minutes.

17. The 3-year-old female child is diagnosed with acute otitis media. Which statement by the parent indicates to the nurse that the parent **needs more teaching**?
1. "I will plan to take my daughter to her follow-up appointment with her doctor."
2. "My son started pulling at his ears, so I gave him some of my daughter's antibiotics."
3. "I will give my daughter all of the medication, even if she starts feeling better."
4. "If my daughter does not get better in 48 hours, I will call her HCP."

18. The mother of a 13-year-old child diagnosed with external otitis tells the nurse her child spends a lot of time swimming. Which information is **most important** for the nurse to discuss with the mother?
1. Insert silicone earplugs before entering the water.
2. Administer a drying agent in the ear canal after swimming.
3. Wear a tight-fitting swim cap, especially in cold water.
4. Tilt the head to allow water to drain from the ear.

19. The 2-year-old child is diagnosed with acute otitis media. Which intervention will help increase the parent's compliance with the medical regimen?
1. Instruct the parent verbally on how to use a calibrated measuring device.
2. Give the parent a sample of the antibiotic therapy to take home.
3. Make an appointment for a follow-up visit in 1 week.
4. Provide written and oral instructions about antibiotic therapy.

20. The primary nurse is administering antibiotic otic drops to a 2-year-old child. Which action by the primary nurse **warrants intervention** by the charge nurse?
1. The primary nurse asks the parent if the child has any known allergies.
2. The primary nurse dons nonsterile gloves before inserting the otic drops.
3. The primary nurse washes their hands before administering medication.
4. The primary nurse gets assistance to restrain the child when giving otic drops.

ANSWERS AND RATIONALES

The correct answer number and rationale are in **boldface blue type.** Rationales for why other answer options are incorrect are also given.

Eye Disorder

1. 1. The client should wash hands before instilling medication to ensure that bacteria do not fall into the eye. This action does not warrant intervention.
2. The client should gently squeeze the nose bridge after administering the medication to prevent systemic absorption of the medication. This action does not warrant intervention.
3. The client should close the eyes for 1 to 2 minutes after instilling ophthalmic eye drops to distribute the medication and enhance medication effectiveness (Hoffman & Sullivan, 2018). This action warrants the nurse correcting the behavior.
4. The client should not touch the eye with the dropper to help prevent trauma to the eye. This action does not warrant intervention.

2. Correct answers are 1, 3, 5, and 6.
1. The ophthalmic medication, latanoprostene bunod (Vyzulta), should be administered in the lower conjunctival sac.
2. The client should wait at least 5 minutes after administering latanoprostene bunod drops before administering another ophthalmic medication.
3. Contact lenses should be removed for medication administration to avoid damage. The lenses may be reinserted 15 minutes after administration.
4. Changes in eyelash length, color, thickness, and number may occur. These changes resolve with medication discontinuation.
5. The medication should be kept refrigerated before opening. Once opened, the bottle may be stored at room temperature for 8 weeks.
6. Latanoprostene may cause a brownish pigmentation of the iris and eyelids due to increased melanin content. It is recommended that these clients be closely monitored for potential long-term effects (Hussar, 2018).

3. 1. Eye pain may indicate an attack of angle-closure glaucoma and must be reported to the HCP immediately.
2. The client should avoid using any over-the-counter (OTC) sinus and cold medications containing pseudoephedrine and phenylephrine, which may accentuate side effects of epinephrine (Epitrate), mydriatic ophthalmic drops.
3. If the client experiences any central nervous system side effects, such as anxiety, nervousness, or muscle tremors, the client should notify the HCP. Depending on side effect severity, the HCP may or may not discontinue the medication.
4. There is no reason the client must lie down for 1 hour after administering epinephrine (Epitrate) mydriatic ophthalmic drops.

4. 1. The nurse does not have to don sterile gloves when applying ophthalmic medication; nonsterile gloves can be used.
2. The client's eyelids should not be shut during surgery. This medication paralyzes the eye during surgery.
3. There is no such thing as an eye catheter that is inserted into the outer canthus of the eye.
4. Cycloplegic medication paralyzes the eye for 1 to 2 days. The client should be aware of this information because most ophthalmic surgery is performed as day surgery. Because the client will be at home, they need to be knowledgeable about the medication.

5. Correct answers are 1, 2, and 5.
1. The client should instill eye ointment into the lower conjunctival sac, which is the inner edge of the lower lid margin.
2. Applying pressure to the nasolacrimal duct will prevent systemic medication absorption.
3. The client does not have to wear gloves when applying ointment to their eyes. The client should be instructed to wash hands before and after applying ointment.
4. The antibiotic ointment should be applied from the inner canthus to the outer canthus, from the nose side of the eye to the outer area.
5. The client should sit with the head slightly tilted back or lie supine when applying ophthalmic ointment or drops to better access the lower conjunctival sac.

MEMORY MEDICATION JOGGER: The nurse must know the correct technique when administering medications. This is considered one of the "rights" of medication administration.

6. 1. If there is no redness, inflammation, or other signs of an infection, the nurse could recommend using artificial tears, an OTC medication. However, this is not the first intervention.
   2. The nurse should first assess the eyes for redness or inflammation to determine if there is any type of infection, which would need an HCP's prescription for antibiotics.
   3. The nurse could use the ophthalmoscope to assess the client's eyes, but the first intervention is a visual inspection.
   4. The nurse could evaluate the client's cardinal fields of vision, but the first intervention is a visual inspection.

7. 1. The client should come to the ED to determine if permanent damage has occurred and be seen by an ophthalmologist, but that is not the first intervention.
   2. Normal saline flush would help cleanse bleach from the eyes, but it is not the first intervention.
   3. Regular antibiotic ointment should not be used in the eye. Bilateral patching is not appropriate for chemical irritation to the eye.
   4. The nurse should instruct the client to rinse the eye with tap water for at least 5 minutes in each eye and then come to the ED. Bleach must be thoroughly removed from the eyes as soon as possible.

8. 1. This medication is prescribed for clients diagnosed with open-angle glaucoma.
   2. There is no contraindication to administering this eye drop to a client in liver failure because the medication should not be absorbed systemically.
   3. There is no contraindication to administering this eye drop to a client who is allergic to sulfa.
   4. Contraindications to using the beta-adrenergic blocker betaxolol (Betoptic) ophthalmic drops include clients who may be receiving beta-blocker therapy, including clients diagnosed with COPD, asthma, heart block, and heart failure.

9. 1. Miotic medications, not mydriatic medications, constrict the pupil and block sympathetic nervous system input, which causes the pupil to dilate in low light and contracts the ciliary muscle.
   2. Mydriatic medications dilate the pupil, reduce aqueous humor production, and increase absorption effectiveness of aqueous humor, reducing intraocular pressure in open-angle glaucoma.
   3. Beta-adrenergic blockers decrease aqueous humor production, which reduces intraocular pressure, but they do not affect pupil size and lens accommodation.
   4. Carbonic anhydrase inhibitors are used as adjunctive therapy to reduce intraocular pressure.

10. 1. The medication should not be administered in the inner canthus because it may increase systemic medication absorption.
   2. The medication should not be administered on the pupil because the medication will not be retained in the eye.
   3. The medication should be administered into the lower conjunctival sac, then the client should close the eye for 1 to 2 minutes, which will help ensure medication stays in the eye.
   4. The medication should not be administered in the outer canthus because it will not be retained in the eye.

Ear Infection

11. **Correct answers are 1, 2, and 4.**
   1. In children older than 3 years, the pinna should be pulled upward and back to straighten the eustachian tube.
   2. Gentle massage of the area immediately anterior to the ear facilitates entry of drops into the ear canal.
   3. This should be done with children younger than 3 years because it will straighten the ear canal. In children older than age 3, the pinna should be pulled upward and back.
   4. After ear drop instillation, the child should remain lying on the unaffected side for a few minutes.
   5. The dropper should be held over the ear canal when instilling ear drops. Inserting the dropper deep into the ear could cause ear injury.

12. 1. The parent should never attempt to place anything inside the ear to clean the canal because the risk of rupturing the tympanic membrane is high.
   2. Cold otic drops cause pain when they contact the tympanic membrane; therefore, otic solutions should be allowed to warm to room temperature before being administered.

3. A heating pad could cause the tympanic membrane to rupture. The parent should not put heat or cold over the ear.
4. The dropper should not be placed in the ear canal. The dropper should be held over the canal when releasing drops into the canal.

13. 1. Any age child can receive antibiotics.
2. This is "passing the buck," and the nurse should answer the parent's question.
3. Otitis media with effusion differs from acute otitis media in that there are no signs of acute infection. If there are no signs of infection, such as fever or pain, the nurse should explain that, with emergence of antimicrobial-resistant organisms, recent recommendations discourage antibiotic use for otitis media with effusion. Most effusions will resolve on their own.
4. Acute otitis media with clinical manifestations is treated with 5 to 7 days of oral antibiotics.

14. 1. There are only so many antibiotics that treat otitis media, and the HCP will not continue using antibiotics because the child can become resistant to antibiotics.
2. This is a therapeutic response, which is not appropriate because the parent needs factual information. This response helps the client express feelings.
3. Dunking the head underwater does not cause ear infections.
4. This is the most appropriate response. A myringotomy with insertion of tympanostomy tubes is performed on children with persistent ear infections despite antibiotic therapy or otitis media with effusion for more than 3 months with associated hearing loss.

15. 1. Acetaminophen (Tylenol) or ibuprofen (Advil, Motrin) can help reduce fever and discomfort in children.
2. Determining the last dose of antibiotic will not help relieve the child's pain.
3. Aspirin should not be given to children because of the possibility of their developing Reye's syndrome.
4. This is a good action to take, but the child needs medication to help ease the pain.

16. Correct order is 3, 1, 4, 2, 5.
3. The nurse should talk to the child and explain the procedure. This will help develop trust with the child. Many nurses talk to the parents and not the child.
1. Bracing the hand helps prevent the child from moving the head.
4. For children older than 3 years, the pinna should be pulled up and back to straighten the ear canal so that drops get to the tympanic membrane.
2. After inserting drops, massaging the tragus (anterior portion) ensures that the drops reach the tympanic membrane.
5. This prevents the medication from spilling out of the ear.

17. 1. This statement indicates the parent understands the medication teaching. Clients should keep all follow-up appointments.
2. Antibiotics are prescribed for a specific condition for a specific client. The parent should not give antibiotics prescribed for their daughter to their son. The parent does not understand the medication teaching.
3. The entire antibiotic prescription should be taken whether the client is feeling better or not.
4. After 2 days of antibiotic therapy, the child should start feeling better. This statement indicates the parent understands the medication teaching.

18. 1. Silicone earplugs can keep water out of the ear without reducing hearing significantly, but it is not the most important information to discuss with the client.
2. A 2% acetic acid solution or 2% boric acid in ethyl alcohol is effective in drying the canal and restoring its normal acidic environment. This is the most important information for the nurse to teach because, although suggesting ways to prevent water from entering is helpful, the client must dry the canal to prevent further external otitis episodes.
3. A swim cap does not prevent water from entering the ear. It protects the ear from the cold and possibly slows the formation of bony growths in the ears. It also protects the ear from debris in the water.
4. Tilting the head to allow water to drain from the ear is helpful, but it does not ensure the ear will be restored to a normal acidic environment.

19. 1. The nurse should have the mother demonstrate how to use the measuring device to ensure the parent knows how to use it. Verbal instructions alone do not ensure that the parent knows how to administer medication correctly.

2. Providing the parent with an antibiotics sample will not ensure compliance.
3. A follow-up visit will not ensure compliance with the medication regimen.
4. **Many times in the HCP's office, the parent may be nervous. The child is in the room, and there are many distractions; therefore, verbal instructions alone may not be thoroughly understood. Written information may increase compliance with the medication regimen.**

20. 1. This indicates the nurse understands the correct procedure for administering otic drops; therefore, this does not warrant intervention by the charge nurse.
2. **This procedure does not warrant wearing nonsterile gloves because the nurse will not come into contact with any blood or body fluids. The nurse should wash their hands and administer medication. This action warrants intervention by the charge nurse.**
3. This is the correct procedure before administering medications; therefore, this action does not warrant intervention by the charge nurse.
4. Assistance in restraining a young child might be necessary; therefore, this would not warrant intervention by the charge nurse.

SENSORY DEFICITS COMPREHENSIVE EXAMINATION

1. The client diagnosed with glaucoma is prescribed oral acetazolamide. Which information should the client discuss with the client?
   1. Administer the medication in the morning.
   2. Instill medication in the lower conjunctival sac.
   3. Wash hands before administering medication.
   4. Hold the eyes shut for 2 minutes after taking medication.

2. The nurse is discussing how to instill artificial tears into the client's eyes. Which information should the nurse discuss with the client? **Select all that apply.**
   1. Do not allow the artificial tear dropper to touch the eye.
   2. Keep the eyes closed 1 to 2 minutes after instilling drops.
   3. Apply pressure to the inner canthus after instilling eye drops.
   4. Wash the hands before instilling the artificial tears into the eyes.
   5. Lie in the prone position when instilling the eye drops.

3. The client diagnosed with glaucoma is prescribed betaxolol ophthalmic drops. Which information should the nurse discuss with the client?
   1. Instruct the client to call the HCP if dizziness occurs when getting up too fast.
   2. Discuss that the drops will cause the vision to get worse initially.
   3. Teach the client how to prevent orthostatic hypotension.
   4. Explain the importance of applying pressure at the outer canthus.

4. The client diagnosed with Meniere's disease, also known as endolymphatic hydrops, is prescribed meclizine. Which statement **best** describes the scientific rationale for this medication?
   1. It will help decrease the whirling sensation experienced in Meniere's disease.
   2. It will help prevent an acute episode of nausea and vomiting.
   3. It will help maintain a lower labyrinthine pressure in the ears.
   4. It will help the ear canal vasoconstrict, reducing ear pressure.

5. The client diagnosed with Meniere's disease is admitted with an acute attack and prescribed IV diazepam. Which intervention should the nurse implement when administering this medication?
   1. Dilute the diazepam to a 10-mL bolus with normal saline.
   2. Administer the diazepam undiluted via a saline lock.
   3. Infuse the diazepam via an IV piggyback (IVPB) over 1 hour.
   4. Question the order because diazepam cannot be given IV push (IVP).

6. The nurse is instructing the adult client diagnosed with external otitis how to instill otic drops. How should the nurse teach the interventions? **Rank in order of performance.**
   1. Loosely place a small piece of cotton in the auditory meatus.
   2. Demonstrate pulling the pinna of the ear up and back when inserting drops.
   3. Warm the medication by holding the container in hand for 5 minutes.
   4. Tilt the head toward the unaffected side when in the sitting position.
   5. Administer the prescribed number of drops into the ear canal.

7. The client calls the clinic and tells the nurse that a live insect is in the client's right ear. Which intervention should the clinic nurse implement?
   1. Encourage the client to get someone to remove the insect.
   2. Instruct the client to put water into the ear canal.
   3. Have the client put mineral oil into the ear canal.
   4. Tell the client to put a medicated cotton ball in the ear.

8. The client diagnosed with nasal congestion is prescribed a nasal solution. Which information should be included in the medication teaching?
   1. Direct the solution toward the base of the nasal cavity.
   2. Tell the client to blow the nose before instilling the solution.
   3. Replace the remaining nasal solution in the dropper back into the bottle.
   4. Have the client squeeze the nostrils shut after instilling nasal solution.

9. The client is diagnosed with allergies and rhinitis. The HCP prescribed OTC fluticasone nasal spray. How should the nurse teach the client to position themselves to administer the nasal spray?
   1. Stand upright, head facing forward.
   2. Sitting, head leaning back.
   3. Bend at the waist, head down.
   4. Supine, head tilted back.

10. After undergoing eye surgery, the client reports being nauseated. Which intervention should the postanesthesia care unit (PACU) recovery room nurse implement?
    1. Administer an IV antiemetic medication.
    2. Determine if the client had anything to eat preoperatively.
    3. Place a cold washcloth under the chin along the client's throat.
    4. Put the client on the left side and insert a rectal antiemetic medication.

11. The pediatric nurse is administering nasal medication to the 13-month-old child. Which intervention should the nurse implement?
    1. Place the child in a prone position with the head to the side.
    2. Gently place the child's chin on the chest using the nondominant hand.
    3. Turn the child's head slightly from side to side and back to midline.
    4. Allow the child to sit up immediately after the medication is instilled.

12. The 3-year-old child diagnosed with an eye infection has an ophthalmic ointment and ophthalmic drops prescribed. Which action by the primary nurse **warrants intervention** by the charge nurse?
    1. The primary nurse applies ophthalmic ointment first.
    2. The primary nurse instills ophthalmic drops in the lower lid.
    3. The primary nurse does not allow the dropper to touch the eye.
    4. The primary nurse instills ophthalmic drops first.

13. The client diagnosed with seasonal allergies is reporting ocular itching. The HCP orders cetirizine ophthalmic solution. Which information should the nurse include when teaching about this medication?
    1. Contact lenses should not be worn until the medication course of treatment is complete.
    2. This medication does not affect wearing of contact lenses.
    3. Contact lenses may be reinserted 10 minutes after medication administration.
    4. Wearing contact lenses during medication administration improves visual acuity.

14. The client diagnosed with a fungal infection of the eye is prescribed natamycin ophthalmic drops. Which medication teaching should the nurse discuss with the client? **Select all that apply.**
    1. Instruct the client to patch both eyes after instilling the medication.
    2. Tell the client to apply cool packs to the eye after instilling the medication.
    3. Explain that the medication may cause temporary blurred vision.
    4. Discuss the need to instill drops once a day before going to sleep.
    5. Teach the client to shake the medication well before using.

15. To which client should the HCP recommend an OTC ceruminolytic?
    1. The client diagnosed with "swimmer's ear"
    2. The client diagnosed with impacted earwax
    3. The client diagnosed with external otitis
    4. The client diagnosed with bilateral cataracts

16. The client diagnosed with otitis media is prescribed clarithromycin 500 mg by mouth every 12 hours for 10 days. Which medication teaching should the nurse discuss with the client?

1. Discuss the need to take the medication with food.
2. Tell the client to wear sunglasses when going outdoors.
3. Instruct the client to get cultures after completing medications.
4. Encourage the client to eat yogurt or buttermilk daily.

17. The client diagnosed with multiple mouth ulcers is prescribed nystatin oral suspension. Which interventions should the nurse implement when administering this medication? **Select all that apply.**

1. Instruct the client to swish medication in the mouth quickly, then spit it out.
2. Encourage the client to swish medication in the mouth for at least 2 minutes.
3. Tell the client to swish the mouth with normal saline after swallowing medication.
4. Apply nystatin medication to the mouth ulcers with a sterile cotton swab.
5. Teach the client to avoid eating for 5 to 10 minutes after using the medication.

18. The nurse is instructing the client on how to instill nasal drops. How should the nurse teach the interventions? **Rank in order of performance.**

1. Discard any remaining solution in the dropper.
2. Remain in position for 5 minutes.
3. Open and breathe through the mouth.
4. Instill the solution laterally toward the nasal septum.
5. Hold the dropper tip just above the nostril without touching the nose.

19. The client diagnosed with glaucoma is prescribed pilocarpine eye drops. Which statement indicates the client **needs more teaching** concerning the medication?

1. "I will use nightlights in the halls and the bathroom."
2. "I will get my wife or son to drive me around at night."
3. "I will avoid doing tasks that require sharp vision."
4. "I will take the eye drops every time I have eye pain."

20. The nurse is administering ophthalmic medication to the client. To which area should the nurse instruct the client to apply pressure for 1 to 2 minutes after instilling the medication?

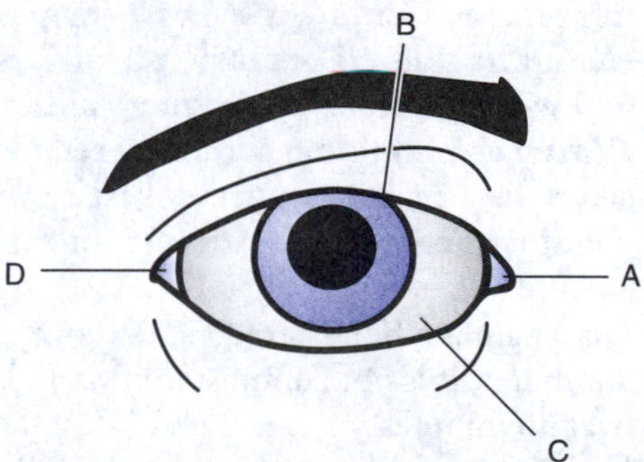

1. A
2. B
3. C
4. D

SENSORY DEFICITS COMPREHENSIVE EXAMINATION ANSWERS AND RATIONALES

1. **1. The oral medication acetazolamide (Diamox), a carbonic anhydrase inhibitor, has a diuretic effect; therefore, it should be taken in the morning to prevent sleep deprivation because of the need to get up to urinate during the night.**
2. This is an oral medication that is used as adjunctive therapy for clients diagnosed with glaucoma. It is not instilled into the eye.
3. This is an oral medication that is used as adjunctive therapy for clients diagnosed with glaucoma. The client does not have to wash hands before taking an oral medication.
4. This is an oral medication that is used as adjunctive therapy for clients diagnosed with glaucoma. It is not instilled into the eye, and there is no reason for the client to hold the eyes shut.

2. Correct answers are 1, 2, and 4.
1. Not letting the dropper touch the eye ensures that the eye will not be injured during artificial tear application.
2. Keeping the eyes shut for a minute or two after instilling drops will enhance medication effectiveness.
3. Applying pressure to the inner canthus is not an appropriate intervention because this prevents systemic medication absorption and artificial tears are not a medication that would cause systemic effects.
4. Washing hands is an appropriate intervention so that bacteria on the hands will not fall into the eye when instilling eye drops.
5. Lying on the stomach (prone position) is not an appropriate intervention to discuss with the client. This position would allow drops to leak out of the eye.

MEDICATION MEMORY JOGGER: "Select all that apply" questions require the test taker to view each option as a True/False question. One option cannot assist the test taker in eliminating another option.

3. 1. Betaxolol (Betoptic) is a beta blocker that, if absorbed systemically, may cause bradycardia and hypotension. The nurse should discuss orthostatic hypotension with the client, but there is no need for the client to call the HCP.
2. If vision worsens, the client should call the HCP because this is an adverse reaction that warrants intervention.
3. Betaxolol (Betoptic) is a beta blocker that may cause bradycardia and hypotension if absorbed systemically. The nurse should discuss ways to prevent orthostatic hypotension.
4. The client should apply pressure at the inner canthus (closest to nose) to help prevent systemic medication absorption.

4. **1. Meclizine (Antivert), an antivertigo medication, helps prevent dizziness and the whirling sensation characteristic of Meniere's disease.**
2. An antiemetic medication, not Antivert, would be prescribed to help prevent nausea and vomiting.
3. An oral diuretic, not Antivert, is prescribed for clients with Meniere's disease to help maintain a lower labyrinthine pressure.
4. Vasoconstriction should be avoided in clients diagnosed with Meniere's disease because it may precipitate an attack. Tobacco products, alcohol, and caffeine should be avoided because they cause vasoconstriction.

5. 1. Diazepam cannot be diluted because it is oil based and will not dissolve with normal saline.
2. Diazepam (Valium), a sedative–hypnotic, cannot be diluted because it is oil based and will not dissolve with normal saline. Diazepam should be administered via a saline lock or at the port closest to the client if administered through an existing IV line.
3. Diazepam is administered via IVP over 2 to 5 minutes; it is not administered via IVPB over 30 minutes.
4. Diazepam can be administered via IVP.

6. Correct order is 3, 4, 2, 5, 1.
3. Warming medications promotes comfort when the ear drops are instilled.
4. Sitting with the head tilted toward the unaffected side allows gravity to move medication to the inner portion of the ear canal.
2. Pulling the pinna up and back straightens the ear canal in adults and allows the medication to travel along the length of the canal.

5. **This ensures the full amount of prescribed medication will be administered to penetrate the canal length and achieve full effectiveness.**
1. **Leaving a small piece of cotton in the auditory meatus for 15 to 20 minutes helps keep medication in the canal.**

7. 1. A live insect cannot be removed from the ear. The insect must be killed before removal.
2. Water should not be inserted into the ear canal because organic foreign bodies such as an insect or bean will swell when water is inserted into the ear canal, which makes removal more difficult.
3. **Mineral oil or topical lidocaine drops are used to immobilize or kill insects before their removal from the ear.**
4. There is no such thing as medicated cotton balls available OTC; therefore, this is not an appropriate action.

8. 1. The solution should be directed laterally toward the midline of the superior concha of the ethmoid bone, not at the base of the nasal cavity, because then it will run down the throat and into the eustachian tube.
2. **The client should blow their nose to clear nasal passages before instilling nasal solution.**
3. The client should discard any solution remaining in the dropper.
4. The client should not squeeze the nostrils but should remain with the head tilted for 5 minutes after instilling nasal solution.

9. 1. Standing upright and head facing forward is not the best position for distributing and absorbing nasal spray.
2. Sitting with the head leaning back is not the best position for distributing and absorbing nasal spray.
3. **The best position for distribution and absorption of nasal spray is to bend at the waist with the head down. The client will be looking at their feet.**
4. Supine with head tilted back is the appropriate position for sinus drops, not for nasal spray.

10. 1. **The nurse must take action as soon as possible to prevent vomiting because vomiting will increase intraocular pressure.**
2. Determining if the client had anything to eat preoperatively should have been done before the client had surgery. It is not pertinent information at this time.
3. A cold washcloth will not help prevent the client from vomiting. The client needs an antiemetic medication.
4. The client in the recovery room would have an IV route. The nurse should administer the antiemetic via the route that would decrease nausea as fast as possible, which would be the IV route.

11. 1. The child should be in the supine position.
2. The nurse should hyperextend the neck slightly by placing a rolled towel or small blanket under the shoulder blades.
3. **Turning the head slightly from side to side and back to the midline position will help disperse medication to the maxillary and frontal sinuses.**
4. The child should be kept in the midline position for at least 3 minutes after the medication is instilled into the nose to allow the medication to reach the ethmoid and sphenoid sinuses.

12. 1. **The nurse should apply the drops first because if the drops are placed after the ointment, the ophthalmic drops will not be absorbed. This action would warrant intervention by the charge nurse.**
2. This is the correct procedure; therefore, this intervention would not warrant intervention by the charge nurse.
3. This is the correct procedure; therefore, this intervention would not warrant intervention by the charge nurse.
4. The ophthalmic drops should be administered first because if ointment is instilled first, ophthalmic drops will not be absorbed. This action would not warrant intervention by the charge nurse.

13. 1. The client may continue to wear contact lenses while taking this medication. The contact lenses should be removed before administration. They may be reinserted 10 minutes after cetirizine solution (Zerviate), an antihistamine, is administered.
2. Cetirizine ophthalmic solution (Zerviate), an antihistamine, contains a preservative that affects contact lenses. The lenses should be removed before administration.
3. **Contact lenses should be removed before administering cetirizine ophthalmic solution (Zerviate), an antihistamine. The contacts may be reinserted 10 minutes after medication administration.**

4. The client should be instructed to remove contacts before medication administration. Decreased visual acuity after instillation of cetirizine ophthalmic solution (Zerviate) is an expected occurrence, not improved visual acuity.

14. Correct answers are 3 and 5.
1. There is no reason for the client to patch the eyes after administering medication.
2. There is no reason for the client to apply cool packs after instilling medication.
3. **The nurse should instruct the client that natamycin (Natacyn) ophthalmic drops may cause temporary vision blurring and may cause transient stinging.**
4. The ophthalmic medication is administered one drop every 2 hours for the first 3 to 4 days. After that, one drop should be administered every 3 hours for 14 to 21 days.
5. **Natamycin (Natacyn) ophthalmic drops should be shaken thoroughly before use.**

15. 1. The client diagnosed with swimmer's ear would need a 2% acetic acid solution or 2% boric acid in ethyl alcohol to help dry the ear canal and restore its normal acidic environment.
2. **A ceruminolytic medication helps to loosen and remove impacted cerumen (earwax) from the ear canal.**
3. This is an inflammation of the external ear that would not require a ceruminolytic.
4. Cataracts are eye disorders, not ear disorders.

16. 1. The medication can be taken with or without food.
2. This medication does not cause photosensitivity.
3. There is no need for the client to get a culture after antibiotic therapy. Otitis media is not diagnosed with a culture but with a visual ear examination.
4. **Yogurt and buttermilk will help maintain intestinal flora, which may be destroyed when receiving clarithromycin (Biaxin) antibiotic therapy. Destruction of intestinal flora will lead to a superinfection, resulting in diarrhea.**

17. Correct answers are 2 and 5.
1. The client should swish medication in the mouth for at least 2 minutes and then swallow the medication, not spit the medication out.
2. **The client should swish medication in the mouth for at least 2 minutes and then swallow the medication.**
3. The client should not swish the mouth with normal saline because medication should remain in the mouth even after the medication is swallowed.
4. This is not the correct procedure for administering this medication.
5. **The client should avoid eating for 5 to 10 minutes after using the medication.**

18. Correct order is 3, 5, 4, 2, 1.
3. **The client should first breathe through the mouth.**
5. **The dropper tip should not touch the nose because this could cause dropper contamination when being replaced into the bottle.**
4. **The solution should be inserted laterally toward the midline of the superior concha of the ethmoid bone, not the base of the nasal cavity, where it will run down the throat and into the eustachian tube.**
2. **The client should remain lying down for 5 minutes so that the solution will not run out of the nose.**
1. **The remaining solution should be discarded to prevent bottle contamination.**

19. 1. Vision is reduced in dim lights; therefore, the client should use a nightlight to prevent falls. This statement indicates the client understands the teaching.
2. Vision is reduced in dim lights; therefore, the client should avoid night driving for the safety of himself and others. This statement indicates the client understands the teaching.
3. Visual acuity may be decreased during therapy initiation; therefore, the client should avoid tasks requiring sharp vision. This statement indicates the client understands the teaching.
4. **This medication should be taken routinely every day to reduce intraocular pressure. Glaucoma is painless, so if the client experiences pain, the client should call the HCP immediately. This statement indicates the client needs more teaching.**

20. 1. Gentle pressure should be applied to the inner canthus (lacrimal sac) for 1 to 2 minutes to increase the local effect and decrease systemic absorption.
2. Gentle pressure to the eyelid is not helpful when instilling ophthalmic medication.
3. Gentle pressure to the lower conjunctival sac is not helpful when instilling ophthalmic medication.
4. Gentle pressure to the outer canthus is not helpful when instilling ophthalmic medication.

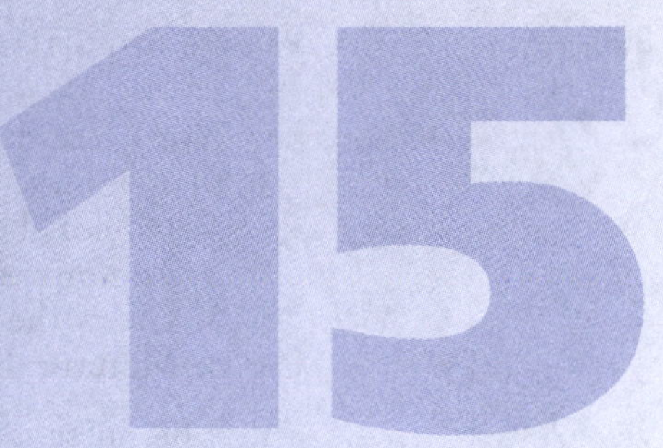

Emergency Nursing

Drug interactions that might have trivial consequences in a young adult can have devastating consequences in an older person.

—Mickey Stanley, Kathryn Blair, and Patricia Beare

QUESTIONS

Shock

1. The nurse is preparing to administer a nitroglycerin drip to a client diagnosed with cardiogenic shock. The client has total parenteral nutrition (TPN) running through a triple lumen catheter. Which intervention should the nurse implement?
   1. Mix the nitroglycerin in 500 mL of lactated Ringer's solution.
   2. Initiate the drip in a separate IV line.
   3. Use regular IV tubing when administering nitroglycerin.
   4. Ensure that the client's nitroglycerin patch is in a hairless area.

2. The nurse is preparing to administer dopamine to a client diagnosed with cardiogenic shock. Which intervention should the nurse implement? **Select all that apply.**
   1. Ensure the client is on a cardiac monitor.
   2. Monitor the blood pressure every 15 minutes.
   3. Evaluate the intake and output every hour.
   4. Instruct the client to report burning at the IV site.
   5. Assess the client's neurological status every hour.

3. The client diagnosed with hypovolemic shock is receiving dextran. Which assessment data **warrants immediate** intervention by the nurse?
   1. The client's blood pressure is 102/78.
   2. The client's pulse oximeter reading is 95%.
   3. The client's lung sounds reveal bilateral crackles.
   4. The client's urine output is 120 mL in 3 hours.

4. The nurse is caring for the client diagnosed with septic shock. The nurse administered the twice-a-day IV ceftriaxone at 0900. At 1100 the health-care provider (HCP) prescribed daily IV vancomycin. Which intervention should the nurse implement?
   1. Administer the vancomycin within 2 hours.
   2. Notify the HCP and question the antibiotic order.
   3. Schedule the vancomycin to be administered at 2100.
   4. Assess the client's white blood cell (WBC) count.

5. The client diagnosed with cardiogenic shock is receiving norepinephrine. Which **priority** intervention should the nurse implement?
   1. Do not abruptly discontinue the medication.
   2. Administer medication on an infusion pump.
   3. Check the client's creatinine and BUN levels.
   4. Monitor the client's blood pressure continuously.

6. The nurse is preparing to administer albumin 5%. Which statement is the scientific rationale for administering this medication?
   1. Albumin acts directly on the smooth muscles to cause vasodilation.
   2. Albumin mimics the fight-or-flight response of the sympathetic nervous system.
   3. Albumin is a blood volume expander that promotes circulatory volume.
   4. Albumin contains dextrose and increases fluid volume in the interstitial space.

7. During the first 15 minutes of administering blood to a client, the client reports shortness of breath, low back pain, and itching all over the body. Which interventions should the nurse implement? **Select all that apply.**
   1. Administer 0.5 mL of epinephrine intravenously.
   2. Assess the client's temperature, pulse, and blood pressure.
   3. Infuse normal saline at 125 mL an hour via a peripheral IV.
   4. Discontinue the blood at the hub of the IV catheter.
   5. Notify the client's HCP of the situation.

8. The primary nurse is preparing to administer dobutamine to a client diagnosed with cardiogenic shock. Which action by the primary nurse **warrants intervention** by the charge nurse?
   1. The primary nurse administers the dobutamine drip via gravity.
   2. The primary nurse attaches a urometer to the client's Foley catheter.
   3. The primary nurse applies a pulse oximeter to the client's finger.
   4. The primary nurse checks the client for any medication allergies.

9. The client diagnosed with cardiogenic shock is receiving dopamine. The peripheral IV site becomes infiltrated. Which intervention should the nurse implement?
   1. Assess the client's blood pressure and apical pulse.
   2. Elevate the arm and apply ice to the infiltrated area.
   3. Inject phentolamine at the site of infiltration.
   4. Discontinue the IV and take no other action.

10. The nurse is caring for a client diagnosed with cardiogenic shock receiving a dopamine drip. Which interventions should the nurse implement? **Select all that apply.**
    1. Aspirate the injection site to avoid injecting directly into the vein.
    2. Do not administer any alkaline solutions in the same tubing as dopamine.
    3. Assess the client's lung sounds, vital signs, and hemodynamic parameters.
    4. Ask if the client has a living will or durable power of attorney for health care.
    5. Administer the dopamine via Y-tubing along with normal saline (0.9%).

Bioterrorism

11. The nurse working in an emergency department (ED) receives a call that the ED will be receiving multiple casualties from a chlorine chemical explosion. Which intervention is **most important** in preparing for the victims?
    1. Prepare to decontaminate clients in a decontamination room.
    2. Refrain from touching the clothing of clients.
    3. Have IV supplies ready to start IV lines.
    4. Prepare to administer oxygen immediately to all casualties.

12. The nurse is discussing bioterrorism threat vectors with a community group. Which information regarding smallpox should be included in the discussion? **Select all that apply.**
 1. The incubation period for smallpox is about 12 days after exposure.
 2. The organism can only live for 5 to 6 minutes outside the host body.
 3. It can spread by direct or indirect contact with an infected person.
 4. The rash begins on the lower half of the body and progresses from there.
 5. A smallpox vaccine is available for anyone in the general population who desires it.

13. The client is suspected of being exposed to anthrax by inhalation. Which **priority** intervention should the nurse implement?
 1. Assess the client's lungs.
 2. Start the IV piggyback (IVPB) antibiotics.
 3. Place the client on respiratory isolation.
 4. Maintain the client's blood pressure.

14. The Homeland Security Office has issued a warning of suspected biological warfare using the *Francisella tularensis* bacteria. Which clinical manifestations **support** the initial diagnosis of tularemia?
 1. Fever, chills, headache, and malaise
 2. Hypotension; red, raised rash; and nasal congestion
 3. Enlarged cervical lymph nodes and polydipsia
 4. Metallic taste and disorientation

15. The client has been diagnosed with botulism. Which isolation procedures should the nurse implement?
 1. Airborne precautions
 2. Standard precautions
 3. Contact precautions
 4. Droplet precautions

16. The client has been exposed to nitrogen mustard gas. Which solution should be used to decontaminate the client?
 1. Normal saline
 2. Milk and dairy products
 3. Soap and water
 4. Diluted baking soda

17. The client working in a chemical plant that processes malathion for agricultural use presents to the ED with profuse sweating, visual disturbances, gastrointestinal disturbances, and bradycardia. Which medication should the nurse prepare to administer?
 1. Phenytoin IV every 4 hours
 2. Methylprednisolone IV every 8 hours
 3. Activated charcoal by mouth (PO) every 2 hours
 4. Atropine IV every 5 minutes

18. The employee health nurse working in an industrial plant that manufactures cyanide detects a bitter almond odor. Which actions should the nurse implement? **Select all that apply.**
 1. Have the workers evacuate the area.
 2. Close off the area in question.
 3. Notify the Office of Emergency Management.
 4. Call the emergency broadcast system to alert the public.
 5. Assess the workers for respiratory distress.

19. The client is diagnosed with acute radiation syndrome (ARS). Which findings would the nurse assess in the **acute** phase?
 1. Elevated blood pressure and bradycardia
 2. Fluid and electrolyte imbalance and shock
 3. Decreased lymphocytes, leukocytes, and erythrocytes
 4. Nausea, vomiting, diarrhea, and fatigue

20. The ED triage nurse notes five clients have been admitted within 6 hours with reports of severe abdominal cramping, nausea, vomiting, and diarrhea. Which intervention should the nurse implement **first**?
1. Notify the public health department of a botulism outbreak.
2. Check the clients' complete blood count (CBC) results.
3. Determine if the clients dined at the same place recently.
4. Discuss the situation with the house supervisor.

Code

21. A code has been called for the client experiencing ventricular fibrillation. Which medication should the nurse prepare to administer to the client?
1. Epinephrine IV push (IVP)
2. Lidocaine IVP
3. Atropine IVP
4. Digoxin IVP

22. The client is experiencing a code resulting from an overdose of tricyclic antidepressants. The client's arterial blood gases (ABGs) are populated in the following laboratory chart.

Arterial Blood Gas	Client Values	Reference Values
pH	7.31	7.35 to 7.45
Pco_2	58	35 to 45 mm Hg
Hco_3	19	22 to 26 mEq/L
Pao_2	60	80 to 95 mm Hg

Which medication should the nurse prepare to administer to the client?
1. Dopamine
2. Sodium bicarbonate
3. Calcium gluconate
4. Adenosine

23. The hospital nurse is administering epinephrine 1 mg to a client in a code. The client has a primary IV line of dextrose 5% in water set to keep open rate. Which intervention should the nurse implement?
1. Administer the medication rapidly into the IV.
2. Flush the IV tubing before and after administering epinephrine.
3. Administer the epinephrine via the intraosseous (IO) route.
4. Dilute the medication with 10 mL normal saline.

24. The HCP orders a lidocaine drip at 3 mg/min for a client who has just converted from ventricular fibrillation to normal sinus rhythm with multiple premature ventricular contractions (PVCs). The IV bag has 2 g of lidocaine in 500 mL normal saline. How would the nurse set the IV rate?

____

25. The client who is coding has the telemetry strip shown below.

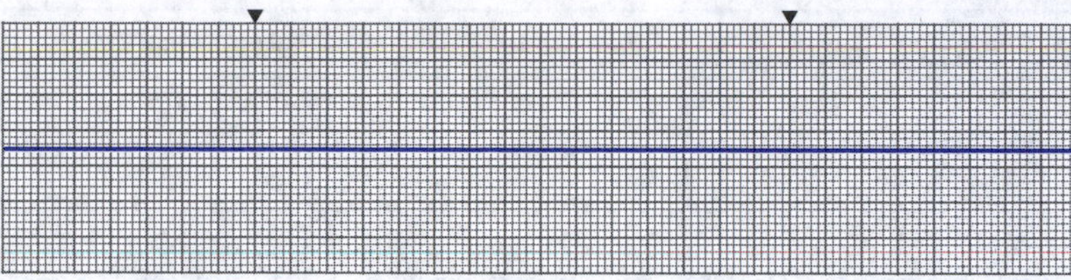

Which interventions should the nurse implement? **Select all that apply.**
1. Prepare to defibrillate the client at 300 joules.
2. Prepare for synchronized cardioversion.
3. Prepare to administer epinephrine IVP.
4. Initiate cardiopulmonary resuscitation (CPR).
5. Determine if the client has a do not resuscitate (DNR) order.

26. The client in a code is in ventricular fibrillation and then converts to a sinus rhythm with PVCs. After taking vital signs the HCP orders a dopamine drip at 3 mg/kg per hour. Which interventions should the nurse implement concerning this medication? **Select all that apply.**
1. Monitor the client's blood pressure every 15 minutes.
2. Assess the client's telemetry reading every hour.
3. Check the client's urine output every hour.
4. Evaluate the client's glucometer readings every 4 hours.
5. Obtain laboratory dopamine levels every day.

27. The client is in a code and is exhibiting the telemetry strip shown below.

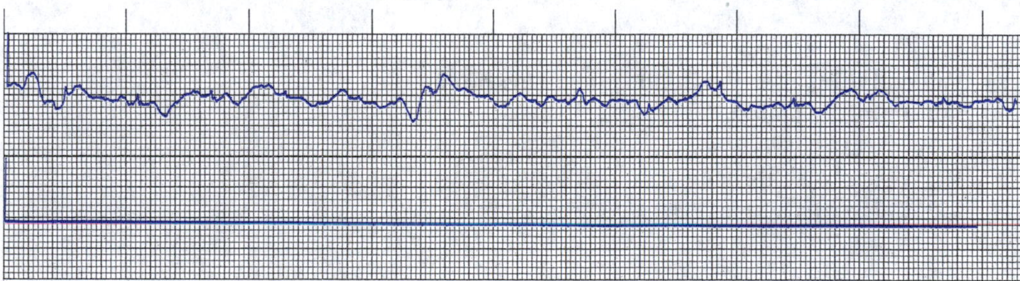

Which medication would the nurse prepare to administer?
1. Dopamine IV drip
2. Amiodarone IVP
3. Procainamide IVP
4. Dobutamine IV drip.

28. The nurse is preparing to hang a dopamine drip for the client who has just been successfully resuscitated. The client is receiving lidocaine 2 mg/min in the existing IV site. Which intervention should the nurse implement when hanging the dopamine drip?
1. Initiate another IV line to administer the dopamine drip.
2. Piggyback the dopamine drip in the lidocaine tubing.
3. Question the order because dopamine cannot be administered with lidocaine.
4. Prepare to help the HCP insert a subclavian line for the dopamine drip.

29. The client has just been successfully resuscitated and has the following ABGs:

Arterial Blood Gas	Client Values	Reference Values
pH	7.35	7.35 to 7.45
Pco_2	46	35 to 45 mm Hg
Hco_3	22	22 to 26 mEq/L
Pao_2	78	80 to 95 mm Hg

Which intervention should the nurse implement?
1. Prepare to administer sodium bicarbonate IVP.
2. Administer oxygen 8 L/min via nasal cannula.
3. Take no action because the ABGs are within normal limits.
4. Assess the client's pulse oximeter reading.

30. The client in a code is experiencing the telemetry strip below.

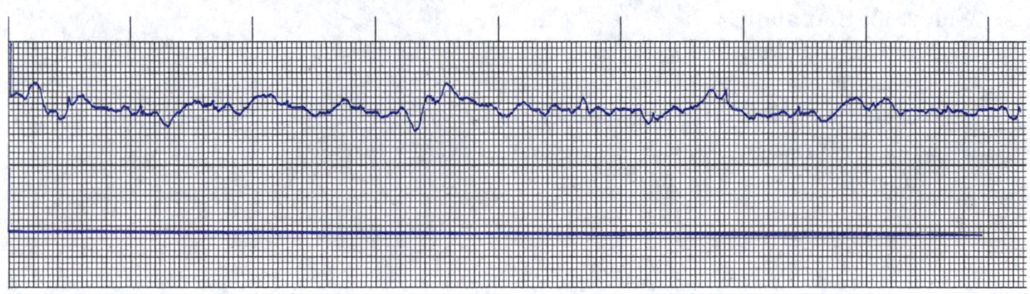

Which HCP order should the nurse **question**?
1. Administer amiodarone.
2. Administer lidocaine.
3. Prepare to defibrillate at 360 joules.
4. Prepare to insert an external pacemaker.

Poisoning

31. A 4-year-old child is brought to the ED as a suspected poisoning victim. Which interventions should the nurse implement? **Select all that apply.**
1. Implement supportive care.
2. Identify the poison.
3. Prevent further poison absorption.
4. Promote poison removal.
5. Administer an antidote.

32. Which statement **best** describes the scientific rationale for administering activated charcoal to a child who has ingested a poison?
1. Charcoal neutralizes toxic substances by changing the pH of the poison.
2. The charcoal binds with the poison and is excreted through the bowel.
3. Charcoal enhances antidotes for better results than antidotes given alone.
4. The charcoal induces vomiting, and the client eliminates much of the poison.

33. The ED is caring for pediatric clients who have ingested poisons. To which client would the nurse **question** administering a gastric lavage?
   1. The 2-year-old child in a coma who took a bottle of acetaminophen
   2. The 3-year-old child who ate a bottle of unknown tablets
   3. The hyperactive 6-year-old child who swallowed motor oil
   4. The 10-year-old child who took prescription painkillers

34. The nurse is caring for a client who swallowed the contents of a large acetaminophen bottle. Which medication would the nurse expect to be ordered for the client?
   1. Paracetamol
   2. Sodium bicarbonate
   3. N-acetylcysteine
   4. Ipecac syrup

35. The 13-year-old child admitted to the intensive care department diagnosed with an overdose of zolpidem is ordered whole bowel irrigation. Which intervention should the nurse implement?
   1. Administer 0.5 L of polyethylene glycol (PEG) with electrolyte every hour.
   2. Administer 1.0 L of PEG with electrolyte every hour.
   3. Administer 1.5 to 2.0 L of PEG with electrolyte every hour.
   4. Administer 2.5 to 3.0 L of PEG with electrolyte every hour.

36. The nurse working in the ED triages a child who has ingested a poison. Which referral agency should be contacted for specific information regarding the poison?
   1. The Material Safety Data information line
   2. The Poison Help line
   3. Child Protective Services (CPS)
   4. The local police department

37. The nurse is admitting a client suspected of poison ingestion to the ED. Which method is **preferred** to aid in the removal of ingested poisons?
   1. Emesis
   2. Gastric lavage
   3. Catharsis
   4. Activated charcoal

38. The HCP has prescribed edetate calcium disodium for a child diagnosed with lead poisoning. Which intervention should the nurse implement? **Select all that apply.**
   1. Administer orally with a large glass of water.
   2. Monitor the client's liver function tests.
   3. Check the client's intake and output.
   4. Tell the child to prepare to vomit.
   5. Prepare the child for x-rays.

39. The nurse administered naloxone to a 7-year-old child who drank a large bottle of narcotic cough syrup. Which interventions should the nurse implement? **Select all that apply.**
   1. Prepare to administer naloxone again in 30 minutes.
   2. Place the child on a negative pressure ventilator.
   3. Assess the client's respiratory status.
   4. Prepare the child for a tracheostomy.
   5. Have the parents discuss the situation with the police.

40. The school-age child is brought to the ED with carbon monoxide poisoning. Which intervention should the nurse implement **first**?
   1. Place the child on a pulse oximeter.
   2. Have respiratory therapy draw ABGs.
   3. Administer oxygen at 10 L per minute.
   4. Prevent chilling by wrapping the child in blankets.

ANSWERS AND RATIONALES

The correct answer number and rationale are in **boldface blue type.** Rationales for why other answer options are incorrect are also given.

Shock

1. 1. Nitroglycerin (Tridil), a coronary vasodilator, should only be mixed with dextrose 5% in water or normal saline (NS).
2. There are compatibility issues with many medications. Nitroglycerin (Tridil) is best running through its own lumen. No medication should be administered through the TPN line.
3. Regular IV tubing can absorb 40% to 80% of the nitroglycerin (Tridil); therefore, this should be administered in special tubing.
4. Nitroglycerin patches should be removed when administering IV nitroglycerin (Tridil) to prevent overdosage.

2. Correct answers are 1, 3 and 4.
1. Clients must be connected to a cardiac monitor before and during dopamine infusion, a beta and alpha agonist, and other cardiotonic drugs. The client in cardiogenic shock will be in the intensive care department.
2. Dopamine, a beta and alpha agonist, is administered to increase blood pressure. Blood pressure should be monitored every 5 to 15 minutes.
3. The client's urinary output should be monitored hourly to ensure the client has at least 30 mL of urine output an hour.
4. Extravasation of dopamine, a beta and alpha agonist, causes severe, localized vasoconstriction, resulting in slough of the tissue and tissue necrosis. The client should report burning at the IV site immediately.
5. Septic shock does not explicitly affect the neurological system; therefore, the nurse does not need to assess this system every hour, just every shift.

3. 1. A blood pressure of 102/78 is a stable blood pressure reading for a client in hypovolemic shock. A blood pressure reading of less than 90/60 would warrant intervention by the nurse.
2. A pulse oximeter reading of greater than 93% indicates the arterial oxygen level is between 80 and 100, which is normal.
3. Because of the ability of all colloids, including dextran, a nonblood colloid, to pull fluid into the vascular space, circulatory overload is a severe adverse outcome. Lung crackles reflect pulmonary congestion, a sign of fluid-volume overload.
4. A urinary output of 120 mL in 3 hours indicates that the client is urinating 40 mL an hour. Urinary output of at least 30 mL of urine output an hour indicates the kidneys are being perfused adequately.

MEDICATION MEMORY JOGGER: If the client verbalizes a symptom, if the nurse assesses data, or if laboratory data indicates an adverse effect secondary to a medication, the nurse must intervene. The nurse must implement an independent intervention or notify the HCP because medications can result in serious or even life-threatening complications.

4. 1. Septic shock is secondary to a blood infection and a broad-spectrum antibiotic, ceftriaxone (Rocephin), is prescribed until cultures and sensitivity results are obtained. The antibiotic specific to the bacteria causing the septic shock—in this case, vancomycin, an aminoglycoside antibiotic—should be administered as soon as possible.
2. There is no reason for the nurse to call the HCP and question this order.
3. The nurse should not wait 10 hours to administer an antibiotic to help save the client's life. Septic shock is life-threatening and must be treated with the appropriate antibiotic as soon as possible.
4. The client's WBC count does not impact the nurse's responsibility to administer vancomycin, an aminoglycoside antibiotic, as soon as possible.

5. 1. Norepinephrine (Levophed), a sympathomimetic, must be tapered, but this is not the priority nursing intervention when administering this medication. Caring for the client is always the priority.
2. Administering medication on an infusion pump is essential, but the priority intervention is caring for the client, not a machine.

3. The nurse should check the client's renal status, but the priority nursing intervention is assessing the data for which the client is receiving the medication.
4. **Norepinephrine (Levophed), a sympathomimetic, is a potent vasoconstrictor; therefore, continuous monitoring of the blood pressure is required to avoid hypertension.**

6. 1. This statement is the scientific rationale for administering vasodilators such as nitroglycerin (Tridil) or nitroprusside (Nipride), not albumin 5% (Albuminar-5) colloid solution.
2. This statement is the scientific rationale for administering adrenergics (sympathomimetics) such as norepinephrine (Levophed), not colloid solutions.
3. **This is the scientific rationale for administering albumin 5% (Albuminar-5), a colloid solution. They are blood volume expanders that promote circulatory volume and tissue perfusion.**
4. Crystalloid solutions, such as isotonic (0.9% normal saline) or hypotonic (0.45% normal saline) solutions, increase fluid volume in the intravascular and the interstitial spaces.

7. Correct answers are 1, 2, 3, 4, and 5.
1. **Shortness of breath, low back pain, and itching all over the body are signs of anaphylactic shock. Epinephrine, an adrenergic, is the drug of choice to treat anaphylaxis.**
2. **The client's assessment data indicates a life-threatening anaphylactic reaction to the blood transfusion. Therefore, the nurse should take action and assess the client.**
3. **The nurse should keep an IV access so that normal saline and medication can be administered to help prevent anaphylactic shock.**
4. **Discontinuing the blood at the hub of the IV catheter is the first intervention because the client is exhibiting signs of an anaphylactic reaction, which can lead to anaphylactic shock if the allergen (blood) is not stopped immediately. Many different allergens can cause anaphylactic shock, including medications, blood administration, latex, foods, snake venom, and insect stings.**
5. **The client is having an allergic reaction to the blood, and the HCP should be notified.**

MEDICATION MEMORY JOGGER: When answering test questions or when caring for clients at the bedside, the nurse should remember that assessing the client may not be the first action to take when the client is in distress. The nurse may need to intervene directly to help the client.

8. 1. **An infusion pump should be used when administering dobutamine (Dobutrex), a beta$_1$-adrenergic agonist, because an overdose, which could occur if a drip via gravity is used, could cause the client's death. This action by the primary nurse would warrant immediate intervention by the charge nurse.**
2. A urometer is a triangular plastic container attached to a Foley catheter that allows the nurse to obtain hourly urinary outputs. This action would not require intervention by the charge nurse.
3. Monitoring the client's peripheral oxygen saturation would be appropriate for a client in cardiogenic shock; therefore, this action would not warrant intervention by the charge nurse.
4. The nurse should always check the client for any types of allergies; therefore, this action would not warrant intervention by the charge nurse.

9. 1. The nurse should address the infiltrated site because of the toxic effects of the medication in the tissue. The blood pressure reading and apical pulse rate will not help the infiltrated site.
2. This is not the appropriate action to take when dopamine, a beta and alpha agonist, infiltrates.
3. **Extravasation of dopamine, a beta and alpha agonist, causes severe, localized vasoconstriction, resulting in a tissue slough and tissue necrosis if not reversed with the antidote phentolamine (Regitine) injections at the infiltration site.**
4. The IV should be discontinued, but the nurse must take further action, or else the IV site may have tissue necrosis.

10. Correct answers are 2 and 3.
1. This would be appropriate when injecting medications intramuscularly or subcutaneously, but dopamine drip, a sympathomimetic, can only be administered intravenously.
2. **Sympathomimetics are incompatible with sodium bicarbonate or alkaline solutions.**

3. **The client in hypovolemic shock is in critical condition, and a thorough assessment must be completed on the client frequently.**
4. This intervention is not specific for the dopamine drip, a sympathomimetic, but a client in cardiogenic shock, taking dopamine, is in critical condition. An advance directive would be an appropriate intervention for this client.
5. Dopamine is not administered via Y-tubing. Blood and blood products are administered via Y-tubing.

MEDICATION MEMORY JOGGER: "Select all that apply" questions require the test taker to view each option as a True/False question. One option cannot assist the test taker in eliminating another option.

Bioterrorism

11. 1. Chlorine is a gas. Although the clothing may have some chlorine on it, decontamination procedures are not required.
2. Chlorine is a gas. Although the clothing may have some chlorine on it, the chlorine in the clothing should not pose a threat to the ED.
3. IV access is important but not as important as supplying clients with oxygen and ventilatory support.
4. **Chlorine gas, when inhaled, separates the alveoli from the capillary bed. Oxygenation and ventilatory support are the most critical interventions.**

12. Correct answers are 1 and 3.
1. **The incubation period is about 12 days.**
2. The organism can survive on clothing and blankets in cool temperatures for at least 24 hours.
3. **Smallpox spreads by direct contact with an infected person, by droplet contact, or by direct contact with a contaminated item of bedding or clothing. During the French and Indian War (1754–1763), smallpox was used as a weapon when contaminated bedding was sent into Indian villages, resulting in a 50% casualty rate.**
4. The rash begins on the face, mouth, pharynx, and forearms and then proceeds to the trunk and the rest of the body.
5. The Centers for Disease Control and Prevention (CDC) does not make the smallpox vaccine available to the public because the disease has been eradicated. However, if a smallpox outbreak were to occur, the CDC has enough vaccines available to vaccinate every person in the United States (CDC, 2016).

13. 1. Assessing is usually the first intervention, but in this case, a delay of any kind in starting antibiotics could result in death.
2. **If antibiotics are initiated within 24 hours of the onset of clinical manifestations from anthrax inhalation, death can be prevented. However, the nurse must keep in mind that the client will have had the symptoms for some hours before seeking medical attention.**
3. Standard precaution procedures are all that are necessary. However, if the client dies, cremation should be the method of body disposal because the body can harbor the spores for decades and pose a threat to mortuary and medical examiner personnel.
4. The client's blood pressure should remain stable unless sepsis overwhelms the client's body, in which case recommended treatment is antibiotics.

MEDICATION MEMORY JOGGER: The nurse must remember that if treatment initiation can prevent a complication (death), then treatment has priority over assessment.

14. 1. **Tularemia is highly contagious and can be contracted by direct contact with infected animals or by breathing aerosolized *F. tularensis* (tularemia) bacteria. It can be used as a biologic weapon. Initial clinical manifestations are sudden onset of fever, fatigue, chills, headache, lower backache, malaise, rigor, coryza (profuse discharge from the mucous membranes of the nose), dry cough, sore throat without adenopathy, and nausea and vomiting.**
2. These are not clinical manifestations of tularemia.
3. These are not clinical manifestations of tularemia.
4. These are not clinical manifestations of tularemia.

15. 1. Airborne precautions are used for clients suspected of having tuberculosis. Hospital staff must use 0.3-micron filtration masks when caring for these clients. This is not needed for clients diagnosed with botulism.
2. **Clients diagnosed with botulism were infected by direct contact with the bacteria. It is not transmitted from human to human. Standard precautions are required for all clients.**

3. Contact precautions are used to prevent contact with bacteria in wounds or infected gastrointestinal secretions. Botulism is not transmitted from human to human.
4. Droplet precautions are used for respiratory illnesses where transmission can occur when in close contact with the client. Botulism is not transmitted from human to human.

16. 1. Wash the chemical off the body with mild soap and water, not with normal saline.
2. Wash the chemical off the body with mild soap and water, not with milk products.
3. Wash the chemical off the body with mild soap and water (CDC, 2018).
4. Wash the chemical off the body with mild soap and water, not diluted baking soda.

17. 1. Diazepam (Valium), a benzodiazepine, is the drug of choice for potential convulsions associated with nerve agent toxicity.
2. Methylprednisolone (Solu-Medrol), a glucocorticosteroid, would not be administered for excessive nerve stimulation.
3. Activated charcoal, an absorbent agent, is administered to prevent absorption of ingested poisons.
4. IV atropine, an anticholinergic, 2 to 4 mg, followed by 2 mg every 3 to 8 minutes for 24 hours, is the drug of choice to reverse toxic drug effects of malathion, a nerve agent. Ingredients in many pesticides bond with acetylcholinesterase so that acetylcholine cannot be removed from the body. The result is hyperstimulation of nerve endings (Agency for Toxic Substances and Disease Registry, n.d.).

MEDICATION MEMORY JOGGER: Atropine, an anticholinergic, is the medication administered for symptomatic bradycardia. This might lead the test taker to choose option 4 as the correct answer.

18. Correct answers are 1, 2, and 5.
1. The smell of bitter almonds is associated with cyanide gas, a deadly poison. The nurse should evacuate the area.
2. The smell of bitter almonds is associated with cyanide gas, a deadly poison. The nurse should attempt to contain the gas in the area in question.
3. The nurse would notify local authorities and plant administration, not federal emergency personnel. Nurses must know and follow emergency procedures and guidelines.
4. Plant administration or the local authorities are responsible for notifying the public. There are procedures designed to limit mass panic.
5. Clinical manifestations of cyanide poisoning include respiratory muscle failure, respiratory or cardiac failure, and death.

19. 1. Elevated blood pressure and bradycardia occur in the last phase of radiation sickness and death occurs soon after.
2. Fluid and electrolyte imbalance and shock occur in the illness phase after 4 or more weeks.
3. Decreased lymphocytes, leukocytes, and erythrocytes occur in the latent phase and can last for 3 weeks or more.
4. Nausea, vomiting, diarrhea, and fatigue are initial presenting clinical manifestations of exposure to radiation occurring within 48 to 72 hours after exposure.

20. 1. This would not be done until it is determined that all clients have botulism, then it is the individual with the responsibility of working with the public health department to notify the agency, not the ED nurse.
2. Clients' CBC results will not indicate if the clients have botulism.
3. Severe abdominal cramping, nausea, vomiting, and diarrhea are clinical manifestations of botulism, but it has not been determined that this is the diagnosis in the triage area. Determining whether clients have eaten in the same place recently is the first step in determining if the client has been exposed to botulism.
4. The person with the responsibility for the facility should be notified whenever there is a potential situation where the press and public will be arriving at the facility, but this is not the first intervention.

Code

21. 1. Epinephrine, an adrenergic agonist, is the first medication administered in a code because it constricts the periphery and shunts the blood to the trunk of the body.
2. Lidocaine, an antiarrhythmic, is administered in ventricular fibrillation, but it is not administered first in a code.
3. Atropine, an antiarrhythmic, is administered for asystole.
4. Digoxin, a cardiac glycoside, is administered for cardiac failure.

22. 1. Dopamine, a vasopressor medication, is administered to increase blood pressure.
2. ABGs indicate the client is in metabolic acidosis, and the drug of choice is sodium bicarbonate, an alkalinizing agent. Sodium bicarbonate is only recommended for cardiac arrest resulting from hypokalemia or overdose of tricyclic antidepressants.
3. Calcium gluconate, an electrolyte replacement, is administered in clients experiencing hypocalcemia.
4. Adenosine, an antiarrhythmic medication, is the drug of choice for supraventricular tachycardia (SVT).

23. 1. The medication should be pushed as fast as possible in a code situation.
2. Epinephrine is compatible with the primary IV line; therefore, there is no reason to flush the tubing before and after administering the medication.
3. Although the Intraosseous route can be used to administer epinephrine, some efficacy of the IO route compared to the IV route is noted in the research. The nurse should administer medication in the existing IV line (Merchant et al., 2020).
4. Epinephrine in the crash cart is diluted in 10 mL of normal saline in a Bristojet and ready for administration; therefore, the nurse should not dilute the medication.

24. 45 mL. Drip rates are set per hour. A drip rate of 3 mg/min is 180 mg/hr. If 500 mL contains 2,000 mg (2 g) of lidocaine, then each milliliter contains 4 mg of lidocaine (2,000 ÷ 500 = 4). To determine how many milliliters per hour are needed, divide 180 mg ÷ 4 = 45. The nurse should set the IV rate at 45 mL.

MEDICATION MEMORY JOGGER: There is a way to remember this in an emergency situation: 1 mg (15 mL), 2 mg (30 mL), 3 mg (45 mL), 4 mg (60 mL). This is the rate if the medication is 2 g in 500 mL, which is how it comes, prepackaged.

25. Correct answers are 3, 4, and 5.
1. The client in asystole would not benefit from defibrillation because there is no heart activity. The client must have some heart activity (ventricular activity) for defibrillation to be successful.
2. Synchronized cardioversion is used for new-onset atrial fibrillation or unstable ventricular tachycardia.
3. Epinephrine is the drug of choice for asystole because it increases blood flow to the heart and increases the heart's ability to generate an electrical impulse.
4. The nurse should initiate and perform CPR on the client in asystole.
5. The nurse should determine if the client has a DNR because if that is the case, CPR should be discontinued.

26. Correct answers are 1 and 3.
1. This medication increases blood pressure, and blood pressure should be monitored every 15 minutes.
2. The client's telemetry reading will not indicate dopamine effectiveness or identify complications secondary to dopamine, a vasopressor; therefore, assessing the client's telemetry reading hourly is not a pertinent intervention for dopamine administration.
3. The client's urine output must be assessed hourly to determine effectiveness of dopamine administration because dopamine, a vasopressor, increases blood pressure. If the client's blood pressure increases, then urine output increases; if the client's blood pressure decreases, then urine output decreases. Kidneys will retain water to help increase blood pressure. The client should have at least 30 mL/hour output.
4. The glucose level is not used when evaluating dopamine effectiveness, nor does it identify complications secondary to dopamine; therefore, this is not a pertinent intervention for dopamine administration.
5. There is not a laboratory test for therapeutic dopamine levels. The medication is titrated to achieve the desired effect.

27. 1. Dopamine, a vasopressor, is used to increase blood pressure.
2. Ventricular fibrillation is a very common arrhythmia in a code situation, and amiodarone, an antiarrhythmic, is the drug of choice to treat this arrhythmia (American Heart Association, 2020).
3. Procainamide is an antiarrhythmic (Class 1A) medication that is used for ventricular and atrial arrhythmias, but it is not the medication the nurse would prepare to administer for this specific arrhythmia.
4. Dobutamine, an inotropic medication, is only used for cardiac failure.

28. 1. **Dopamine, a vasopressor, is incompatible with all other IV fluids; therefore, the nurse must initiate another IV line to infuse dopamine in a separate line.**
2. Dopamine is incompatible with all other IV fluids; therefore, it cannot be piggybacked with lidocaine.
3. The nurse does not need to question the order because the nurse can start another saline lock without talking to the HCP.
4. The dopamine drip does not have to be administered via a subclavian line as long as it is not piggybacked with any other medication.

29. 1. ABGs do not indicate metabolic acidosis, so sodium bicarbonate should not be administered.
2. **PaO_2 is low (normal is 80 to 100); therefore, the nurse should administer oxygen via nasal cannula. Oxygen is considered a medication.**
3. ABGs are not normal and intervention is needed.
4. The client's ABGs reveal a low arterial oxygen level and do not need to be verified by a pulse oximeter reading.

30. 1. Amiodarone, an antiarrhythmic, suppresses ventricular ectopy and is the drug of choice for this arrhythmic. The nurse would not question this order.
2. Lidocaine, an antiarrhythmic, suppresses ventricular ectopy. The nurse would not question this order.
3. Defibrillation is the treatment of choice for a client in ventricular fibrillation.
4. **Pacemakers are used for clients diagnosed with symptomatic sinus bradycardia or asystole. This client is in ventricular fibrillation; therefore, the nurse would question this order.**

Poisoning

31. Correct answers are 1, 2, 3, 4, and 5.
1. **The child must receive supportive care to maintain life until the poison can be identified and further specific measures can be implemented.**
2. **Treatment is facilitated by identifying the specific poison and amount ingested; then specific treatment can be instituted.**
3. **Limiting amount of poison absorbed by the body can limit damage.**
4. **Measures to eliminate poison from the body prevent further absorption.**
5. **An antidote is administered to counteract the poison's effects.**

32. 1. Charcoal does not change the pH of a substance.
2. **Charcoal binds with poison to form an inert substance that can be eliminated through the bowel because the body is incapable of absorbing charcoal molecules. The charcoal must be administered within 60 minutes of ingesting poison. After that, the feces will be black (Juurlink, 2016).**
3. Charcoal can absorb the antidote. Charcoal should not be administered before, with, or immediately after the antidote.
4. Charcoal does not cause emesis. An emetic such as ipecac would induce vomiting.

33. 1. Gastric lavage would not be contraindicated for a 2-year-old child in a coma who ingested the contents of a bottle of acetaminophen (Tylenol).
2. Gastric lavage would not be contraindicated for a 3-year-old child who ate a bottle of unknown tablets.
3. **Although rarely used today, gastric lavage should not be attempted when there has been ingestion of caustic agents, high-viscosity petroleum products, or sharp objects. Antidotes, supportive care, and aspiration prevention are implemented if gastric lavage is not to be performed.**
4. Gastric lavage would not be contraindicated for a 10 year old who took prescription painkillers.

34. 1. Paracetamol is the name for acetaminophen in Europe. It would not be administered for acetaminophen overdose.
2. Sodium bicarbonate is used in the treatment of salicylate poisoning but not in acetaminophen overdose.
3. **N-acetylcysteine, the antidote for acetaminophen toxicity, is given orally or IV to minimize hepatotoxicity.**
4. Ipecac syrup is not recommended to manage acetaminophen toxicity because it can interfere with other antidotal therapies. Ipecac syrup is no longer recommended by the poison control center.

35. 1. 0.5 L of PEG with electrolyte (GoLYTELY) every hour is the dose for children younger than 6 years old.
2. 1.0 L of PEG with electrolyte (GoLYTELY) every hour is the dose for children 6 to 12 years old.
3. 1.5 to 2.0 L of PEG with electrolyte (GoLYTELY) is the dose for clients 12 years old or older. Whole-bowel irrigation is effective after ingestion of lead, lithium, iron, and sustained-release medications.
4. This dosage is not recommended for any client.

36. 1. Material Safety Data information is required for every chemical in a health-care facility, but it is not an agency to contact regarding specific poisons and antidotes.
2. The National Poison Control Hotline (1-800-222-1222) is the equivalent of dialing 911 locally. The hotline can be dialed from anywhere in the United States, and the organization's representative will connect the nurse with the local poison control agency.
3. CPS will not be able to help the nurse with information regarding the poison.
4. The police department will not be able to help the nurse with information regarding the poison.

MEDICATION MEMORY JOGGER: In an emergency situation, the client must be cared for first, and then other agencies such as CPS or the police may be notified.

37. 1. Ipecac is not the preferred method for poison removal because it should not be given to clients experiencing convulsions or who have a reduced level of consciousness or otherwise cannot protect their airway.
2. Gastric lavage is not the preferred method of removal of an ingested poison because of the potential for aspiration of stomach contents into the lungs.
3. Catharsis (administration of harsh stimulant laxatives) may help to remove the poison, but this method has not been shown to improve clinical outcomes.
4. Activated charcoal and whole-bowel irrigation are preferred methods of removal of ingested poisons from the body. Activated charcoal binds with the poison, and the body cannot absorb charcoal, so the poison is eliminated in the feces.

38. Correct answers are 3 and 5.
1. Calcium EDTA, a chelating agent, is administered intramuscularly or intravenously because it is poorly absorbed through the gastrointestinal tract.
2. The drug and lead will be excreted through glomerular filtration; therefore, kidney function is monitored, not liver function.
3. Edetate calcium disodium (Calcium EDTA), a chelating agent, and lead will be excreted through glomerular filtration. The nurse should ensure adequate renal function before administering the medication.
4. Calcium EDTA is not an emetic medication.
5. A child treated with calcium EDTA may need to have x-rays to determine the amount of circulating lead in the body.

39. Correct answers are 1 and 3.
1. Narcotic antagonist naloxone (Narcan) has a short half-life and could wear off before the effects of the narcotic cough syrup. The nurse should observe for signs of returning respiratory depression and be ready to intervene.
2. Negative-pressure ventilators (the old iron lung) are no longer used. Currently, positive-pressure ventilation is preferred.
3. The narcotic cough syrup has depressed the client's respiratory status; therefore, the nurse should assess the child.
4. The child would have an endotracheal tube placed first, not a tracheostomy, for a few days until it is determined if the child needs permanent ventilatory support because of brain damage.
5. This is not the nurse's responsibility. The nurse would report the case to CPS, who could call the police if necessary.

40. 1. A pulse oximeter would give an inaccurately high reading because the blood is saturated with carbon monoxide.
2. ABGs are not a priority.
3. The client should receive high levels of oxygen. Carbon monoxide binds to the hemoglobin molecule with a greater affinity than oxygen. It is imperative to get oxygen to the client as quickly as possible.
4. The child should be prevented from chilling, but oxygen is the priority.

EMERGENCY NURSING COMPREHENSIVE EXAMINATION

1. The mother of a 2-year-old child calls the ED and reports that the child has swallowed a bottle of prenatal vitamins. Which question is **most important** for the nurse to ask the mother?
   1. "How much does your daughter weigh?"
   2. "Are the prenatal vitamins with iron or without iron?"
   3. "Have you called the Poison Control Center?"
   4. "When did you purchase the prenatal vitamins?"

2. The client is admitted to the ED diagnosed with heatstroke. The client has a temperature of 104°F (40°C) and hot, dry skin. Which intervention should the nurse implement? **Select all that apply.**
   1. Start an IV to infuse IV fluids.
   2. Administer acetaminophen for elevated temperature.
   3. Encourage the client to drink cold water.
   4. Cover with wet sheets and place the client in front of a fan.
   5. Administer chlorpromazine to control shivering.

3. The ED nurse notifies the Poison Control Center concerning an accidental poisoning of a 4-year-old child. Which action by the ED nurse **warrants intervention** by the charge nurse?
   1. The ED nurse tells the Poison Control Center the type of poison ingested.
   2. The ED nurse tells the Poison Control Center the type and estimated time the poison was taken.
   3. The ED nurse informs the Poison Control Center of the client's vital signs.
   4. The ED nurse tells the Poison Control Center the age and weight of the child who ingested the poison.

4. Which document protects the nurse from liability as long as no grossly negligent care or willful misconduct is provided that deliberately harms a person outside the hospital?
   1. The American First Aid Association mission
   2. The Board of Nurse Examiners First Aid section
   3. The Good Samaritan Act
   4. The Lay Rescuer Administration Act

5. The nurse has just completed administering medication to a client diagnosed with a cerebrovascular accident (CVA) via a gastrostomy tube. As the nurse is leaving the room, the client starts vomiting. Which action should the nurse implement **first**?
   1. Ask the client if they can speak.
   2. Assist the client to sit on the side of the bed.
   3. Place the client in the side-lying position.
   4. Assess the client's bowel sounds.

6. The school nurse is administering treatment to a 14-year-old student who stepped on a rusty nail that punctured the skin. How should the nurse implement the interventions? **Rank in order of performance.**
   1. Cleanse the puncture site with soap and water.
   2. Put sterile, nonadhesive dressings on the wound.
   3. Apply an antibiotic ointment to the puncture site.
   4. Determine when the child last had a tetanus shot.
   5. Ask the student if he or she is allergic to any antibiotic.

7. The client diagnosed with type 2 diabetes is being discharged from the ED after sustaining a head injury. Which statement indicates the client **needs more teaching** before discharge?
   1. "I should not take my insulin if I am unable to eat."
   2. "I should take acetaminophen if I have a headache."
   3. "If I become nauseated or start vomiting, I will call my doctor."
   4. "I will not take any type of sedative medications."

8. The client who has a history of peptic ulcer disease (PUD) presents to the ED. The client's vital signs are populated in the following vital sign flow sheet.

Vital Sign Flowsheet	Client Values	Reference Values
Pulse	128 bpm	60 to 100 beats/min
Blood pressure	86/42 mm Hg	100 to 119 mm Hg systolic 60 to 80 mm Hg diastolic

   Which intervention should the nurse implement **first**?
   1. Administer dopamine by IV constant infusion.
   2. Request a stat CBC, Chem 7, and type and crossmatch.
   3. Prepare to administer IV pantoprazole.
   4. Initiate an IV with lactated Ringer's solution with an 18-gauge angiocath.

9. Which medication should the nurse administer **first** to the client experiencing cardiac arrest?
   1. Epinephrine
   2. Oxygen
   3. Lidocaine
   4. Atropine

10. The client presented to the ED diagnosed with a rattlesnake bite on the left foot 2 hours ago. Which intervention should the nurse implement **during** the administration of the antivenom?
   1. Take the client's vital signs every 15 minutes.
   2. Administer diphenhydramine.
   3. Monitor the circumference of the left leg every 2 hours.
   4. Administer cimetidine.

11. The 22-year-old college student is admitted to the medical department with a diagnosis of an overdose of sleeping pills. Which task should the registered nurse (RN) delegate to the unlicensed assistive personnel (UAP)?
   1. Ask the UAP to assess the stool for color.
   2. Have the UAP reset the rate on the IV pump.
   3. Instruct the UAP to sit with the client.
   4. Have the UAP evaluate the client's Glasgow Coma Scale score.

12. The nurse is caring for a client diagnosed with a severe burn. The prescribed medication for administration is in the following medication administration record.

Client: Mr. A.C.	MR# 1234567	Date: Today
Medication	**0701–1900**	**1901–0700**
Pantoprazole 40 mg IV every day	0900	
PCN 5 million units IVPB every 6 hours	0900 1500	2100 0300
Lorazepam 3 mg PO every 12 hours	0900	2100
Morphine sulfate 5 mg IM every 1 to 2 hours PRN pain		

Which medication should the nurse **question** administering?
1. Pantoprazole
2. Penicillin (PCN)
3. Lorazepam
4. Morphine

13. The client tells the triage nurse in the ED she has food poisoning similar to others who recently ate at a local restaurant. The client has been vomiting and has had diarrhea for the past 6 hours and needs help. Which medication should the nurse administer **first**?
1. Diphenoxylate orally
2. Ceftriaxone IVPB
3. Pantoprazole IVPB
4. Promethazine intramuscularly

14. The client who is being discharged from the ED after being raped is offered the medication levonorgestrel. Which statement **best** describes the scientific rationale for administering this medication?
1. Levonorgestrel will help prevent the client from getting a sexually transmitted disease.
2. Levonorgestrel is known as a morning-after pill and helps prevent pregnancy.
3. Levonorgestrel will help decrease the client's anxiety and nervousness.
4. Levonorgestrel will promote the healing process of the vaginal tissues.

15. The client is diagnosed with an open fracture of the right forearm. Which interventions should the ED nurse implement? **Select all that apply.**
1. Administer a prophylactic antibiotic.
2. Apply a warm pack to the right forearm.
3. Evaluate effectiveness of the pain medication.
4. Prepare to administer the preoperative medication on call.
5. Explain the surgical procedure to the client and family.

16. The client diagnosed with type 1 diabetes is brought to the ED by the family. The client is belligerent, confused, and uncooperative. Which interventions should the nurse implement? **Select all that apply.**
1. Administer 1 amp of dextrose 50%.
2. Give the client 2 cups of orange juice.
3. Determine when the client took the last insulin shot.
4. Inject glucagon subcutaneously in the abdomen.
5. Obtain a glucose level via a glucometer.

17. The HCP is preparing to suture a laceration on the client's right hand. Which question is **most important** for the nurse to ask the client?
1. "Are you right- or left-handed?"
2. "Do you have any allergies?"
3. "How did you cut yourself?"
4. "Are you afraid of needles?"

18. The elderly client diagnosed with chronic hypertension is brought to the ED by the caregiver. The client has a blood pressure of 198/120 and has multiple contusions on the abdomen and forearms. Which question is **most important** for the nurse to ask the client?
1. "How did you get the bruises on your abdomen and forearm?"
2. "Has anyone forced you to sign papers against your will?"
3. "When was the last time you took your blood pressure medication?"
4. "You seem frightened. Are you afraid of anyone in your home?"

19. The Homeland Security Office has issued a warning of suspected biological warfare using the *F. tularensis* (tularemia) bacteria. Which intervention should the charge nurse implement?
1. Initiate the hospital's external emergency disaster plan.
2. Instruct the staff to prepare the decontamination area.
3. Prepare to administer the antitoxin intravenously.
4. Check on the supply of oral doxycycline.

20. The client diagnosed with botulism poisoning is prescribed gentamycin. The medication is available in 250 mL of normal saline. At which rate should the nurse set the IV pump?

____

EMERGENCY NURSING COMPREHENSIVE EXAMINATION ANSWERS AND RATIONALES

1. 1. The weight of the child is pertinent information, but it is not the most important question.

2. If the prenatal vitamins have iron, this is a life-threatening situation. The child can hemorrhage because of the ulcerogenic effects of unbound iron, causing shock. As few as 10 tablets of ferrous sulfate (3 g) taken at one time can be fatal within 12 to 48 hours. This is the most important question to ask to determine what treatment the child should have for the accidental overdose.

3. Because the mother has called the ED, it is not a priority to know if she called the Poison Control Center.

4. Determining if the vitamins may have lost potency because they were purchased months ago is not as high a priority as determining if the prenatal vitamins have iron.

2. Correct answers are 1, 4, and 5.

1. The nurse should start an IV and infuse fluids, which will help rehydrate the client.

2. Antipyretic medication, acetaminophen (Tylenol), will not help decrease the temperature when hyperpyrexia is secondary to a heatstroke.

3. The client should be kept nothing by mouth (NPO) to prevent vomiting and possible aspiration.

4. Cooling measures such as immersion in a cool bath or placing wet sheets on the client and putting the client in front of a fan should be initiated.

5. Cooling measures can cause shivering in the client. Shivering should be controlled with chlorpromazine (Thorazine) intravenously to avoid the temperature increase that occurs in the body from shivering.

3. 1. The Poison Control Center needs to know the type of poison ingested; therefore, this would not warrant intervention by the charge nurse.

2. The Poison Control Center needs to know the type and estimated time the poison was taken; therefore, this would not warrant intervention by the charge nurse.

3. The Poison Control Center does not need to know the client's vital signs; therefore, this would warrant intervention by the charge nurse. The center's responsibility is to inform the nurse of the antidote and treatment to decrease the possibility of life-threatening complications secondary to the poisoning.

4. The Poison Control Center needs to know the child's age and weight to determine the severity of the poisoning; therefore, this would not warrant intervention by the charge nurse.

4. 1. There is no American First Aid Association.

2. The Board of Nurse Examiners does not have a section addressing emergency care outside the hospital.

3. The Good Samaritan Act protects nurses and lay rescuers when caring for individuals outside the hospital. Nurses are held to a different standard because they have received teaching on first aid.

4. There is no Lay Rescuer Administration Act.

5. 1. Asking the client if he or she can speak is the correct action if the client is choking, not vomiting.

2. Because the client had a CVA, the client may not be able to sit on the side of the bed.

3. The client should be lying on the side to help prevent aspirating vomit contents into the lungs.

4. The client is vomiting; therefore, assessing the bowel sounds is not an appropriate nursing intervention.

MEDICATION MEMORY JOGGER: When answering test questions or when caring for clients at the bedside, the nurse should remember that assessing the client may not be the first action to take when the client is in distress. The nurse may need to intervene directly to help the client.

6. Correct order is 1, 5, 3, 2, 4.

1. The nurse must cleanse the area with soap and water to remove any debris.

5. The nurse should make sure the student is not allergic to any type of antibiotics before applying ointment. Topical medication can cause allergic reactions.

3. **The nurse should then apply antibiotic ointment to help prevent a wound infection.**
2. **A dressing should be applied over the wound to help prevent infection.**
4. **The nurse should then check the last tetanus shot administration date to determine the student's need for a booster.**

7. 1. **Physiologic stress, such as stress that might occur after a head injury, increases blood glucose level; therefore, the client must take insulin as prescribed but needs glucose (carbohydrates) to prevent hypoglycemia. Therefore, the client should drink the amount of carbohydrates in the prescribed American Diabetes Association diet, including Popsicles, regular Jell-O, or regular cola. This statement indicates the client needs more teaching before discharge.**
2. The client can take acetaminophen (Tylenol) for a headache secondary to a head injury. The client does not need more teaching.
3. Nausea and vomiting are signs of increasing intracranial pressure, and the client should call the HCP. This statement indicates the client does not need more teaching.
4. The client should not take any type of sedative, which may cause further neurologic deficit. The client does not need more teaching before discharge.

8. 1. Dopamine, a sympathomimetic, is administered to increase the client's blood pressure, but the client must have an IV route. Because the client does not have an IV route, this is not the nurse's first intervention.
2. Laboratory tests are important, but not more important than preventing circulatory collapse, which is inevitable in a client in hypovolemic shock, as this client is.
3. Pantoprazole (Protonix), a proton-pump inhibitor (PPI), is administered to decrease gastric acid production, but the client must have an IV route; therefore, this is not the first intervention.
4. **The client's vital signs indicate shock, and with the history of PUD, the nurse should suspect hypovolemic shock; however, no matter what type of shock, the nurse must first initiate IV therapy because of the low blood pressure and increased heart rate.**

9. 1. Epinephrine, a sympathomimetic, is the first medication administered intravenously or intratracheally, but oxygen should be administered when CPR is instituted.
2. **Oxygen is the first medication administered to all clients experiencing cardiac arrest. It will be administered through an Ambu-bag via a face mask until the client is intubated (American Heart Association, 2020).**
3. Lidocaine, an antidysrhythmic, is the drug of choice for ventricular dysrhythmias, but the client must be monitored by telemetry to determine the specific rhythm.
4. Atropine, an antidysrhythmic, is the drug of choice for asystole, but the client must be monitored by telemetry to determine the specific rhythm.

10. 1. **The client's vital signs must be monitored every 15 minutes throughout the 6-hour IV infusion because of the great potential for a life-threatening reaction to the antivenin.**
2. Diphenhydramine (Benadryl), an H_1 antagonist, must be administered before the initiation of the antivenom infusion to decrease allergic response to the antivenom. This is an H_1 antihistamine.
3. Leg circumference should be measured every 30 to 60 minutes for 48 hours after the infusion.
4. Cimetidine (Tagamet), an H_2 histamine blocker, must be administered before initiation of the antivenom infusion to decrease allergic response to the antivenom. This is an H_2 antihistamine.

11. 1. The UAP can assist the client to the bathroom, but the UAP does not have the knowledge to determine if the stool color is normal for this client. If the client received charcoal, the stool should be black.
2. IV fluids are considered medications, and the nurse cannot delegate medication administration to a UAP.
3. **An overdose of sleeping pills should be considered a suicide attempt until proved otherwise. The client should be on one-to-one suicide precautions. A UAP could sit with the client.**
4. The Glasgow Coma Scale assesses the client's neurologic status, and this cannot be delegated to a UAP.

12. 1. Pantoprazole is given to burn clients to decrease stomach acid and reduce ulceration risk. The nurse would not question this medication.
 2. Penicillin is given for streptococcal infections. The nurse would not question this medication.
 3. Lorazepam can be administered to burn clients to help reduce anxiety. The nurse would not question this medication.
 4. Morphine is the drug of choice for pain control with severe burn injuries. However, morphine should not be administered intramuscularly because of impaired medication absorption due to edema and decreased peripheral perfusion with severe burns. The nurse should question this order and recommend continuous IV dosing (Hoffman & Sullivan, 2020).

13. 1. The client will not be able to tolerate oral medications until nausea is controlled; therefore, diphenoxylate (Lomotil), an antidiarrheal, will not be administered. The client needs to rid the body of the offending substance; therefore, diarrhea is not stopped.
 2. Antibiotics are not administered to clients diagnosed with food poisoning.
 3. Pantoprazole (Protonix), a PPI, is administered to decrease gastric acid and may or may not be given to the client, but it is not the first medication administered.
 4. Measures to control nausea and vomiting will prevent further fluid and electrolyte loss; therefore, promethazine (Phenergan), an antiemetic, is the first medication that should be administered.

14. 1. Levonorgestrel is an emergency contraceptive pill and does not prevent an STI (sexually transmitted infection).
 2. Levonorgestrel (Plan B One-Step), an emergency contraceptive pill is most effective if taken within 3 to 5 days after unprotected sexual intercourse. Levonorgestrel works by inhibiting ovulation and altering the uterus lining to prevent fertilized ovum implantation.
 3. Antianxiety medications, not levonorgestrel, would be prescribed for anxiety and nervousness.
 4. Levonorgestrel does not promote wound healing.

15. Correct answers are 1, 3, and 4.
 1. The client diagnosed with an open fracture will be receiving antibiotics to prevent infection.
 2. The nurse should apply ice, not heat, to an acute injury.
 3. The client diagnosed with a fracture will have pain; therefore, the nurse should evaluate effectiveness of the medication given for pain.
 4. The client diagnosed with an open fracture will have to go to surgery; therefore, preparing to administer the preoperative medication is an appropriate intervention.
 5. The HCP or surgeon is responsible for explaining the surgical procedure. This is not within the realm of the nurse's responsibility.

16. Correct answers are 1, 3, and 5.
 1. Dextrose 50% is the drug of choice to treat hypoglycemia if the client is in a comatose state or not able to cooperate. This client exhibits signs of hypoglycemia.
 2. The uncooperative client may refuse fluids or choke when being belligerent. If the client were cooperative, the family could have given the client juice.
 3. The nurse should determine how much and when the client last took insulin and last ate any foods.
 4. Glucagon is provided in an emergency kit to be used by significant others at home to treat hypoglycemic reactions. It takes longer to elevate the client's glucose level and is dependent on the client's glycogen stores.
 5. The nurse should obtain a glucose level as soon as possible.

17. 1. Determining if the client is right- or left-handed does not matter because the sutures must be placed in the hand with the laceration.
 2. The nurse should determine the client's allergies.
 3. The history of how the accident occurred is not the most essential information.
 4. The question could initiate an anxiety reaction, and the nurse cannot do anything if the client is afraid of needles.

18. 1. This question is appropriate if the nurse suspects elder abuse, but the client's physiological status is a priority at this time.

2. This question is appropriate if the nurse suspects elder abuse, but the client's physiological status is a priority at this time.

3. This client's blood pressure is extremely high and could lead to a life-threatening condition if antihypertensive medications are not administered immediately. The nurse should suspect elder abuse, including unfilled medication prescriptions and other forms of neglect. According to Maslow's Hierarchy of Needs, physiological needs are a priority over potential other problems.

4. This question is appropriate if the nurse suspects elder abuse, but the client's physiological status is the priority at this time.

19. 1. This is a warning, not an actual event; therefore, the nurse should not initiate the disaster plan.

2. Tularemia is not contagious from human-to-human contact; it is acquired through direct contact with infected animals or by inhaling aerosolized bacteria. There is no decontamination for this.

3. Antitoxins are available for botulism but not for tularemia.

4. For persons exposed to this biologic bacterium, doxycycline is recommended for 14 days. The nurse should ensure that a supply of doxycycline, an antibiotic, is available.

20. 250 mL. The nurse must know that aminoglycoside antibiotics such as gentamicin are very ototoxic and nephrotoxic and must be administered via an infusion pump over a minimum of 1 hour. The IV pump is regulated to infuse mL/hour.

16 Nonprescribed Medications

Curiosity has its own reason for existing.

—Albert Einstein

QUESTIONS

Herbs

1. The female client tells the perioperative nurse that she takes dong quai for menstrual cramps. Which intervention should the nurse implement **first**?
1. Assess the client for any abnormal bleeding.
2. Determine when the client took the last dose.
3. Document the finding in the client's EHR.
4. Notify the client's surgeon that the client takes this herb.

2. The client asks the nurse, "My grandmother puts aloe vera on her burns when she is cooking. Is that all right?" Which statement is the nurse's **best** response?
1. "Aloe vera juice is safe to use for minor burns, but not for deep burns."
2. "Aloe is approved by the FDA as a laxative."
3. "Any type of herbal product or remedy has potential complications."
4. "Aloe should not be used on any type of burns. Flush the burn with cool water."

3. The client tells the clinic nurse that she is taking St. John's wort for her depression. Which information should the nurse discuss with the client?
1. Discuss the need to avoid tyramine-rich foods.
2. Instruct the client to avoid touching the eyes after taking the medication.
3. Tell the client to apply sunscreen freely when outdoors.
4. Explain that this medication often causes liver damage.

4. The client diagnosed with endometriosis is discussing herbal and vitamin supplements used on a daily basis. Which supplement should the nurse **question**? **Select all that apply.**
1. Milk thistle
2. Fish oil
3. Soy
4. Folic acid
5. Raspberry leaves

5. The client taking valerian root to decrease anxiety tells the nurse the medication has a pungent odor that smells like "dirty socks" and it makes her drowsy. Which action should the nurse take?
1. Tell the client to quit taking the medication immediately.
2. Warn the client that valerian root is highly addictive.
3. Explain that the odor is related to the dried plant and is normal.
4. Determine if the client has discussed the drowsiness with the HCP.

6. The nurse is presenting a lecture on herbs to a community group. Which guidelines should the nurse discuss with the group? **Select all that apply.**
   1. Do not take herbs if you are pregnant or attempting to get pregnant.
   2. Administer smaller amounts of herbs to babies and young children.
   3. Store the herbal remedy in a cool, dry, dark place.
   4. Advise against belief in herbs being "miracle cures."
   5. Think of herbs as medicines—more is not necessarily better.

7. The client diagnosed with atherosclerosis tells the nurse, "I would really like to take herbs instead of medications for my atherosclerosis." Which statement is the nurse's **best** response?
   1. "You should not take any herbs to treat your atherosclerosis."
   2. "Garlic has been shown to decrease the 'stickiness' of platelets."
   3. "Horehound has sometimes been used to decrease atherosclerosis."
   4. "Taking low-dose aspirin daily helps to decrease atherosclerosis."

8. The client is taking *Echinacea purpurea (E. purpurea)*. Which statement by the client would indicate to the nurse that the herb has been **effective**?
   1. "It has prevented me from getting diarrhea since I have been taking antibiotics."
   2. "Since I started taking echinacea I do not get nauseated in the morning anymore."
   3. "The fungal infection on my feet is getting better since I started taking echinacea."
   4. "This medication is the reason I have not had a cold the entire winter."

9. With which client would the nurse discuss taking hawthorn?
   1. The client diagnosed with congestive heart failure (CHF)
   2. The client diagnosed with hypertension
   3. The client diagnosed with Alzheimer's disease
   4. The client diagnosed with diabetes mellitus

Vitamins and Minerals

10. The client is taking vitamin A. Which assessment data indicates to the nurse that the client is experiencing vitamin A toxicity?
    1. Nausea, vomiting, and diarrhea
    2. Tingling and numbness of extremities
    3. Dermatitis, fatigue, and dementia
    4. Bleeding gums and gingivitis

11. The client is prescribed folic acid. Which information should the nurse discuss with the client?
    1. "Do not use any laxatives that contain mineral oil."
    2. "Avoid drinking any type of alcoholic beverage."
    3. "See the ophthalmologist periodically."
    4. "Increase your intake of milk and milk products."

12. The client diagnosed with anemia is taking an iron tablet daily. Which statement indicates the client **understands** the medication teaching?
    1. "I will call my HCP if my stools become black or dark green."
    2. "I must take my iron tablet with meals and one glass of milk."
    3. "I will sit upright for 10 minutes after taking my iron tablet."
    4. "I will have to take an iron tablet for the rest of my life."

13. The client diagnosed with pernicious anemia is prescribed cyanocobalamin. Which intervention should the nurse implement?
    1. Administer the intramuscular injection via Z-track.
    2. Instruct the client to sip medication through a straw.
    3. Double-check the dose with another registered nurse.
    4. Monitor the client's serum potassium level.

14. The female client having her annual physical exam tells the clinic nurse, "I take vitamins daily, but I have not had the money to buy any for the past week." Which response is **most appropriate** for the nurse?
    1. "I will have the HCP give you a prescription for some vitamins."
    2. "As long as you eat a balanced diet you do not need to take vitamins."
    3. "Daily vitamins are necessary, so please get them as soon as possible."
    4. "This should not hurt you because vitamin deficiencies do not occur for some time."

15. The client asks the clinic nurse, "Vitamin E is a primary antioxidant. What does that mean?" Which statement is the nurse's **best response**?
    1. "Antioxidants minimize damage and keep your body's cells healthy."
    2. "Vitamin E is essential for general growth and development."
    3. "Antioxidants prevent free radical formation in your muscles and skin."
    4. "Antioxidants are vitamins that help the blood clot."

16. The health-care provider (HCP) has recommended the client take 100 mg of zinc a day. Which statement **best supports** the scientific rationale for taking zinc daily?
    1. Zinc is needed for the formation of connective tissue.
    2. Zinc is vital for hemoglobin (Hgb) regeneration in the client's body.
    3. Zinc is thought to help alleviate the common cold.
    4. Zinc aids in iron absorption and in folic acid conversion.

17. The nurse is discussing vitamins with a group of women at a community center. The nurse is discussing water-soluble vitamins and fat-soluble vitamins. Which vitamins are **fat-soluble vitamins**? **Select all that apply.**
    1. Vitamin A
    2. Vitamin D
    3. Vitamin E
    4. Vitamin C
    5. Folic acid

18. The nurse is taking the male client's medication history. The client informs the nurse he takes mega doses of vitamin C daily, a daily aspirin, and an iron tablet. Which statement is the nurse's **best** response?
    1. "I am glad you take mega doses of vitamin C because it prevents the common cold."
    2. "Taking aspirin and mega doses of vitamin C may cause crystals in your urine."
    3. "Mega doses of vitamins and a balanced diet will help prevent you from getting sick."
    4. "You should take megavitamins—not just mega doses of vitamin C alone."

Self-Prescribed OTC Medications

19. The client tells the clinic nurse that they have been taking the over-the-counter (OTC) medication omeprazole for heartburn. Which statement is the nurse's **best** response?
    1. "You should not take medications without notifying the HCP."
    2. "Have you also had breathing difficulties, especially at night?"
    3. "Be sure to limit taking the medication to less than 1 week."
    4. "OTC cimetidine is cheaper and works better than omeprazole."

20. The adolescent client has been admitted to the intensive care unit for an acetaminophen overdose. Which laboratory data should the nurse monitor for **long-term** complications?
    1. Arterial blood gases (ABGs)
    2. Liver function tests
    3. Hemoglobin A_{1c} levels
    4. Complete blood count (CBC)

21. The elderly client has been diagnosed with compression fractures of the vertebrae and has been taking large doses of ibuprofen for pain. Which intervention should the nurse implement?
    1. Teach the client not to take the medication on an empty stomach.
    2. Have the HCP order PTT/PT and INR laboratory tests.
    3. Ask the HCP to prescribe a narcotic medication for the client.
    4. Determine why the client thinks they need so much medication.

22. The parent of a 1-year-old child calls the clinic to ask about medications that can be administered to reduce fever. Which medications should the nurse discuss with the parent? **Select all that apply.**
    1. Acetylsalicylic acid
    2. Diphenhydramine
    3. Docosanol
    4. Docusate sodium
    5. Ibuprofen

23. The client diagnosed with hypertension reports a cold and a runny nose. Which information about OTC medications should the nurse teach the client? **Select all that apply.**
    1. Avoid medications with caffeine.
    2. Avoid medications high in sodium.
    3. Avoid medications containing phenylephrine.
    4. Avoid medications containing pseudoephedrine.
    5. Avoid medications containing oxymetazoline.

24. The client calls the clinic nurse to discuss problems concerning not being able to sleep at night. Which OTC medications are taken to assist with sleep? **Select all that apply.**
    1. Acetaminophen
    2. Ibuprofen
    3. Diphenhydramine
    4. Zolpidem
    5. Melatonin

25. The HCP has instructed the 21-year-old female client diagnosed with allergies to take the OTC medication pseudoephedrine. Which specific information should the nurse tell the client? **Select all that apply.**
    1. "An expected side effect is drowsiness, so plan for rest periods."
    2. "Plan to use a second method of birth control while taking this medication."
    3. "The medication will cause a developing fetus to become deformed."
    4. "Take a driver's license to the pharmacy when purchasing this medication."
    5. "Do not take pseudoephedrine for more than 7 days."

ANSWERS AND RATIONALES

The correct answer number and rationale are in **boldface blue type.** Rationales for why other answer options are incorrect are also given.

Herbs

1. 1. Dong quai increases risk of bleeding postoperatively, but the nurse would not need to assess for abnormal bleeding preoperatively.
   2. The American Society of Anesthesiologists recommends that all herbal products be stopped at least 2 to 3 weeks before surgery to avoid potential complications of herbal use. The client should have been NPO (nothing by mouth) since midnight; therefore, determining when the client last took the herb is the nurse's first intervention.
   3. The client's medications should be documented in the chart, but assessment is the first step of the nursing process. The nurse should first determine when the client last took the herb.
   4. The nurse should first determine when the client last took the herb before notifying the surgeon.

2. **1. Aloe vera juice is used externally for treatment of minor burns, insect bites, and sunburn. It is a safe herb to use externally and will not hurt the client.**
   2. Aloe taken internally is a powerful laxative, but the client is asking about burns, not about using aloe as a laxative. Also, the U.S. Food and Drug Administration (FDA) (2015) does not approve herbal supplements; however, they are regulated as dietary supplements.
   3. This is a true statement about many herbal supplements, but topical aloe does not have any known complications that would prevent it from being used for minor burns.
   4. This is a false statement. Aloe can be used externally for treating minor burns. Many lotions have aloe as an ingredient.

3. 1. Users of St. John's wort do not need to avoid tyramine-rich foods. These types of foods should be avoided in clients taking monoamine oxidase inhibitors for depression.
   2. This would be appropriate when applying capsicum or cayenne pepper lotion. St. John's wort is a pill or it can be taken in tea form.
   3. St. John's wort can cause photosensitization dermatitis; therefore, the client should use sunscreen when outside.
   4. Many herbal supplements are hepatotoxic, but St. John's wort is not one that causes liver damage.

4. **Correct answers are 1 and 3.**
   1. Milk thistle simulates estrogen effects, which can cause endometriosis growth. The nurse should question this supplement.
   2. Omega-3 fatty acids in fish oil have been found to reduce inflammation associated with endometriosis. The nurse would not question this supplement.
   3. Soy can increase estrogen levels, which can cause the growth of endometriosis; therefore, the nurse should question this supplement.
   4. Folic acid deficiency has been linked to endometriosis exacerbations. The nurse would not question this supplement.
   5. Raspberry leaves have been shown to decrease endometriosis pain. The nurse would not question this supplement.

5. 1. There is no reason to quit taking the medication because of the odor.
   2. There is a theoretical risk of habituation or addiction with valerian root when taken with alcohol or benzodiazepines (National Institutes of Health [NIH], 2013).
   3. The "dirty socks" odor is related to the dried plant. Valerian root, an herbal product, is promoted as a mild sedative and a treatment for nervous tension and insomnia but results from clinical trials are inconclusive. Valerian has no hangover effect (NIH, 2013).
   4. The pungent odor and drowsiness are expected with this medication, and there is no reason to discuss this with the HCP.

6. **Correct answers are 1, 3, 4, and 5.**
   1. This is a guideline for prudent use of herbs.
   2. According to guidelines for prudent use of herbs, babies and young children should not be given any types of herbs.
   3. Herbs exposed to sunlight and heat may lose potency.
   4. This is a guideline for prudent use of herbs. Dietary supplements cannot legally be described as a cure (NIH, 2020).

5. This is a guideline that consumers and HCPs must be aware of when using herbal therapy.

7. 1. The nurse should not be judgmental when clients request information about herbal therapy.
2. Garlic is one of the best-studied herbs. It has been shown to decrease total cholesterol and low-density lipoprotein (LDL) cholesterol levels, thus producing an anticoagulant effect that is useful in treating atherosclerosis (National Center for Complementary and Integrative Health, 2020b).
3. Horehound or *Marrubium vulgare L.* has been used as an herbal remedy for the treatment of respiratory disorders, including asthma, bronchitis, whooping cough, and tuberculosis, but not atherosclerosis.
4. This is a true statement, but aspirin is a medical treatment and is not considered an herb.

8. 1. *Lactobacillus acidophilus*, not *E. purpurea*, is used to restore or to maintain normal intestinal flora during antibiotic therapy.
2. Ginger is one of the best-studied herbs and is used for treating nausea caused by motion sickness, pregnancy morning sickness, and postoperative procedures.
3. Goldenseal is an herb that when used topically is purported to be of value in treating bacterial and fungal skin infections, and oral conditions such as gingivitis and thrush.
4. Some substances in *Echinacea* appear to have antiviral activity; thus, the herb is sometimes taken to reduce risk of catching the common cold (National Center for Complementary and Integrative Health, 2020).

MEDICATION MEMORY JOGGER: The nurse determines medication effectiveness by assessing for the clinical manifestations, or lack thereof, for which the medication was prescribed.

9. 1. Clients taking cardiac glycosides should avoid hawthorn, an herb, because it has the ability to decrease cardiac output. The client diagnosed with CHF would be taking cardiac glycosides.
2. Hawthorn, an herb, has been purported to lower blood pressure after 4 weeks or longer of therapy; therefore, the nurse would not question the client diagnosed with hypertension taking this medication.
3. Hawthorn is not recommended for a client diagnosed with Alzheimer's disease. Ginkgo biloba is the herb that is recommended for clients diagnosed with Alzheimer's disease.
4. Hawthorn, an herb, is not recommended for a client diagnosed with diabetes mellitus. Stevia, an herb indigenous to Paraguay, may be helpful to people diagnosed with diabetes because it is used as a sweetener.

Vitamins and Minerals

10. **1. Clinical manifestations of vitamin A overdose include nausea, vomiting, anorexia, dry skin and lips, headache, and loss of hair. The nurse should instruct the client to quit taking vitamin A immediately.**
2. Paresthesia is not a sign of vitamin A toxicity. It may be a sign of thiamine deficiency, along with neuralgia and progressive loss of feeling and reflexes.
3. Dermatitis, fatigue, and dementia are clinical manifestations of advanced niacin deficiency.
4. Bleeding gums and gingivitis are signs of vitamin C deficiency.

11. 1. This is appropriate information for the client who is taking vitamin A. Mineral oil inhibits vitamin A absorption.
2. The client should avoid drinking alcohol because it inhibits folic acid absorption (NIH, 2021).
3. This is appropriate information for the client who is taking vitamin A. Vitamin A may cause miosis, papilledema, and nystagmus.
4. Milk and milk products are good sources of vitamin D, not folic acid.

MEDICATION MEMORY JOGGER: Alcohol consumption is always discouraged when taking any prescribed or OTC medication because of adverse interactions. The nurse should encourage the client not to drink alcoholic beverages.

12. 1. Iron turns the stool a harmless black or dark green color. This statement indicates the client does not understand the medication teaching.
2. The iron tablet should be taken between meals and with 8 ounces of water to promote absorption. The iron tablet should not be taken within 1 hour of ingesting antacid, milk, ice cream, or other milk products such as pudding. This statement indicates the client does not understand the medication teaching.

3. Sitting upright will prevent esophageal corrosion from reflux. This statement indicates the client understands the medication teaching.
4. Drug treatment for anemia is generally less than 6 months. This statement indicates the client does not understand the medication teaching.

13. 1. Intramuscular iron, not vitamin B_{12}, must be administered Z-track to prevent skin staining.
2. Cyanocobalamin does not stain the teeth and therefore does not need to be administered through a straw. Liquid iron must be administered through a straw.
3. This is required when administering insulin or digoxin IV push, but it is not required when administering this medication.
4. Because conversion to normal red blood cell (RBC) production—the purpose of giving cyanocobalamin (Cyanabin), vitamin B_{12}—increases the need for potassium, hypokalemia is a possible side effect of this medication, especially during the first 48 hours that the medication is administered.

14. 1. Vitamins are usually OTC medications. If the client does not have money for OTC medications, she would not have money for a prescription.
2. A balanced diet can provide all vitamins a client needs daily, but if the client was taking a daily vitamin, the nurse should not discourage her from taking the vitamins.
3. Vitamin supplements are not necessary if the person is healthy and receives proper nutrition on a regular basis.
4. Clinical manifestations of vitamin deficiencies will not occur if the client has not taken the vitamins in more than a week. Vitamin deficiencies may take months to occur, and if the client is eating a well-balanced diet, vitamin deficiencies will not occur.

15. 1. Vitamin E is a primary antioxidant that prevents formation of free radicals that damage cell membranes and cellular structure (NIH, 2021b).
2. This is vitamin A's role in the body. It is essential for general growth and development.
3. This statement includes medical jargon that the client probably would not understand. The nurse needs to explain information in layman's terms.
4. Vitamin K, not the antioxidant vitamin E, is required by the body to help the blood clot.

16. 1. Copper is needed for formation of RBCs and connective tissue.
2. Iron is vital for Hgb regeneration. More than 60% of the iron in the body is found in Hgb.
3. Zinc is an essential mineral important in immune function. Zinc is thought to alleviate clinical manifestations of the common cold and can be found in lozenges and cold remedies (NIH, 2021c).
4. Vitamin C aids in iron absorption and in folic acid conversion.

17. Correct answers are 1, 2, and 3.
1. Vitamin A is a fat-soluble vitamin that is essential for maintenance of epithelial tissues, skin, eyes, hair, and bone growth.
2. Vitamin D is a fat-soluble vitamin that has a major role in regulating calcium and phosphorus metabolism, and is needed for calcium absorption from the intestines.
3. Vitamin E is a fat-soluble vitamin that has antioxidant properties that protect cellular components from being oxidized and RBCs from hemolysis.
4. Vitamin C is a water-soluble vitamin that aids in iron absorption and folic acid conversion.
5. Folic acid is a water-soluble vitamin that is essential for body growth. It is needed for DNA synthesis. Without folic acid there is a disruption in cellular division.

18. 1. Most authorities believe that vitamin C does not cure or prevent the common cold. Rather, it is believed that vitamin C has a placebo effect. This would not be appropriate information to share with the client.
2. Megadoses of vitamin C taken with aspirin or sulfonamides may cause crystalluria, or crystal formation in the urine.
3. Megadoses of vitamins can cause toxicity and might result in a minimal desired effect.
4. Megavitamin therapy use, or massive doses of vitamins, is questionable at best. The nurse should not recommend this action.

Self-Prescribed OTC Medications

19. 1. Most adult clients self-medicate for minor problems, such as a headache or indigestion, and only seek medical attention if the clinical manifestations are unrelieved. This is not the best response for the nurse to make.

2. **The esophagus and trachea are in close proximity. An adult-onset asthma relationship with heartburn is caused by gastroesophageal reflux disease (GERD). Therefore, the nurse should assess what other clinical manifestations are occurring.**
3. The medication is taken for up to 2 weeks per package instructions. Many clients have been prescribed omeprazole (Prilosec) for many months to years.
4. Histamine$_2$ blockers, such as cimetidine (Tagamet), ranitidine (Zantac), or famotidine (Pepcid), may or may not be more effective than omeprazole (Prilosec). It depends on the individual's response to medication. Most clients report better symptom control with proton-pump inhibitors.

20. 1. ABGs would give information about the immediate situation, not long-term problems.
2. **Acetaminophen (Tylenol) is toxic to the liver, and liver function tests should be monitored in the hospital and in the HCP's office afterward to determine if there is permanent liver damage.**
3. Hemoglobin A_{1c} levels monitor long-term glycemic control in diabetics, not long-term issues from acetaminophen toxicity (Vallerand & Sanoski, 2019).
4. Acetaminophen (Tylenol) does not damage bone marrow. It is not necessary to monitor the CBC.

21. 1. NSAIDs interfere with prostaglandin production in the stomach, resulting in the client being susceptible to ulcer formation. To prevent stomach lining erosion, the client should not take the medication on an empty stomach.
2. NSAIDs will not affect the partial thrombin time/prothrombin time/International Normalized Ratio (PTT/PT/INR) results.
3. If NSAIDs are effective, there is no reason for the HCP to prescribe a narcotic.
4. The priority is to prevent medication complications. The client is taking the medication because bone fractures are painful.

22. Correct answers are 1 and 5.
1. **The parent should be taught never to administer aspirin to a child because of the association of acetylsalicylic acid (Aspirin) with Reye's syndrome (Vallerand & Sanoski, 2019). Acetaminophen (Tylenol) or ibuprofen (Motrin) may be administered to a child for a fever.**
2. Diphenhydramine (Benadryl), an antihistamine, can make the child drowsy and will help nasal congestion, but it will not treat a fever.
3. Docosanol (Abreva), an anti-infective, is a topical medication for cold sores, not for fever.
4. Docusate sodium (Colace) is a stool softener, not an antipyretic.
5. **Ibuprofen (Motrin) or acetaminophen (Tylenol) may be administered to a child for a fever.**

23. Correct answers are 1, 2, 3, 4, and 5.
1. **OTC medications that contain caffeine can raise blood pressure.**
2. **Many OTC medications contain high doses of sodium, which can raise blood pressure.**
3. **Phenylephrine is a decongestion, present in some OTC cold and flu medications that can cause vasoconstriction and increase the client's blood pressure.**
4. **Pseudoephedrine is a decongestant, present in some OTC cold and flu medications that can cause vasoconstriction and increase the client's blood pressure.**
5. **Oxymetazoline is a decongestant, present in some OTC cold and flu medications that can cause vasoconstriction and increase the client's blood pressure. Many cold and flu medications are available OTC that are formulated for clients with hypertension. The nurse should instruct the client to read labels carefully (American Heart Association, 2021).**

24. Correct answers are 3 and 5.
1. Acetaminophen (Tylenol) is an analgesic. It is not formulated with ingredients that induce sleep. Tylenol PM contains diphenhydramine. This medication can be taken to aid in sleep.
2. Ibuprofen (Motrin) is an analgesic and antipyretic, not a sleeping medication.
3. **Diphenhydramine (Benadryl) is an antihistamine that has the side effect of causing drowsiness. This is the main ingredient in OTC sleep aids.**
4. Zolpidem (Ambien) is not an OTC medication.
5. **Melatonin is a synthetic dietary supplement that can assist with sleep.**

25. Correct answers are 4 and 5.
1. Pseudoephedrine can cause insomnia, not drowsiness. It is the ability to rev people up that makes it an ingredient in "uppers."

2. Oral or topical contraceptive hormone products interact with antibiotics, not pseudoephedrine.
3. This is a class C medication. Its use during pregnancy is questionable, but it is not known to be teratogenic.
4. **The federal government enacted a law limiting the purchase of products containing pseudoephedrine to adults (at least 18 years of age) and to no more than 9 grams per month, such as two 15-dose boxes of Claritin D or six 24-dose boxes of Sudafed. The client should be able to prove her age when purchasing the products at the pharmacy.**
5. **Pseudoephedrine is effective in cases of acute congestion. If clinical manifestations persist longer than 7 days, this indicates chronic congestion, and the client should be evaluated by their HCP.**

NONPRESCRIBED MEDICATIONS COMPREHENSIVE EXAMINATION

1. The client diagnosed with anemia is taking an iron tablet. Which assessment data indicates the medication is **effective**?
   1. The client denies night blindness.
   2. The client has not had a cold this winter.
   3. The client's potassium level is 4.5 mEq/L.
   4. The client's Hgb level is 12.

2. The 50-year-old female client tells the nurse that she has been having frequent episodes of suddenly feeling hot and flushed and asks the nurse if there is any medication that can help her clinical manifestations. Which statement is the nurse's **best** response?
   1. "There is really nothing except time that helps these clinical manifestations."
   2. "I would suggest taking a vitamin that has soy in it to help the problem."
   3. "The HCP can prescribe hormone replacement therapy for you."
   4. "Are you concerned about having clinical manifestations of menopause?"

3. The nurse is discussing vitamins with a group of women at a community center. The nurse is discussing water-soluble vitamins and fat-soluble vitamins. Which vitamins are water-soluble vitamins? **Select all that apply.**
   1. Vitamin C
   2. Vitamin D
   3. Folic acid
   4. Vitamin B_{12}
   5. Vitamin K

4. The 60-year-old client who is postmenopausal tells the nurse she is taking the herb chasteberry. Which data indicates the herb is **effective**?
   1. The client reports decreased pain with sexual intercourse.
   2. The client reports less bleeding and a more regular menstrual cycle.
   3. The client reports an increase in hot flashes and mood swings.
   4. The client reports less bloating and breast fullness.

5. The 27-year-old female client tells the nurse she is taking melatonin to help her sleep better at night. Which response is **most appropriate** by the nurse?
   1. "Melatonin has not shown any efficacy in helping people sleep."
   2. "Is there any chance you may be pregnant or trying to get pregnant?"
   3. "This natural hormone may help you to sleep better at night."
   4. "You should really take a prescription medication to help you sleep."

6. The client tells the nurse, "My grandmother gives me licorice tea to help my stomach ulcers. Is this bad for me?" Which response is **most appropriate** for the nurse?
   1. "Yes, it is bad for you because it increases gastric acid production."
   2. "Pure licorice root is the best type to take to help heal your ulcer."
   3. "The best thing for a stomach ulcer is an antacid such as Maalox."
   4. "No, it is not bad. It is one of the most effective herbs for stomach protection."

7. The nurse is teaching a class on herbal therapy to a community group. Which information should the nurse share with group members?
   1. Dandelion is an herb that can be used externally to help heal minor burns.
   2. Peppermint is an herb that exerts a protective effect on the liver.
   3. Cascara is an herb that can be used as a laxative if the client is constipated.
   4. Witch hazel is an herb that is used as a long-term antidepressant.

8. The wife of a client diagnosed with Alzheimer's disease is requesting information about any herbal therapy that may help with her husband's memory. Which herb should the nurse discuss with the client?
   1. St. John's wort
   2. Ginkgo biloba
   3. Psyllium
   4. Sarsaparilla

9. The female client tells the clinic nurse that she has frequent vaginal yeast infections and uses an OTC preparation to cure infections. Which statement is the nurse's **first** response?
   1. "How often do you use OTC yeast medications?"
   2. "You should tell the HCP about the frequent infections."
   3. "You should take lactic acidophilus when you take antibiotics."
   4. "Have you tried eating yogurt daily to prevent infections?"

10. The nurse is discussing the importance of antioxidants in the body. Which vitamins and minerals help neutralize the free-radical assault and keep the client's body cells healthy? **Select all that apply.**
    1. Vitamin C
    2. Vitamin D
    3. Vitamin E
    4. Selenium
    5. Copper

11. The nurse is preparing to administer the following medications. Which medication should the nurse **question** administering?
    1. Cyanocobalamin to a client diagnosed with end-stage chronic obstructive pulmonary disease
    2. Ferrous sulfate to a client who is 22 weeks pregnant and is 2 days postoperative appendectomy
    3. Phytonadione to a client who has an INR of 4.0
    4. Calcium citrate to a client who has a serum calcium level of 4.0 mEq/L

12. The nurse is discussing nutritional supplements with a client recently diagnosed with cancer. Which supplement should the nurse recommend for the client at this time?
    1. PulmoCare, a supplement formulated for clients with lung diseases
    2. Glucerna, a supplement formulated for clients with diabetes mellitus
    3. Boost, a supplement formulated with added fiber
    4. None. The client should try milkshakes and other foods first

13. The client diagnosed with cancer tells the oncology clinic nurse that an employee of a health food store suggested that he take 50,000 mg of vitamin C every day to treat the cancer. Which information is **most important** for the nurse to discuss with the client?
    1. Excessive amounts of water-soluble vitamins are excreted by the body.
    2. Too much acid could result in the client developing mouth ulcers.
    3. This is an alternative treatment to taking chemotherapy or radiation.
    4. The individual at the store wanted to sell the vitamins to the client.

14. The pregnant client tells the clinic nurse that she has been using phenylephrine and cocoa butter hemorrhoid ointment. Which information should the nurse teach the client? **Select all that apply.**
    1. "Apply the ointment after a bath but before drying the area."
    2. "Do not use the medication because of possible harm to the fetus."
    3. "Suppositories may be used up to four times a day for symptom relief."
    4. "Witch hazel-glycerin works better than phenylephrine and cocoa butter for hemorrhoids."
    5. "Avoid having a bowel movement for 3 hours after insertion of medication."

15. The client is diagnosed with mild psoriasis of the scalp. Which shampoo should the nurse recommend to the client? **Select all that apply.**
 1. Head and Shoulders shampoo
 2. T-Gel, a tar shampoo
 3. Scalpicin, an anti-itch shampoo
 4. Nizoral (ketoconazole), a psoriasis shampoo
 5. Any gentle or mild hair shampoo

16. The female client tells the clinic nurse that she has been having urinary frequency, lower abdominal cramping, and burning on urination. The client has been using an OTC urinary antispasmodic, but reports that the burning has not gone away. Which intervention should the nurse implement?
 1. Tell the client to continue taking the antispasmodic.
 2. Encourage the client to decrease her amount of fluid intake.
 3. Make an appointment for the client to see the HCP.
 4. Have the client start drinking cranberry juice daily.

17. Which medications and supplies can be purchased OTC to treat diabetes mellitus? **Select all that apply.**
 1. Glargine insulin
 2. Regular insulin
 3. Glucose tablets
 4. Glucose-monitoring strips
 5. Insulin isophane

18. The school nurse assesses lice and nits (lice eggs) in the hair of a child attending the elementary school. Which instructions should the nurse include when talking with the parent? **Select all that apply.**
 1. Apply permethrin topically to the scalp twice a day for 1 week.
 2. Ask the HCP for a prescription for a shampoo to treat the lice.
 3. It is fine to allow the child to continue attending class while being treated.
 4. Shampoo the hair with pyrethrin with piperonyl butoxide and comb the nits out.
 5. All household members should be checked for head lice.

19. Which OTC medication would the nurse caution use of for a client diagnosed with an allergy to the numbing medication used in dental offices? **Select all that apply.**
 1. Benzocaine
 2. Benzalkonium and lidocaine
 3. Dibucaine
 4. Mineral oil
 5. Miconazole

20. The client diagnosed with macular degeneration asks the nurse why the HCP would prescribe OTC supplements of CoQ10 and flaxseed oil. Which statement **best describes** the scientific rationale for the nurse's response?
 1. This is an unproven folk remedy that the HCP thinks might work.
 2. This is an antioxidant that will support arterial functioning.
 3. This is an omega-3 fatty acid that decreases risk of heart attack.
 4. This combination of medications has been shown to cure eye problems.

NONPRESCRIBED MEDICATIONS COMPREHENSIVE EXAMINATION ANSWERS AND RATIONALES

1. 1. This would indicate that vitamin A therapy is effective.
2. This would indicate zinc therapy is effective.
3. The potassium level would not indicate that iron therapy was effective.
4. **Effectiveness of iron therapy can be determined by a normal Hgb level and by the client denying fatigue or shortness of breath.**

MEDICATION MEMORY JOGGER: The nurse determines medication effectiveness by assessing for the clinical manifestations, or lack thereof, for which the medication was prescribed.

2. 1. These clinical manifestations and the client's age suggest that she is having "hot flashes" associated with menopause. There are OTC preparations and hormone replacement therapy (HRT) that help with clinical manifestations of menopause.
2. **Many women believe some natural estrogen enhancers such as soy (e.g., soy milk, some vitamins containing soy) help with clinical manifestations of menopause. This is the best response.**
3. In some instances, the HCP will prescribe HRT for a woman experiencing menopause, but this is rarely done now because current research indicates that, although HRT protects against osteoporosis and treats clinical manifestations of menopause, it also increases risk of heart attack, stroke, and breast cancer.
4. The client is asking for information, not expressing a need to discuss feelings.

3. Correct answers are 1, 3, and 4.
1. **Vitamin C is a water-soluble vitamin that aids in iron absorption and folic acid conversion.**
2. Vitamin D is a fat-soluble vitamin that plays a major role in regulating calcium and phosphorus metabolism and is needed for intestinal calcium absorption.
3. **Folic acid is a water-soluble vitamin that is essential for body growth. It is needed for DNA synthesis. Without folic acid, there is a disruption in cellular division.**
4. **Vitamin B_{12} is a water-soluble vitamin that, like folic acid, is essential for DNA synthesis. It aids in folic acid conversion to its active form.**
5. Vitamin K is a fat-soluble vitamin that is needed for prothrombin synthesis and clotting factors VII, IX, and X.

4. 1. **Chasteberry exerts effects similar to those of progesterone. When used during menopause and postmenopause, it may help reverse vaginal changes and diminished libido.**
2. The client is postmenopausal; therefore, the client does not have regular menstrual cycles.
3. The client would have a decrease in hot flashes and mood swings if the herb was helping decrease menopausal discomforts.
4. This would indicate the herb was helping a client diagnosed with premenstrual syndrome.

5. 1. Melatonin, a natural hormone, decreases alertness and body temperature, both of which make sleep more inviting; therefore, this is a false statement.
2. **Melatonin should not be taken by clients who are pregnant because there is a lack of studies that indicate its safety. Large doses of melatonin, a natural hormone, have been shown to inhibit ovulation, so women trying to conceive should reconsider taking melatonin. This is the most appropriate response from the nurse.**
3. Melatonin does show efficacy for helping the client sleep, but because the client is 27 years old, the nurse's best response is to discuss pregnancy.
4. OTC medications, herbs, and natural hormones have been proved to help clients sleep; therefore, prescription medication is not absolutely necessary.

MEDICATION MEMORY JOGGER: The test taker should question administering any medication to a client who is pregnant or may become pregnant. Many medications cross the placental barrier and could affect the fetus.

6. 1. Licorice does not increase gastric acid production.
   2. Frequent use of pure licorice root can contribute to sodium and water retention, hypertension, and other ill effects; therefore, this is not the nurse's best response.
   3. The client is not asking what is best to treat a stomach ulcer. The nurse's best response is to answer the client's question.
   4. **Licorice, a weak-tasting herb, contains substances that protect the stomach lining. It has been shown in several studies to help heal ulcers. It protects the stomach by increasing mucus production and blood flow through the membranes.**

7. 1. Dandelion, an herb, is used as a digestive aid, laxative, diuretic, and liver and gallbladder protectant, and it prevents iron-deficiency anemia. It is not used to heal minor burns.
   2. Peppermint helps soothe the stomach. It has a direct spasmolytic action on the smooth muscles of the digestive tract.
   3. **Cascara is used as a laxative. It stimulates peristalsis.**
   4. Witch hazel is used as an astringent, not as an antidepressant.

8. 1. St. John's wort is used for its antidepressant effects.
   2. **Ginkgo biloba has been shown to improve mental functioning and stabilize Alzheimer's disease.**
   3. Psyllium is used as a laxative.
   4. The herb sarsaparilla is best used as a flavoring agent in soft drinks.

9. 1. **This is an assessment question to determine the extent of the client's problem. This is the first question.**
   2. The nurse should assess the problem before making this statement.
   3. This is a true statement, especially for clients diagnosed with chronic illness, but it is not the first statement.
   4. Eating yogurt daily will prevent most yeast infections when the client is taking prescribed antibiotics, but assessing the extent of the problem should be the nurse's first response.

MEDICATION MEMORY JOGGER: Whenever the question asks for a "first" intervention, even when discussing medications, assessing is usually the correct answer.

10. **Correct answers are 1, 3, and 4.**
   1. **Antioxidants protect the body from damage caused by harmful molecules called free radicals. This damage is a factor in atherosclerosis development. Vitamin C captures the free radical and neutralizes it before it causes damage.**
   2. Vitamin D is not an antioxidant. It is a fat-soluble vitamin that plays a major role in regulating calcium and phosphorus metabolism and is needed for intestinal calcium absorption.
   3. **Vitamin E is a chain-breaking antioxidant. Whenever vitamin E is sitting on a cell membrane, it breaks the chain reaction before free radicals cause damage.**
   4. **Selenium is an antioxidant that has shown efficacy in decreasing the risk for lung, prostate, and colorectal cancers.**
   5. Copper is a mineral, but it is not an antioxidant. Copper is needed for formation of RBCs and connective tissue.

11. 1. **Cyanocobalamin (Cyanabin), vitamin B_{12}, is contraindicated in clients diagnosed with severe pulmonary disease and is used cautiously in clients with heart disease. Clients with these conditions may develop pulmonary edema and heart failure. The nurse should question administering this medication.**
   2. Prenatal vitamins with iron are part of a pregnant woman's routine medications. Ferrous sulfate is Pregnancy Category A, which means it has been proven safe for the fetus. The nurse would not question administering this medication.
   3. The normal INR is 2 to 3; therefore, the nurse would not question administering this medication because it is the antidote for overdose of Coumadin.
   4. Hypocalcemia occurs when a serum calcium level falls below 4.5 mEq/L; therefore, the nurse would not question administering this medication to the client whose serum calcium level is low.

12. 1. Pulmocare is a supplement recommended for clients diagnosed with chronic lung disease because the supplement does not have as much carbon dioxide as a byproduct of its metabolism as do other supplements; however, the stem did not state the client had lung disease.

2. Glucerna is the supplement recommended for clients who have diabetes because this supplement has a slower release of carbohydrates and provides more controllable blood glucose, but the stem did not state that the client has diabetes.
3. Because of the added fiber, Boost would be the supplement recommended for clients diagnosed with cancer who have significant pain and are taking narcotic pain medications, but this client is newly diagnosed and pain was not mentioned in the question stem.
4. **Newly diagnosed clients should try homemade supplements to support their diets. Supplements are expensive (ranging from $2 to more than $8 per can), and if the client develops an aversion to the taste, then it is unlikely that anyone else in the family will want to drink the supplement. The nurse should suggest the client try to make milkshakes and use canned soups to supplement the diet first.**

13. 1. This is true, but this is not the most important information to provide the client.
2. **Nutrition is an important consideration for clients diagnosed with cancer and undergoing treatment. Many antineoplastic medications can cause stomatitis, and a combination of huge amounts of vitamin C and chemotherapy could result in a serious complication for the client.**
3. There are many alternative treatments that should be encouraged for use by clients diagnosed with different diseases. This is not one of them.
4. This is true, but it is not the most important information for the nurse to teach the client.

14. Correct answers are 3 and 5.
1. The ointment and suppositories should be used after the area is cleaned and patted dry.
2. Preparation H (phenylephrine and cocoa butter), an OTC medication, will not harm the fetus.
3. **Labeling directions for Preparation H (phenylephrine and cocoa butter), an OTC medication, state four times a day as part of the safe administration guidelines. The phenylephrine shrinks the size of the hemorrhoids and provides relief from pain and burning, and cocoa butter provides some emollient relief for expelling feces.**
4. Witch hazel-glycerin (Tucks) will provide relief from burning and itching, but will not shrink hemorrhoids. Tucks may initially sting when applied to the area.
5. **For maximum effectiveness, the client should avoid having a bowel movement for 1 to 3 hours after using the medication.**

15. Correct answers are 2, 3, and 4.
1. Head and Shoulders is a dandruff shampoo. It is not effective in controlling psoriasis.
2. **T-Gel is a shampoo formulated with coal tar and is recommended for clients with mild psoriasis.**
3. **Scalpicin has hydrocortisone and is marketed for mild psoriasis clinical manifestations.**
4. **Ketoconazole is an antifungal medication that has some efficacy for psoriasis.**
5. Psoriasis is a painful skin problem accompanied by intense itching. A mild shampoo without some other ingredient will not be effective for this client.

MEDICATION MEMORY JOGGER: Nurses are frequently asked to provide information about OTC medications and preparations. The test taker could eliminate option 5 in the previous question because of the psoriasis diagnosis.

16. 1. The OTC antispasmodic is masking some of the client's clinical manifestations. The nurse should recognize clinical manifestations of a urinary tract infection (UTI). The client should see the HCP and have a urine culture performed.
2. The client should increase her amount of fluid intake when there is suspicion of a UTI.
3. **The client has clinical manifestations of a UTI and should see the HCP for a urine culture and antibiotic prescription.**
4. Cranberry juice is helpful in preventing UTIs, but this client already has clinical manifestations of a UTI.

17. Correct answers are 2, 3, 4, and 5.
1. Glargine (Lantus), a steady-state insulin, is not available OTC. A prescription is required.

2. **Humulin R, N, L, and U are all available OTC, but they are usually kept behind the counter with the pharmacist. These insulins can be purchased without a prescription. In some states, syringes may be purchased without prescription. A prescription is only required if the client has insurance that will pay part of the cost.**
3. **Glucose tablets are recommended for clients to carry with them in case of a hypoglycemic reaction and may be purchased without prescription.**
4. **Glucose-monitoring devices and strips may be purchased without prescription; however, if the client has insurance that will pay for the equipment, a prescription is required.**
5. **Humulin R, N, and L are all available OTC. They are kept behind the counter with the pharmacist, but can be purchased without a prescription. In some states, syringes may be purchased without prescription. A prescription is only required if the client has insurance that will pay part of the cost.**

18. **Correct answers are 3, 4, and 5.**
    1. Permethrin (Nix) is applied once, and the clean hair is combed to get rid of the nits.
    2. Permethrin (Nix) and pyrethrin with piperonyl butoxide (RID) are OTC medications that treat lice.
    3. **The Centers for Disease Control and Prevention states that head lice is a nuisance but has not been shown to cause disease. The American Academy of Pediatrics and the National Association of School Nurses advocate that "no-nit" policies should be discontinued; therefore, the child should be allowed to attend school during treatment.**
    4. **This is the correct procedure for treating lice.**
    5. **Head lice is spread by direct contact with infected hair; therefore, all household members and close contacts should check for lice or nits.**

19. **Correct answers are 1, 2, and 3.**
    1. **The most common local anesthetic used in dental procedures is a "-caine" medication, procaine (Novocaine); therefore, a client allergic to procaine (Novocaine) could be allergic to benzocaine (Lanacane), a topical preparation for sunburns.**
    2. **The most common local anesthetic used in dental procedures is a "-caine" medication, lidocaine; therefore, a client allergic to procaine (Novocaine) could be allergic to benzalkonium and lidocaine (Bactine), an antiseptic/pain reliever.**
    3. **The most common local anesthetic used in dental procedures is a "-caine" medication, dibucaine (Nupercainal); therefore, a client allergic to procaine (Novocaine) could be allergic to dibucaine (Nupercainal), for the pain, itching, and burning of hemorrhoids.**
    4. Mineral oil, a lubricant laxative used as a preparation for a radiologic exam, is not a "-caine" medication; therefore, the nurse would not caution the client using this medication.
    5. Miconazole (Monistat) vaginal cream, for a client diagnosed with a yeast infection, is not a "-caine" medication; therefore, the nurse would not caution the client using this medication.

MEDICATION MEMORY JOGGER: If the test taker was not familiar with the local anesthetic procaine (Novocaine), the test taker could possibly still get this question correct by reading the ending of the generic medication names in the first three options.

20. 1. There is evidence that CoQ10 in combination with fish oil (omega-3 fatty acid) or flaxseed oil will reduce damage to blood vessels and may delay macular degeneration.
    2. **CoQ10 is a fat-soluble antioxidant found in almost every cell in the body. Flaxseed oil (or omega-3 fatty acid) is taken in conjunction with CoQ10 to help the body use CoQ10. Antioxidants are supportive of arterial health by decreasing fat deposits in the vessels.**
    3. CoQ10 is not an omega-3 fatty acid.
    4. There is no cure for macular degeneration. An injection, Ranibizumab (Lucentis), has been approved by the U.S. Food and Drug Administration for use by some clients with macular degeneration. The medication is injected into the eye monthly.

Administration of Medications

Whether you think you can or think you can't, you're right.

—Henry Ford

QUESTIONS

Administering Medications

1. The nurse is teaching the client the correct use of a metered-dose inhaler. How should the nurse teach the interventions? **Rank in order of performance.**
   1. Shake the inhaler canister.
   2. Hold breath as long as possible, then exhale through pursed lips.
   3. Wait one minute before taking another dose.
   4. Push the top of the canister while taking a deep breath.
   5. Breathe out slowly and completely.

2. The primary nurse is at the bedside and is preparing to administer 3 mL of medication into the deltoid muscle. Which intervention should the charge nurse implement?
   1. Take no action because this is an acceptable standard of practice.
   2. Ask the primary nurse to come to the nurse's station.
   3. Tell the nurse not to inject the medication into the deltoid muscle.
   4. Complete an occurrence report documenting the behavior.

3. The nurse is administering digoxin 0.25 mg IV push (IVP) medication to the client. Which interventions should the nurse implement? **Select all that apply.**
   1. Administer the medication in a calibrated syringe.
   2. Insert the needle in the port closest to the client's IV site.
   3. Pinch off the IV tubing below the port.
   4. Inject the medication quickly and at a steady rate.
   5. Disinfect the IV port with alcohol before administration.

4. The nurse is adding a medication to an IV bag. Which action indicates the nurse **needs more teaching** in performing this procedure?
   1. The nurse clamps the roller clamp on the tubing attached to the IV solution.
   2. The nurse inserts the needle into the center of the medication port.
   3. The nurse avoids rotating the solution after administering the medication.
   4. The nurse writes the name and dose of the medication on the medication label.

5. Which interventions should the nurse implement when withdrawing medication from an ampule? **Select all that apply.**
   1. Do not use if the ampule was opened more than 30 days ago.
   2. Ensure that all the medication is in the upper chamber of the ampule.
   3. Snap the neck of the ampule so that it opens toward the nurse.
   4. Insert the needle into the center of the opening of the ampule.
   5. Use a filter needle to withdraw medication from the ampule.

6. Which action by the primary nurse **warrants intervention** by the charge nurse?
   1. The charge nurse observes the primary nurse carrying a used needle to the medication room.
   2. The charge nurse observes the primary nurse using two methods to identify the client who is receiving medications.
   3. The charge nurse observes the primary nurse injecting air into a vial when preparing an intramuscular (IM) injection.
   4. The charge nurse observes the primary nurse documenting the removal of meperidine from the narcotics box.

7. The nurse is administering an unpleasant-tasting liquid medication to a 2-year-old child. Which intervention should the nurse implement?
   1. Prepare the medication in the child's favorite food.
   2. Tell the child the medication will not taste bad.
   3. Put the medication in 4 ounces of apple juice.
   4. Use a dropper to place the medication between the gum and cheek.

8. The nurse administers medication to a client, and 30 minutes later the client tells the nurse he is starting to itch. The nurse notes a red rash over the client's body. Which intervention should the nurse implement **first**?
   1. Have the crash cart brought to the room.
   2. Assess the client's apical pulse and blood pressure.
   3. Notify the health-care provider (HCP) immediately.
   4. Prepare to administer diphenhydramine.

9. The nurse is preparing to administer 15 mL of aluminum hydroxide/magnesium hydroxide/simethicone from a bottle to a client. Which intervention should the nurse implement?
   1. Determine the correct amount at the sides of the cup.
   2. Measure the medication at the base of the meniscus.
   3. Avoid shaking the bottle of medication.
   4. Draw the medication into a 20-mL syringe.

10. The nurse is preparing to administer 0.1 mL of medication intradermally to the client. How much medication would the nurse draw up in the tuberculin (1.0-mL) syringe?

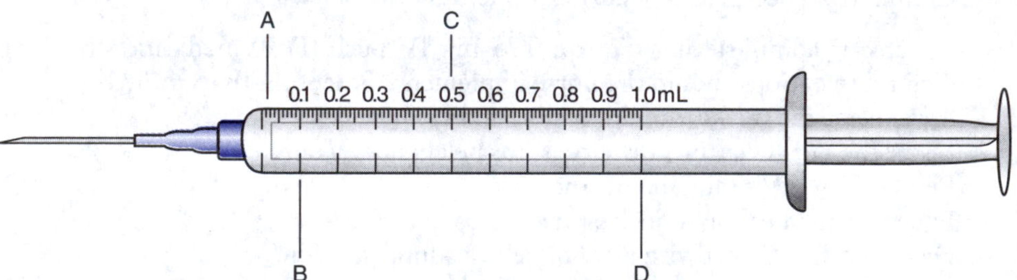

   1. A
   2. B
   3. C
   4. D

Computing Math to Administer Medications

11. The client who has had abdominal surgery has an IV of Ringer's lactate solution infusing at 150 mL/hour. The nurse is hanging a new bag of fluid. The IV administration set delivers 10 gtt/mL. At what rate would the nurse set the infusion?

____

12. The nurse is preparing to administer vancomycin IV piggyback (IVPB) via an infusion pump. The IVPB is delivered in 250 mL of normal saline. At what rate should the nurse set the pump?

____

13. The order is penicillin 2 million units IM. The medication comes in a powder form of 5 million units per vial with directions to reconstitute with 3.2 mL of sterile diluent to produce 3.5 mL of solution. How many milliliters will the nurse administer?

____

14. The order is to administer acetaminophen 15 mg/kg as needed (PRN) every 6 hours to an infant weighing 33 pounds. How many milligrams of acetaminophen could the infant receive in a 24-hour time period?

____

15. The client's medication administration record (MAR) reads:

Client: A.C.	MR# 1234567	Date: Today
Age: 35 years	Allergies: NKDA	Diagnosis:
Medication	0701–1900	1901–0700
Heparin 40,000 units in 500 mL D_5W infuse per protocol		2400 @ 15 mL/hr NN
For PTT results: <50 increase rate by 4 mL/hr and redraw PTT in 4 hours		
For PTT results: <60 increase rate by 2 mL/hr and redraw PTT in 4 hours		
For PTT results: 60–90 maintain rate and redraw PTT in 4 hours × 2		0400 PTT 69 NN
For PTT results: >90 decrease rate by 2 mL/hr and redraw PTT in 4 hours		
Nurse Initials/Credentials	DN/RN	NN/RN

At 0800 the client's partial thromboplastin time (PTT) result is 58. How many units per hour will the client receive for the next 6 hours?

____

16. The client is receiving a heparin infusion at 24 mL/hour via an infusion pump. The medication comes 25,000 units in 500 mL of D_5W. How much heparin is the client receiving during a 12-hour shift?

____

17. The client is to receive a preoperative medication of morphine 10 mg and promethazine 25 mg IM on call to the operating room. The medication comes as morphine 15 mg/mL and promethazine 25 mg/mL. How many milliliters of medication will the nurse administer?

____

18. The nurse is preparing to administer an IVPB of 40 mEq of potassium in 200 mL of IV solution over 4 hours. At what rate would the nurse set the pump?

____

19. The client is to receive 1.5 g of a medication every morning. The medication comes 1,000 mg per tablet. How many tablets would the nurse administer?

____

20. The HCP has ordered 3 mcg/kg per minute of dopamine 2 G/500 mL of D_5W to be administered to a client in the intensive care unit. The client weighs 165 pounds. At which rate would the nurse set the IV pump in mL/hour?

____

ANSWERS AND RATIONALES

The correct answer number and rationale are in **boldface blue type.** Rationales for why other answer options are incorrect are also given.

Administering Medications

1. **Correct order is 1, 5, 4, 2, 3.**
   1. **The nurse should instruct the client to shake the inhaler canister.**
   5. **The client should take a deep breath and breathe out slowly.**
   4. **The client should press the top of the canister to dispense the medication while taking a deep breath.**
   2. **The client should hold their breath for as long as possible, then exhale through pursed lips.**
   3. **The nurse should teach the client to wait one minute before administering a second dose to allow for medication to be absorbed and canister to be recharged (Treas et al., 2018).**

2. 1. This is not the acceptable standard of practice. The ventrogluteal muscle (on the side of the hip between the trochanter and ischium) is the injection site of choice because it is a large muscle mass free of major nerves and adipose tissue.
   2. **This is the correct action to take because the charge nurse should not correct the primary nurse in front of the client. The deltoid muscle (in the upper arm) should not be used to administer 3 mL of medication IM because the muscle is small and can only accommodate small doses of medications, no more than 0.5 to 1 mL of medication (Treas et al., 2018).**
   3. The charge nurse should not correct the primary nurse at the bedside in front of the client. This embarrasses the primary nurse and will make the client lose confidence in the primary nurse.
   4. An occurrence report should not be completed because the charge nurse stopped the action before the client received the injection in the incorrect muscle. The charge nurse would want to discuss the correct site for administering IM medication with the primary nurse.

3. **Correct answers are 1, 2, and 5.**
   1. **The medication can be given diluted with normal saline or undiluted. The syringe selected should be calibrated to allow for accurate measurement of the medication dosage.**
   2. **Using the closest port ensures the least resistance to the flow of medication into the client and helps to control the rate at which the medication reaches the client's bloodstream.**
   3. The nurse should pinch off the tubing above the port, not below, to ensure that the medication flows into the client's vein and not upward into the IV tubing.
   4. The medication should be injected slowly over 5 minutes (2 minutes for most IV medications) and at a steady rate because a rapid injection could cause speed shock. Speed shock is a sudden adverse physiological reaction secondary to an IVP medication where the client develops a flushed face, headache, a tight feeling in the chest, irregular pulse, loss of consciousness, and possible cardiac arrest.
   5. **The port should be disinfected with an alcohol prep pad before administering the IVP medication (CDC, 2019).**

4. 1. The roller clamp should be closed on the tubing to prevent fluid loss from the IV bag. The nurse does not need more teaching.
   2. The medication should be inserted into the center of the port to prevent accidental puncture of the sides of the port or the IV bag. The nurse does not need more teaching.
   3. **This indicates the nurse needs more teaching because the IV bag should be gently rotated to distribute the medication evenly throughout the IV solution.**
   4. The label must clearly identify what the nurse added to the IV solution. The nurse does not need more teaching.

5. **Correct answers are 1, 4, and 5.**
   1. **This is appropriate because an ampule is a one-time use container and should not be used if already opened.**
   2. All medication should be in the lower chamber of the ampule. The nurse should tap the upper chamber to ensure all medicine is in the lower chamber.
   3. The ampule should be snapped away from the nurse so any glass fragments are directed away from the nurse to prevent injury.

4. **The nurse should not allow the needle to touch the ampule rim because the rim is considered contaminated. The correct procedure is to insert the needle in the center of the ampule opening.**
5. **The nurse should use a filter needle to draw up the medication to remove any glass particles that could be present from opening the glass ampule (Treas et al., 2018).**

6\. 1. **The primary nurse must discard the used needle in the sharps container in the client's room and, according to the Occupational Safety and Health Administration (OSHA), cannot remove a used or "dirty" needle from the client's room. This action would require intervention from the charge nurse.**
2. The Joint Commission mandates that the nurse use two forms of identification when administering medications to a client to ensure that the correct client is given the prescribed medication. This action would not warrant intervention by the charge nurse.
3. Air should be injected into a vial to create a positive pressure inside the vial to ease medication withdrawal and prevent a vacuum when withdrawing medication. This action would not warrant intervention by the charge nurse.
4. Narcotics must be documented and accounted for when removed from the narcotics box or container. This action would not warrant intervention by the charge nurse.

7\. 1. Do not use a favorite food or essential dietary item when administering a medication because the child may refuse the food in the future. The medication will cause the favorite food to taste bad or "funny."
2. The nurse should be honest with the child and the parent or guardian and tell the truth. Not telling the truth will damage the parent's trust in the nurse. Even if a 2-year-old does not understand, the child gagging or spitting out the medication indicates it is unpleasant tasting, and the parent will know the nurse lied about the medication.
3. The nurse should not use large volumes of fluid because if the child does not drink the entire amount, then the nurse cannot determine if the entire dose has been taken.
4. **This action promotes swallowing and prevents medication from being aspirated or spit out.**

8\. 1. The client appears to be having an anaphylactic reaction. Bringing the crash cart to the bedside is an appropriate intervention, but it is not the first intervention.
2. The client is in distress. Taking vital signs will not help an allergic reaction.
3. **The HCP should be notified so an order for a medication to counteract the anaphylactic reaction can be obtained; therefore, this is the first intervention.**
4. The nurse can prepare to administer medication, but the HCP determines if the client is having an allergic reaction and then orders the appropriate medication. Very few clients have a PRN order in place from the HCP for a possible allergic reaction, so this is not the first intervention.

9\. 1. This is not the correct way to determine the prescribed amount when using a calibrated measuring cup.
2. **The liquid aluminum hydroxide/magnesium hydroxide/simethicone (Maalox) must be poured into a calibrated measuring cup and measured at the meniscus base to ensure the correct dose.**
3. The aluminum hydroxide/magnesium hydroxide/simethicone (Maalox) bottle must be shaken vigorously to ensure the medication is well dispersed in the bottle.
4. A syringe is primarily used to give liquid medications to children to ensure accurate dosing. It is not used to administer antacids to an adult.

10\. 1. If the nurse drew up this much medication, then the dose would be 10 times less than the prescribed dose.
2. **This is the correct amount of medication to administer to the client intradermally. This is the prescribed dose when administering a purified protein derivative (PPD) intradermal injection to a client who is being tested for possible exposure to tuberculosis (TB).**
3. This is five times the prescribed dose of medication.
4. If the nurse drew up this much medication, then the dose would be 10 times too much medication. This much medication intradermally would cause damage to the intradermal layer of skin.

Computing Math to Administer Medications

11\. **25 gtt/minutes. The nurse should divide 150 mL/hour by 60 minutes to get 2.5 mL/minute. Then multiply 2.5 mL/minute by 10 gtt/mL to get 25 gtt/minute as the rate to set the infusion.**

12. 250 mL/hour. Vancomycin, an aminoglycoside antibiotic, is administered over a minimum of 1 hour. Pumps deliver fluids at an hourly rate. The nurse should set the pump to deliver the 250 mL of fluid over 1 hour.

13. 1.4 mL will be administered IM. To set up this equation the nurse would write:
5,000,000 units: 3.5 mL = 2,000,000 units: X mL
Cross-multiply to get: 7,000,000 = 5,000,000 X
To solve for X, divide both sides of the equation by 5,000,000
X = 1.4 mL

14. 900 mg/24-hour time period. The nurse must first determine the infant's weight in kilograms. To do this, divide 33 pounds by 2.2 conversion factor = 15 kg of body weight. Then, multiply 15 kg times 15 mg per kg to equal 225 mg per dose. The medication can be administered every 6 hours. The question asks how many milligrams could be administered within 24 hours. To find out the number of potential dosing times, divide 24 by 6, which equals 4. Multiply 225 mg per dose times 4 doses to obtain 900 mg of acetaminophen (Tylenol) administered in a 24-hour time period.

15. 1,360 units of heparin per hour. The heparin mixture is 40,000 per 500 mL of fluid. The first step in solving this problem is to find out how many units of heparin are in each mL of fluid. Divide 40,000 by 500 = 80 units of heparin per milliliter of IV fluid. The current rate is 15 mL per hour, but the client should have the IV infusion rate increased by 2 mL per hour per the protocol = 17 units per hour. Multiply 80 units per mL times 17 = 1,360 units of heparin per hour for the next 6 hours.

16. 14,400 units of heparin per 12-hour shift. The first step in solving this problem is to find out how many units are in each milliliter of IV fluid. To do this, divide 25,000 units by 500 mL of IV fluid = 50 units per milliliter of IV fluid. The next step is to multiply the number of units per milliliter times the number of milliliters per hour the client is receiving: 15 × 24 = 1,200 units of heparin infusing per hour. Many math problems will ask for the number of units per hour. If this is the question, then 1,200 units is the answer, but this question is asking the cumulative shift total of medication. Multiply 1,200 times 12 = 14,400 units per 12-hour shift.

17. 1.67 mL. To find out how many milliliters of morphine should be administered:
15 : 1 = 10 : X
Then cross-multiply:
10 = 15 X
To solve for X, divide both sides of the equation by 15
$$\frac{10}{15} = \frac{15X}{15}$$
10 divided by 15 = 0.666 or 0.67 mL of morphine
For promethazine (Phenergan), the dose is 25 mg. Promethazine (Phenergan) comes as 25 mg/mL, so 1 mL contains the dose prescribed.
Then add the two:
1 mL + 0.67 mL = 1.67 mL

18. 50 mL per hour. The nurse would divide the amount of fluid—200 mL—by the number of hours—4—to infuse the medication. 200 ÷ 4 = 50 mL per hour. Pumps are always set at the rate per hour to infuse.

19. 1-1/2 tablets. To set up this problem, convert grams to milligrams. There are 1,000 mg in 1 g, so 1.5 g equals 1,500 mg. Then set up the problem:
1,000 : 1 = 1,500 : X
Then cross-multiply
1,000 X = 1,500
To solve for X, divide each side of the equation by 1,000
$$\frac{1{,}000X}{1{,}000} = \frac{1{,}500}{1{,}000}$$
X = 1.5

20. 3.4 mL per hour. This is a multistep problem. The first step is to find out how many kilograms the client weighs. Divide 165 pounds by 2.2 conversion factor to equal 75 kg of body weight. Then multiply 3 times 75 = 225 mcg/minute infusion rate. Multiply 225 times 60 equals 13,500 mcg per hour to infuse. Pumps are set at an hourly rate in mL/hour. Next convert the milligrams of medication to mcg: multiply 2 g times 1,000 = 2,000 mg, and then multiply 2,000 times 1,000 = 2,000,000 mg (or 2 g times 1,000,000).
13,500 : X = 2,000,000 : 500
2,000,000 X = 6,750,000
$$\frac{2{,}000{,}000X}{2{,}000{,}000} = \frac{6{,}750{,}000}{2{,}000{,}000}$$
3.375 or 3.4 mL per hour. Most pumps in an intensive care unit can be set in increments of tenths of a milliliter.

ADMINISTRATION OF MEDICATIONS COMPREHENSIVE EXAMINATION

1. Which interventions should the nurse implement when administering sublingual medication? **Select all that apply.**
   1. Place the medication between the gum line and the cheek.
   2. Assess the client's ability to swallow the medication.
   3. Instruct the client to allow the tablet to dissolve completely.
   4. Wear gloves when administering sublingual medication.
   5. Remain with the client until the medication has dissolved.

2. The nurse is preparing to administer medication via a nasogastric tube. Which intervention should the nurse implement **first**?
   1. Assess and verify tube placement.
   2. Check the residual volume.
   3. Elevate the foot of the client's bed.
   4. Pour medication into the syringe barrel.

3. The nurse is administering a tablet to the client. How should the nurse implement the interventions? **Rank in order of performance.**
   1. Offer a glass of water to facilitate swallowing the medication.
   2. Assess that the client is alert and has the ability to swallow.
   3. Open the medication and place in the medication cup.
   4. Check the client's identification band and date of birth.
   5. Remain with the client until all medication is swallowed.

4. The charge nurse is making rounds and notices that the primary nurse left a medication cup with three tablets at the client's bedside. Which intervention should the charge nurse implement?
   1. Administer the client's medications.
   2. Remove the medication cup from the room.
   3. Request the primary nurse come to the room.
   4. Leave the cup at the bedside and talk to the primary nurse.

5. The nurse is preparing to administer a rectal suppository to a client. Which interventions should the nurse implement? **Select all that apply.**
   1. Insert the suppository beyond the anal–rectal ridge.
   2. Instruct the client to lie in the supine position.
   3. Lubricate the suppository with a water-soluble lubricant.
   4. Apply a sterile glove on the dominant hand.
   5. Encourage the client to retain the suppository for 30 minutes.

6. Which action indicates the nurse **needs more teaching** when administering a transdermal medication to a client?
   1. The nurse rotates the site when administering the transdermal patch.
   2. The nurse removes the previous transdermal patch and cleans the area.
   3. The nurse applies the transdermal patch using nonsterile gloves.
   4. The nurse applies the transdermal patch to a dry, hairy area.

7. The nurse is administering heparin via the subcutaneous route. Which interventions should the nurse implement? **Select all that apply.**
   1. Prepare the medication using a 20-gauge, 1.5-inch needle.
   2. After injecting the needle, aspirate and observe for blood.
   3. After removing the needle, massage the area gently.
   4. Check previous injection sites and administer in another area.
   5. After drawing up the correct dose, add 0.2 mL of air to the syringe.

8. Which interventions should the nurse implement when administering medication via the intradermal route? **Select all that apply.**
   1. Insert the needle with the bevel up at a 5- to 15-degree angle in the skin.
   2. Prepare the medication in a 3-mL syringe using a 23-gauge, 1-inch needle.
   3. Hold the skin taut between the thumb and index finger of the nondominant hand.
   4. Quickly inject the medication to avoid forming a wheal or bleb.
   5. Cover the injection site with an adhesive bandage.

9. The nurse is administering ophthalmic drops to the client. How should the nurse implement the interventions? **Rank in order of performance.**
   1. Firmly press the lacrimal duct for 5 minutes after instilling drops.
   2. Cleanse the eyelid from the inner to the outer canthus.
   3. Wash hands and apply nonsterile gloves.
   4. Administer ophthalmic drops in the lower conjunctival sac.
   5. Position the eyedropper 1.5 to 2 cm above the client's eye.

10. The charge nurse is observing the primary nurse administering otic drops to a 2-year-old child by pulling down and back on the auricle. Which action should the charge nurse take?
    1. Stop the primary nurse and ask the nurse to step out of the room.
    2. Demonstrate inserting the otic drops by pulling up and back on the auricle.
    3. Take no action because this is the correct way to administer the ear drops.
    4. Allow the nurse to administer the otic drops and then discuss the technique with the nurse.

11. Which action indicates the nurse **needs more teaching** when administering nasal drops to the client?
    1. Instruct the client to blow the nose before administering the nasal drops.
    2. Have the client keep the head tilted back for 5 minutes after instilling drops.
    3. During administration have the client tilt the head back and to the affected side.
    4. Place a sterile cotton ball into the nostril where the nasal spray was administered.

12. The nurse prepared 2 mg of morphine IV for a client who is reporting pain. When the nurse enters the room, the client tells the nurse, "I don't want to take a shot. I would like to have a pain pill." Which action should the nurse take?
    1. Explain that the medication must be administered because it has been drawn up.
    2. Ask another nurse to watch the medication being wasted in the sink.
    3. Place the syringe in the sharps container in the client's room.
    4. Notify the pharmacy that a narcotic was not administered to the client.

13. The nurse is preparing to administer morning medications to a group of clients in a medical department. Which intervention should the nurse implement **first**?
    1. Compare the medication with the MAR.
    2. Take the medication and MAR to the bedside.
    3. Check the client's identification band with the MAR.
    4. Wash the hands with soap and warm water for at least 30 seconds.

14. The nurse is administering medications through a gastrostomy tube (GT). Which intervention should the nurse implement **first**?
    1. Place the crushed pills in the GT.
    2. Flush the gastrostomy with at least 30 mL of tap water.
    3. Use the plunger to push the medication into the GT.
    4. Clamp the GT closed.

15. The nurse is preparing to administer IV fluids to a 2-year-old child. Which intervention is **most important** for the nurse to implement?
    1. Use a volume-controlled chamber to administer IV fluids.
    2. Ensure that the IV catheter is securely taped to the child's skin.
    3. Request that an adult hold the child's hand when hanging IV fluid.
    4. Check the IV solution type with another nurse before administering.

16. The nurse is preparing to administer 3 mL of a medication IM. Which muscle is the **best** site to administer the medication?
1. The deltoid muscle
2. The dorsogluteal muscle
3. The ventrogluteal muscle
4. The vastus lateralis muscle

17. The client is prescribed vaginal cream. Which information should the nurse discuss with the client?
1. Instruct the client to lie down for 10 to 15 minutes after inserting medication.
2. Tell the client not to use a perineal pad after administering the medication.
3. Teach the client not to insert the vaginal applicator very far into the vagina.
4. Discuss the need to douche 30 minutes before inserting the vaginal cream.

18. The nurse is preparing to administer a liquid-form oral medication. How should the nurse implement the interventions? **Rank in order of performance.**
1. Place the lid of the bottle right side up, so the outer surface is up.
2. Assist the client to an upright position, if possible.
3. Hold the medication cup at eye level when reading the proper dose.
4. Pour the liquid into the bottle with the label against the hand.
5. Check to see if the liquid should be shaken before opening the container.

19. The nurse on a medical unit is providing discharge instructions to a client who is prescribed a glucocorticoid, fluticasone, and a metered-dose inhaler. Which statement by the client **warrants intervention**?
1. "I will use a spacer when using my inhaler."
2. "I will hold the medication in my mouth for 10 seconds."
3. "I will wait a few minutes between puffs."
4. "I will notify my HCP if I get mouth sores."

20. The nurse is preparing to administer 14 units of regular insulin and 28 units of intermediate insulin. How much insulin would the nurse draw up in the insulin syringe?

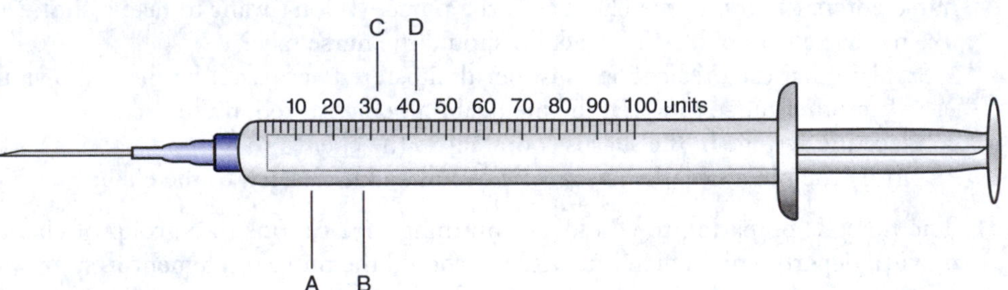

1. A
2. B
3. C
4. D

ADMINISTRATION OF MEDICATIONS COMPREHENSIVE EXAMINATION ANSWERS AND RATIONALES

1. **Correct answers are 3, 4, and 5.**
   1. The medication should be placed under the tongue, not between the gum line and the cheek (buccal).
   2. The medication should be placed under the tongue, not swallowed.
   3. **Sublingual medication is placed under the tongue and should be kept there until the tablet is completely dissolved before swallowing saliva.**
   4. **The nurse will need to don gloves to administer this medication if the client cannot place the medication under their tongue.**
   5. **The nurse should remain at the bedside until medication is dissolved to ensure the client has received the full dose.**

2. 1. **Assessment is the first intervention. Verifying that the tube is in the stomach is the priority when administering medications via the nasogastric tube.**
   2. If the residual is greater than 100 mL for an adult, the medication should not be administered because this indicates the client is not digesting the feedings.
   3. The head of the client's bed should be elevated to prevent aspiration. The foot of the bed should not be elevated.
   4. The medication should not be poured into the syringe until tube placement is verified, residual is checked, and the head of the bed is elevated.

3. **Correct order is 4, 2, 3, 1, 5.**
   4. **The nurse must first check to make sure the right client is getting the right medication.**
   2. **The nurse should determine if the client can swallow the medication.**
   3. **The nurse should check the medication against the MAR, open the medication package, and place it in the medication cup at the bedside. If the client cannot swallow or refuses the medication, the package can be sent back to the pharmacy if it has not been opened, preventing an unnecessary charge to the client.**
   1. **The nurse should offer water so that the client can swallow the medication.**
   5. **The nurse should remain with the client until the medication is swallowed.**

4. 1. The charge nurse cannot administer these medications without verifying the medications against the MAR.
   2. **The nurse should take the medication cup back to the medication room and discuss this situation with the primary nurse. Medications should never be left at the bedside.**
   3. The charge nurse should not correct the primary nurse in front of the client; therefore, this would not be an appropriate intervention.
   4. The charge nurse should not leave the medications at the bedside. Medication should never be left at the bedside.

5. **Correct answers are 1, 3, and 5.**
   1. **Inserting the suppository beyond the anal–rectal ridge will ensure the suppository is retained.**
   2. The client should lie on the left side (Sims' position).
   3. **A water-soluble lubricant will ensure the suppository is inserted without trauma to the rectal area and will allow the suppository to dissolve.**
   4. The nurse should wear nonsterile gloves on both hands, not just on the dominant hand.
   5. **Thirty minutes will allow for medication absorption.**

6. 1. Rotating sites prevents skin irritation. The nurse understands the correct way to apply a transdermal patch and does not need more teaching.
   2. The old patch must be removed and the area must be cleansed to prevent further medication absorption. The nurse does not need more teaching.
   3. The nurse should use nonsterile gloves to prevent absorption of the medication through the nurse's hands. The nurse does not need more teaching.
   4. **The patch should be applied to a clean, dry, hairless area to ensure adherence and proper medication absorption. Because the nurse is applying the medication to a hairy area, the nurse needs more teaching.**

7. **Correct answers are 4 and 5.**
   1. The nurse should prepare the medication using a 25-gauge, 3/8- to 5/8-inch needle.

2. For heparin, do not aspirate for blood because this can damage surrounding tissue and cause bruising.
3. Do not massage after injecting heparin because this may cause bruising or bleeding.
4. The nurse should not administer heparin in the same site because this may cause tissue necrosis or other tissue damage.
5. Add 0.2 mL of air to the syringe after drawing up the correct heparin dose. Air will ensure the medication is injected into the subcutaneous tissue and not the superficial tissue surrounding the injection site (Treas et al., 2018).

8. Correct answers are 1 and 3.
1. The nurse should insert the needle, bevel up, at a 5- to 15-degree angle, advancing the needle approximately 3 mm (1/8 inch) (Treas et al., 2018).
2. The medication should be administered in a tuberculin or 1-mL syringe using a 25- to 27-gauge, 3/8- to 5/8-inch needle.
3. The nurse should use the thumb and index finger of the nondominant hand to spread the skin taut.
4. The medication should be injected slowly to form a small wheal or bleb.
5. An adhesive bandage can irritate the injection site and interfere with the intradermal skin test.

9. Correct order is 3, 2, 5, 4, 1.
3. The nurse should wash hands and don nonsterile gloves before administering ophthalmic drops.
2. The nurse should remove any discharge by gently wiping out from the inner canthus, using a separate cloth for each eye.
5. The eyedropper should be positioned 1.5 to 2 cm (1/2 to 3/4 inch) above the client's eye for medication administration. Do not allow the eyedropper to touch the eye.
4. Medication placed directly on the cornea can cause discomfort or damage, which is why the medication is placed in the lower conjunctival sac.
1. The nurse should gently press on the lacrimal duct for 1 to 2 minutes to prevent systemic absorption through the lacrimal canal.

10. 1. The nurse is administering the ear drops correctly, so there is no reason to stop the nurse from administering ear drops.
2. This is the correct way to administer ear drops to an adult, but not to a young child.
3. The nurse should administer ear drops to a child younger than age 3 in this manner. This is done because of the child's short Eustachian tube. The charge nurse need not take action.
4. This is the correct way to administer ear drops to a 2-year-old child; therefore, the charge nurse does not need to discuss the administration technique with the primary nurse.

11. 1. The nurse should have the client blow the nose before instilling nasal drops to clear the nasal passage. Instructing the client to blow the nose indicates the nurse does not need more teaching.
2. This action allows the drops to have time to work effectively. The nurse does not need more teaching.
3. The client should tilt the head back for the drops to reach the frontal sinus, and tilt the head to the affected side to reach the ethmoid sinus. This action indicates the nurse knows the correct administration of nasal drops and does not need more teaching.
4. Some nasal drops require the client to close one nostril and tilt the head to the closed side or to hold the breath or breathe through the nose for 1 minute. None of the nasal drops requires a sterile cotton ball to be inserted into the nostril. The nurse needs more teaching.

12. 1. The client has the right to refuse medication; therefore, the nurse cannot force the client to take the medication.
2. This nurse must have a witness when wasting a narcotic.
3. Legally the nurse must have someone witness the narcotic being wasted.
4. The pharmacy does not need to be notified that a narcotic was wasted. It must be witnessed and documented on the narcotics log.

13. 1. The nurse must compare the medication with the MAR to make sure it is the right medication, but this is not the nurse's first intervention.
2. The nurse must take the MAR to the bedside with medication to make sure the medication is being administered to the correct client, but this is not the nurse's first intervention.
3. The nurse must check the MAR with at least two forms of identification, one of which can be the client's identification band, but this is not the nurse's first intervention.

4. Washing the hands is essential to avoid contaminating the medication. Although it seems like an obvious step, it is often neglected by the nurse as a result of being busy and in a hurry.

14. 1. Only crushed or liquid medication should be administered through the GT, but this is not the first intervention the nurse should implement.

2. The nurse should first flush the gastrostomy with tap water to ensure that it is patent before putting any medication into the GT.

3. The medication can be administered via gravity or a plunger can be used, if needed, but this is not the nurse's first intervention.

4. After the medication is administered, the nurse should flush the GT with tap water to make sure all medication is in the stomach and not in the tubing.

15. 1. A volume-controlled chamber (Buretrol), along with an IV administration pump, should be used when administering IV fluids to children to ensure that the child does not experience fluid-volume overload. Fluid-volume overload in a child could cause death.

2. The IV catheter should be secured, but this is not the most important intervention because even if it is not secured the child would not experience fluid-volume overload, which is a potentially life-threatening complication of IV fluid therapy.

3. Having the mother or father at the bedside is an appropriate intervention because the child will be frightened, but it is not the most important intervention.

4. Double-checking a routine IV fluid is not necessary, but the nurse should double-check medication according to the child's weight.

16. 1. The deltoid muscle (in the upper arm) should not be used to administer 3 mL of medication IM because the muscle is small and can only accommodate small doses, no more than 0.5 to 1 mL, of medication.

2. The dorsogluteal (the buttocks) is not recommended for IM injections because the sciatic nerve may be injured if the nurse fails to identify proper landmarks to ensure missing it.

3. The ventrogluteal muscle on the side of the hip between the trochanter and ischium is the injection site of choice because it is a large muscle mass free of major nerves and adipose tissue to ensure medication goes in the muscle.

4. The vastus lateralis muscle (lateral side of the thigh) can be used for administering IM injections, but the client often reports that this is more painful than other areas.

17. 1. The client should lie down for 10 to 15 minutes so that all medication can melt and coat the vaginal walls.

2. The client may need to use a perineal pad to catch any drainage or prevent undergarment staining.

3. The filled vaginal applicator should be inserted as far into the vaginal canal as possible, and then the client should push the plunger, depositing medication in the vagina.

4. The client should not douche before administering vaginal cream because douching removes the vagina's normal flora.

18. Correct order is 2, 5, 1, 4, 3.

2. Assist the client to an upright position.

5. Check to see if the medication should be shaken before pouring into the medication cup.

1. Place the bottle lid right side up, so the outer surface is up.

4. Pour liquid into the bottle with the label against the hand.

3. Hold the medication cup at eye level when reading the proper dose (Treas et al., 2018).

19. 1. Use of a spacing device increases the amount of medication reaching the lungs with less medication being deposited in the mouth and throat. This is the correct procedure, and the nurse would not have to correct the information.

2. The site of action for inhalers is the lungs. The client should not hold the medication in the mouth because this will increase the likelihood of the client developing a fungal infection of the mouth. The client should inhale deeply and hold the breath after medication is in the lung. The nurse should correct this misinformation.

3. Pausing between puffs allows the lungs to absorb more medication. This is correct information.

4. Mouth sores may indicate a fungal mouth infection as a result of medication, and the HCP should be notified. This is correct information.

20. 1. This point indicates the amount of regular insulin only—14 units.
2. This point indicates the amount of intermediate insulin only—28 units.
3. This point is 32 units, which is the incorrect dosage.
4. The nurse would first draw up 14 units of regular-acting insulin and have another nurse check the dosage. Then the nurse should draw up 28 units of intermediate-acting insulin to total 42 units of insulin and verify the dosage with another nurse. Drawing up regular insulin first ensures that the intermediate-acting insulin does not accidentally get inserted into the regular insulin, thereby altering the regular insulin's peak time.

MEDICATION MEMORY JOGGER: Remember "clear to cloudy" when combining regular-acting and intermediate-acting insulin.

18 Comprehensive Examination

I was gratified to be able to answer promptly. I said, "I don't know."

—Mark Twain

QUESTIONS

1. The client diagnosed with cardiac disease is prescribed amiodarone orally. For each intervention, specify if the intervention is **indicated or not indicated** for the client's care.

Potential Nursing Intervention	Indicated	Not Indicated
1. Notify the HCP of dyspnea, fatigue, and cough.		
2. Take the medication before going to bed.		
3. Do not take the medication if apical pulse <60 bpm.		
4. The medication may cause the stool to turn black.		
5. Avoid grapefruit juice while taking the medication.		
6. Permanent bluish facial discoloration can occur.		
7. Wear sunscreen and protective clothing during therapy.		
8. If a dose is missed, do not take the dose at all.		

2. The nurse is administering 0900 medications to the following clients. To which client should the nurse **question** administering the medication?
   1. The client receiving a calcium channel blocker after drinking a full glass of water
   2. The client receiving a beta blocker with blood pressure (BP) of 96/70
   3. The client receiving a nitroglycerin patch reporting a headache
   4. The client receiving an antiplatelet medication with a platelet count of 33,000

3. The client diagnosed with a head injury is ordered a computed tomography (CT) scan of the head with contrast dye. Which intervention should the nurse include when discussing this procedure?
   1. Instruct the client not to take any of the routine medications.
   2. Inform the client an IV line will be started before the procedure.
   3. Ask about any allergies to nonsteroidal anti-inflammatory medication.
   4. Explain that the client will be given sedatives before the procedure.

4. The obstetric clinic nurse is discussing folic acid with a client trying to conceive. Which information should the nurse discuss with the client when taking this medication?
   1. "Do not use any laxatives containing mineral oil when taking folic acid."
   2. "Drink one glass of red wine daily to potentiate the medication."
   3. "This medication will help prevent spina bifida in the unborn child."
   4. "Notify the health-care provider (HCP) if your vision becomes blurry."

5. Which statement **best describes** the scientific rationale for prescribing pioglitazone?
   1. This medication increases glucose uptake in the skeletal muscles and adipose tissue.
   2. This medication allows carbohydrates to pass slowly through the large intestine.
   3. This medication will decrease hepatic production of glucose from stored glycogen.
   4. This medication stimulates beta cells to release more insulin into the bloodstream.

6. The client is experiencing ventricular tachycardia and has a weak, thready apical pulse. Which medication should the nurse prepare to administer to the client?
   1. Epinephrine IVP
   2. Amiodarone IVP
   3. Atropine IVP
   4. Digoxin IVP

7. The client diagnosed with major depressive disorder is prescribed fluoxetine. Which information should the nurse discuss with the client? **Select all that apply.**
   1. Tell the client it will take 2 to 3 weeks for the medication to be effective.
   2. Instruct the client not to eat any type of tyramine-containing foods such as wines or cheeses.
   3. Tell the client to notify the HCP if they become anxious or have an elevated temperature.
   4. Tell the client not to stop taking fluoxetine abruptly; the medication should be weaned.
   5. Explain to the client that tremors and sweating are initial expected side effects.
   6. Advise the client to chew gum or suck on hard candy to minimize dry mouth.
   7. Inform the client that fluoxetine can cause an increased libido.
   8. Teach the client to notify the HCP for continued weight loss.

8. The client, after abdominal surgery, has an IV of Ringer's lactate solution infusing at 100 mL/hour. The nurse is hanging a new bag of fluid. Which rate should the nurse set the pump to infuse the Ringer's lactate solution?

   ____

9. The client admitted for diagnosis of an acute exacerbation of reactive airway disease is receiving IV theophylline. The client's serum theophylline level is 18 mcg/mL. Which intervention should the nurse implement **first**?
   1. Continue to monitor the theophylline drip.
   2. Assess the client for nausea and restlessness.
   3. Discontinue the theophylline drip.
   4. Increase infusion rate by 2 mcg/mL per protocol.

10. The nurse is administering 0800 medications. Which medication should the nurse **question**?
1. Misoprostol to a 29-year-old male client diagnosed with an NSAID-produced ulcer
2. Omeprazole to a 68-year-old male client diagnosed with a duodenal ulcer
3. Furosemide to a 56-year-old male client with a potassium level of 3.0 mEq/L
4. Acetaminophen to an 84-year-old male client diagnosed with a frontal headache

11. The elderly client calls the clinic and reports being constipated and having abdominal discomfort. Which interventions should the nurse implement? **Select all that apply.**
1. Instruct the client to take an over-the-counter (OTC) laxative as recommended on the label.
2. Recommend the client drink clear liquids only, such as tea or broth.
3. Determine when the client last had a bowel movement.
4. Tell the client to go to the emergency department (ED) as soon as possible.
5. Ask the client what other medications are currently being taken.

12. The nurse is administering morning medications on a medical floor. Which medication should the nurse administer **first**?
1. Regular insulin sliding scale to an elderly client diagnosed with type 1 diabetes mellitus
2. Methylprednisolone to a client diagnosed with systemic lupus erythematosus (SLE)
3. Morphine to a client diagnosed with Guillain-Barré syndrome
4. Etanercept to a client diagnosed with rheumatoid arthritis (RA)

13. The registered nurse (RN) is caring for clients diagnosed with AIDS. Which action by the unlicensed assistive personnel (UAP) **warrants immediate action** by the nurse?
1. The UAP uses nonsterile gloves to empty a client's urinal.
2. The UAP is helping a client take OTC herbs brought from home.
3. The UAP provides a tube of moisture barrier cream to a client.
4. The UAP fills a client's water pitcher with ice and water.

14. Which interventions should the nurse implement when administering filgrastim subcutaneously? **Select all that apply.**
1. Do not shake the vial before preparing the injection.
2. Apply a warm washcloth after administering the medication.
3. Discard any unused portion of the vial after withdrawing the correct dose.
4. Keep the medication vials in the refrigerator until preparing to administer.
5. Instruct the client to take acetaminophen before and 24 hours after the injection.

15. The elderly client diagnosed with coronary artery disease has been taking acetylsalicylic acid daily for more than a year. Which data **warrants notifying** the HCP?
1. The client has lost 5 pounds in the past month.
2. The client has trouble hearing low tones.
3. The client reports having a funny taste in the mouth.
4. The client is reporting bleeding gums.

16. The nurse is reviewing laboratory data of a client receiving chemotherapy. The client's laboratory values are populated in the chart below.

Laboratory Test	Client Values	Reference Values
White blood cell (WBC) count	7.4	4.5 to 11.1 x 10^3/microL
Red blood cell (RBC) count	2.0	Male: 4.21 to 5.81 (10^6 cells/microL) Female: 3.61 to 5.11 (10^6 cells/microL)
Hemoglobin (Hgb)	6.6	Male: 14 to 17.3 g/dL Female: 11.7 to 15.5 g/dL
Hematocrit (Hct)	19.2	Male: 42% to 52% Female: 36% to 48%
	~~83~~	~~81–96 mg/m^3~~
~~MCHC~~	~~31~~	~~33–36 g/dL~~
~~RDW~~	~~12~~	~~11%–14.5%~~
~~Reticulocyte~~	~~1.4~~	~~0.5%–1.5%~~
Platelets	110	140 to 400 × 10^3/microL
DIFFERENTIAL		
Neutrophils	40	40% to 75%
Lymphocytes	50	20% to 50%
Monocytes	2	1% to 10%
Eosinophils	6	0% to 6%
Basophils	2	0% to 2%

Which intervention should the nurse implement?
1. Assess for an infection.
2. Assess for petechiae.
3. Assess for shortness of breath.
4. Assess for rubor.

17. The client experienced a full-thickness burn to 45% of the body, including the chest area. The HCP ordered fluid resuscitation. Which data indicates the fluid resuscitation has been **effective**?
1. The client's urine output is less than 30 mL/hr.
2. The client has a productive cough and clear lungs.
3. The client's BP is 110/70.
4. The client's urine contains sediment.

18. Which statement **best describes** the scientific rationale for administering a miotic ophthalmic medication to a client diagnosed with glaucoma?
1. It constricts the pupil, which causes the pupil to dilate in low light.
2. It dilates the pupil to reduce aqueous humor production.
3. It decreases aqueous humor production but does not affect the eye.
4. It is used as adjunctive therapy primarily to reduce intraocular pressure.

19. The nurse is administering medications to clients on an orthopedic unit. Which medication should the nurse **question**?
   1. Ibuprofen 600 mg PO to a client diagnosed with back pain, rated a "5" on a pain scale of 1–10.
   2. Morphine 2 mg IV to a client diagnosed with back pain rated a "2" on a pain scale of 1–10.
   3. Methocarbamol 1500 mg PO three times daily to a client diagnosed with chronic back pain.
   4. Acetaminophen 500 mg PO q 6 hours to a client diagnosed with mild back pain.

20. Which is the scientific rationale for prescribing decongestants for a client diagnosed with a cold?
   1. Decongestants vasoconstrict blood vessels, reducing nasal inflammation.
   2. Decongestants decrease bacterial growth in the sputum.
   3. Decongestants activate viral receptors in the body's immune system.
   4. Decongestants loosen secretions, which prevent organisms from binding to epithelial cells of the nose.

21. The nurse is caring for clients on the telemetry unit. Which medication should the nurse administer **first**?
   1. Digoxin to the client diagnosed with congestive heart failure (CHF) with digoxin level 1.9 mg/dL
   2. Morphine IVP to the client diagnosed with pleuritic chest pain that is rated a "7" on a pain scale of 1–10
   3. Lidocaine to the client exhibiting two unifocal premature ventricular contractions (PVCs) per minute
   4. Lisinopril to the client diagnosed with hypertension (HTN) and BP of 130/68

22. The nurse is preparing to administer medications to the following clients. Which medication should the nurse **question** administering?
   1. Furosemide to the client with a serum potassium level of 4.2 mEq/L
   2. Mannitol to the client with a serum osmolality of 280 mOsm/kg
   3. Digoxin to the client with a digoxin level of 1.2 mg/dL
   4. Phenytoin to the client with a phenytoin level of 24 mcg/mL

23. The nurse is administering digoxin 0.25 mg IV push (IVP) medication to the client. For each intervention, specify if the intervention is **indicated or not indicated** for the client's care.

Potential Nursing Intervention	Indicated	Not Indicated
1. Administer the medication undiluted.		
2. Check the client's serum potassium level.		
3. Pinch off the IV tubing above the port.		
4. Inject medication over 5 minutes at a steady rate.		
5. Explain that experiencing a yellow haze is an expected side effect.		

24. Which client should the nurse expect the HCP to prescribe chlordiazepoxide?
   1. A client diagnosed with a cocaine addiction
   2. A client diagnosed with a heroin addiction
   3. A client diagnosed with an amphetamine addiction
   4. A client diagnosed with an alcohol addiction

25. The client is discussing wanting to quit smoking cigarettes with the clinic nurse. Which intervention is **most successful** in helping the client to quit smoking cigarettes?
1. Encourage the client to attend a smoking cessation support group.
2. Discuss tapering the number of cigarettes smoked daily.
3. Instruct the client to use varenicline.
4. Explain that clonidine can be taken daily to help decrease withdrawal symptoms.

26. Each client is diagnosed with a head injury. To which client would the nurse **question** administering mannitol?
1. The 34-year-old client diagnosed as HIV positive
2. The 84-year-old client diagnosed with glaucoma
3. The 68-year-old client diagnosed with CHF
4. The 16-year-old client diagnosed with cystic fibrosis (CF)

27. The nurse is caring for a client with the following telemetry strip.

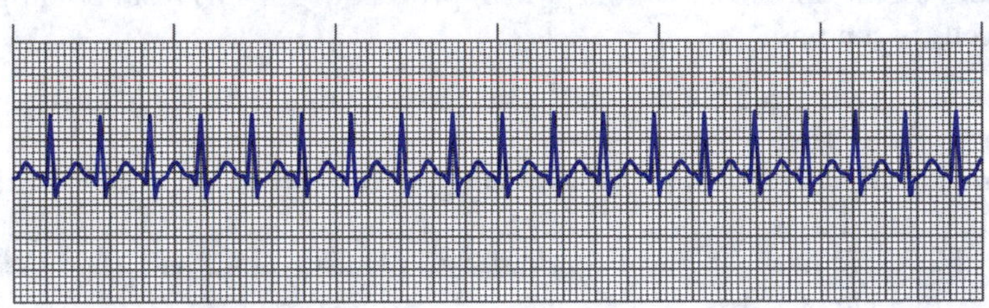

Which antidysrhythmic medication should the nurse administer?
1. Lidocaine
2. Atropine
3. Adenosine
4. Epinephrine

28. The client diagnosed with coronary artery disease is prescribed atorvastatin. Which statement by the client indicates the medication is **effective**?
1. "I really haven't changed my diet, but I am taking my medication every day."
2. "I am feeling good because my doctor told me my cholesterol level came down."
3. "I am swimming at the local pool about three times a week for 30 minutes."
4. "Because I have been taking this medication, the swelling in my legs is better."

29. The nurse is preparing to administer medications on a pulmonary unit. Which medication should the nurse administer **first**?
1. Prednisone for a client diagnosed with chronic bronchitis
2. Ceftriaxone, IV piggyback (IVPB), an initial dose
3. Lactic acidophilus to a client receiving IVPB antibiotics
4. Cephalexin by mouth (PO) to a client being discharged

30. The client diagnosed with chronic obstructive pulmonary disease (COPD) is prescribed methylprednisolone IVP. The client's laboratory values are populated in the chart below.

Laboratory Test	Client Values	Reference Values
White blood cell (WBC) count	15	4.5 to 11.1 × 10^3/microL
Hemoglobin (Hgb)	13	Male: 14 to 17.3 g/dL Female: 11.7 to 15.5 g/dL
Hematocrit (Hct)	39%	Male: 42% to 52% Female: 36% to 48%
Glucose	238 mg/dL	Fasting: <100 mg/dL Random: <200 mg/dL
Creatinine	1.1 mg/dL	Male: 0.61 to 1.21 mg/dL Female: 0.51 to 1.11 mg/dL
Potassium	3.9 mEq/L	3.5 to 5.3 mEq/L or mmol/L

Which laboratory data **warrants intervention** by the nurse? **Select all that apply.**
1. White blood cell count
2. Hemoglobin level
3. Hematocrit level
4. Blood glucose
5. Creatinine level
6. Potassium level

31. The client's arterial blood gas (ABG) results are populated in the following chart.

Laboratory Test	Client Values	Reference Values
pH	7.35	7.35 to 7.45
Po_2	75	80 to 95 mm Hg
Pco_2	35	35 to 45 mm Hg
Hco_3	24	22 to 26 mmol/L

Which intervention is **most appropriate** for this client?
1. Administer oxygen 10 L/min via nasal cannula.
2. Administer an antianxiety medication.
3. Administer 1 amp of sodium bicarbonate IVP.
4. Administer 30 mL of an antacid.

32. Which data indicates the antibiotic therapy has been **successful** for a client diagnosed with bacterial pneumonia?
1. The client's Hct level is 45%.
2. The client is expectorating thick green sputum.
3. The client's lung sounds are clear to auscultation.
4. The client reports pleuritic chest pain.

33. Which statement is the scientific rationale for administering an antacid to a client diagnosed with gastrointestinal reflux disease (GERD)?
1. Antacids neutralize gastric secretions.
2. Antacids block H_2 receptors on parietal cells.
3. Antacids inhibit the enzyme that generates gastric acid.
4. Antacids form a protective barrier against acid and pepsin.

34. The client diagnosed with a severe acute exacerbation of Crohn's disease is prescribed total parenteral nutrition (TPN). Which interventions should the nurse implement when administering TPN? **Select all that apply.**
1. Monitor the client's glucose level daily.
2. Administer TPN via an IV pump.
3. Assess the subclavian line insertion site.
4. Check TPN according to medication rights before administering.
5. Encourage the client to eat all of the food offered at meals.

35. The client is prescribed a stool softener. Which statement **best describes** the scientific rationale for administering this medication?
1. The medication acts by lubricating the stool and the colon mucosa.
2. Stool softeners irritate the bowel to increase peristalsis.
3. The medication causes more water and fat to be absorbed into the stool.
4. Stool softeners absorb water, adding size to the fecal mass.

36. The nurse is preparing to administer medications to the following clients. To which client should the nurse **question administering** the medication?
1. Lactulose to a client with an ammonia level of 10 mcg/dL
2. Furosemide to a client with a potassium level of 3.7 mEq/L
3. Spironolactone to a client with a potassium level of 3.5 mEq/L
4. Vasopressin to a client with a serum sodium level of 137 mEq/L

37. The nurse administered 25 units of insulin isophane to a client diagnosed with type 1 diabetes at 0700. For each intervention, specify if the intervention is **indicated or not indicated** for the client's care.

Potential Nursing Intervention	Indicated	Not Indicated
1. Assess the client for hypoglycemia around 1800.		
2. Ensure the client eats the nighttime snack.		
3. Check client's blood glucose level via a glucometer.		
4. Determine how much food the client ate at lunch.		
5. Monitor client for low blood glucose around 1500.		

38. The nurse is administering insulin lispro at 0730 to a client diagnosed with type 1 diabetes. Which intervention should the nurse implement?
1. Ensure the client eats at least 90% of the food on the lunch tray.
2. Do not administer unless the breakfast tray is in the client's room.
3. Check the client's blood glucose level 1 hour after receiving insulin.
4. Have 50% dextrose in water at the bedside for emergency use.

39. The client diagnosed with hypothyroidism is prescribed levothyroxine. Which assessment data supports the client is taking **too much** medication? **Select all that apply.**
1. The client has a 2-kg weight gain.
2. The client reports being too hot.
3. The client's radial pulse rate is 110 beats per minute (bpm).
4. The client reports having diarrhea.
5. The client has fine tremors in the hands.

40. The client diagnosed with chronic pancreatitis is reporting steatorrhea. Which medication should the nurse prepare to administer?
1. Insulin lispro intravenously, then monitor glucose levels
2. Pancrelipase sprinkled on the client's food with meals
3. Insulin regular subcutaneously after assessing the blood glucose level
4. Famotidine orally before meals

41. The client diagnosed with end-stage renal disease is receiving oral sodium polystyrene sulfonate. Which assessment data indicates the medication is **not effective**?
1. The client's serum potassium level is 5.8 mEq/L
2. The client's serum sodium level is 135 mEq/L
3. The client's serum potassium level is 4.2 mEq/L
4. The client's serum sodium level is 147 mEq/L

42. The registered nurse (RN) observes the UAP performing nursing tasks. Which action by the UAP **requires immediate intervention**?
1. The UAP increases the saline irrigation rate for a client after transurethral prostate resection.
2. The UAP tells the nurse that a client on strict bedrest has green, funny-looking urine in the bedpan.
3. The UAP encourages the client to drink a glass of water after the nurse administers the oral antibiotic.
4. The UAP assists the client diagnosed with a urinary tract infection to the bedside commode every 2 hours.

43. The client is diagnosed with herpes simplex 2 viral infection and is prescribed valacyclovir. For each teaching intervention, specify if the intervention is **indicated or not indicated** for the client's care.

Potential Nursing Intervention	Indicated	Not Indicated
1. Medication will dry the lesions within a day or two.		
2. Valacyclovir is taken once a day to control outbreaks.		
3. Condom use will increase herpes spread.		
4. After lesions are gone, the client will not transmit the virus.		
5. Wash hands frequently to prevent virus transmission.		
6. Drink plenty of water while taking valacyclovir.		

44. The client is 38 weeks pregnant, diagnosed with preeclampsia, and admitted to the labor and delivery area. The HCP has prescribed IV magnesium sulfate. Which data indicates the medication is **not effective**?
1. The client's deep tendon reflexes are 4+.
2. The client's BP is 148/90.
3. The client's deep tendon reflexes are 2 to 3+.
4. The client's deep tendon reflexes are 0.

45. The client diagnosed as postmenopausal is prescribed alendronate to help prevent osteoporosis. Which information should the nurse discuss with the client?
1. "Chew the tablet thoroughly before swallowing."
2. "Eat a meal before taking the medication."
3. "Take the medication at night before going to sleep."
4. "Remain upright for 30 minutes after taking the medication."

46. The client is prescribed methotrexate for psoriasis. Which intervention should the nurse teach the client?
1. Teach the client that the urine may turn a red-orange color.
2. Have the client drink Ensure to increase nutritional status.
3. Tell the client to notify the HCP if a fever develops.
4. Encourage the client to increase green, leafy vegetables in the diet.

47. With which client should the nurse use caution when applying mafenide acetate to a burned area?
1. A client with a creatinine level of 2.8 mg/dL
2. A client diagnosed with CHF
3. A client with a pulse oximeter reading of 95%
4. A client diagnosed with type 2 diabetes taking insulin

48. The long-term care nurse is administering botulinum toxin type A to a client diagnosed with a cerebrovascular accident (CVA). Which statement **best describes** the scientific rationale for administering this medication?
1. This medication is administered for the cosmetic effect to reduce wrinkles.
2. This medication reduces muscle spasticity associated with strokes.
3. This medication will improve the client's residual limb strength.
4. This medication will decrease the pain associated with neuropathy.

49. The client is diagnosed with second- and third-degree burns to 40% of the body. The HCP writes an order for 8,000 mL of fluid to be infused over the next 24 hours. The order reads that one-half of the total amount should be administered in the first 8 hours with the other half being infused over the remaining 16 hours. At what rate would the nurse set the IV pump for the first 8 hours?

____

50. The client has a severe anaphylactic reaction to insect bites. Which **priority** discharge intervention should the nurse discuss with the client?
1. "Wear an insect repellent on exposed skin."
2. "Keep prescribed antihistamines with you."
3. "Keep an injectable epinephrine in the refrigerator at all times."
4. "Wear a MedicAlert identification bracelet."

51. Which statement is the scientific rationale for prescribing the highly active antiretroviral therapy (HAART) regimen to clients diagnosed with HIV infection?
1. HAART will cure clients diagnosed with HIV infection.
2. HAART poses less toxicity risk than other regimens.
3. HAART can decrease HIV to undetectable levels.
4. HAART is less costly than other medication regimens.

52. The client diagnosed with rheumatoid arthritis (RA) is prescribed hydroxychloroquine sulfate. Which statement indicates the client **understands** the medication teaching?
1. "I will get my eyes checked yearly."
2. "I can only have two beers a week."
3. "It is important to take this medication with milk."
4. "I will call my HCP if the pain is not relieved in 2 weeks."

53. The nurse is preparing to administer morning medications on an oncology floor. Which medication should the nurse administer **first**?
1. An analgesic to a client diagnosed with a headache rated a "3" on a pain scale of 1–10
2. An anxiolytic to a client with a concern of becoming anxious
3. A mucosal barrier agent to a client diagnosed with peptic ulcer disease
4. A biologic response modifier to a client with low red blood cell (RBC) counts

54. The client calls the nursing station and requests pain medication. When the nurse enters the room with the narcotic medication, the nurse finds the client laughing and talking with visitors. Which action should the nurse implement **first**?
1. Administer the client's prescribed pain medication.
2. Assess the client's pain perception on a 1–10 scale.
3. Wait until the visitors leave to administer any medication.
4. Check the MAR to see if a nonnarcotic medication is ordered.

55. The nurse administered a narcotic pain medication 30 minutes ago to a client diagnosed with cancer. Which data indicates the medication was **effective**?
1. The client keeps their eyes closed and the drapes are drawn.
2. The client uses guided imagery to help with pain control.
3. The client is snoring lightly when the nurse enters the room.
4. The client is lying as still as possible in the bed.

56. The client has received chemotherapy 2 days a week every 3 weeks for the past 8 months. The client's laboratory values are populated in the chart below.

Laboratory Test	Client Values	Reference Values
Hemoglobin (Hgb)	10.3 g/dL	Male: 14 to 17.3 g/dL Female: 11.7 to 15.5 g/dL
Hematocrit (Hct)	31%	Male: 42% to 52% Female: 36% to 48%
White blood cell (WBC) count	2	4.5 to 11.1 × 10^3/microL
Neutrophils	50%	40 to 75%
Platelets	189	140 to 400 × 10^3/microL

Which information should the nurse teach the client? **Select all that apply.**
1. "Avoid individuals with colds or other infections."
2. "Maintain nutritional status with supplements."
3. "Do not eat raw fruit or have plants or flowers in the room."
4. "Plan for periods of rest to prevent fatigue."
5. "Use a soft-bristled toothbrush and electric razor."

57. The nurse is preparing to administer lithium to a client diagnosed with bipolar disorder. The lithium level is 3.5 mEq/L. Which intervention should the nurse implement **first**?
1. Administer the medication.
2. Hold the medication.
3. Notify the HCP.
4. Verify the lithium level.

58. The 8-year-old child newly diagnosed with attention-deficit hyperactivity disorder (ADHD) is prescribed methylphenidate. In the following table, does the statement by the parent indicate the teaching interventions performed by the nurse are **effective or not effective?**

Statement by Parent	Effective	Not Effective
1. "I will keep the medication in a safe place."		
2. "I will give my child this medication every 12 hours."		
3. "It may cause my child to have growth spurts."		
4. "My child will probably experience insomnia."		
5. "I will notify the HCP if my child reports finger pain."		

59. The client diagnosed with bilateral conjunctivitis is prescribed antibiotic ophthalmic ointment. Which medication teaching should the nurse discuss with the client? **Select all that apply.**
1. "Apply a thin line of ointment evenly along the inner edge of the lower lid margin."
2. "Press the nasolacrimal duct after applying the antibiotic ointment."
3. "Don nonsterile gloves before administering medication."
4. "Apply antibiotic ointment from the outer canthus to the inner canthus."
5. "Sit with the head slightly tilted back or lie supine."

60. The nurse has administered an ophthalmic medication to the client. Which area should the nurse put pressure on to prevent systemic absorption?

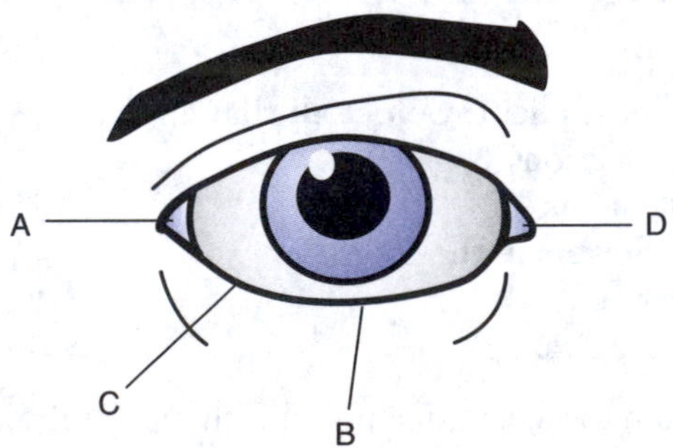

1. A
2. B
3. C
4. D

61. The client diagnosed with hypovolemic shock is receiving normal saline by rapid IV infusion. Which assessment data **warrants immediate intervention** by the nurse?
1. The client's BP is 89/48.
2. The client's pulse oximeter reading is 95%.
3. The client's lung sounds are clear bilaterally.
4. The client's urine output is 120 mL in 3 hours.

62. The client is exhibiting the following telemetry strip and is coding.

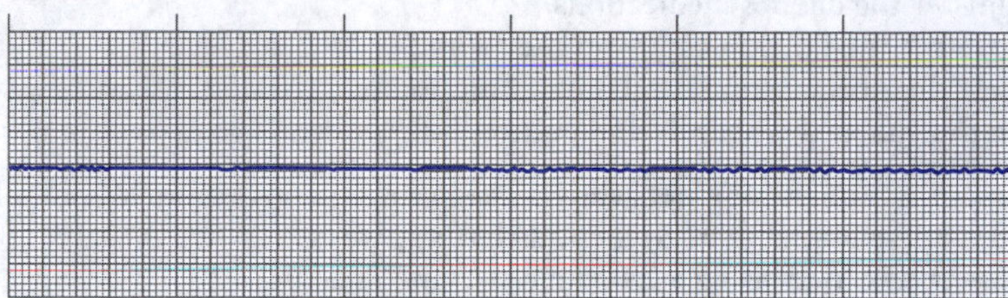

Which intervention should the nurse implement **first**?
1. Prepare to defibrillate the client at 360 joules.
2. Prepare for synchronized cardioversion.
3. Prepare to administer epinephrine IVP.
4. Prepare to administer amiodarone.

63. Which statement **best describes** the scientific rationale for administering acetylcysteine to a child brought to the ED for accidental ingestion of a substance?
1. Acetylcysteine neutralizes toxic substances by changing the pH of the poison.
2. Acetylcysteine binds with bleach and is excreted through the bowel.
3. Acetylcysteine is the antidote for acute acetaminophen poisoning.
4. Acetylcysteine induces vomiting, and the client eliminates much of the narcotics.

64. The parent of a 2-year-old child calls the ED and reports that the child drank some dishwashing detergent. Which question is **most important** for the nurse to ask the parent?
1. "How much does your child weigh?"
2. "Is your child reporting a stomachache?"
3. "Have you called the Poison Control Center?"
4. "Where did you keep the dishwashing soap?"

65. The client admitted to the medical floor for a pneumonia diagnosis of pneumonia informs the nurse of taking acetylsalicylic acid every day. Which intervention should the nurse implement?
1. Assess the client's BP and pulse.
2. Check the client's urine for ketones.
3. Monitor for an elevated temperature.
4. Document the information in the electronic health record (EHR).

66. The client diagnosed with anemia is taking an iron tablet daily. Which statement indicates the client **needs more medication teaching**?
1. "I will not call my HCP if my stools become black or dark green."
2. "I must take my iron tablet with meals and one glass of milk."
3. "I will sit upright for 30 minutes after taking my iron tablet."
4. "I will have to take an iron tablet for about 6 months."

67. Which statement **best explains** the scientific rationale for a client taking antioxidants?
1. Antioxidants will increase oxygen availability to the heart muscle.
2. Antioxidants will help prevent platelet aggregation in the arteries.
3. Antioxidants decrease atherosclerotic plaque build-up in the arteries.
4. Antioxidants decrease oxygen demands of the peripheral tissues.

68. The nurse is presenting a lecture on herbs to a community group. Which guideline should the nurse discuss with the group?
1. Administer smaller amounts of herbs to babies and young children.
2. Store the herbal remedy in a sunny, warm, moist area.
3. Encourage clients to use herbs as an alternative to other medications.
4. Consumers should think of herbs as medicines; more is not necessarily better.

69. The UAP is making rounds and notices that the RN left a medication cup with three tablets at the client's bedside. Which action should the UAP implement?
1. Administer the client's medications.
2. Remove the medication cup from the room.
3. Request the primary nurse to come to the room.
4. Leave the cup at the bedside and do nothing.

70. The nurse is administering heparin via the subcutaneous route. Which interventions should the nurse implement? **Select all that apply.**
1. Prepare medication using a 25-gauge, 1/2-inch needle.
2. After injecting medication, do not aspirate.
3. Check the client's PTT before administering medication.
4. After removing the needle, massage the area gently.
5. Administer the medication in the client's "love handles."

71. The nurse is administering therapeutic heparin for a client diagnosed with deep vein thrombosis (DVT). Which laboratory value should the nurse monitor?
1. International normalized ratio (INR)
2. Prothrombin time (PT)
3. Partial thromboplastin time (PTT)
4. Platelet count

72. The ED nurse is providing discharge instructions to the client diagnosed with a concussion. For each intervention, specify if the intervention is **indicated or not indicated** for the client's care.

Potential Nursing Intervention	Indicated	Not Indicated
1. Instruct client to take acetaminophen for a headache.		
2. Tell client to stay on a clear liquid diet for the next 24 hours.		
3. Instruct client to take one hydrocodone for pain.		
4. Recommend client take acetylsalicylic acid for any physical discomfort.		
5. Tell client to return to the ED if experiencing nausea and vomiting.		
6. Encourage client to maintain strict bedrest for 24 hours.		
7. Advise client to avoid alcohol until fully recovered.		
8. Teach client to remain awake for the next 12 hours.		

73. The nurse is preparing to administer the following anticonvulsant medications. Which medication should the nurse **question administering**?
1. Carbamazepine to the client with carbamazepine serum level of 22 mcg/mL
2. Clonazepam to the client with clonazepam serum level of 0.6 mcg/mL
3. Phenytoin to the client with phenytoin serum level of 19 mcg/mL
4. Ethosuximide to the client with ethosuximide serum level of 45 mcg/mL

74. Which information should the nurse teach the client and family of a client prescribed donepezil?
1. Donepezil may delay progression of Alzheimer's disease for 6 months to a year.
2. Donepezil will repair brain damage for clients diagnosed with Alzheimer's disease.
3. Donepezil is still experimental as to how it treats Alzheimer's disease.
4. Donepezil is difficult for clients to tolerate because of the many side effects.

75. Which statement is the scientific rationale for prescribing dexamethasone to a client diagnosed with a primary brain tumor?
1. Dexamethasone will prevent metastasis to other parts of the body.
2. Dexamethasone is a potent anticonvulsant and will prevent seizures.
3. Dexamethasone increases serotonin uptake in the brain tissues.
4. Dexamethasone decreases intracranial pressure by decreasing inflammation.

76. The HCP in the ED has prescribed alteplase for a client reporting new onset of slurred speech, difficulty swallowing, and paralysis of the left arm. In which situations should the nurse **question** administering the medication? **Select all that apply.**
1. The client has the comorbid condition of CHF.
2. The client had abdominal surgery 6 weeks ago for a bleeding ulcer.
3. The client has not had a CT scan done.
4. The client is taking warfarin.
5. The client has a history of DVT with pulmonary embolism (PE).

77. The ED nurse received a client on warfarin with an INR of 1.5. Which intervention should the nurse implement?
1. Prepare to administer protamine sulfate.
2. Document the laboratory result and take no action.
3. Prepare to administer vitamin K.
4. Notify the client's HCP.

78. The nurse is preparing to administer a nitroglycerin patch to a client diagnosed with coronary artery disease. Which interventions should the nurse implement **first**?
1. Date and time the nitroglycerin patch.
2. Remove the old patch.
3. Apply the nitroglycerin patch.
4. Check the patch against the MAR.

79. The client diagnosed with CHF is taking digoxin. Which data indicates the medication is **ineffective**?
1. The client's BP is 110/68.
2. The client's apical pulse rate is 68 bpm.
3. The client's potassium level is 4.2 mEq/L.
4. The client's lungs have crackles bilaterally.

80. The client is exhibiting the following telemetry strip and has no pulse.

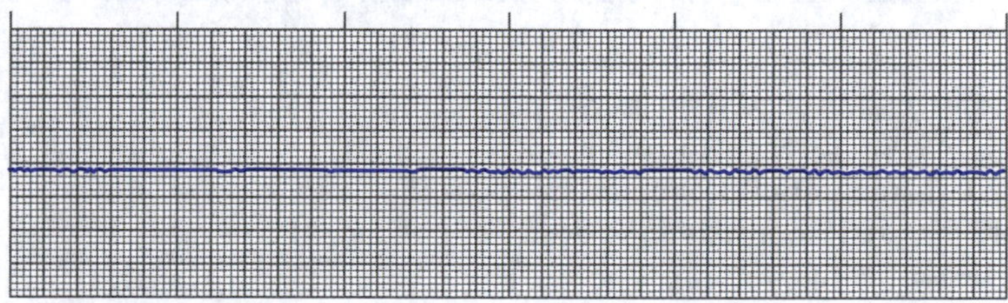

Which medication should the nurse administer **first**?
1. Amiodarone
2. Atropine
3. Adenosine
4. Epinephrine

81. The nurse is preparing to administer medications to the following clients. To which client should the nurse **question administering** the medication?
1. The client receiving losartan with BP of 168/94.
2. The client receiving diltiazem with 2+ pitting edema.
3. The client receiving terazosin with regular apical pulse of 56 bpm.
4. The client receiving hydrochlorothiazide and reporting a headache.

82. The nurse is discharging a client diagnosed with COPD. Which discharge instructions should the nurse provide regarding the client's prednisone? **Select all that apply.**
1. "The prednisone must be tapered when discontinuing."
2. "Take prednisone with food to prevent gastrointestinal upset."
3. "Stop taking prednisone if a noticeable weight gain occurs."
4. "Keep prednisone in a dark-colored bottle at all times."
5. "The medication will increase the risk of developing an infection."

83. Which assessment data **best indicates** the client diagnosed with reactive airway disease has **not achieved** "good" control with the medication regimen?
1. The client's peak expiratory flow rate (PEFR) is greater than 80% of their personal best.
2. The client's lung sounds are clear bilaterally, both anteriorly and posteriorly.
3. The client has only had three acute exacerbations of asthma in the past month.
4. The client's monthly serum theophylline level is 18 mcg/mL.

84. The nurse is preparing to administer the following medications. To which client should the nurse **question administering** the medication?
1. The client receiving prednisone with a glucose level of 140 mg/dL
2. The client receiving ceftriaxone with a WBC count of 15,000
3. The client receiving heparin with a PTT of 108 seconds with a control of 39
4. The client receiving theophylline with a theophylline level of 12 mcg/dL

85. The nurse is preparing to administer warfarin. The client's laboratory values are populated in the chart below.

Laboratory Test	Client Values	Reference Values
Prothrombin time (PT)	48 Control 12.9	10 to 13 seconds
Partial thromboplastin time (PTT)	40 Control 36	25 to 35 seconds
International Normalized Ratio (INR)	4.2	0.9 to 1.1 without anticoagulation therapy 2 to 3 with therapy 2.5 to 3.5 if the client has a mechanical heart valve

Which intervention should the nurse implement?
1. Question administering the medication.
2. Prepare to administer protamine sulfate.
3. Notify the HCP to increase the dose.
4. Administer the medication as ordered.

86. The nurse is caring for a client diagnosed with pneumonia. Which data indicates the antibiotic therapy has been **effective**?
1. The white blood cell (WBC) count is 7.2×10^3/microL.
2. The culture and sensitivity (C&S) show gram-negative rods.
3. The client completed taking all prescribed antibiotics.
4. The client reports pleurisy.

87. The nurse is administering 0800 medications. Which medication should the nurse **question**?
1. Ibuprofen to a 49-year-old client diagnosed with a peptic ulcer
2. Omeprazole to an 18-year-old client diagnosed with a duodenal ulcer
3. Digoxin to a 76-year-old client with a potassium level of 4.2 mEq/L
4. Magaldrate oral to a 67-year-old client diagnosed with CHF and reporting indigestion

88. The client diagnosed with inflammatory bowel disease (IBD) is prescribed a mesalamine suppository. Which statement indicates the client **needs more** medication teaching?
1. "I should retain the suppository for at least 15 minutes."
2. "The suppository may stain my underwear or clothing."
3. "I should store my medication in my medicine cabinet."
4. "I should have an empty rectum when applying the suppository."

89. The client postgastrectomy has a patient-controlled analgesia (PCA) pump. Which data indicates the client and family **understand** the instructions regarding the PCA pump?
1. The family pushes the PCA button whenever the time limit has expired.
2. The client uses the PCA before turning, coughing, and deep breathing.
3. The family discourages the client from using the PCA pump.
4. The client pushes the PCA button when the pain is an "8" or "9" on a pain scale of 1 to 10.

90. The elderly client diagnosed with diverticulosis tells the nurse about taking bisacodyl daily. Which teaching is **most important** for the nurse to provide the client?
1. "You don't need to have a bowel movement every day."
2. "You need to increase fluids to prevent dehydration when taking this medication."
3. "You should use a bulk laxative when taking laxatives daily."
4. "You will need to increase the laxative dose if you do not get good results."

91. The UAP notified the RN that the client is reporting being jittery and nervous and is diaphoretic. The client is diagnosed with diabetes mellitus. Which interventions should the primary nurse implement **first**?
1. Have the UAP check the client's glucose level.
2. Tell the UAP to get the client some orange juice.
3. Check the client's MAR.
4. Immediately go to the room and assess the client.

92. The nurse is administering medications to a client diagnosed with type 1 diabetes. The client's 1100 glucometer reading is 299. Which intervention should the nurse implement?

Client: A.C.	MR# 1234567	Date: Today
Age: 65 years	Allergies: NKDA	Diagnosis: Type 1 Diabetes
Medication	0701–1900	1901–0700
Regular insulin by bedside glucose sliding scale SQ ac and hs <60 notify HCP <150 0 units 151–200 2 units 201–250 4 units 251–300 6 units 301–350 8 units 351–400 10 units >400 notify HCP	0730 DN BG 142 0 units	
Nurse Initials/Credentials	DN/RN	NN/RN

1. Have the laboratory verify the glucose results.
2. Notify the HCP of the results.
3. Administer six units of regular insulin subcutaneously.
4. Recheck the client's glucometer reading at 1130.

93. The client diagnosed with chronic pancreatitis is prescribed pancrease. Which data indicates the medication is **effective**?

1. No bowel movement for 3 days
2. Fatty, frothy, foul-smelling stools
3. Brown, soft, formed stools
4. Normal bowel sounds in four quadrants

94. The client diagnosed with diabetes insipidus (DI) is receiving desmopressin intranasally. Which assessment data **warrants** the client **notifying** the HCP?

1. The client reports being thirsty all the time.
2. The client can sleep through the night.
3. The client has lost 1 pound in the past 24 hours.
4. The client has to urinate at least five times daily.

95. The client diagnosed with Addison's disease is being discharged. Which statement indicates the client **understands** the medication discharge teaching?

1. "I will be sure to keep my dose of steroid constant and not vary."
2. "I may have to take two forms of steroids to remain healthy."
3. "It is normal to become weak and dizzy when taking this medication."
4. "I must take prophylactic antibiotics before getting my teeth cleaned."

ANSWERS AND RATIONALES

The correct answer number and rationale are in **boldface blue type.** Rationales for why other answer options are incorrect are also given.

1.

Potential Nursing Intervention	Indicated	Not Indicated
1. Notify the HCP of dyspnea, fatigue, and cough.	X	
2. Take medication before going to bed.		X
3. Do not take medication if apical pulse <60 bpm.		X
4. Medication may cause the stool to turn black.		X
5. Avoid grapefruit juice while taking the medication.	X	
6. Permanent bluish facial discoloration can occur.		X
7. Wear sunscreen and protective clothing during therapy.	X	
8. If a dose is missed, do not take the dose at all.	X	

1. **These adverse effects would cause the HCP to discontinue this medication. Amiodarone (Cordarone), an antidysrhythmic, can cause pulmonary toxicity, which is progressive dyspnea, cough, fatigue, and pleuritic pain.**
2. **The medication can be taken at the client's convenience. Amiodarone (Cordarone), an antidysrhythmic, should be taken at the same time each day.**
3. **The client checks the radial pulse at home, not the apical pulse, which requires a stethoscope.**
4. **This medication does not cause the stool to turn black. Iron supplements make the client's stool turn black.**
5. **The client should avoid drinking grapefruit juice. Grapefruit juice interferes with amiodarone absorption, causing increased medication levels and toxicity risk.**
6. **Bluish discoloration of the face, neck, and arms can occur with prolonged use of amiodarone. This side effect is usually reversible and will fade over time.**
7. **Photosensitivity reactions can occur on amiodarone therapy. The client should be instructed to wear sunscreen and protective clothing.**
8. **If a dose is missed, the client should not take the dose at all. If two doses are missed, the client should notify the HCP.**

2. 1. The client receiving a calcium channel blocker can take the medication with water; therefore, the nurse would not question administering this medication.
2. This BP is above 90/60; therefore, the nurse would not question administering this medication.
3. Headache is a side effect of nitroglycerin; therefore, the nurse would not question administering this medication, but could administer acetaminophen (Tylenol) or a nonnarcotic analgesic.
4. **The client's platelet count is not monitored when administering antiplatelet medication. Still, if the nurse is aware that the client has a low platelet count, the nurse would question administering any medication that would inactivate the platelets.**

3. 1. Antihypertensive medications do not interfere with the contrast dye used when performing a CT scan. Glucophage may be held before or after the procedure until a normal creatinine level can be established.
2. **The client will have an IV line to administer the contrast dye.**
3. The contrast dye is iodine-based, so an allergy to shellfish would be important, but there is no contraindication to taking an NSAID.
4. Sedatives are not administered for this procedure; however, if the client is anxious about the machine, sometimes an antianxiety medication is administered.

4. 1. Mineral oil will not affect folic acid, but it will inhibit vitamin A absorption.
   2. The client should avoid drinking alcohol products because they increase folic acid requirements.
   3. Research has proved that decreased stores of folic acid, a vitamin, in the maternal body directly affect spina bifida development in the fetus.
   4. This would be significant if a client is at risk for developing gestational HTN, but not when taking folic acid, a vitamin.

5. **1. This is the scientific rationale for administering the thiazolidinediones pioglitazone (Actos) or rosiglitazone (Avandia).**
   2. This is the scientific rationale for administering an alpha-glucosidase inhibitor, acarbose (Precose) or miglitol (Glyset).
   3. This is the scientific rationale for administering metformin (Glucophage). It diminishes the increase in serum glucose after a meal and blunts the degree of postprandial hyperglycemia.
   4. This is the scientific rationale for administering meglitinides, repaglinide (Prandin), sulfonylureas, or nateglinide (Starlix).

6. 1. Epinephrine, an adrenergic agonist, is the first medication administered in a code because it constricts the periphery and shunts the blood to the body's trunk.
   2. Amiodarone, an antidysrhythmic, is a drug of choice for treating ventricular dysrhythmias.
   3. Atropine, an antidysrhythmic, is administered for asystole.
   4. Digoxin, a cardiac glycoside, is administered for cardiac failure.

7. **Correct answers are 1, 3, 4, 6, and 8.**
   1. An antidepressant often takes 2 to 4 weeks to build up its effect and work fully.
   2. This would be appropriate for monoamine oxidase inhibitors (MAOIs).
   3. Serotonin syndrome (SES) is a serious complication of selective serotonin reuptake inhibitors (SSRIs) that produce mental changes (confusion, anxiety, and restlessness), HTN, tremors, sweating, hyperpyrexia (elevated temperature), and ataxia. Conservative treatment includes stopping the SSRI fluoxetine (Prozac) and using supportive treatment. If untreated, it can lead to death.
   4. The SSRI fluoxetine (Prozac) has to be weaned because the client may develop some withdrawal symptoms. The dose is usually gradually reduced before stopping entirely at the end of a course of treatment.
   5. These are additional findings of serotonin syndrome and should be reported to the HCP.
   6. Fluoxetine can cause dry mouth. The client should chew gum, suck on hard candy, or use mouth rinses to minimize dry mouth. The HCP can prescribe saliva substitutes.
   7. Fluoxetine can cause a decrease in libido and erectile dysfunction.
   8. The client's appetite and nutritional intake should be monitored, and the client should notify the HCP if continued weight loss occurs.

8. **100 mL. The pump is set at the rate to be administered per hour; therefore, the nurse should set the rate at 100 mL.**

9. **1. The therapeutic level for theophylline (Aminophylline) is 10 to 20 mcg/mL; therefore, the nurse should continue to monitor the theophylline because this is within the therapeutic range.**
   2. If the serum theophylline level rises above 20 mcg/mL, the client will experience nausea, vomiting, diarrhea, insomnia, and restlessness. This theophylline level may result in serious effects such as convulsion and ventricular fibrillation; therefore, the client should not be assessed first.
   3. The nurse should not discontinue the aminophylline because the client's blood level is within the therapeutic range.
   4. There is no reason to increase the theophylline infusion rate because the theophylline level is within the therapeutic range.

10. **1. The client diagnosed with an ulcer would be prescribed a medication that decreases gastric acid secretion. Females of childbearing age should not receive this medication because it can cause an abortion; therefore, the nurse would question administering misoprostol (Cytotec), a prostaglandin analog.**
   2. Omeprazole (Prilosec), a proton-pump inhibitor (PPI), is prescribed to treat duodenal and gastric ulcers; the nurse would not question this medication.

3. The potassium level is only slightly high (3.5 to 5.3 mEq/L); therefore, the nurse should not question furosemide (Lasix), a loop diuretic.
4. Acetaminophen (Tylenol), a nonnarcotic analgesic, is frequently administered for headaches; therefore, the nurse would not question this medication.

11. Correct answers are 1, 3, and 5.
1. The nurse can recommend the client take OTC medication to help relieve constipation.
2. The client should be encouraged to eat high-fiber foods and increase fluid intake, preferably water.
3. The nurse should determine when the last bowel movement was to take appropriate action to resolve constipation.
4. The client does not need to go to the ED because constipation should resolve with medication, but the client may need to be seen in the clinic if there is still no bowel movement within several days.
5. The nurse should determine the client's other medications because constipation can be a side effect of many prescribed and OTC medications.

12. **1. Regular insulin sliding scale is administered before meals; therefore, this medication should be administered first.**
2. Methylprednisolone, a glucocorticoid, can be administered within the 30-minute acceptable time frame.
3. A pain medication such as morphine, a narcotic analgesic, is a priority, but it can be administered after the sliding scale.
4. Etanercept (Enbrel), a biologic response modifier, can be administered within the 30-minute acceptable time frame.

13. 1. This is a standard precaution and does not require intervention by the nurse.
2. Herbs are considered medications, and the UAP cannot administer medications to the client even if they are from home. Many herbs will interact with prescribed medications, and the registered nurse (RN) must be aware of what the client is taking.
3. The client can apply their own moisture barrier protection cream. This does not warrant immediate intervention by the nurse.
4. This is a comfort measure and does not warrant intervention by the nurse.

14. Correct answers are 1, 3, 4, and 5.
1. Do not shake the vial because shaking may denature the glycoprotein, rendering it biologically inactive.
2. The nurse should apply ice to numb the injection site, not a warm washcloth.
3. The nurse should only use the vial for one dose. The nurse should not reenter the vial and discard any unused portion because the vial contains no preservatives.
4. The biologic response modifier filgrastim (Neupogen) should be stored in the refrigerator and warmed to room temperature before administering medication.
5. The biologic response modifier filgrastim (Neupogen) can cause bone pain; therefore, the nurse should encourage the client to take acetaminophen (Tylenol) before and after the injection to decrease pain.

15. 1. A 5-pound weight loss in 1 month would not make the nurse suspect the client is experiencing any long-term complications from taking daily acetylsalicylic acid (Aspirin).
2. Elderly clients often have a hearing loss, but it is not a complication of long-term aspirin use.
3. Elderly clients often lose taste buds, which may cause a funny taste in their mouth, but it is not a complication of taking daily aspirin.
4. A complication of long-term acetylsalicylic acid (Aspirin) use is gastric bleeding, resulting in bleeding gums. This data would warrant further intervention.

16. 1. The WBC count is within the normal range; therefore, the nurse would not need to assess for infection.
2. The client's platelet count is less than normal (150,000) but still greater than 100,000. Less than 100,000 is thrombocytopenia. Critical values begin at 50,000, which would cause the client to have petechiae.
3. The client's Hgb is critically low; therefore, the client might fatigue quickly because of oxygen demands on the body and have shortness of breath.
4. The client would not have rubor (redness); the client would be pale.

17. 1. This would not indicate that fluid resuscitation is effective.
2. This would indicate that the respiratory system is functioning but not that fluid resuscitation is effective.

3. **The client's BP indicates that fluid resuscitation is effective and can maintain an adequate BP to perfuse the vital organs.**
4. This would indicate that fluid resuscitation is not effective because this is a finding of decreased urine output.

18. 1. **This is the scientific rationale for miotic medications, which constrict the pupil and block sympathetic nervous system input, causing the pupil to dilate in low light and contract the ciliary muscle.**
2. This is the scientific rationale for mydriatic medications, which dilate the pupil, reducing aqueous humor production, and increase absorption effectiveness, reducing intraocular pressure in open-angle glaucoma.
3. This is the scientific rationale for beta-adrenergic blockers, which reduce intraocular pressure but do not affect pupil size and lens accommodation.
4. This is the scientific rationale for carbonic anhydrase inhibitors, which reduce intraocular pressure.

19. 1. NSAIDs are appropriate interventions for clients diagnosed with back pain. They decrease pain and inflammation.
2. **Opioid analgesics are administered for pain. The client is in the mild pain range. The nurse would question administering morphine, an opioid analgesic, because of its addictive properties. A less potent analgesic should be administered.**
3. Muscle relaxant medications are administered to clients diagnosed with back pain to relax muscles and decrease pain. The nurse would administer methocarbamol (Robaxin), a muscle relaxant.
4. Acetaminophen, an analgesic and antipyretic, can be administered to decrease pain. The nurse would administer this medication.

20. 1. **Decongestants vasoconstrict the blood vessels, resulting in decreased inflammation in the nasal passages. This vasoconstriction is why OTC cold medications are labeled not to be used by clients diagnosed with HTN and diabetes.**
2. Decongestants do not decrease the immune system's response to the virus.
3. Activating viral receptors would increase cold symptoms.
4. This is the rationale for zinc. Theoretically, zinc blocks the virus from binding to the nasal epithelium. Research has shown that increased amounts of zinc can prevent rhinovirus binding and development.

21. 1. The digoxin level is within the therapeutic range; therefore, the nurse could administer the cardiotonic digoxin, but it is a routine medication and can be administered at any time.
2. **Pleuritic pain involves the thoracic pleura, and pain rated a "7" should be treated with the narcotic morphine before routine medications are dispensed.**
3. A client with two unifocal PVCs in a minute would be considered normal, and no intervention would be needed at this time.
4. This BP is within normal limits, and the angiotensin-converting enzyme (ACE) inhibitor lisinopril (Vasotec) could be given within the 30-minute time frame.

22. 1. The normal serum potassium level is 3.5 to 5.3 mEq/L; therefore, the nurse would administer the loop diuretic furosemide (Lasix).
2. The normal serum osmolality is 275 to 295 mOsm/kg; therefore, the nurse would administer the osmotic diuretic mannitol (Osmitrol).
3. The normal digoxin level is 0.5 to 2 mg/dL; a digoxin level of 1.2 mg/dL is within therapeutic range. The nurse would administer the cardiac glycoside digoxin (Lanoxin).
4. **The therapeutic serum level of Dilantin is 10 to 20 mcg/mL; therefore, the nurse should question administering the anticonvulsant phenytoin (Dilantin).**

23.

Potential Nursing Intervention	Indicated	Not Indicated
1. Administer medication undiluted.	X	
2. Check client's serum potassium level.	X	
3. Pinch off the IV tubing above the port.	X	
4. Inject medication over 5 minutes at a steady rate.	X	
5. Explain that experiencing a yellow haze is an expected side effect.		X

1. The digoxin (Lanoxin) can be administered undiluted or can dilute 1 mL digoxin with 4 mL sterile water, dextrose 5% in water, or normal saline.
2. Hypokalemia may potentiate digoxin toxicity; therefore, the nurse should check the client's potassium level.
3. The nurse should pinch off the tubing above the port to ensure that digoxin (Lanoxin) flows into the client's vein and not upward into the IV tubing.
4. Digoxin (Lanoxin) should be injected slowly over 5 minutes (2 minutes for most IV medications, except for medications that act directly on the cardiovascular system and narcotics) and at a steady rate because a rapid injection could cause speed shock. Speed shock is a sudden adverse physiological reaction secondary to an IVP medication wherein the client develops a flushed face, headache, a tight feeling in the chest, irregular pulse, loss of consciousness, and possible cardiac arrest.
5. A yellow haze, nausea, vomiting, and anorexia are clinical manifestations of digoxin toxicity and should be reported to the HCP.

24. 1. Chlordiazepoxide (Librium), a benzodiazepine, would not help a client addicted to cocaine.
2. Methadone, not Librium, blocks the heroin craving.
3. Librium would not help a client addicted to amphetamines.
4. Chlordiazepoxide (Librium), a benzodiazepine, is the drug of choice to prevent neurological complications and delirium tremens (DTs), a life-threatening complication of alcohol withdrawal.

25. 1. A smoking cessation support group may be helpful, but nicotine involves a physical withdrawal, and medication should help with withdrawal symptoms.
2. Tapering the daily number of cigarettes is not the most successful method to quit smoking cigarettes.
3. Research has shown that 44% of smokers were able to quit smoking at the end of 12 weeks with varenicline, a smoking cessation medication, compared to other smoking cessation medications, which have a 30% chance of success. It reduces the urge to smoke. The makers of varenicline (Chantix) recalled the medication in 2021 due to high levels of nitrosamines. The FDA, however, has approved the generic varenicline for production in the United States because nitrosamine levels are within acceptable ranges (U.S. Food & Drug Administration, 2021).
4. Clonidine is used to help prevent DTs for clients diagnosed with alcohol dependence.

26. 1. The osmotic diuretic mannitol (Osmitrol) would not be contraindicated for a client diagnosed with HIV.
2. Mannitol, an osmotic diuretic, would not be contraindicated for a client diagnosed with glaucoma. The osmotic diuretic medication Diamox is administered to clients diagnosed with glaucoma.
3. Because the osmotic diuretic mannitol (Osmitrol) will pull fluid off the brain by osmosis into the circulatory system, it can lead to a circulatory overload, which the heart could not handle because the client already has a diagnosis of CHF. This client would need an order for a loop diuretic to prevent serious cardiac complications.
4. The client is 16 years old, and even diagnosed with CF, the client's heart should be able to handle the fluid-volume overload.

27. 1. Lidocaine suppresses ventricular ectopy and is used to treat ventricular dysrhythmias if amiodarone is not available.
2. Atropine decreases vagal stimulation, which increases the heart rate and is the drug of choice for asystole, complete heart block, and symptomatic bradycardia.
3. Adenosine is the drug of choice for terminating paroxysmal supraventricular tachycardia by decreasing automaticity of the sinoatrial (SA) node and slowing conduction through the atrioventricular (AV) node.
4. Epinephrine constricts the periphery and shunts the blood to the central trunk, and is the first medication administered for a coding client diagnosed with asystole.

28. 1. The client should adhere to a low-fat, low-cholesterol diet, but this does not indicate the medication is effective.
2. Atorvastatin (Lipitor), an HMG-CoA reductase inhibitor, is prescribed to help decrease the client's cholesterol level; therefore, this statement indicates it is effective.
3. A sedentary lifestyle is a risk factor for developing atherosclerosis; therefore, exercising should be praised, but it does not indicate effective medication.

4. Atorvastatin (Lipitor), an HMG-CoA reductase inhibitor, is not administered to decrease edema; therefore, this statement does not indicate the medication is effective.

29. 1. Prednisone, a glucocorticoid, is an oral preparation and one that can be given daily. This is not the first medication to be administered.
2. An initial dose of Ceftriaxone (Rocephin), an IV antibiotic, is a priority because the client must be started on the medication as soon as possible to prevent the client from becoming septic.
3. Lactic acidophilus (Lactinex) is administered to replace the good bacteria in the body destroyed by the antibiotic, but it does not need to be administered first.
4. Cephalexin (Keflex) PO is an oral antibiotic, but this client is being discharged, indicating the client's condition has improved. This client could wait until the initial dose of an IV antibiotic is administered.

30. Correct answer is 1 and 4.
1. WBCs are monitored to detect presence of an infection. An elevated WBC count is a finding of infection that would warrant intervention. Steroids such as methylprednisolone (Solu-Medrol), a glucocorticoid, mask infection.
2. The Hgb level is monitored to detect blood loss, not for steroid therapy.
3. The Hct level is monitored to detect blood loss, not steroid therapy.
4. Steroid therapy interferes with glucose metabolism and increases insulin resistance. The blood glucose levels should be monitored to determine if an intervention is needed. A glucose level of 238 would warrant intervention.
5. The creatinine level is monitored to determine renal status and is within normal limits. The adrenal glands produce cortisol.
6. The client's potassium level is within normal limits; therefore, this does not warrant intervention.

31. 1. This client has normal ABGs, but the oxygen level is below normal (80 to 95); therefore, the nurse should administer oxygen.
2. The client has normal ABGs; therefore, an antianxiety medication does not need to be administered. The client needs oxygen.
3. Sodium bicarbonate is the drug of choice for metabolic acidosis, and this client has normal ABGs except for hypoxia.
4. The client has normal ABGs with hypoxia.

32. 1. This Hct is normal but does not indicate that the client is responding to the antibiotics.
2. Thick green sputum is a finding of pneumonia, indicating that antibiotic therapy is ineffective. If the sputum were changing from thick green sputum to thinner, lighter-colored sputum, it would indicate an improvement in the condition.
3. The clinical manifestations of pneumonia include crackles and wheezing in the lung fields. Clear lung sounds indicate an improvement in pneumonia and that the medication is effective.
4. Pleuritic chest is a symptom of pneumonia and does not indicate the medication is effective. Lack of symptoms indicates the medication is effective.

33. 1. This is the mechanism of action for antacids.
2. This is the mechanism of action for histamine$_2$ blockers.
3. This is the mechanism of action for PPIs.
4. This is the mechanism of action for mucosal barrier agents.

34. Correct answers are 2, 3, and 4.
1. TPN is 50% dextrose; therefore, the client's blood glucose level should be checked every 6 hours, and sliding-scale insulin coverage should be ordered.
2. TPN should always be administered using an IV pump and not by gravity. Fluid volume and increased glucose resulting from a TPN overload could cause a life-threatening fluid volume or hyperglycemic crisis.
3. TPN must be administered via a subclavian line, and any infection may lead to endocarditis; therefore, the nurse should assess the site.
4. TPN is considered a medication and should be administered as any other medication.
5. The client diagnosed with severe acute exacerbation of Crohn's is nothing by mouth (NPO) to rest the bowel. When clients are on TPN, they are usually NPO because TPN provides all necessary nutrients; therefore, the nurse would not encourage eating food.

35. 1. This is the rationale for administering mineral oil.
2. This is the rationale for administering stimulants.
3. Stool softeners or surfactants have a detergent action to reduce surface tension, permitting water and fats to penetrate and soften the stool.
4. This is the rationale for bulk-forming agents.

36. 1. The normal plasma ammonia level is 15 to 45 mcg/dL (varies with method); this is below normal. The client diagnosed with end-stage liver failure would be receiving lactulose (Cephulac), a laxative, and the client does not need to receive a laxative that will cause diarrhea.
2. The normal serum potassium level is 3.5 to 5.3 mEq/L; therefore, the nurse should administer furosemide (Lasix), a loop diuretic, because the potassium level is within normal limits.
3. The normal serum potassium level is 3.5 to 5.3 mEq/L; therefore, the nurse should not question administering spironolactone (Aldactone), a potassium-sparing diuretic, because the potassium level is within normal limits.
4. Hyponatremia (normal sodium: 135 to 145 mEq/L) may occur when the client is taking vasopressin therapy. This sodium level is within normal limits; therefore, the nurse would not question administering vasopressin (Pitressin).

37.

Potential Nursing Intervention	Indicated	Not Indicated
1. Assess the client for hypoglycemia around 1800.		X
2. Ensure the client eats the nighttime snack.		X
3. Check client's blood glucose level via a glucometer.	X	
4. Determine how much food the client ate at lunch.	X	
5. Monitor client for low blood glucose around 1500.	X	

1. Insulin isophane (Humulin N) is an intermediate-acting insulin that will peak 6 to 8 hours after administration; therefore, the client would experience hypoglycemia symptoms around 1300 to 1500.
2. The nurse must ensure the client eats the nighttime (HS) snack to help prevent nighttime hypoglycemia if the insulin isophane (Humulin N) is administered at 1600. This insulin has been administered at 0700, so the nurse should ensure that the client eats lunch or a mid-afternoon snack for this administration time.
3. The client should have the blood glucose checked. It should be done with a glucometer at the bedside.
4. Eating the food from the lunch tray will help prevent a hypoglycemic reaction because insulin isophane (Humulin N) is an intermediate-acting insulin that peaks in 6 to 8 hours.
5. The insulin isophane (Humulin N) peaks in 6 to 8 hours; therefore, the nurse should assess the client for hypoglycemia around 1500.

38. 1. Insulin lispro (Humalog), fast-acting insulin, will not be working 4 to 5 hours after being administered.
2. Insulin lispro (Humalog), fast-acting insulin, peaks 15 to 20 minutes after being administered; therefore, the meal should be at the bedside before administering this medication.
3. The glucose level should be checked before meals, not after meals.
4. This medication is administered when a client is unconscious secondary to hypoglycemia and should not be kept at the bedside. Orange juice or some type of simple glucose should be kept at the bedside.

39. Correct answers are 2, 3, 4, and 5.
1. Weight gain indicates the client is not taking enough medication.
2. Intolerance to heat indicates the client is not taking too much medication.
3. Tachycardia, a heart rate greater than 100, is a finding of hyperthyroidism and indicates the client is taking too much levothyroxine (Synthroid).
4. Increased metabolism and diarrhea indicate the client is taking too much levothyroxine (Synthroid), a thyroid hormone.

5. **Fine hand tremors indicate the client is taking too much levothyroxine (Synthroid), a thyroid hormone. This is a finding of hyperthyroidism.**

40. 1. Insulin lispro (Humalog), fast-acting insulin, is not administered intravenously, and glucose levels should be monitored before insulin administration.
2. **Steatorrhea is fatty, frothy stools that indicate pancreatic enzymes are not sufficient for digestive purposes. The nurse should be prepared to administer pancrelipase (Cotazym), a pancreatic enzyme.**
3. Insulin regular (Humulin R) is administered by a sliding scale to decrease blood glucose levels. Clients diagnosed with pancreatitis should be monitored for development of diabetes mellitus.
4. Famotidine (Pepcid), a $histamine_2$ receptor blocker, would not treat the client's symptoms.

41. 1. **Sodium polystyrene sulfonate (Kayexalate), a cation exchange resin, is a medication that is administered to decrease an elevated serum potassium level; therefore, elevated serum potassium (5.5 mEq/L) would indicate the medication is not effective.**
2. Kayexalate is not used to alter the serum sodium level.
3. Sodium polystyrene sulfonate (Kayexalate), a cation exchange resin, is a medication that is administered to decrease an elevated serum potassium level; therefore, a potassium level within the normal range of 3.5 to 5.3 mEq/L indicates the medication is effective.
4. Kayexalate is not used to alter the serum sodium level.

42. 1. **The saline irrigation is being instilled into the bladder and requires nursing judgment; therefore, this nursing task requires immediate intervention.**
2. The UAP reporting abnormal data is appropriate. A green-blue color indicates the client is taking bethanechol (Urecholine), a urinary stimulant used for clients diagnosed with a neurogenic bladder. This is an expected color.
3. The client should be encouraged to drink fluids. The registered nurse (RN) would not intervene to stop this action.
4. This action encourages bowel and urine continence and is part of a fall prevention protocol. The nurse would not intervene to stop this action.

43.

Potential Nursing Intervention	Indicated	Not Indicated
1. Medication will dry the lesions within a day or two.		X
2. Valacyclovir is taken once a day to control out-breaks.	X	
3. Condom use will increase herpes spread.		X
4. After lesions are gone, the client will not transmit the virus.		X
5. Wash hands frequently to prevent virus transmission.	X	
6. Drink plenty of water while taking valacyclovir.	X	

1. **The time for lesions to heal depends on several factors, including immune status of the individual infected and amount of stress the individual is experiencing at the time. It usually requires several days to more than a week to heal from an outbreak.**
2. **Suppressive therapy with valacyclovir (Valtrex) is once daily, every day. This is an advantage of Valtrex over other antiretroviral medications, which require twice-a-day dosing.**
3. **Condom use may prevent spread of herpes infections; it does not increase virus spread.**
4. **It is possible to transmit the virus to a sexual partner with no visible findings of a lesion being present. Valacyclovir (Valtrex) will not prevent virus spread. It will treat an outbreak and decrease transmission risk.**
5. **The client should be taught to wash hands frequently to prevent infection transmission.**
6. **Clients should be taught to drink plenty of fluids while taking valacyclovir to lessen the impact on kidney function.**

44. 1. **If the client's deep tendon reflexes are 4+, indicating the client may have a seizure at any time, this indicates that magnesium sulfate, an anticonvulsant medication, is not effective.**
    2. Magnesium sulfate is not administered to treat the client's BP; therefore, this data cannot be used to evaluate medication effectiveness.
    3. Magnesium sulfate is administered to prevent seizure activity and is determined to be effective and in the therapeutic range when the client's deep tendon reflexes are normal, which is 2+ to 3+ on a 0 to 4+ scale.
    4. A 0 deep tendon reflex indicates the client has received too much magnesium sulfate, but the client would not have seizure activity; therefore, it is effective. The client is at risk for respiratory depression.

45. 1. The client should swallow the medication. The client should not crush, chew, or suck the medication.
    2. The medication should be taken on an empty stomach at least 30 minutes before eating or drinking any liquid. Foods and beverages significantly decrease the effect of Fosamax.
    3. Alendronate (Fosamax), a bisphosphonate, will irritate the stomach and esophagus if the client lies down; therefore, the medication should be taken when the client can remain upright for at least 30 minutes.
    4. **Alendronate (Fosamax), a bisphosphonate, can be taken daily or weekly. Still, because of the high risk of esophageal complications, if the client does not take Fosamax exactly as prescribed, most HCPs prescribe the medication to be taken once a week. The client must take the medication on an empty stomach and remain upright for a minimum of 30 minutes.**

46. 1. Urine does not change color when the client takes methotrexate (Rheumatrex), an antineoplastic agent.
    2. The client should be encouraged to eat a balanced diet; drinking a supplement is unnecessary.
    3. **Methotrexate (Rheumatrex), an antineoplastic agent, suppresses the bone marrow, resulting in decreased numbers of WBCs. The client should notify the HCP if a fever develops, indicating an infection.**
    4. There is no reason to increase the green, leafy vegetables consumed when taking this medication.

47. 1. **Mafenide acetate (Sulfamylon), a topical antimicrobial agent, affects the acid-base balance in the body and should not be administered to clients diagnosed with renal disease. A 2.8 mg/dL serum creatinine level indicates renal insufficiency; therefore, the nurse would use caution with this client.**
    2. Clients diagnosed with CHF would not be affected by this medication.
    3. This client has adequate respiratory status; therefore, the nurse would not need to use caution with this client.
    4. There is no reason a client diagnosed with diabetes could not be prescribed mafenide acetate (Sulfamylon), a topical antimicrobial agent.

48. 1. Botulinum toxin type A (Botox) will reduce wrinkles, but that is not why it is administered to a client diagnosed with a cerebrovascular accident (CVA). Paralysis of the facial muscles lasts 3 to 6 months.
    2. **Botulinum toxin type A (Botox), an antispasmodic, produces partial chemical denervation of the muscle, resulting in localized reduction in muscle activity and spasticity.**
    3. This medication will not improve limb weakness.
    4. Botulinum toxin type A (Botox), an antispasmodic, does not help with pain secondary to neuropathy.

49. **500 mL/hr. The nurse should divide 8,000 mL by 2, which equals 4,000 mL. The 4,000 must be divided by 8, which equals 500 mL/hr. There are formulas that are used to determine the client's fluid-volume resuscitation. The formulas specify that the total amount of fluid must be infused in 24 hours, 50% in the first 8 hours followed by the other 50% over the other 16 hours. This is a large amount of fluid, but it is not uncommon in clients diagnosed with full-thickness burns over greater than 20% total body surface area.**

50. 1. Wearing insect repellent is an appropriate intervention, but if the client has an insect bite, repellent will not help prevent anaphylaxis; therefore, this is not the priority intervention.
    2. Antihistamines are used for clients diagnosed with anaphylaxis. Still, it takes at least 30 minutes for the medication to work, and if the client has an insect bite, it is not the priority medication.

3. Clients with documented severe anaphylaxis should carry an EpiPen, a prescribed epinephrine injectable device that clients can administer to themselves in case of an insect bite. Keeping the medication in the refrigerator does not allow it to be available to the client at all times.
4. The client should wear a MedicAlert identification bracelet because even if the client uses insect repellent, a sting could occur. The bracelet indicates the client is at risk for an anaphylactic reaction; therefore, this is the priority intervention.

51. 1. There is no cure for HIV infection; HIV is a retrovirus that never dies as long as the host is alive.
2. HAART is complex and expensive and poses a risk of toxicity and serious drug interactions.
3. Because of HAART, plasma levels of HIV can be reduced to undetectable levels with current technology.
4. HAART medications are very expensive.

52. 1. Hydroxychloroquine sulfate (Plaquenil), a disease-modifying antirheumatic drug (DMARD), can cause pigmentary retinitis and vision loss, so the client should have a thorough vision examination every 6 months; therefore, the client does not understand the medication teaching.
2. Plaquenil may increase liver toxicity risk when administered with hepatotoxic drugs, so alcohol use should be eliminated during therapy; therefore, the client does not understand the medication teaching.
3. Hydroxychloroquine sulfate (Plaquenil), a DMARD, should be taken with milk to decrease gastrointestinal upset. This statement indicates the client understands the medication teaching.
4. The medication takes 3 to 6 months to achieve the desired response; therefore, the client needs more medication teaching.

53. 1. A "3" is considered mild pain and could wait until the client with more emergent needs is medicated.
2. An antianxiety medication is not a priority over a client required to take their medication on an empty stomach. This is a potential anxiety attack over a physiological problem.
3. The medication must be administered before a meal. Administering a mucosal barrier agent after a meal places medication in the stomach to coat the food, not the stomach lining. This medication should be administered first.
4. This medication stimulates the bone marrow to produce RBCs; the medication's full effect will not be seen for 30 to 90 days. It could be administered after the antianxiety medication and the analgesic.

54. 1. The nurse should not administer pain medication until after assessing the client's pain.
2. The first action is always to assess the client in pain to determine if the client has a complication that requires medical intervention rather than PRN pain medication.
3. The nurse should assess the client, then administer the pain medication, whether the client has visitors or not.
4. The nurse should first assess the client's pain.

55. 1. Keeping the eyes closed and drapes drawn would not indicate the pain medication is effective. These actions may be the client's way of dealing with the pain.
2. Using guided imagery is an excellent method to assist with the control of pain, but its use does not indicate medication effectiveness.
3. Light snoring indicates the client is asleep, which would mean the medication is effective.
4. This action may be the client's way of dealing with the pain, but it does not indicate the medication is effective.

56. Correct answers are 1 and 3.
1. The client's WBC count is low, and the absolute neutrophil count is 1,100, which indicates the client is immunosuppressed; therefore, the client should not be exposed to people with active infections.
2. This is good information to teach, but it is not based on laboratory values. The client may develop mouth ulcers as a result of chemotherapy administration, and the nurse should discuss methods of maintaining nutrition for this reason, not the laboratory values.
3. The client's WBC count is low and the absolute neutrophil count is 1,100, indicating the client is immunosuppressed; therefore, the client should avoid contact with live plants or flowers (soil and standing water germs).
4. This is good information to teach, but it is not based on laboratory values. Cancer and treatment-related fatigue are real and should be addressed. Hgb and Hct levels of around 8 and 24, respectively, could cause fatigue, but at the current level, this is not indicated.

5. A platelet count of less than 100,000 is the definition of thrombocytopenia; therefore, this client is not at risk for bleeding.

57. 1. This level is above the therapeutic range; therefore, the nurse should not administer the medication.

2. The therapeutic serum level is 0.6 to 1.2 mEq/L; therefore, the first intervention is to hold the lithium (Eskalith), an antimania medication.

3. After holding the medication, the nurse should notify the HCP.

4. The nurse should first hold the lithium (Eskalith), an antimania medication, and then verify the level later.

58.

Statement by Parent	Effective	Not Effective
1. "I will keep the medication in a safe place."	X	
2. "I will give my child this medication every 12 hours."		X
3. "It may cause my child to have growth spurts."		X
4. "My child will probably experience insomnia."		X
5. "I will notify the HCP if my child reports finger pain."	X	

1. All medication must be kept in a safe place to prevent accidental poisoning of children.

2. The last medication should be administered no later than 1400 in the afternoon or the child will not sleep at night. Methylphenidate (Ritalin) is a central nervous system (CNS) stimulant. This statement indicates the mother does not understand the medication teaching.

3. Growth rate may be stalled in response to nutritional deficiency caused by anorexia; it does not cause growth spurts. This statement indicates the mother does not understand the medication teaching.

4. Insomnia is an adverse reaction to methylphenidate (Ritalin), a CNS stimulant; CNS stimulants may disrupt normal sleep patterns. This statement indicates that medication teaching has not been effective.

5. Methylphenidate can cause Raynaud's phenomenon, characterized by tingling or pain in the fingers or toes when exposed to cold temperatures or a skin color change in the toes or fingers. This statement indicates that medication teaching has been effective.

59. Correct answers are 1, 2, and 5.

1. The client should instill eye ointment into the lower conjunctival sac, which is the inner edge of the lower lid margin.

2. This pressure will prevent systemic medication absorption.

3. The client does not have to wear gloves when applying the ointment to their eyes. The client should be instructed to wash hands before and after using the ointment.

4. The antibiotic ointment should be applied from the inner canthus to the outer canthus, from the nose side of the eye to the outer area.

5. The client should be in this position when applying ophthalmic ointment or drops to better access the lower conjunctival sac.

60. 1. The outer canthus does not have access to the systemic system; therefore, the nurse would not hold pressure in this area.

2. The nurse should not hold pressure under the eyelid because the medication will not be retained in the eye.

3. The nurse cannot hold pressure in the lower conjunctival sac because this would be painful for the client and would not prevent systemic medication absorption.

4. The lacrimal duct is located in the inner canthus area and systemic medication absorption can occur if the nurse does not apply light pressure to the area.

61. 1. This is a low BP reading for a client in hypovolemic shock. A BP less than 90/60 warrants intervention by the nurse and indicates fluid resuscitation is not effective.

2. A pulse oximeter reading of greater than 93% indicates the arterial oxygen level is between 80 and 100, which is normal.

3. The client's lungs are clear, which indicates the client is not in fluid-volume overload; therefore, this does not warrant immediate intervention.

4. If the client has at least 30 mL of urine output an hour, the kidneys are being perfused adequately. This indicates the client is urinating 40 mL an hour.

62. 1. The client in asystole would not benefit from defibrillation because there is no heart activity. The client must have some heart activity (ventricular activity) for defibrillation to be successful.
2. Synchronized cardioversion is used for new-onset atrial fibrillation or unstable ventricular tachycardia.
3. Epinephrine is given IV or IO to increase blood flow during cardiopulmonary resuscitation with asystole.
4. Amiodarone, an antidysrhythmic, is administered in life-threatening ventricular dysrhythmias, not asystole.

63. 1. Acetylcysteine, an antidote, does not neutralize substances by changing their pH.
2. Acetylcysteine is not used to treat bleach poisonings. Charcoal binds with poisons to form an inert substance that can be eliminated through the bowel because the body cannot absorb charcoal molecules.
3. This is the scientific rationale for administering acetylcysteine, an antidote.
4. Acetylcysteine does not cause emesis. An emetic such as ipecac would induce vomiting.

64. 1. The child's weight is pertinent information, but it is not the most important question.
2. Most dishwashing liquids are vegetable-based products that produce osmotic diarrhea when ingested; therefore, the nurse should ask about abdominal cramping. The soap is not poisonous, but the child may become dehydrated and be uncomfortable.
3. Because the parent has called the ED, it is not a priority to know if they called the Poison Control Center.
4. Determining where the soap was will not help the child.

65. 1. Acetylsalicylic acid (Aspirin) does not affect BP and pulse; therefore, the nurse would not need to implement this intervention.
2. Aspirin will not cause a breakdown of fat, which results in increased ketone production.
3. Daily acetylsalicylic acid (Aspirin) is taken as an antiplatelet medication, not as an antipyretic.
4. This information should be documented in the EHR, and no further action should be taken.

66. 1. Iron turns the stool a harmless black or dark green. This statement indicates the client understands the medication teaching.
2. The iron tablet, a mineral, should be taken between meals and with 8 ounces of water to promote absorption. The iron tablet should not be taken within 1 hour of ingesting antacid, milk, ice cream, or other milk products such as pudding. This statement indicates the client does not understand the medication teaching.
3. Sitting upright will prevent esophageal corrosion from reflux. This statement indicates the client understands the medication teaching.
4. The drug treatment for anemia generally lasts less than 6 months. This statement indicates the client understands the medication teaching.

67. 1. This is the scientific rationale for a coronary vasodilator.
2. This is the scientific rationale for antiplatelet medications.
3. Antioxidants are being prescribed to help prevent cardiovascular diseases.
4. Rest is the only action that will help decrease oxygen demands of the peripheral tissues.

68. 1. According to guidelines for prudent use of herbs, babies and young children should not be given any types of herbs.
2. Herbs exposed to sunlight and heat may lose their potency.
3. When presenting information as a nurse, the nurse must encourage a discussion with an HCP when substituting herbs for prescribed medications.
4. This is a guideline that consumers and HCPs must know when using herbal therapy.

69. 1. The UAP cannot administer medications, and medications should not be left at the bedside. Medication aides are permitted in some states to practice in long-term care facilities. This was not stated in the stem. Regardless, no one should administer a medication dispensed by another person.
2. The UAP should take the medication cup back to the medication room and tell the registered nurse (RN). Medications should never be left at the bedside.

3. The UAP should not correct the RN in front of the client; therefore, this would not be an appropriate intervention. This is not in the realm of a UAP's duties. The person over the nurse is the one to confront the nurse.
4. The UAP is a vital part of the health-care team and is expected to maintain client safety.

70. **Correct answers are 1 and 2.**
   1. **The nurse should prepare the medication using a 25-gauge, 1/2- to 5/8-inch needle.**
   2. **The nurse should not aspirate for blood when administering heparin, an anticoagulant, because this can damage surrounding tissue and cause bruising.**
   3. The client's PTT is not monitored for subcutaneous heparin administration because the heparin must be administered intravenously to increase the PTT level.
   4. The nurse should not massage after injecting heparin because this may cause bruising or bleeding.
   5. Heparin is administered in the lower abdominal area at least 2 inches from the umbilicus. Lovenox is administered in the "love handles," located anterolateral to the upper abdomen.

71. 1. The INR is monitored for oral anticoagulant therapy, warfarin (Coumadin).
   2. The PT is not directly monitored for oral anticoagulant therapy but will be elevated in clients receiving oral anticoagulants.
   3. **The PTT should be 1.5 to 2.0 times the normal PTT of a control to determine if IV heparin, an anticoagulant, is therapeutic.**
   4. The platelet count is not monitored during heparin therapy.

72.

Potential Nursing Intervention	Indicated	Not Indicated
1. Instruct client to take acetaminophen for a headache.	X	
2. Tell client to stay on a clear liquid diet for the next 24 hours.		X
3. Instruct client to take one hydrocodone for pain.		X
4. Recommend client take acetylsalicylic acid for any physical discomfort.		X
5. Tell client to return to the ED if experiencing nausea and vomiting.	X	
6. Encourage client to maintain strict bedrest for 24 hours.		X
7. Advise client to avoid alcohol until fully recovered.	X	
8. Teach client to remain awake for the next 12 hours.		X

1. **The client can take nonnarcotic analgesics if experiencing a headache. Acetaminophen (Tylenol) would be appropriate to take for a headache.**
2. **The client can eat anything after experiencing a concussion.**
3. **Narcotic analgesics should not be taken after a head injury because of further depression of the neurological status.**
4. **The client should not take acetylsalicylic acid (Aspirin) because it may cause bleeding, increasing intracranial pressure.**
5. **Any nausea, vomiting (especially projectile), or blurred vision could be increasing intracranial pressure; therefore, the client should return to the ED for further evaluation.**
6. **The client does not have to remain in bed for 24 hours, although the client should be instructed to avoid exercise, lifting weights, or other heavy activity.**
7. **The client should avoid alcohol until fully recovered to decrease chances of another injury.**
8. **The client does not need to remain awake for 12 hours after discharge. Still, the HCP may ask someone to wake the client every 2 to 3 hours during this period to ensure the client is not experiencing confusion or other neurological changes.**

73. **1. The therapeutic serum level of carbamazepine (Tegretol) is 4 to 12 mcg/mL; therefore, the nurse should question administering this medication.**
2. The therapeutic serum level of clonazepam (Klonopin) is 0.02 to 0.08 mcg/mL; therefore, the nurse should administer this medication.
3. The therapeutic serum level of phenytoin (Dilantin) is 10 to 20 mcg/mL; therefore, the nurse should administer this medication.
4. The therapeutic serum level of ethosuximide (Zarontin) is 40 to 100 mcg/mL; therefore, the nurse should administer this medication.

74. **1. Donepezil (Aricept) and other cholinesterase inhibitors can potentially delay the progression of Alzheimer's disease. The client and family should be told that it only lasts for 6 months to a year, although it offers them hope.**
2. Aricept does not repair the brain tissue; no medication repairs lost brain tissue.
3. Donepezil (Aricept), a cholinesterase inhibitor, is not an experimental medication. Aricept works by preventing acetylcholine (Ach) breakdown by acetylcholinesterase and thereby increases Ach availability at the cholinergic synapses.
4. Aricept is the best tolerated of the cholinesterase inhibitors because it has fewer side effects.

75. 1. Primary brain tumors rarely metastasize outside of the cranium because they kill by occupying space and increasing intracranial pressure.
2. Dexamethasone (Decadron), a glucocorticoid, is not an anticonvulsant; it may reduce the chance of seizures by decreasing intracranial pressure, but the client may still have a seizure while taking Decadron.
3. Decadron does not affect serotonin uptake.
4. Dexamethasone (Decadron), a glucocorticoid, decreases the inflammatory response of tissues. It is mainly used for edema (swelling) of brain tissues.

76. Correct answers are 2, 3, and 4.
1. Administration of alteplase (Activase) is not contraindicated for clients diagnosed with CHF.
2. Surgery and bleeding ulcers are both reasons for not administering thrombolytic therapy to the client.
3. A CT scan must be done before administering alteplase (Activase) to ensure that the CVA is not caused by an intracranial hemorrhage. There are three types of stroke: thrombotic, embolic, and hemorrhagic. If the client is experiencing a hemorrhagic stroke, administering a medication that dissolves clots could initiate more bleeding and cause death.
4. The client receiving anticoagulants cannot receive thrombolytic therapy due to increased bleeding time secondary to the anticoagulant therapy.
5. This history would indicate the client has experienced a DVT and may have been on anticoagulants but is not on them at this time; therefore, the client can receive thrombolytic therapy.

77. 1. Protamine sulfate is the antidote for heparin toxicity.
2. The therapeutic range for INR is 2 to 3; therefore, the nurse should document the results and take no action.
3. Vitamin K is the antidote for warfarin (Coumadin) toxicity, which is supported by an elevated INR greater than 3.
4. The nurse does not need to notify the HCP of a normal laboratory value.

78. 1. After opening the medication, the nurse should date and time the patch before putting it on the client so that the nurse does not press the client when writing on the patch.
2. The old patch should be removed but not before checking the MAR.
3. The nurse should administer the patch in a clean, dry, nonhairy place while wearing gloves.
4. The nurse should implement the Rights of Medication Administration, and the first ones are to make sure it is the right medication and the right client.

79. 1. Digoxin (Lanoxin), a cardiac glycoside, does not affect the client's BP; therefore, it cannot be used to determine medication effectiveness.
2. The client's apical pulse must be assessed before administering digoxin (Lanoxin), a cardiac glycoside, but it is not used to determine medication effectiveness.
3. The client's potassium level must be assessed before administering digoxin (Lanoxin), a cardiac glycoside, but it is not used to determine medication effectiveness.

4. Clinical manifestations of CHF are crackles in the lungs, jugular vein distention, and pitting edema; therefore, digoxin (Lanoxin), a cardiac glycoside, is not effective.

80. 1. Amiodarone suppresses ventricular ectopy and is the first-line drug for the treatment of ventricular dysrhythmias, but it is not the first medication to be administered in a code.

2. Atropine decreases vagal stimulation, which increases the heart rate and is the drug of choice for complete heart block and symptomatic bradycardia.

3. Adenosine is the drug of choice for terminating paroxysmal supraventricular tachycardia by decreasing automaticity of the SA node and slowing conduction through the AV node.

4. Epinephrine constricts the periphery, shunts blood to the central trunk, and is the first medication administered to a client in a code. The client does not have a pulse (asystole); therefore, the nurse must call a code.

81. 1. The nurse would want to give this antihypertensive medication to a client with an elevated BP. The nurse would question the angiotensin receptor blocker losartan (Cozaar) if BP was low.

2. The client diagnosed with 2+ pitting edema would not be affected by diltiazem (Cardizem), a calcium channel blocker.

3. The nurse should question the alpha blocker terazosin (Hytrin) if the apical rate is less than 60 bpm.

4. A headache is not an adverse effect of the thiazide diuretic hydrochlorothiazide (HCTZ); therefore, the nurse would not question administering this medication.

82. Correct answers are 1, 2, and 5.

1. Steroids (glucocorticoids) cannot be abruptly discontinued because the adrenal glands stop producing cortisol (a steroid) when the client is taking them exogenously, and the client could experience a hypotensive crisis.

2. Prednisone, a glucocorticoid, can produce gastric distress. It is given with food to minimize gastric discomfort.

3. Weight gain is a side effect of steroid therapy; the client should not stop taking the medication. This medication must be tapered off if the client can discontinue the medication at all.

4. Prednisone, a glucocorticoid, is not affected by light, so it does not have to be kept in a dark-colored bottle. Sublingual nitroglycerin needs to be stored in a dark-colored bottle.

5. Prednisone, a steroid, suppresses the body's immune system response, increasing risk of developing an infection.

83. 1. The PEFR is defined as the maximal rate of airflow during expiration. It can be measured with a relatively inexpensive, handheld device. More frequent monitoring should be done if the peak flow is less than 80% of the client's personal best. The PEFR should be measured every morning.

2. A normal respiratory assessment does not indicate that the medication regimen is effective and has "good" or "bad" control.

3. Three asthma attacks in the past month would not indicate the client has "good" control of the reactive airway disease.

4. A serum theophylline level between 10 and 20 mcg/mL indicates the medication is within the therapeutic range. Still, it is not the best indicator of the client's control of clinical manifestations.

84. 1. Steroids increase insulin resistance; this would be an expected effect of prednisone, a glucocorticoid. The nurse would not question administering this medication.

2. This WBC count is elevated and indicates an infection. Antibiotics are administered for bacterial infections. The nurse would not question administering ceftriaxone (Rocephin), an antibiotic.

3. The therapeutic range for this control would be 59 to 78 seconds. This is an extremely high PTT level, and the client is at risk for bleeding. The heparin should be discontinued immediately. The nurse would question heparin, an anticoagulant.

4. This theophylline level is therapeutic (10 to 20 mcg/dL). The nurse would not question administering theophylline (Theo-Dur).

85. 1. The INR is outside of the therapeutic range; therefore, the nurse should question administering warfarin (Coumadin), an anticoagulant.

2. Vitamin K is the antidote for Coumadin toxicity. Protamine sulfate is the antidote for heparin toxicity.

3. There is no reason to notify the HCP to request an increase in the dose; the dose should be discontinued. The HCP should be notified of this abnormal laboratory data.
4. When the nurse is administering Coumadin, the INR must be monitored to determine the therapeutic level, which is 2 to 3. Because the INR is 4.2, the nurse should not administer warfarin (Coumadin), an anticoagulant.

86. 1. The client's WBC count shows a normal value, which would indicate the medication is effective.
2. This culture indicates there is still infection; therefore, the medication is not effective.
3. This indicates medication compliance, not medication effectiveness.
4. Pleurisy is noncardiac chest pain, which indicates that the medication is not effective.

87. 1. NSAIDs decrease prostaglandin and increase the client's risk for ulcer disease. They are contraindicated in clients diagnosed with ulcer disease. The nurse should question ibuprofen (Motrin), an NSAID.
2. Omeprazole (Prilosec), a PPI, is prescribed to treat duodenal and gastric ulcers; therefore, the nurse would not question this medication.
3. Hypokalemia can increase digoxin toxicity. This potassium level is within the normal range (3.5 to 5.3 mEq/L); therefore, the nurse would not question digoxin (Lanoxin), a cardiotonic.
4. Magaldrate oral suspension (Riopan), an antacid, is a low-sodium antacid and is the antacid of choice for clients diagnosed with CHF. The nurse would not question this medication.

88. 1. The suppository should be retained for 1 to 3 hours, if possible, to get the maximum benefit of mesalamine (Asacol) suppository, an aspirin product. This statement indicates the client does not understand the medication teaching.
2. The client should use caution when using the suppository because it may stain clothing, flooring, painted surfaces, vinyl, enamel, marble, granite, and other surfaces. This statement indicates the client understands the teaching.
3. Mesalamine (Asacol) suppository, an aspirin product, should be stored at room temperature away from moisture and heat. This indicates the client understands the teaching.
4. The client should empty the bowel just before inserting the rectal suppository. This statement indicates the client understands the teaching.

89. 1. No one but the client should push the PCA button. If the client has pain, the client should push the button. Family members administering doses could overdose the client. This statement indicates the client and family do not understand the correct use of the PCA.
2. The client should premedicate with the PCA so that effective coughing, deep breathing, and turning can be performed with some degree of comfort. This indicates the client understands the teaching.
3. The family should let the client decide when they are in pain, and the client should use the PCA at that time. This statement indicates the family does not understand the correct use of the PCA.
4. The client should use the PCA before the pain reaches this level. This statement indicates the client does not understand the correct use of the PCA.

90. 1. This is true, but the client is using stimulant laxatives daily. This is not the most important teaching.
2. Fluids are increased when taking bulk laxatives so that fluid is available to increase stool volume.
3. If the client insists on taking a laxative daily, it should be a bulk-forming laxative such as Metamucil. This type of laxative encourages the bowel to perform its normal job and will not harm bowel integrity. Bisacodyl (Dulcolax) is a stimulant laxative. Stimulant laxative use over time causes a narrowing of the lumen of the bowel and will increase likelihood of obstipation and bowel obstruction.
4. Increasing the amount of bisacodyl (Dulcolax), a stimulant laxative, will increase potential for serious complications related to laxative abuse.

91\. 1. The registered nurse (RN) cannot delegate the care of an unstable client, and hypoglycemia is a complication of treatment for diabetes mellitus.

2. The treatment of choice for a conscious client experiencing a hypoglycemic reaction is to administer food or a source of glucose, but it is not the first intervention. Orange juice is a source of glucose, and the UAP can get it.
3. The nurse should check the MAR to determine when the last dose of insulin or oral hypoglycemic medication was administered, but it is not the first intervention.
4. **These are clinical manifestations of a hypoglycemic reaction, and the nurse should assess the client immediately; therefore, this is the first intervention.**

92\. 1. According to the sliding scale, blood glucose results should be verified when less than 60 or greater than 400.

2. The HCP does not need to be notified unless the blood glucose is greater than 400.
3. **The client's reading is 299; therefore, the nurse should administer six units of regular insulin as per the HCP's order.**
4. There is no reason for the nurse to recheck the results.

93\. 1. Constipation does not determine pancrease effectiveness of a pancreatic enzyme.

2. Steatorrhea (fatty, frothy, foul-smelling stools) or diarrhea indicates lack of pancreatic enzymes in the small intestines. This would indicate the dosage is too small and needs to be increased.
3. **Normal bowel movements indicate pancrease, a pancreatic enzyme, effectively prevents steatorrhea.**
4. Normal bowel sounds would not indicate the medication is effective.

94\. 1. **The major clinical manifestation with DI is polyuria resulting in polydipsia (extreme thirst); therefore, the client's thirst indicates that desmopressin (DDAVP), a pituitary hormone, is ineffective and would warrant notifying the HCP.**

2. If the client can sleep throughout the night, this indicates the client is not up urinating due to polyuria; therefore, the medication is effective.
3. A weight loss of 1 pound would not warrant notifying the HCP.
4. The client only urinating five times a day indicates DDAVP, a pituitary hormone, is effective; therefore, the client would not have to notify the HCP.

95\. 1. The corticosteroid dose may have to be increased during the stress of infection or surgery; therefore, this statement indicates the client does not understand the discharge teaching.

2. **This statement indicates the client understands the discharge teaching. The client may be prescribed both mineral and glucocorticoid medications.**
3. If the client gets weak or dizzy, it may indicate a medication underdosing; therefore, the client does not understand the discharge teaching.
4. The client does not have to take prophylactic antibiotics before invasive procedures.

Appendix A: Drug Charts

Classifications	Uses	Selected Interventions
ADRENERGICS (SYMPATHOMIMETICS) albuterol epinephrine metaproterenol (Alupent) terbutaline (Brethine)	Dilates bronchial smooth muscles to relieve bronchospasm. Helps manage cardiac arrest. Vasoconstricts the periphery and shunts blood to the trunk of the body when a client is coding.	• Teach the client using an inhaler to exhale forcefully, use their lips to form a tight seal around the inhaler, press the top of the inhaler, inhale deeply, and hold their breath as long as possible. Instruct the client to wait 3–5 minutes before taking a second inhalation. • Instruct the client that nervousness, anxiety, insomnia, tachycardia, palpitations, and headache may occur. • Monitor blood pressure (BP), pulse, electrocardiogram (EKG), and respiratory rate frequently. • The 1:10,000 solution can be administered undiluted. • The medication can be injected directly into the bronchial tree via endotracheal tube.
ADRENERGICS, INOTROPICS, VASOPRESSORS dopamine	Adjunct to standard measures to improve BP, cardiac output, urine output in treatment of shock unresponsive to fluid replacement.	• Monitor vital signs every 5–15 minutes; monitor EKG and cardiac output. • Monitor urine output continuously (hourly outputs) during administration. Report decrease in urine output. • Report a change in the quality of peripheral pulses or if extremities become cold or mottled. • Rate of infusion should be decreased or temporarily discontinued until BP is decreased. • Extravasation may cause severe irritation, necrosis, and tissue sloughing.
ADRENOCORTICAL STEROID INHIBITORS aminoglutethimide (Cytadren) ketoconazole (Nizoral) mitotane (Lysodren)	Decreases cortisol production. Reduces hyperadrenalism caused by ectopic adrenocorticotropic hormone secretion by a tumor that cannot be totally eradicated.	• Administer in divided doses to reduce nausea and vomiting, and instruct the client to continue taking the medication despite discomfort. • Inform the client to take safety precautions because the medication may cause drowsiness and orthostatic hypotension.

Continued

Classifications	Uses	Selected Interventions
ALKALINIZING AGENTS sodium citrate with citric acid (Bicitra) sodium bicarbonate	Elevates the plasma pH, thereby causing potassium to move into the cells and lower serum potassium levels. Management of metabolic acidosis. Alkalinizes urine and promotes excretion of certain drugs in overdose situations (phenobarbital, aspirin).	• Obtain and monitor arterial blood gases (ABGs) for signs of metabolic acidosis or alkalosis, especially in emergency situations. • Administer by rapid bolus via prefilled syringe to ensure accurate dose. • Flush IV line before and after administration to prevent incompatible medications. • Observe client for metabolic acidosis and metabolic alkalosis. • Avoid extravasation, as tissue irritation or cellulitis may occur.
ALOE VERA	Treats skin problems, heals wounds, and treats intestinal issues. Contains a component that acts against viruses such as the flu, chickenpox, and herpes, and can also kill bacteria. Stops bowels from absorbing water. This speeds the passage and volume of the bowel's contents, resulting in a laxative effect. Possesses external healing properties and speeds healing of skin injuries such as poison ivy, ulcerations, hives, and burns.	• Notify the health-care provider (HCP) before taking any herbal remedies if taking prescription or over-the-counter (OTC) medications, if pregnant or breastfeeding, having surgery, or younger than 18 or older than 65. • Do not exceed recommended dosages or take the herb longer than recommended. • Check alerts and advisories, including those of the National Center for Complementary and Integrative Health (NCCIH; formerly the National Center for Complementary and Alternative Medicine; NCCAM), the Office of Dietary Supplements, and the U.S. Food and Drug Administration (FDA).
ALPHA-GLUCOSIDASE INHIBITORS acarbose (Precose)	Slows digestion of some carbohydrates; after-meal blood glucose peaks are not as high.	• Instruct the client to take medication daily and continue other measures (diet, exercise) to decrease blood glucose levels. • Advise the client that insulin may be needed during times of increased stress. • Forewarn the client that possible adverse effects may include hypoglycemia.
ANALGESICS–ANTIPYRETICS: NSAIDS acetaminophen (Tylenol) acetylsalicylic acid (Aspirin) ibuprofen (Motrin) indomethacin (Indocin) ketorolac (Toradol) naproxen (Aleve)	Relieves pain, fever, and inflammation.	• Instruct the client to take medication with a full glass of water and just after food. • Warn the client that gastrointestinal (GI) symptoms (nausea, vomiting, bleeding, ulceration) can occur when taking these medications on a long-term basis, and symptoms should be reported to the HCP. • Teach the client to report tinnitus (ringing in ears), a sign of aspirin toxicity. • Inform the client that medication may have an anticoagulant effect. • Caution the client that overdose may be toxic to the liver.

Classifications	Uses	Selected Interventions
ANALGESICS, OPIOID codeine hydrocodone (Vicodin) hydromorphone (Dilaudid) morphine	Relieves pain by reducing pain sensation, producing sedation, and decreasing emotional upset often associated with pain; often schedule II drugs.	• Assess type, locations, and intensity of pain using a 1–10 pain scale. • Rule out any complications before administering pain medication requiring notifying the HCP. • Evaluate effectiveness of pain medication in 30 minutes. • Ensure client safety: bed in the low position, call light within reach, instruct the client to get assistance to ambulate. • Avoid overdosing, which can lead to tolerance and dependence. • Monitor the client's respiratory function. • Explain proper use of the patient-controlled analgesia (PCA) machine if used. • Monitor for bowel elimination; may cause constipation.
ANGIOTENSIN-CONVERTING ENZYME INHIBITORS captopril (Capoten) enalapril (Vasotec) lisinopril (Zestril)	Prevents angiotensin I from converting to angiotensin II, a potent vasoconstrictor, thereby decreasing peripheral vascular resistance. Blocks secretion of aldosterone from adrenal gland.	• Monitor the client's BP; if less than 90/60 mm Hg, hold and question the order. Notify HCP when holding the medication because it is cardioprotective and the drug may be given for reasons other than BP. HCP will provide a set of parameters for holding. • Instruct client to report any type of barky, goosy cough. Medication will be discontinued or changed to a different drug. • Teach the client about orthostatic hypotension. • Instruct the client not to discontinue abruptly. • Monitor potassium levels; this can cause a rise in potassium.
ANGIOTENSIN II RECEPTOR ANTAGONISTS (BLOCKERS) losartan (Cozaar) valsartan (Diovan)	Blocks angiotensin II at the receptor sites, thereby decreasing peripheral vascular resistance. Blocks secretion of aldosterone from the adrenal gland.	• Monitor the client's BP; if less than 90/60 mm Hg, hold and question the order. Notify HCP when holding because it is cardioprotective and the drug may be given for reasons other than BP. HCP will provide a set of parameters for holding. • Teach the client about orthostatic hypotension. • Instruct the client not to discontinue abruptly.
ANTACIDS aluminum hydroxide (Amphojel) calcium carbonate (Tums) magaldrate (Riopan)	Neutralizes hydrochloric acid secreted by the stomach.	• Instruct the client to take 1 and 3 hours after meals and at bedtime. • Instruct the client to avoid taking them with other medications. • Instruct the client to chew antacid tablets (not swallow them whole) and shake liquids before taking them.

Continued

Classifications	Uses	Selected Interventions
ANTIANXIETY AGENTS ***BENZODIAZEPINES*** diazepam (Valium) lorazepam (Ativan)	Treats generalized anxiety disorder and panic disorder. Acts at many levels of the central nervous system (CNS) to produce anxiolytic effects.	• Avoid use of alcohol and other CNS depressants. • Avoid drinking grapefruit juice. • These agents may cause drowsiness or dizziness; caution to avoid driving and activities requiring alertness. • Inform client that antianxiety medications are prescribed for short-term therapy and do not cure underlying problems. • Antianxiety medications have potential addictive behavior.
ANTI-ARRHYTHMICS Class IA—quinidine (Quindex), procainamide Class IB—lidocaine, phenytoin (Dilantin) Class IC—flecainide (Tambocor) Class II—propranolol Class III—amiodarone Class IV—diltiazem (Cardizem) verapamil (Calan) Miscellaneous adenosine atropine digoxin (Lanoxin)	Reduces automaticity, slows conduction of electrical impulses through the heart, and prolongs refractory period of myocardial cells.	• Take apical pulse rate before administering the drug. Notify the HCP if the rate falls below 60 beats per minute (bpm). Teach the client to monitor and record pulse. • Make sure the client is closely monitored on telemetry, with frequent BP monitoring; when administering IV, do not leave the client. • Monitor serum drug levels to maintain therapeutic range.
ANTIBIOTICS amoxicillin (Amoxil) cefazolin (Kefzol) erythromycin gentamicin penicillin (PCN) streptomycin tetracycline tobramycin (Tobrex) vancomycin	For treatment and prophylaxis of bacterial infections. Kills bacteria or inhibits growth of bacteriostatic-susceptible pathogenic bacteria.	• Check the client's history for drug allergies before administering, and check whether culture has been obtained. • After multiple doses, assess the client for superinfection (thrush, yeast, and diarrhea); notify HCP if these occur. • Notify HCP if fever and diarrhea occur. Do not treat until contacting HCP. May be developing *Clostridium difficile (C. diff)*, a potentially life-threatening complication. • Assess insertion site for phlebitis if antibiotics are being administered IV. • To assess effectiveness of antimicrobial therapy, monitor the client's white blood cell (WBC) count, temperature, or wound for redness, warmth, and drainage. • Monitor peaks and troughs for aminoglycosides to evaluate for nephrotoxicity and ototoxicity. • Aminoglycosides are administered on a pump to prevent rapid infusion. • Instruct client to take all medication around the clock until finished, even if feeling better.

Classifications	Uses	Selected Interventions
ANTIBIOTICS, TOPICAL clindamycin (Cleocin) erythromycin gentamicin	Treats eye infections.	• Administer from inner canthus to outer canthus. • Advise the client to wash hands before and after application.
ANTICHOLINERGICS atropine benztropine propantheline (Pro-Banthine) scopolamine (Transderm-Scop)	Treats sinus bradycardia and heart block by increasing heart rate. Blocks effects of vagus nerve stimulation. Inhibits actions of acetylcholine at cholinergic receptor sites, thereby decreasing gastric secretions.	• Rapid administration (1 mg or less over 1 minute) may be used in cardiac arrest. • Caution when glaucoma or urine retention is present. • Assess vital signs and EKG tracings frequently in IV drug therapy. • It is possible to administer endotracheal tube followed by several positive pressure ventilations. • Advise the client that adverse effects include drowsiness and dry mouth. • Encourage increased fluid intake to prevent constipation. • Caution the client to avoid activities such as driving that require alertness and concentration until effects of the drug are known.
ANTICHOLINESTERASE AGENTS neostigmine (Prostigmin) pyridostigmine (Mestinon)	Inhibits breakdown of acetylcholine (a substance associated with muscle tone).	• Administer medication at same time daily to ensure maximum strength available for activity. • Administer medication with food to minimize GI distress. • In case of an overdose, have the antidote atropine on hand.
ANTICOAGULANTS IV heparin oral warfarin (Coumadin)	Prevents recurrence of emboli (do not affect emboli that are already present).	• For heparin therapy, monitor partial thromboplastin time (PTT), for which the therapeutic range should be 1.5 to 2 times the normal PTT or control. The antidote is protamine sulfate. • For Coumadin therapy, monitor the international normalized ratio (INR), the therapeutic level of 2 to 3. The antidote is AquaMEPHYTON (vitamin K). • Instruct the client to report bruising, unexplained bleeding, or dark, tarry stools; use a soft-bristle toothbrush; be cautious when using sharp objects and machinery; wear a MedicAlert bracelet; and notify HCPs (dentist, pharmacist) that the client is on an anticoagulant. • If bleeding occurs, instruct the client to apply direct pressure to the wound; if bleeding does not stop after 5 minutes, get medical help.

Continued

Classifications	Uses	Selected Interventions
ANTICOAGULANTS, DIRECT THROMBIN INHIBITORS dabigatran (Pradaxa) rivaroxaban (Xarelto)	Helps prevent strokes or serious blood clots for clients diagnosed with atrial fibrillation without heart valve disease. Works by preventing blood clots from forming in the body.	• Notify HCP if any unusual bruising or bleeding. • Notify HCP if having surgery, including dental surgery; tell the doctor or dentist. • Monitor renal function closely. • It is not necessary to monitor prothrombin time, INR, and PTT.
ANTICOAGULANTS, LOW-MOLECULAR-WEIGHT HEPARIN enoxaparin (Lovenox)	Prophylactically prevents deep vein thrombosis (DVT). Low-molecular-weight molecules are short and preferentially inactivate newly formed factor Xa.	• Administer subcutaneously in left and right anterolateral and posterolateral abdomen. • Monitor platelets. Hold if <100. • Do not aspirate; do not massage. • It is not necessary to monitor activated PTT because of short half-life. • Instruct the client to report bruising, unexplained bleeding, or dark, tarry stools.
ANTICONVULSANTS carbamazepine (Tegretol) phenobarbital phenytoin (Dilantin)	Controls seizure activity by an unknown mechanism.	• Inform the client that the medication may cause drowsiness, and advise avoiding activities that require mental alertness and coordination. • Caution the client not to stop the medication abruptly because doing so may trigger seizure activity. • Teach the client to perform regular oral hygiene and seek regular dental care to control gingival problems and other adverse oral effects. • Urge the client to carry medical identification. • Instruct the client to report signs of serious adverse effects, such as rash or flu-like symptoms. • Monitor therapeutic serum drug levels.
ANTIDEPRESSANTS, MONOAMINE OXIDASE INHIBITORS (MAOIS) phenelzine (Nardil)	Treats various forms of atypical depression and is sometimes helpful in Parkinson's disease.	• If taking MAOIs, avoid OTC drugs, foods, and beverages containing tyramine; any of these can cause a hypertensive crisis.
ANTIDEPRESSANTS, SELECTIVE SEROTONIN REUPTAKE INHIBITORS (SSRIS) citalopram (Celexa) duloxetine (Cymbalta) fluoxetine (Prozac)	Treats various forms of endogenous depression. Antidepressant activity is most likely due to preventing reuptake of dopamine, norepinephrine, and serotonin by presynaptic neurons.	• Monitor mental status and affect. • Assess the client for suicidal tendencies. • Restrict amount of medication available to the client. • Administer medication at night to avoid excessive drowsiness.
ANTIDEPRESSANTS, TRICYCLIC amitriptyline (Elavil) imipramine (Tofranil)	Treats depression, panic, and anxiety.	• These can cause dry mouth, blurred vision, urinary retention, and hypertension. • Avoid alcohol and other CNS depressants. • Some are pregnancy class C medications; fetal harm is a possibility.

Classifications	Uses	Selected Interventions
ANTIDIARRHEALS diphenoxylate and atropine (Lomotil) loperamide (Imodium) bismuth subsalicylate (Pepto-Bismol)	Absorbs excess water from the stool.	• To assess medication effectiveness, record the number and consistency of stools. • Monitor intake and output, daily weight, and serum electrolyte levels. • There is a maximum of 8 tablets per 24 hours of Lomotil to prevent cardiovascular effects of atropine.
ANTIDIURETIC HORMONE REPLACEMENT AGENTS desmopressin (DDAVP) vasopressin (Pitressin)	Conserves renal water by increasing urine osmolality and decreasing urine flow rate.	• These agents may be administered intranasally; instruct the client to notify the HCP if nasal stuffiness occurs. • Intramuscular (IM) injection must be administered deep IM; be sure to warm oil-based medications. • Instruct the client to report signs of water intoxication (drowsiness, lethargy, headache, sudden weight gain, severe nasal congestion); caution against adjusting dosage without consulting HCP.
ANTIDOTES, ADSORBENT activated charcoal	Acute management of many oral poisonings after emesis or lavage.	
ANTIEMETICS chlorpromazine HCl (Thorazine) droperidol (Inapsine) hydroxyzine (Atarax) metoclopramide (Reglan) ondansetron (Zofran) promethazine (Phenergan)	Relieves nausea and vomiting by inhibiting medullary chemoreceptor triggers; drug choice depends on the cause of vomiting. Zofran can be given sublingually for fast results.	• Advise the client that this medication may cause drowsiness. • Instruct the client on safety issues. • Because the medication may cause chemical irritation, administer deep IM injection into a large muscle mass. • Measure emesis and maintain accurate intake and output; monitor for dehydration.
ANTIFUNGALS amphotericin B (Fungizone) clotrimazole (Lotrimin) griseofulvin (Fulvicin) miconazole (Monistat) nystatin suspension (Nystatin)	Treats superficial mycosis (fungal infection) or systemic fungal infections.	• If administered orally, absorption is enhanced by taking the drug with a fatty meal. • Monitor IV administration closely. • Be alert for clinical manifestations of renal damage. • Monitor the client's potassium, calcium, magnesium, and liver enzyme levels regularly. • Teach the client taking oral medication to clean their mouth before taking the medication and to swish and swallow. • Instruct the client to wash her hands before and after applying vaginal medication. • Tell the client to continue medication as prescribed to prevent infection (usually 1 to 2 weeks after symptoms subside). • With oral suspension, instruct the client to rinse their mouth with water to cleanse it, "swish and swallow" to coat the oral mucosa, and hold the suspension in the mouth for at least 2 minutes.

Continued

Classifications	Uses	Selected Interventions
ANTIHISTAMINES dimenhydrinate (Dramamine) meclizine (Antivert)	Treats Meniere's disease by suppressing vestibular activity, thereby decreasing vertigo, nausea, and vomiting.	• Instruct the client to avoid hazardous activities. • Instruct the client to take medication with food to decrease GI distress. • Instruct the client to chew sugarless gum to relieve dry mouth.
ANTIHISTAMINES, ALLERGY/COLD/COUGH cetirizine (Zyrtec) diphenhydramine (Benadryl) fexofenadine (Allegra) loratadine (Claritin)	Inhibits histamine release by binding selectively to H_1 receptors.	• Teach the client to avoid alcohol, driving, or engaging in hazardous activities because the medication may cause drowsiness. (Some antihistamines are not sedating. Make sure the client is knowledgeable of the medication's adverse effects.) • Encourage sucking on hard candy or ice chips to relieve dry mouth.
ANTI-INFECTIVES AND ANTIPROTOZOALS metronidazole (Flagyl)	Attacks amoebas at intestinal and other tissue sites; also treats trichomoniasis.	• Advise the client that sexual partners also must be treated. • Caution the client that even small amounts of alcohol cause adverse effects, such as nausea, vomiting, and headache.
ANTILIPEMIC AGENTS BILE ACID SEQUESTRANTS cholestyramine (Questran)	Lowers serum cholesterol level by binding bile salts in the bowel and forming an insoluble complex that is excreted in the stool.	• Monitor the client's cholesterol level; it should be <200 mg/dL. • Mix medication with 60 mL of water or fruit juice to mask the unpleasant flavor. • Instruct the client to increase fluid intake to prevent constipation.
ANTIPARKINSON AGENTS levodopa (Carbidopa) pramipexole (Mirapex) entacapone (Comtan)	Improves transmission of voluntary nerve impulses to the motor cortex by stimulating dopamine receptors.	• Instruct the client to report overdose signs, such as muscle or eye twitching, at once. • Tell the client not to take medication with food but to eat food 30 minutes after the dose to minimize GI distress. • Discuss precautions to prevent or minimize orthostatic hypotension.
ANTIPLATELET AGENTS acetylsalicylic acid (Aspirin) dipyridamole (Persantine) ticlopidine (Ticlid) clopidogrel (Plavix)	Inhibits aggregation of platelets to form plug; platelets do not initiate thrombus formation as readily when taking antiplatelet agents.	• Instruct the client to take medication with food to decrease gastric irritation. • Remind the client to inform the HCP that they are taking these medications and to be careful when taking OTC medications. • Instruct the client to report bruising, bleeding gums, nosebleeds, or bleeding in the stools.
ANTIPRURITIC AGENTS, TOPICAL STEROIDS, OR TOPICAL ANESTHETICS diphenhydramine (Benadryl) hydrocortisone (Cortisol) benzocaine (Lanacane) dibucaine (Nupercainal) lidocaine and prilocaine (EMLA cream)	Relieves or prevents itching (may be topical steroids or anesthetics). Prevents initiation and transmission of nerve impulses, thereby decreasing itching.	• Advise the client to wash hands before and after application. • Instruct the client to clean affected area with warm water before application.

Classifications	Uses	Selected Interventions
ANTIPSYCHOTICS prochlorperazine (Compazine) clozapine (Clozaril) haloperidol (Haldol) risperidone (Risperdal)	Treats acute and chronic psychoses, particularly when accompanied by increased psychomotor activity. Blocks dopamine receptors in the brain.	• Assess the client's mental status (orientation, mood, behavior) during therapy. • Monitor for akathisia, parkinsonian behavior, dystonia, extrapyramidal tardive dyskinesia, neuroleptic malignancy, and agranulocytosis. • Advise client to wear sunscreen and protective clothing to prevent photosensitivity reaction. • Instruct client not to drink alcohol or take CNS depressants.
ANTIRESORPTIVE THERAPIES, BISPHOSPHONATES alendronate (Fosamax) Hormonal Agents calcitonin salmon (Miacalcin)	Decreases bone absorption of calcium. Inhibits bone resorption by osteoclasts. Inhibits osteoclastic bone resorption.	• Instruct the client to continue with other therapies to help prevent and control complications of osteoporosis. • Instruct the client to take medication before breakfast with a full glass of water. • Instruct the client to remain upright for at least 30 minutes after breakfast.
ANTIRETROVIRALS, NONNUCLEOSIDE REVERSE TRANSCRIPTASE INHIBITORS nevirapine (Viramune)	Causes direct inhibition of HIV by binding to active center of reverse transcriptase.	• Instruct the client to take medication 1 hour before or after food or antacids. • Inform the client to notify HCP if a rash occurs.
ANTIRETROVIRALS, NUCLEOSIDE REVERSE TRANSCRIPTASE INHIBITORS zidovudine AZT (azidothymidine, Invirase)	Suppresses synthesis of viral DNA by reverse transcriptase. First drugs used against HIV. Remains a mainstay of treatment.	• The client must adhere closely to the prescribed dosing schedule. • All medications are oral, except IV zidovudine, which must be administered slowly.
ANTIRETROVIRALS, PROTEASE INHIBITORS lopinavir (Kaletra)	Binds to the active site of HIV protease, thereby preventing the enzyme from cleaving HIV polyproteins; the virus remains immature and noninfectious. When used in combination with reverse transcriptase inhibitors, viral load is reduced to a level undetectable by current assays.	• Instruct the client to follow proper instructions when taking the medication; some must be taken on an empty stomach, and others must be taken with food. • Inform the client that all protease inhibitors may cause diabetes. (Inform the client of clinical manifestations of diabetes and to notify HCP if these occur.)
ANTIRHEUMATICS, DISEASE-MODIFYING ANTIRHEUMATIC DRUGS (DMARDS) etanercept (Enbrel) adalimumab (Humira)	Manages symptoms of rheumatoid arthritis. Slows down joint destruction and preserves joint function.	• Discontinue medication if the client develops an infection. Assess for signs of fungal infection (fever, malaise, weight loss, cough, dyspnea). • Administer tuberculin skin test before starting medication. • Tell client not to receive live vaccines when taking medication. • Pregnancy class B or C medications are not safe for a client wishing to become pregnant; fetal harm is a possibility with these medications.

Continued

Classifications	Uses	Selected Interventions
ANTISPASMOTICS dicyclomine hydrochloride (Bentyl)	Relaxes smooth muscle of the GI tract without anticholinergic effects.	• Instruct the client to take doses before meals and at bedtime, unless a timed-release form is used.
ANTITHYROID AGENTS propylthiouracil (PTU)	Interferes with conversion of iodine into thyroglobulin, thereby inhibiting thyroid hormone synthesis.	• Advise the client to report flu-like symptoms and fever immediately; they may be drug induced. • Tell the client to report clinical manifestations of hyperthyroidism or hypothyroidism. • Caution the client not to use or eat products containing iodine, such as cough medicines, iodized salt, or shellfish; tell the client to notify HCP if taking products containing these substances. • Monitor thyroid hormone levels.
ANTITUBERCULIN rifampin (Rifaldazine) ethambutol (Myambutol) isoniazid (INH)	Inhibits RNA synthesis. Always administered with other antitubercular agents. Acts against tubercle bacilli. Treats tuberculosis by inhibiting bacterial wall synthesis.	• Inform the client that urine, feces, sputum, tears, and sweat will turn red-orange. • Instruct the client to notify HCP if jaundice, anorexia, malaise, fatigue, or nausea occurs (signs of hepatotoxicity). • Medications are administered alone or in combination for a 9- to 18-month course. • Instruct the client to notify HCP if changes in visual acuity, perception, and color interpretation occur (signs of optic neuritis). • Some states require that an HCP directly observe the client taking medication daily; direct observation therapy (DOT). • Instruct the client to notify HCP if tingling, numbness, or pain of the hands and feet occur (a sign of peripheral neuropathy).
ANTITUSSIVE AGENTS, EXPECTORANTS, AND MUCOLYTICS dextromethorphan (Robitussin) hydrocodone acetylcysteine (Mucomyst) benzonatate (Tessalon Perles) guaifenesin	Suppresses cough. Facilitates sputum expectoration for disorders characterized by thick, resistant secretions.	• Instruct the client to read OTC product labels to ensure the medication is appropriate for symptoms. • Instruct the client to stay well hydrated and avoid smoking. • Instruct the client to take syrups undiluted and not to eat or drink anything for at least 15 minutes after taking the medication. • Instruct the client not to chew benzonatate perles, which must be swallowed whole.
ANTIVIRALS amantadine (Symmetrel) acyclovir (Zovirax)	Suppresses viral growth (exact mechanism not clearly understood). Also used for prophylaxis and treatment of infections caused by influenza type A. Inhibits viral replication. Treats herpes simplex virus types 1 and 2.	• Instruct the client on how to prevent orthostatic hypotension. • Instruct the client to notify HCP if shortness of breath and edema in extremities occur. • Inform the client that medication can decrease severity and disorder duration, but does not cure, and may exacerbate, the viral infection.

Classifications	Uses	Selected Interventions
		• Instruct the client to increase fluid intake to 3,000 mL/day. • When applying topical agents, always use gloves to prevent contamination and wash hands before and after administration. • Teach self-administration of vaginal creams, suppositories, and irrigants; advise the client to lie down for 30 minutes after insertion and wear a perineal pad to prevent soiling clothes. • For IV administration, dilute medication and administer over 1 hour on a pump. • Teach that transmission may still occur even if no outward signs of infection are visible.
BETA ADRENERGICS dobutamine (beta only) dopamine (alpha or beta) epinephrine	Increases myocardial contractility and heart rate, which raises BP; alpha-plus beta-adrenergic activity. Short-term (<48 hours) management of heart failure caused by depressed contractility from organic heart disease or surgical procedures.	• Monitor vital signs, EKG, and cardiac output. • Report a change in the quality of peripheral pulses or if extremities become cold or mottled. • Monitor BP at least every 5 to 15 minutes. • Epinephrine is administered IV push (IVP).
BETA BLOCKERS atenolol (Tenormin) carvedilol (Coreg) labetalol (Normodyne) metoprolol (Toprol-XL) nebivolol (Bystolic)	Decreases the heart rate and contraction force and reduces vasoconstriction by antagonizing beta-receptors in the myocardium and vasculature.	• Monitor pulse; if apical pulse falls below 60 bpm, hold and question the order. • Monitor BP; if less than 90/60 mm Hg, hold and question the order. • Taper medication when discontinuing to prevent cardiac effects of withdrawal. • Teach the client about orthostatic hypotension.
BETA BLOCKERS, OPTIC betaxolol HCL (Betoptic)	Treats glaucoma by decreasing aqueous humor production.	• Monitor the client's heart rate and BP. • Instruct the client about correct administration of eye drops.
BIGUANIDES metformin (Glucophage)	Keeps the liver from releasing too much glucose.	• Instruct the client to take medication daily and to continue other measures (diet, exercise) to decrease blood glucose levels. • Advise the client that insulin may be needed during times of increased stress. • Teach the client that concurrent administration of IV contrast medium and Glucophage may be nephrotoxic. • Glucophage should be held for 48 hours before a scheduled IV contrast test. • Creatinine level must be within normal limits before performing a computed tomography scan.

Continued

Classifications	Uses	Selected Interventions
BRONCHODILATORS, XANTHINE DERIVATIVES theophylline (Aminophylline, Slo-Phyllin, Theo-Dur)	Relaxes bronchial smooth muscle.	• Monitor serum level of theophylline (therapeutic level is 10 to 20 mg/mL). • Provide medication at regular intervals, before meals, and with a full glass of water. • Instruct the client to notify HCP of irritability, restlessness, headache, insomnia, dizziness, tachycardia, palpitations, or seizures. • Tell the client not to crush the sustained-release medication.
CALCIUM CHANNEL BLOCKERS amlodipine (Norvasc) diltiazem (Cardizem) nifedipine (Procardia) verapamil (Calan)	Inhibits calcium ions from crossing myocardial and vascular smooth muscle, thereby producing vasodilation and decreased myocardial contractility.	• Monitor pulse; if apical pulse falls below 60 bpm, hold and question the order. • Monitor BP; if less than 90/60 mm Hg, hold and question the order. • Teach the client about orthostatic hypotension.
CALCIUM SUPPLEMENTS parenteral calcium salts (calcium gluconate, chloride, gluceptate)	Strengthens skeletal system by supplementing calcium intake.	• Assess for hypocalcemia by checking for Chvostek's and Trousseau's signs. • Explain to the client that vitamin D increases calcium absorption in the GI tract. • Increase dietary intake of calcium (milk products, green leafy vegetables).
CARBONIC ANHYDRASE INHIBITORS acetazolamide (Diamox)	Treats glaucoma by lowering intraocular pressure by decreasing aqueous humor production.	• Inform the client that this medication may cause malaise, anorexia, and fatigue, and continue medication if these adverse effects occur. • Instruct the client to administer medication orally as prescribed.
CARDIAC GLYCOSIDES digitoxin digoxin (Lanoxin)	Increases force of myocardial contractions and slows heart rate and conduction through the atrioventricular node and bundle of His.	• Monitor pulse; if apical pulse falls below 60 bpm, hold and question order. • Monitor digoxin level (therapeutic level is 0.8 to 2). • Monitor potassium level (normal level is 3.5 to 5.5 mEq/L); hypokalemia potentiates digoxin toxicity (clinical manifestations include anorexia, nausea and vomiting, and yellow haze).
CENTRAL ALPHA AGONISTS clonidine (Catapres)	Stimulates alpha-adrenergic receptors in the CNS, resulting in decreased sympathetic outflow.	• If apical pulse rate falls below 60 bpm, hold and question the order. • Monitor BP; if less than 90/60 mm Hg, hold and question the order. • Teach the client about orthostatic hypotension.
CENTRAL NERVOUS SYSTEM STIMULANTS methylphenidate (Ritalin)	Treats attention deficit-hyperactivity disorder (ADHD). Symptomatic of narcolepsy.	• Report weight loss to HCP. Monitor weight two to three times a week. • The stimulants may cause drowsiness or blurred vision. • Avoid using caffeine-containing beverages with medication. • Take early in the day to avoid insomnia.

Classifications	Uses	Selected Interventions
CHASTEBERRY	Stimulates hormone release, which stimulates progesterone production. Regulates and normalizes hormone levels and menstrual cycles. Reduces symptoms of menopause, which include hot flashes, sweating, and vaginal dryness.	• Notify HCP before taking any herbal remedies if taking prescription or OTC medications, if pregnant or breastfeeding, having surgery, or younger than 18 or older than 65. • Instruct the client not to exceed recommended dosages or take the herb longer than recommended. • Check alerts and advisories, including those of the NCCIH, Office of Dietary Supplements, and FDA.
CHELATING AGENT Edetate calcium disodium (Calcium EDTA)	Reduces concentration of free metal ions in solution by complexing it. Combines with metal ions to form stable ring structures.	• Obtain serum levels of heavy metals (e.g., lead, iron) before initiation of therapy and again at termination of the therapy. • Measure intake and output to ensure that the kidney is adequately functioning. • Assess the following: blood urea nitrogen (BUN), serum creatinine, calcium, and protein in the urine.
CHOLESTEROL ABSORPTION INHIBITORS ezetimibe (Zetia)	Reduces absorption of dietary and biliary cholesterol through intestines. Decreases amount of intestinal cholesterol delivered to the liver.	• Use in conjunction with low-fat, low-cholesterol diet.
CHOLINERGICS pilocarpine (Isopto Carpine)	Treats glaucoma by constricting pupils and promoting outflow of aqueous humor.	• Warn the client that visual acuity is decreased in environments with low lighting. • Use caution for clients diagnosed with a urinary tract obstruction. • Instruct the client about correct administration of eye drops.
COLLOIDAL SOLUTION albumin 5%	Expands plasma volume and maintenance of cardiac output in situations associated with fluid volume deficit, including shock, hemorrhage, and burns. Increases intravascular fluid volume.	• Assess for signs of vascular overload, including rales and crackles, dyspnea, hypertension, and jugular venous distention during and after administration. • Administer through a large bore gauge needle (at least 20 gauge). • Record lot number of medication in client's electronic health record. • Solution should be clear amber; do not administer solutions that are discolored or contain particulate matter.
COENZYME Q (COQ10)	Helps in cardiovascular conditions, especially heart failure, cancer, muscular dystrophy, and periodontal disease, and boosts energy and speeds recovery from exercise.	• Dietary supplements may cause side effects, trigger allergic reactions, or interact with prescription and nonprescription medicines or other supplements that the client might be taking. • Check alerts and advisories, including those of the NCCIH, Office of Dietary Supplements, and FDA.

Continued

Classifications	Uses	Selected Interventions
CORONARY VASODILATORS nitroglycerin (Tridil)	Adjunct treatment of acute myocardial infarction. Increases coronary blood flow by dilating coronary arteries and improving collateral flow to ischemic regions.	• IV administration requires continuous monitoring of EKG, BP, and pulse. • Use glass bottles only and special tubing provided by the manufacturer when administering IV. • Inform the client that a headache is a common side effect and is treated with acetaminophen.
CORTICOSTEROIDS Oral dexamethasone (Decadron) hydrocortisone (Cortisol) methylprednisolone (Medrol) prednisone (Deltasone) Intravenous hydrocortisone sodium succinate (Solu-Cortef) methylprednisolone (Solu-Medrol) dexamethasone (Decadron) Injectable betamethasone (Celestone) Inhaled fluticasone (Flonase) beclomethasone (Beconase) Topical desoximetasone (Topicort) hydrocortisone triamcinolone (Kenacort)	Combats severe immune or inflammatory responses. Strengthens biologic membrane, which inhibits capillary permeability and prevents leakage of fluid into the injured area and development of edema (exact mechanism unknown).	• Instruct the client to take medication exactly as directed and to taper it rather than stop it abruptly, which could cause serious withdrawal symptoms (adrenal insufficiency, shock, death). • Forewarn the client that the medication may cause reportable cushingoid effects (weight gain, moon face, buffalo hump, and hirsutism) and may mask clinical manifestations of infection. • The medication will increase glucose levels. • Administer IV delivery during times of acutely increased intracranial pressure. • Caution the client not to exceed the maximum daily dose of four sprays per nostril. • Instruct the client to rinse mouth after each use to prevent nasal candidiasis.
COX-2 INHIBITORS celecoxib (Celebrex) nabumetone (Relafen)	Decreases inflammation for clients diagnosed with severe arthritic conditions by inhibiting formation of substances that can cause joint and connective tissue problems.	• Inform the client to notify HCP of all prescription and OTC medications. • Instruct the client to report tinnitus, which is a sign of aspirin toxicity, to HCP.
D-PHENYLALANINE DERIVATIVES nateglinide (Starlix)	Stimulates insulin release from beta cells.	• Instruct the client to administer at least 30 minutes before meals. • Instruct the client to omit when skipping a meal.
DECONGESTANTS pseudoephedrine HCL (Sudafed)	Treats nasal decongestion by causing blood vessels to constrict, thereby relieving congestion.	• Instruct the client to read product labels to ensure appropriate OTC medications for symptom control. • Instruct the client to inform HCPs about use of OTC medications.

Classifications	Uses	Selected Interventions
DIURETICS, LOOP furosemide (Lasix)	Decreases blood volume, which decreases the heart's workload.	• Monitor potassium level; do not administer if the client is hypokalemic or hyperkalemic. • Monitor intake and output; increase fluid intake.
DIURETICS, OSMOTIC Mannitol (Osmitrol)	Decreases cerebral edema in head trauma by drawing water across intact membranes, thereby reducing brain volume and extracellular fluid.	• Monitor fluid and electrolyte balance. • Maintain accurate intake and output records. • Observe IV preparation for crystals before use; always use a filter needle.
DIURETICS, THIAZIDE chlorothiazide (Diuril)	Decreases reabsorption of sodium and chloride in the kidneys.	• Teach the client to weigh daily and report weight gain of more than 2 pounds in 1 day. • Question order if the client is dehydrated.
DONG QUAI	A sexual stimulant for women. Purifies blood. Aids in relieving insomnia and hypertension. Lowers BP. Strengthens the reproductive system. Assists the body in using hormones. Treats menopause problems, such as hot flashes, vaginal dryness, headaches, breast soreness, premenstrual gas, and irritability.	• Notify HCP before taking any herbal remedies if taking prescription or OTC medications, if pregnant or breastfeeding, if having surgery, or if younger than 18 or older than 65. • Tell the client not to exceed recommended dosages or take the herb longer than recommended. • Check alerts and advisories, including those of the NCCIH, Office of Dietary Supplements, and FDA.
ECHINACEA PURPURA	The most effective blood and lymphatic cleanser in the botanical kingdom. A natural antibiotic that increases production and activity of WBCs; stimulates the immune system; removes toxins from the blood; acts as an immune stimulant that helps the body fight off illness by bolstering its natural defenses; fights inflammation; and can stop a cold, flu, and other infectious illnesses before they can spread in the body.	• Notify HCP before taking any herbal remedies if taking prescription or OTC medications, if pregnant or breastfeeding, having surgery, or younger than 18 or older than 65. • Tell the client not to exceed recommended dosages or take the herb for longer than recommended. • Check alerts and advisories, including those of the NCCIH, Office of Dietary Supplements, and FDA.
ELECTROLYTE REPLACEMENTS calcium gluconate	Maintains capillary integrity and normal functioning of the nervous, muscular, and skeletal systems.	• Administer the amount prescribed slowly through a large vein to avoid infiltration, which may cause severe necrosis and tissue sloughing. • Keep the client on bed rest at least 1 hour after drug administration to prevent orthostatic hypotension. • Keep medication at the bedside with the necessary IV equipment.

Continued

Classifications	Uses	Selected Interventions
ERYTHROPOIETIN epoetin alfa (Epogen)	Aids in production of red blood cells (RBCs).	• This may be administered IV or subcutaneously for clients not receiving dialysis. • Monitor BP, complete blood count with differential BUN, and platelet counts.
FOLIC ACID	Supplements folic acid intake; the minimum daily requirement is 50 g (folic acid is found in most meats, fresh vegetables, and fresh fruits, but is destroyed when cooked for more than 15 minutes). Helps the body make RBCs. Also needed to make DNA.	• Warn the client that these medications cause drowsiness initially but diminish with continued use. • Instruct the client to avoid hazardous activities; do not mix these medications with alcohol or other depressants. • Taper baclofen (Lioresal) to prevent rebound seizures. • Liver, dried beans and other legumes, green leafy vegetables, asparagus, and orange juice are good sources of this vitamin. So are fortified bread, rice, and cereals.
GINKGO BILOBA	A vascular dilator that promotes blood and oxygen circulation to the brain, which in return helps short-term memory, promotes mental alertness, sharpens mental focus and concentration, offers significant protection against Alzheimer's disease, supplies blood nourishment to every part of the body, and helps prevent strokes by preventing blood clot formation.	• Notify HCP before taking any herbal remedies if taking prescription or OTC medications, if pregnant or breastfeeding, if having surgery, or if younger than 18 or older than 65. • Tell the client not to exceed recommended dosages or take the herb for longer than recommended. • Check alerts and advisories, including those of the NCCIH, Office of Dietary Supplements, and FDA.
HAWTHORN	Treats indigestion and is widely known as a diuretic. Used to treat various heart conditions and today is believed to lower BP and cholesterol levels, decrease fat deposit levels, reduce arterial plaque, strengthen vein and capillary structure, and aid in relieving physical symptoms of emotional stress.	• Notify HCP before taking any herbal remedies if taking prescription or OTC medications, if pregnant or breastfeeding, if having surgery, or if younger than 18 or older than 65. • Tell the client not to exceed recommended dosages or take the herb for longer than recommended. • Check alerts and advisories, including those of the NCCIH, Office of Dietary Supplements, and FDA.
HISTAMINE-2 RECEPTOR ANTAGONISTS cimetidine (Tagamet) famotidine (Pepcid)	Blocks receptors that control secretion of hydrochloric acid by parietal cells.	• Instruct the client to continue taking medication regularly, even after pain subsides. • When administering IV, dilute the medication and monitor the client closely. • Emphasize the importance of adhering to all aspects of therapy.
HMG-COA REDUCTASE INHIBITORS (STATINS) lovastatin (Mevacor) simvastatin (Zocor) rosuvastatin (Crestor)	Lowers cholesterol by slowing down the body's ability to make cholesterol.	• Notify the HCP if the client develops muscle tenderness during therapy; if creatine kinase levels are > 10 times the upper limit of normal or if myopathy occurs, medication should be discontinued.

Classifications	Uses	Selected Interventions
		• Instruct the client to take medication at night due to enzyme that metabolizes cholesterol. • Avoid large amounts (>200 mL/day) of grapefruit juice during therapy because it may increase toxicity.
HORMONES clomiphene (Clomid) depot medroxyprogesterone (Depo-Provera) leuprolide (Lupron Depot) human chorionic gonadotropin (HCG) menotropin testosterone pellets (Testopel)	Treats infertility, menstrual problems, and hormonal imbalances.	• The HCP should regularly monitor medications. • Instruct the client to report hypersensitivity or adverse reactions.
HYPEROSMOTICS glycerin (Glycerol) mannitol	Treats angle-closure glaucoma by elevating plasma osmolality and enhancing water flow into the extracellular fluid, thereby reducing intraocular pressure.	• Because angle-closure glaucoma is a medical emergency, try to calm and reassure the client. • Instruct the client to administer orally as prescribed.
HYPNOTICS/SEDATIVES ***BARBITURATES*** phenobarbital	Hypnotics are used to manage insomnia; sedatives are used to provide sedation. Causes generalized CNS depression. These agents have no analgesic properties.	• Caution the client that alcohol and other drugs, such as antihistamines, potentiate tranquilizer effects. • Ensure the client's safety, put bed in a low position and call light within reach, and instruct the client to get assistance to ambulate. • Assess sleep patterns throughout therapy. • Supervise ambulation and client transfer. • Avoid use of alcohol and other CNS depressants.
IMMUNOGLOBULINS gamma globulin Rho (D) immune globulin	Provides passive immunity through immunoglobulin G antibodies to protect against infection.	• Before administering, obtain client's allergy and immunization response history. • After administering, monitor the client closely for clinical manifestations of allergic reactions.
INSULINS <u>Rapid-acting</u> Insulin lispro (Humalog) <u>Short-acting</u> Insulin regular (Humulin R) <u>Intermediate-acting</u> insulin isophane (Humulin N, Novolin) insulin NPH (NPH) <u>Long-acting—steady state</u> insulin glargine (Lantus) insulin detemir (Levemir)	Replaces endogenous insulin and maintains blood glucose levels by regulating protein, carbohydrate, and fat metabolism.	• Answer five questions before administering insulin: 1) When does insulin peak? Humalog acts within 15 minutes; rapid-acting peaks in 2 to 4 hours; intermediate-acting in 6 to 8 hours; long-acting in 16 to 24 hours; this is when hypoglycemic reaction may occur. 2) What meal covers the peak time? Glucose or food is the antidote for insulin (e.g., 7 a.m. regular insulin is covered by breakfast). 3) Is the client receiving nothing by mouth? If so, question the insulin order.

Continued

Classifications	Uses	Selected Interventions
		4) What is the client's blood glucose level? If below 90 mg/dL, question the insulin order. 5) Where will the medication be injected? Absorption is best in the abdomen.
INSULIN MIXES 70/30 (70% NPH and 30% R), 60/40, 50/50 75/25 (Humalog Mix)		• Teach and demonstrate preparation; administration techniques; injection sites and rotation; insulin and equipment care, storage, and disposal.
IODINE-CONTAINING AGENTS	Inhibits release of stored thyroid hormone and retards hormone synthesis.	• Administer for a short term before thyroidectomy; medication has a short half-life. • Dilute oral iodine solution in juice or beverage of choice; administer through a straw with fluids to prevent teeth staining.
ION EXCHANGE RESINS sodium polystyrene sulfonate (Kayexalate)	Exchanges a sodium ion for a potassium ion in the intestinal tract.	• If administered by retention enema, the client should retain for 30 minutes. • Sorbitol is often administered with medication to induce a diarrhea-type effect. • Monitor serum potassium level.
IRON ferrous sulfate (Ferralyn)	Helps RBCs carry oxygen to all parts of the body. Clinical manifestations of iron-deficiency anemia include weakness and fatigue, lightheadedness, and shortness of breath.	• Iron-rich foods include red meat, pork, fish and shellfish, poultry, lentils, beans and soy foods, green leafy vegetables, and raisins. Some flours, cereals, and grain products are also fortified with iron. • Inform client that stool will become black in color, and constipation is common. Increase fluid intake, fiber, and exercise.
IRON SUPPLEMENTS Oral—ferrous sulfate Parenteral—iron dextran	Synthesizes heme, the essential protein of hemoglobin.	• Inform the client that the stool will be dark and tarry; instruct on ways to prevent constipation. • Tell the client to notify the HCP of adverse effects, such as diarrhea, constipation, GI upset, or nausea and vomiting that becomes severe or intolerable. • Forewarn the client that liquid iron may stain teeth. • Suggest diluting iron and administering it through a straw or dropper placed at the back of the tongue. • Administer using the Z-track technique to avoid leakage into subcutaneous tissues. • Caution the client that preparation may discolor skin and cause local pain. • Be alert for a possible anaphylactic reaction.
LAXATIVES <u>Bulk</u> psyllium (Metamucil) <u>Stimulant</u> bisacodyl (Dulcolax)	Absorbs water and increases fecal bulk. Stimulates peristalsis through mucosal irritation. Eases stool passage by facilitating mixing water with fecal mass.	• Administer a bulk laxative with fluid and give it immediately before it congeals. • Avoid overuse of stimulant laxatives, which causes laxative dependence.

Classifications	Uses	Selected Interventions
Saline (osmotic) magnesium hydroxide (Ex-Lax) Stool Softeners docusate calcium (Colace)	Retains and increases water in the feces.	• Inform the client that a daily bowel movement is unnecessary for normal bowel elimination. • Encourage exercise to help prevent constipation.
LEUKOTRIENE RECEPTOR ANTAGONISTS montelukast (Singulair)	Reduces inflammation in airways. Used for prophylactic and maintenance drug therapy for chronic asthma.	• Instruct the client to take medication in the evening without food. • Explain that the medication is not for acute asthma attacks.
LICORICE	Stimulates adrenal glands, which produce energy. Contains glycyrrhizin, which has anti-inflammatory, antiviral, and anti-allergic properties. Stimulates production of cortisone and aldosterone, which reduces inflammation, helpful for arthritis. Used to rejuvenate liver cells and restore liver function. Normalizes enzymes and inhibits liver damage produced by a buildup of toxic chemicals.	• Notify the HCP before taking any herbal remedies if taking prescription or OTC medications, if pregnant or breastfeeding, if having surgery, or if younger than 18 or older than 65. • Tell the client not to exceed recommended dosages or take the herb for longer than recommended. • Check alerts and advisories, including those of the NCCIH, Office of Dietary Supplements, and FDA.
MAGNESIUM SULFATE	Electrolyte replacement effective in decreasing muscular excitability. Acts as an anticonvulsant to prevent and control seizures in preeclampsia and to decrease uterine activity. Useful in preterm labor.	• Monitor BP, respiratory rate, deep tendon reflexes, and urinary output frequently during IV administration. • Antidote is calcium gluconate. • Adverse reactions include CNS depression, respiratory depression, and hypotension.
MAST CELL INHIBITORS cromolyn (Intal)	Inhibits mast cells, thereby releasing chemical mediators that result in bronchodilation and decreased airway inflammation.	• Teach the client to insert capsule in the nebulizer device, exhale completely, place mouthpiece between the lips, inhale deeply, hold breath for 10 seconds, and then exhale. • Instruct the client that the inhaler is to be used prophylactically before exercise, not for an acute asthma attack.
MINERALOCORTICOIDS fludrocortisone (Florinef)	Replaces hormones. Major effect, sodium-retaining activity associated with potassium loss.	• Explain that additional doses may be needed in times of stress. • Instruct the client to report weight gain and severe headaches.
MOOD STABILIZERS lithium (Lithobid, Lithate) Anticonvulsants used as mood stabilizers	Prevents and decreases incidence of acute mania episodes and associated bipolar disorder manic episodes. Contraindicated for clients requiring sodium or fluid restriction.	• Assess the client's mental status (orientation, mood, behavior) during therapy. • Monitor therapeutic serum lithium levels 0.5–1.5 mEq/L.

Continued

Classifications	Uses	Selected Interventions
carbamazepine (Tegretol) lamotrigine (Lamictal) valporic acid (Depakote)	Periodic monitoring of blood lithium levels is required. Acute toxicity is closely related to serum drug levels that are close to therapeutic range. Dose should be maintained between 0.8 and 1.4 mEq/L.	• Low sodium levels may predispose client to toxicity; drink 2,000–3,000 mL of fluid daily. • Avoid activities causing excessive diaphoresis, which leads to sodium loss.
MUCOSAL PROTECTIVE AGENTS misoprostol (Cytotec) sucralfate (Carafate)	Protects ulcer from destructive action of the digestive enzyme pepsin by changing stomach acid into viscous material that binds to proteins in ulcerated tissue.	• Instruct the client to take medication 30–60 minutes before meals and bedtime. • Advise the client to take medication 1 hour before or after taking an antacid. • Tablets may be difficult to chew; liquid preparations are available.
NARCOTIC ANTAGONIST naloxone (Narcan)	Reverses CNS depression and respiratory depression because of suspected opioid overdose.	• Monitor vital signs, EKG, and level of consciousness frequently for 3–4 hours after expected peak of blood concentrations. • Monitor respiratory rate closely because some effects of opioids may last longer than effects of naloxone; repeat doses may be necessary. • Resuscitation equipment, oxygen, vasopressors, and mechanical ventilation should be available to supplement naloxone therapy as needed.
NITRATES Short-acting Nitroglycerin sublingual Long-acting isosorbide dinitrate nitroglycerin topical nitroglycerin patch nitroglycerin tablet nitroglycerin IV (Tridil)	Reduces myocardial oxygen demand by promoting vasodilation and by increasing oxygen supply to myocardial tissue.	• For acute chest pain, instruct client to stop any activity, take one tablet sublingual, wait 5 minutes; if no pain relief, administer another sublingual, wait 5 minutes; if no pain relief, take another sublingual tablet and obtain medical attention immediately (call 911). • Keep sublingual medication in a brown bottle; will lose potency with sunlight. • Inform the client that a headache is a common side effect. • Monitor BP; teach client about orthostatic hypotension. • For topical administration, be sure to wear gloves, remove the old patch, apply to a hairless area, and date and time the new patch. • For IV administration, dilute drug and administer by continuous infusion, with constant monitoring of BP and pulse.
OTHER TOPICAL AGENTS (E.G., COAL TAR PRODUCTS) anthralin preparations	Slows pathologic processes. Retards overactive epidermis without affecting other tissues.	• Apply with a tongue blade or gloved hand; do not apply to normal skin. • Caution the client that anthralin, a coal tar derivative, temporarily stains skin and clothing.

Classifications	Uses	Selected Interventions
OXYTOCICS oxytocin (Pitocin) prostaglandin dinoprostone (Cervidil) carboprost tromethamine (Hemabate)	Stimulates smooth muscle contractions of the uterus used in labor induction or augmentation. Has antidiuretic and vasopressor properties. Synthetic prostaglandin with oxytocic properties. Hormone helpful in dilating pregnant cervix.	• When administering IV, dilute medication, give via infusion pump, and titrate based on uterine contraction pattern. Can be given IM postpartum. • Provide continuous fetal monitoring during administration. • Monitor for drowsiness, confusion, headache, and decreased urine output (indicates water intoxication).
PHOSPHATE-BINDING AGENTS aluminum hydroxide (Amphojel)	Decreases absorption of phosphate from intestines, thereby decreasing serum phosphate levels.	• Instruct the client to restrict sodium intake, drink plenty of fluids, and follow a low-phosphate diet.
PROTON-PUMP INHIBITORS omeprazole (Prilosec) pantoprazole (Protonix)	Prevents final transport of hydrogen into the gastric lumen by binding an enzyme on gastric parietal cells.	• Instruct the client to take medication regularly as prescribed by the HCP. • Instruct the client to avoid products that may cause GI irritation. • Administer IV pantoprazole IV piggyback (IVPB) or IVP.
SEDATIVES phenobarbital	Depresses CNS activity, thereby reducing restlessness and agitation, as in clients diagnosed with cerebral aneurysms.	• Administer IV medication by a large vein to avoid extravasation. • Monitor vital signs closely because sedative drugs depress CNS and respiratory activity and may mask decreasing levels or consciousness. • Institute safety precautions—side rails up and call light within reach.
SKELETAL MUSCLE RELAXANTS carisoprodol (Soma) cyclobenzaprine (Flexeril) methocarbamol (Robaxin)	Relieves pain-producing muscle spasms and spasticity.	• Caution the client that alcohol and other drugs, such as antihistamines, potentiate muscle relaxant effects. • Ensure the client's safety: bed in low position, call light within reach, instruct the client to get assistance to ambulate.
ST. JOHN'S WORT	Nature's "Prozac" contains hypericin, a natural mood-booster that also has germicidal and anti-inflammatory properties. Treats depression, anxiety, nervous disorders, and eating disorders. Controls viral infections, such as staph, human papillomavirus, and HIV viral strains. Reduces and controls tumor growths. Effective in treating insomnia and "mental burnout" conditions, such as chronic fatigue syndrome.	• Notify the HCP before taking any herbal remedies if taking prescription or OTC medications, if pregnant or breastfeeding, if having surgery, or if younger than 18 or older than 65. • Tell the client not to exceed recommended dosages or take the herb for longer than recommended. • Check alerts and advisories, including those of the NCCIH, Office of Dietary Supplements, and FDA.

Continued

Classifications	Uses	Selected Interventions
SULFONYLUREAS chlorpropamide (Diabinese) glipizide (Glucotrol) glyburide (Diabeta)	Reduces blood glucose levels by stimulating pancreatic insulin production and makes cell receptor sites more receptive to circulating insulin.	• Instruct the client to take medication daily and continue other measures (diet, exercise) to decrease blood glucose levels. • Advise the client that insulin may be needed during times of increased stress. • Forewarn the client that possible adverse effects may include hypoglycemia.
THIAZOLIDINEDIONES pioglitazone (Actos) rosiglitazone maleate (Avandia)	Makes muscle cells more sensitive to insulin, decreasing blood glucose levels.	• Instruct the client to take medication daily and to continue other measures (diet, exercise) to decrease blood glucose levels. • Advise the client that insulin may be needed during times of increased stress. • Forewarn the client that possible adverse effects may include hypoglycemia.
THROMBOLYTIC AGENTS alteplase (Activase) streptokinase (Streptase)	Dissolves thrombi or emboli in the coronary or cerebral arteries with preservation of ventricular function.	• Follow hospital protocol when administering a thrombolytic agent. • Clients must begin therapy within 4–6 hours after onset of symptoms. • Monitor for internal bleeding every 15–30 minutes for the first 8 hours and then every 4 hours throughout therapy. • Monitor for reperfusion dysrhythmias indicating medication is effective. • If administering for a cerebrovascular accident (CVA), then must have confirmatory evidence that the CVA is thrombotic or embolic and not hemorrhagic.
THYROID HORMONE levothyroxine (Synthroid)	Raises metabolic rate, promotes gluconeogenesis, increases use of stored glycogen, stimulates protein synthesis, and affects protein and carbohydrate metabolism and cell growth.	• Administer in the morning to avoid bedtime insomnia. • Instruct the client to notify HCP of clinical manifestations of hypothyroidism and hyperthyroidism. • Monitor cardiac response to increased metabolic rate and oxygen requirements.
VALERIAN ROOT	A "natural valium" that acts as a mild tranquilizer by calming the nerves. Eases muscle spasms; relieves menstrual cramps and premenstrual syndrome; relaxes muscles in the digestive system; treats insomnia; hastens sleep, improves sleep quality, and reduces nighttime awakenings; treats anxiety, panic attacks, tension, and headaches; improves circulation and reduces cold-related mucus; relieves irritable bowel syndrome; lowers BP.	• Notify HCP before taking any herbal remedies if taking prescription or OTC medications, if pregnant or breastfeeding, if having surgery, or if younger than 18 or older than 65. • Tell the client not to exceed recommended dosages or take the herb for longer than recommended. • Check alerts and advisories, including those of the NCCIH, Office of Dietary Supplements, and FDA.

Classifications	Uses	Selected Interventions
VASODILATORS hydralazine (Apresoline) nitroprusside sodium (Nipride) sildenafil (Viagra)	Decreases preload by acting directly on blood vessels to cause dilation and decrease vascular resistance. Eectile dysfunction agent.	• Monitor BP; if less than 90/60 mm Hg, hold and question the order. • For IV administration, have the client on a cardiac monitor. • Keep the client on bed rest, with safety precautions instituted. • Avoid concurrent use of erectile dysfunction agents with nitrates; may cause severe hypotension.
VASOPRESSORS metaraminol (Aramine) norepinephrine	Rapidly restores BP in anaphylaxis by producing vasoconstriction and stimulating the heart.	• Monitor the client's vital signs, intake and output, mental status, peripheral pulses, and skin color. • The client should be on telemetry and monitored continuously.
VITAMIN A	Prevents eye problems. Promotes healthy immune system. Essential for cell growth and development.	• Good sources of vitamin A are milk, eggs, liver, fortified cereals, dark-colored orange or green vegetables (such as carrots, sweet potatoes, pumpkin, and kale), and orange fruits (such as cantaloupe, apricots, peaches, papayas, and mangos).
Topical tretinoin (Retin-A)	Keeps skin healthy. Seeds cellular turnover, thereby clearing keratin plugs from pilosebaceous ducts.	• Caution the client to avoid sun exposure. • Explain to the client that noticeable improvement may take 8–12 weeks, during which time skin redness and peeling are common.
VITAMIN B_{12} cyanocobalamin (Cyanabin) vitamin B_{12} injection	Helps to make RBCs and is important for nerve cell function. Stimulates a key reaction in the synthesis of thymidylate, a DNA component. Deficiency results in release of too few blood cells.	• This vitamin is found naturally in fish, red meat, poultry, milk, cheese, and eggs; and is also added to some breakfast cereals. • This vitamin must be given IM to bypass intestines for systemic absorption. • Vitamin B_{12} injections are virtually free of adverse effects. • This vitamin is initially taken by daily injections and then monthly throughout life.
VITAMIN C	Needed to form collagen, a tissue that helps to hold cells together. Essential for healthy bones, teeth, gums, and blood vessels. Helps body absorb iron and calcium. Aids in wound healing. Contributes to brain function.	• This vitamin is found in red berries, kiwi, red and green bell peppers, tomatoes, broccoli, spinach, and juices made from guava, grapefruit, and orange.
VITAMIN D	Strengthens bones because it helps the body absorb bone-building calcium.	• The body manufactures vitamin D when skin is exposed to sunlight. • This vitamin is found in egg yolks, fish oils, and fortified foods like milk.

Continued

Classifications	Uses	Selected Interventions
VITAMIN E	An antioxidant that helps protect cells from damage. Also important for RBC health.	• This vitamin is found in many foods, such as vegetable oils, nuts, and green leafy vegetables. • Avocados, wheat germ, and whole grains are also good sources.
VITAMIN K AquaMEPHYTON	Promotes clotting by providing fat-soluble vitamins necessary for clotting mechanism. Allows blood to clot normally. Helps protect bones from fracture. Helps prevent postmenopausal bone loss. Prevents artery calcification. Provides protection against liver and prostate cancer.	• Vitamin K may be administered IM, subcutaneously, or IV; however, IV administration is dangerous and should only be used as a last resort. • Explain to the client that green leafy vegetables are high in vitamin K; and are provided in parsley, kale, spinach, Brussels sprouts, green beans, asparagus, broccoli, mustard and turnip greens, collard greens, romaine lettuce, cabbage, and celery. • Too much vitamin K causes excessive bleeding, including heavy menstrual bleeding, gum bleeding, bleeding within the digestive tract, or nose bleeding; as well as easy bruising. • There can be problems with bone fracture or bone weakening with lack of the vitamin.
ZINC	Important for normal growth, strong immunity, and wound healing.	• This mineral is found in red meat, poultry, oysters and other seafood, nuts, dried beans, soy foods, milk and other dairy products, whole grains, and fortified breakfast cereals.

Glossary of English Words Commonly Encountered on Nursing Examinations

Abnormality — defect, irregularity, anomaly, oddity

Absence — nonappearance, lack, nonattendance

Abundant — plentiful, rich, profuse

Accelerate — go faster, speed up, increase, hasten

Accumulate — build up, collect, gather

Accurate — precise, correct, exact

Achievement — accomplishment, success, reaching, attainment

Acknowledge — admit, recognize, accept, reply

Activate — start, turn on, stimulate

Adequate — sufficient, ample, plenty, enough

Angle — slant, approach, direction, point of view

Application — use, treatment, request, claim

Approximately — about, around, in the region of, more or less, roughly speaking

Arrange — position, place, organize, display

Associated — linked, related

Attention — notice, concentration, awareness, thought

Authority — power, right, influence, clout, expert

Avoid — keep away from, evade, let alone

Balanced — stable, neutral, steady, fair, impartial

Barrier — barricade, protection, blockage, obstruction, obstacle

Best — most excellent, most important, greatest

Capable — able, competent, accomplished

Capacity — ability, capability, aptitude, role, power, size

Central — middle, mid, innermost, vital

Challenge — confront, dare, dispute, test, defy, face up to

Characteristic — trait, feature, attribute, quality, typical

Circular — round, spherical, globular

Collect — gather, assemble, amass, accumulate, bring together

Commitment — promise, vow, dedication, obligation, pledge, assurance

Commonly — usually, normally, frequently, generally, universally

Compare — contrast, evaluate, match up to, weigh or judge against

Compartment — section, part, cubicle, booth, stall

Complex — difficult, multifaceted, compound, multipart, intricate

Complexity — difficulty, intricacy, complication

Component — part, element, factor, section, constituent

Comprehensive — complete, inclusive, broad, thorough

Conceal — hide, cover up, obscure, mask, suppress, secrete

Conceptualize — form an idea

Concern — worry, anxiety, fear, alarm, distress, unease, trepidation

Concisely — briefly, in a few words, succinctly

Conclude — make a judgment based on reason, finish

Confidence — self-assurance, certainty, poise, self-reliance

Congruent — matching, fitting, going together well

Consequence — result, effect, outcome, end result

Constituents — elements, component, parts that make up a whole

Contain — hold, enclose, surround, include, control, limit

Continual — repeated, constant, persistent, recurrent, frequent

Continuous — constant, incessant, nonstop, unremitting, permanent

Contribute — be a factor, supply, add, give

Convene — assemble, call together, summon, organize, arrange

Convenience — expediency, handiness, ease

Coordinate — organize, direct, manage, bring together

Create — make, invent, establish, generate, produce, fashion, build, construct

Creative — imaginative, original, inspired, inventive, resourceful, productive, innovative

Critical — serious, grave, significant, dangerous, life-threatening

Cue — signal, reminder, prompt, sign, indication

Curiosity — inquisitiveness, interest, desire to learn

Damage — injure, harm, hurt, break, wound

Deduct — subtract, take away, remove, withhold

Deficient — lacking, wanting, underprovided, scarce, faulty

Defining — important, crucial, major, essential, significant, central

Defuse — resolve, calm, soothe, neutralize, rescue, mollify

Delay — hold up, wait, hinder, postpone, slow down, hesitate, linger

Demand — insist, claim, require, command, stipulate, ask

Describe — explain, tell, express, illustrate, depict, portray

Design — plan, invent, intend, aim, propose, devise

Desirable — wanted, pleasing, sought after, attractive, advantageous

Detail — feature, aspect, element, factor, facet

Deteriorate — worsen, decline, weaken

Determine — decide, conclude, resolve, agree on

Dexterity — skillfulness, handiness, agility, deftness

Dignity — self-respect, self-esteem, decorum, formality, poise

Dimension — aspect, measurement

Diminish — reduce, lessen, weaken, detract, moderate

Discharge — drain, fluid secretion, release, dismiss, set free

Discontinue — stop, cease, halt, suspend, terminate, withdraw

Disorder — complaint, problem, confusion, chaos

Display — show, exhibit, demonstrate, present, put-on view

Dispose — get rid of, arrange, order, set out

Dissatisfaction — displeasure, discontent, unhappiness, disappointment

Distinguish — separate and classify, recognize

Distract — divert, side track, entertain

Distress — suffering, trouble, anguish, agony, concern

Distribute — deliver, spread out, hand out, issue, dispense

Disturbed — troubled, unstable, concerned, distressed, anxious

Diversion — distraction, deviation

Don — put on, dress oneself in

Dramatic — spectacular, marked, substantial

Drape — cover, wrap, dress, swathe

Dysfunction — abnormal, impaired

Edge — perimeter, boundary, periphery, brink, border, rim

Effective — successful, useful, helpful, valuable

Efficient — not wasteful, effective, competent, resourceful, capable

Elasticity — stretch, spring, suppleness, flexibility

Eliminate — get rid of, eradicate, abolish, remove, purge

Embarrass — make uncomfortable, make self-conscious, humiliate, mortify

Emerge — appear, come, materialize, become known

Emphasize — call attention to, accentuate, stress, highlight

Ensure — make certain, guarantee

Environment — setting, surroundings, location, atmosphere, milieu, situation

Episode — event, incident, occurrence, experience

Essential — necessary, fundamental, vital, important, crucial, critical, indispensable

Etiology — assigned cause, origin

Exaggerate — overstate, inflate

Excel — stand out, shine, surpass, outclass

Excessive — extreme, too much, unwarranted

Exertion — intense or prolonged physical effort

Exhibit — show signs of, reveal, display

Expand — get bigger, enlarge, spread out, increase, swell, inflate

Expect — wait for, anticipate, imagine

Expectation — hope, anticipation, belief, prospect, probability

Experience — knowledge, skill, occurrence, know-how

Expose — lay open, leave unprotected, reveal, disclose, exhibit

External — outside, exterior, outer

Facilitate — make easy, make possible, help, assist

Factor — part, feature, reason, cause, think, issue

Focus — center, focal point, hub

Fragment — piece, portion, section, part, splinter, chip

Function — purpose, role, job, task, perform, action

Furnish — supply, provide, give, deliver, equip

Further — additional, more, extra, added, supplementary

Generalize —take a broad view, simplify, make inferences from particulars

Generate — make, produce, create

Gentle — mild, calm, tender

Girth — circumference, bulk, weight

Highest — uppermost, maximum, peak, main

Hinder — hold back, delay, hamper, obstruct, impede

Humane — caring, kind, gentle, compassionate, benevolent, civilized

Ignore — pay no attention, disregard, overlook, discount

Imbalance — unevenness, inequality, disparity

Immediate — insistent, urgent, direct

Impair — damage, harm, weaken

Implant — insert, embed, inseminate, graft, prosthesis, fixture

Impotent — powerless, weak, incapable, ineffective, unable

Inadvertent — unintentional, chance, unplanned, accidental

Include — comprise, take in, contain

Indicate — point out, sign of, designate, specify, show

Ineffective — unproductive, unsuccessful, useless, vain, futile

Inevitable — predictable, expected, unavoidable, foreseeable

Influence — power, pressure, sway, manipulate, affect, effect

Initiate — start, begin, open, commence, instigate

Insert — put in, add, supplement, introduce

Inspect — look over, check, examine

Inspire — motivate, energize, encourage, enthuse

Institutionalize — standardize, systematize, place in a facility for treatment

Integrate — put together, mix, add, combine, assimilate

Integrity — honesty, cohesion, stability, wholeness, soundness

Interfere — get in the way, hinder, obstruct, impede, hamper

Interpret — explain the meaning of, make understandable

Intervention — intervention, intercession, mediation, action, activity

Intolerance — impatience, annoyance, bigotry, prejudice

Involuntary — instinctive, reflex, unintentional, automatic, uncontrolled

Irreversible — permanent, irrevocable, irreparable, unalterable

Irritability — sensitivity to stimuli, fretful, quick excitability

Justify — advocate, confirm, defend, explain in accordance with reason

Likely — probably, possible, expected

Liquefy —change into fluid, make more fluid

Logical — rational, analytical, using reason

Longevity — durability, potency, long life

Lowest — minimum, least, inferior in rank

Maintain — continue, uphold, preserve, sustain, retain

Majority — most, preponderance, the greater part of

Mention — talk about, refer to, state, cite, declare, point out

Minimal — least, smallest, nominal, negligible, token

Minimize — reduce, diminish, lessen, curtail, decrease to smallest possible

Mobilize — activate, organize, assemble, gather together, rally

Modify — change, adapt, adjust, revise, alter

Moist — slightly wet, damp

Multiple — many, numerous, several, various

Natural — normal, ordinary, unaffected

Negative — no, none, harmful, downbeat, pessimistic

Negotiate — bargain, talk, discuss, consult, cooperate, settle

Notice — become aware of, see, observe, discern, detect

Notify — inform, tell, alert, advise, warn, report

Nurture — care for, raise, rear, foster

Obsess — preoccupy, consume

Occupy — live in, inhabit, reside in, engage in

Occurrence — event, incident, happening

Odorous — scented, stinking, aromatic

Offensive — unpleasant, distasteful, nasty, disgusting

Opportunity — chance, prospect, break

Organize — put in order, arrange, sort out, categorize, classify

Origin — source, starting point, cause, beginning, derivation

Pace — speed, rate, stride, tempo

Parameter — limit, factor, limitation, issue

Participant — member, contributor, partaker, applicant

Perspective — viewpoint, view, perception

Position — place, location, point, spot, situation

Practice — do, carry out, perform, apply, follow

Precipitate —crystalize, cause to happen, bring on, hasten, abrupt, sudden

Predetermine — fix or set beforehand

Predictable — expected, knowable

Preference — favorite, liking, first choice

Prepare — get ready, plan, make, train, arrange, organize

Prescribe — set down, stipulate, order, recommend, impose

Previous — earlier, prior, before, preceding

Primarily — first, above all, mainly, mostly, largely, principally, predominantly

Primary — first, main, basic, chief, most important, key, prime, major, crucial

Priority — main concern, giving first attention to, order of importance

Production — making, creation, construction, assembly

Profuse — plentiful, copious, abundant, generous, prolific, bountiful

Prolong — extend, delay, put off, lengthen, draw out

Promote — encourage, support, endorse, sponsor

Proportion — ratio, amount, quantity, part of, percentage, section of

Provide — give, offer, supply, make available

Rationalize — explain, reason, justify

Realistic — practical, sensible, reasonable

Receive — get, accept, take delivery of, obtain

Recognize — acknowledge, appreciate, identify, aware of

Recovery — healing, mending, improvement, recuperation, renewal

Reduce — decrease, lessen, ease, moderate, diminish

Reestablish — reinstate, restore, return, bring back

Regard — consider, look upon, relate to, respect

Regular — usual, normal, ordinary, standard, expected, conventional

Relative — comparative, family member

Relevance — importance, significance, pertinence

Reluctant — unwilling, hesitant, disinclined, indisposed, adverse

Reminisce — recall, review, remember experiences

Remove — take away, dispose, eliminate, eradicate

Reposition — move, relocate, change position

Require — need, want, necessitate

Resist — oppose, defend against, keep from, refuse, defy

Resolution — decree, solution, decision, ruling, promise

Resolve — make up your mind, solve, determine, decide

Response — reply, answer, reaction, retort

Restore — reinstate, reestablish, bring back, return, refurbish

Restrict — limit, confine, curb, control, contain, hold back, hamper

Retract — take back, draw in, withdraw, apologize

Reveal — make known, disclose, divulge, expose, tell, make public

Review — appraisal, reconsider, evaluation, assessment, examination, analysis

Ritual — custom, ceremony, formal procedure

Rotate — turn, go around, spin, swivel

Routine — standard, ordinary, usual, habit, custom, practice

Satisfaction — approval, fulfillment, pleasure, happiness

Satisfy — please, convince, fulfill, make happy, gratify

Secure — safe, protected, fixed firmly, sheltered, confident, obtain

Sequential — chronological, in order of occurrence

Significant — important, major, considerable, noteworthy, momentous

Slight — small, slim, minor, unimportant, insignificant, insult

Source — basis, foundation, starting place, cause

Specific — exact, particular, detail, explicit, definite

Stable — steady, even, constant

Statistics — figures, data, information, evidence, analysis

Subtract — take away, deduct

Success — achievement, victory, accomplishment

Surround — enclose, encircle, envelop, contain

Suspect — think, believe, suppose, guess, deduce, infer, distrust, doubtful

Sustain — maintain, carry on, prolong, continue, nourish, suffer

Synonymous — same as, identical, equal, tantamount

Systemic — pervasive, extensive, affecting the entire organism

Thorough — careful, detailed, methodical, systematic, meticulous, comprehensive

Tilt — tip, slant, slope, lean, angle, incline

Translucent — see-through, transparent, clear

Unique — one and only, sole, exclusive, distinctive

Universal — general, widespread, common, worldwide

Unoccupied — vacant, not busy, empty

Unrelated — unconnected, unlinked, distinct, dissimilar, irrelevant

Unresolved — unsettled, uncertain, unsolved, unclear, in doubt

Utilize — make use of, employ

Various — numerous, variety, range, mixture, assortment

Verbalize — express, voice, speak, articulate, vent

Verify — confirm, make certain, prove, attest to, validate, substantiate, corroborate, authenticate

Vigorous — forceful, strong, brisk, energetic

Volume — quantity, amount, size

Withdraw — remove, pull out, take out, extract

Index

A